Clinical Thoracic Anesthesia

Jayashree Sood • Shikha Sharma
Editors

Clinical Thoracic Anesthesia

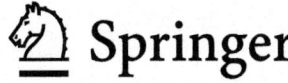

Editors
Jayashree Sood
Institute of Anaesthesiology
Pain and Perioperative Medicine
Sir Ganga Ram Hospital
New Delhi
India

Shikha Sharma
Institute of Anaesthesiology
Pain and Perioperative Medicine
Sir Ganga Ram Hospital
New Delhi
India

ISBN 978-981-15-0748-9   ISBN 978-981-15-0746-5 (eBook)
https://doi.org/10.1007/978-981-15-0746-5

© Springer Nature Singapore Pte Ltd. 2020
This work is subject to copyright. All rights are reserved by the Publisher, whether the whole or part of the material is concerned, specifically the rights of translation, reprinting, reuse of illustrations, recitation, broadcasting, reproduction on microfilms or in any other physical way, and transmission or information storage and retrieval, electronic adaptation, computer software, or by similar or dissimilar methodology now known or hereafter developed.
The use of general descriptive names, registered names, trademarks, service marks, etc. in this publication does not imply, even in the absence of a specific statement, that such names are exempt from the relevant protective laws and regulations and therefore free for general use.
The publisher, the authors, and the editors are safe to assume that the advice and information in this book are believed to be true and accurate at the date of publication. Neither the publisher nor the authors or the editors give a warranty, expressed or implied, with respect to the material contained herein or for any errors or omissions that may have been made. The publisher remains neutral with regard to jurisdictional claims in published maps and institutional affiliations.

This Springer imprint is published by the registered company Springer Nature Singapore Pte Ltd.
The registered company address is: 152 Beach Road, #21-01/04 Gateway East, Singapore 189721, Singapore

Preface

Thoracic surgery, although a very specialized branch, is now being done in several tertiary care hospitals. This book is an endeavor to help those anesthesiologists who are dealing with these patients. It has taken into consideration all the practical aspects which will help them to perfect their skills.

The authors have been practicing thoracic anesthesia for several years. Their practical points will go a long way in helping the young anesthesiologists who are aiming to practice this specialty.

We hope that reading this book would be a help, whether you are a postgraduate student, a fellow, a consultant, or anyone involved in the care of thoracic surgery patients. The increase in the understanding of this branch of anesthesia will aid in the better management of their patients.

New Delhi, India
Jayashree Sood
Shikha Sharma

Acknowledgment

The editing of this book has been a herculean task and for this I would like to acknowledge the hard work and contribution of all the authors. The publishing of the book has been possible only because of their dedication and perseverance.

Thanks to Dr. Shikha Sharma, the coeditor, who has worked tirelessly to edit the book.

A book on 'Clinical Thoracic Anaesthesia' could be written only because of the enormous practical experience that all contributors gained due to the high volume of thoracic surgeries performed by our thoracic surgeon, Dr. Arvind Kumar. His contribution is highly appreciated.

A special thanks to Dr. D. S. Rana, Chairman, Board of Management, Sir Ganga Ram Hospital, for his keen interest in academics that has encouraged all of us to pursue our academic interests.

I am particularly grateful to Dr. V. P. Kumra, Emeritus Consultant and Advisor to our department, for his mentorship to all of us.

The secretarial assistance of Ms. Silvi Philip and Mr. Prakash Bisht is highly appreciated. They worked for several days overtime to ensure timely completion of the book.

This book would not have been possible without the constant inspiration and support of my husband, Dr. Subhash Sood and my blue-eyed children Rahul, Ruchi, Dheeraj, and Kanika, and my grandchildren 'Ayra', 'Samaira,' and 'Aryaveer'.

Jayashree Sood

It is an immense satisfaction to present this book to the readers. Looking back at the journey, I would, at the outset, like to thank my coeditor Dr. Jayashree Sood as the force behind this book. Dr. Chand Sahai, one of the authors, for her constant and continuous encouragement. I take immense pride in presenting the other authors and our journey together.

Thanks are due to Dr. Arvind Kumar, Chairperson, Department of Thoracic Surgery, for his confidence in all of us. Special thanks are due to Mr. Prakash Bisht for his untiring and ever smiling support with manuscript correction and Ms. Silvy Philip for her support.

Thanks are due to my family for their understanding and support in the journey of thoracic anesthesia and this book.

Shikha Sharma

Contents

Part I Preoperative Considerations

1. History of Thoracic Surgery and Anesthesia 3
   Chand Sahai

2. Ethical and Philosophical Considerations in
   Thoracic Anesthesia 21
   Amitabh Dutta

3. Functional Anatomy of Thorax 33
   Ajay Sirohi

4. Lung Physiology Relevant to Thoracic Anesthesia 47
   Anil Kumar Jain

5. Thoracic Anesthesia Equipment 61
   Shvet Mahajan and Akhil Kumar

6. Preoperative Assessment of Thoracic Surgery Patient 83
   Jayashree Sood and Nitin Sethi

7. Patient Positioning in Thoracic Surgery.................... 95
   Bhuwan Chand Panday

8. Monitoring in Thoracic Surgery 99
   Bhuwan Chand Panday

Part II Anesthesia for Operative Procedures

9. Fluid Management 113
   Shikha Sharma

10. Lung Isolation Techniques 121
    Namrata Ranganath and Kavitha Lakshman

11. Ventilation Strategies for Thoracic Surgery................. 139
    Nitin Sethi

12. Anesthesia for Lung Resection and Pleural Surgery.......... 149
    Himani Chabra and Shikha Sharma

13	**Mediastinal Masses**........................ 163 Mahinder Singh Baansal
14	**Anesthesia Considerations for Tracheal Reconstruction** ...... 181 Ashwin Marwaha
15	**Awake/Non-intubated Thoracic Surgery** .... 203 Mahinder Singh Baansal
16	**Anesthetic Considerations for Procedures in Bronchoscopy Suite**........................ 215 Naresh Dua
17	**Overview of Lung Transplant** .... 231 Akhil Kumar
18	**Pediatric Thoracic Anesthesia and Challenges**............... 251 Deepanjali Pant and Archna Koul
19	**Anesthesia for Oesophageal Surgeries** .... 263 Ajay Sirohi and Jayashree Sood
20	**Anesthetic Management of Thoracic Trauma** .... 275 Sudeep Goyal and Bhuwan Chand Panday

Part III Postoperative Management

21	**General Principles of Postoperative Care**.................. 285 Bimla Sharma and Samia Kohli
22	**Postoperative Management of Thoracic Surgery Patients: A Surgeon's Perspective** .... 295 Belal Bin Asaf, Harsh Vardhan Puri, and Arvind Kumar
23	**Enhanced Recovery After Thoracic Surgery** .... 303 Samia Kohli and Jayashree Sood
24	**Postoperative Complications Following Thoracic Surgery**..... 315 Anjeleena Kumar Gupta
25	**Pain Management in Thoracic Surgery** .... 335 Manish Kohli and Pradeep Jain

About the Editors

Jayashree Sood (MD, FFARCS, PGDHHM, FICA) graduated from BJ Medical College, Pune, India, and completed postgraduate training at the Postgraduate Institute of Medical Education and Research (PGIMER), Chandigarh, India. She also qualified as an FFARCS in the UK. She holds a postgraduate degree in Hospital & Healthcare Management (PGDHHM) from Pune, India. She is currently the chair of the Institute of Anaesthesiology, Pain and Perioperative Medicine at Sir Ganga Ram Hospital, New Delhi, India. She has published more than 100 papers and has delivered several lectures at various national and international conferences. She received the IMA Mediko Healthcare Excellence Award 2019 for Excellence in Anesthesia Management in Hyderabad, India, as well as the Best Teacher Award 2018 and Best Academician Award from Sir Ganga Ram Hospital, New Delhi, India. She is also the CEO of the Indian College of Anesthesiologists. She has edited the books *Anesthesia in Laparoscopic Surgery* and *Anesthesia for Transplant Surgery* and authored an atlas of procedures in neonate and pediatric practice.

Shikha Sharma graduated from Sawai Man Singh Medical College, Jaipur, India, and completed her postgraduate training at Banaras Hindu University, Varanasi, India. She also underwent training in lung transplant and thoracic anesthesia at Toronto General Hospital and the University of Alabama Hospital, Birmingham, USA. She is currently a senior consultant in charge of thoracic anesthesia at Sir Ganga Ram Hospital, New Delhi, India, and her team has been involved in more than 2900 major thoracic cases to date.

Part I
Preoperative Considerations

History of Thoracic Surgery and Anesthesia

Chand Sahai

"The farther backward you can look, the farther forward you are likely to see."

—Winston Churchill

Conflict between nations and communities has resulted in war throughout history: from ancient times (Persian wars, Gallic wars) to the World Wars and the more recent Gulf wars. Strangely enough, these hostilities have contributed to the evolution of medicine, especially of the surgical specialties. Hippocrates put it very succinctly: "He who would become a surgeon should join the army and follow it."

Mortality from thoracic war wounds before the First World War was more than 50%. It reduced to 25% during the First World War, was down to 10% in WWII, and 5% during the Korean War. At the time of the Vietnam War, the mortality rate was 2–4%. The bloody fields of WWI gave birth to thoracic surgery, as a result of experience gained with chest trauma and the type of weapons that an army was using on its foe [1].

The evolution of anesthesia for thoracic surgery was a long time in the making for several reasons, the principal one being the unique problems associated with the opening of the thorax; so while surgeons had worked out how to operate on diverse areas of the body, such as the abdomen, the thorax was still a no man's land [2].

Modern thoracic surgery was possible only because of the concurrent evolution of anesthesia, for there were problems (and solutions) inherent to the surgery of this unique section of the human body: open thorax, lateral decubitus position, manipulation of major organs, sharing of the airway, potential for heavy bleeding, lung isolation, confirmation of DLT by auscultation, and fiberoptic endoscopy (large margin of error if fiberscope not used) [3, 4].

The right path had been shown many centuries earlier in the masterpiece *De humani corporis fabrica libri septem* by Andreas Vesalius, the Flemish anatomist, who illustrated this using the letter Q, which encloses cherubs performing a tracheostomy on a sow.

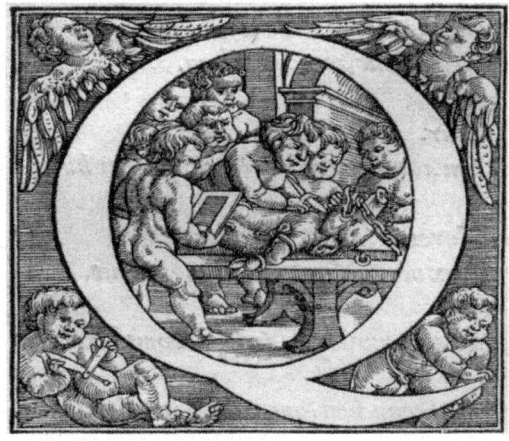

Courtesy: The Thomas Fisher Rare Book Library, University of Toronto

C. Sahai (✉)
Institute of Anaesthesiology, Pain and Perioperative Medicine, Sir Ganga Ram Hospital, New Delhi, India

Vesalius, in 1543, after opening the chest of an animal watched the lungs collapse, followed by the heart beating irregularly before it stopped completely. He wrote, "But that life may in a manner of speaking be restored to the animal, an opening must be attempted in the trunk of the trachea, into which a tube of reed or cane should be put; you will then blow into this, so that the lung may rise again and the animal take in air. Indeed, with a slight breath in the case of this living animal the lung will swell to the full extent of the thoracic cavity, and the heart become strong ... for when the lung, long flaccid, has collapsed, the beat of the heart and arteries appears wavy, creepy, twisting, but when the lung is inflated, it becomes strong again. And as I do this, and take care that the lung is inflated at intervals, the motion of heart and arteries does not stop...."

1.1 Negative Pressure, Positive Pressure Ventilation, and Endotracheal Tubes

Rudolph Matas (1860–1957), a great pioneer of surgery, caught the essence of the problem when he said, "Until the danger of seriously interfering with the respiratory functions, by inducing acute collapse of the lungs, is clearly eliminated or is reduced to a safe minimum, the analogy between the pleura and the peritoneum from the surgical point of view will never exist" [5].

In another article, Matas wrote "The procedure that promises the most benefit in preventing pulmonary collapse in operations on the chest is the artificial inflation of the lung and the rhythmical maintenance of artificial respiration by a tube in the glottis directly connected with a bellows. Like other discoveries, it is not only elementary in its simplicity, but the fundamental ideas involved in this important suggestion have been lying idle before the eyes of the profession for years. It is curious that surgeons should have failed to apply for so long a time the suggestions of the physiological laboratory, where bellows and tracheal tubes have been in constant use from the days of Magendie (1783–1855) to the present, in practising artificial respiration on animals." [6]

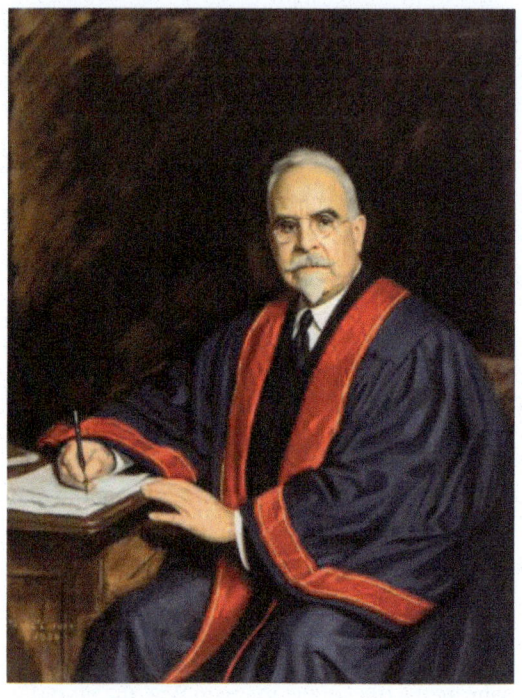

Image of Rudolph Matas courtesy of the Archives of the American College of Surgeons

As early as 1887, in Buffalo, USA, George Fell used a bellows which was connected to a mask or a tracheostomy to generate intermittent positive pressure to treat the respiratory depression caused by morphine poisoning [7].

Subsequently, O'Dwyer modified Fell's method and used a foot bellows connected to a tracheal tube [8]. But it was that brilliant surgeon Rudolph Matas who realized that the Fell–Dwyer apparatus could be the solution to the pneumothorax problem, adapting it for use in removing a tumor from the chest wall in 1889 [9].

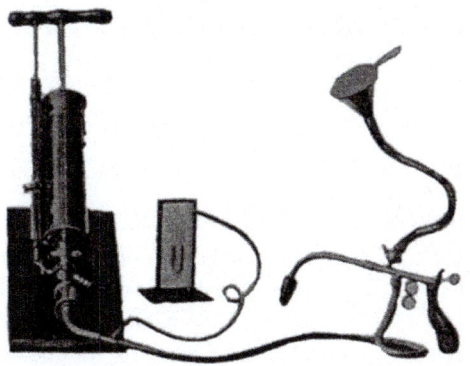

The Matas-Smythe modified Fell-O'Dwyer apparatus for artificial respiration during surgery. From the original manuscript of –and illustrated by– Dr Rudolph Matas [9]. Image reproduced from [10] with permission of Wolters Kluwer

Despite this successful use, the apparatus was not used widely for another four decades. This was due to the influence of Prof Ferdinand Sauerbruch who with Johannes von Mikulicz introduced a negative pressure operating chamber in 1904, which was used on animals at first and later on a woman for sternal removal of a tumor [11]. Sauerbruch demonstrated his chamber in an operation theater in 1908 in Chicago [12]. Although the cuffed endotracheal tube had been invented around this time, its use was limited to oropharyngeal and facial surgery. Sauerbruch deemed these tubes for controlling the airway unnecessary and even dangerous. His influence was such that positive pressure ventilation and endotracheal tubes did not enter mainstream anesthesia until the 1930s [11].

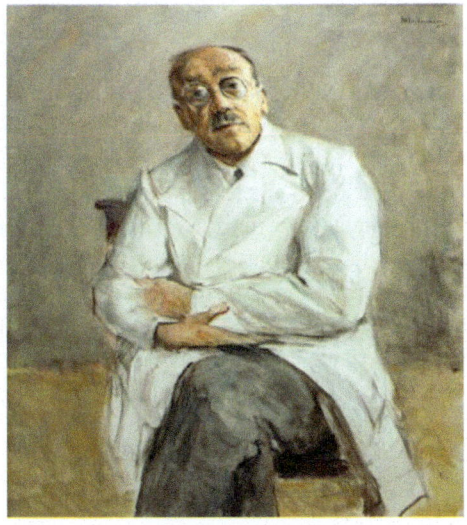

Ferdinand Sauerbruch URL: https://commons.wikimedia.org/w/index.php?title=File:1932_Liebermann_Der_Chirurg_Ferdinand_Sauerbruch_anagoria.JPG&oldid=313509243

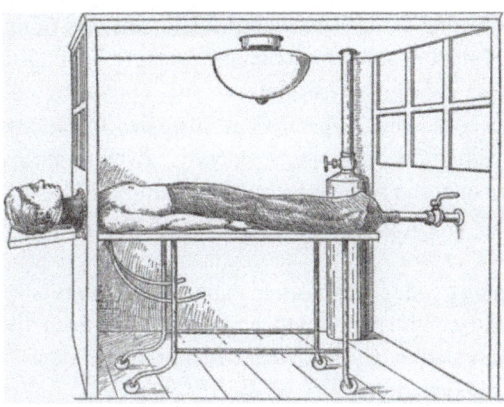

Negative pressure chamber at the Breslau Clinic. Image from: W Meyer M, Transthoracic resection of the lower end of the oesophagus in a dog. *Ann Surg*. 1905 May; 41 [5]: 667–685. With permission

1.2 The Biggest Obstacle in the Way of Successful Thoracic Surgery

One of the major stumbling blocks in the advancement of thoracic surgery has been the pneumothorax problem. The consequences of opening the chest wall have been known for a very long time; a large opening in the chest wall into the pleural cavity led to the demise of the injured individual. The soldiers in the Roman army infantry were trained to inflict penetrating injuries to the chest during combat. What happened was that the stab penetrated the pleura, leading to lung collapse, because the physiological dead space was moving to and fro between the two lungs (known as *pendelluft*) and, in a person breathing spontaneously, this would lead to carbon dioxide accumulation, mediastinal shift, and respiratory and circulatory collapse, and death would ensue shortly. The harmful effects were directly proportional to the size of the wound [13]. About two millennia ago, the Roman encyclopedia author Celsus described the effects of pneumothorax by noting that the abdomen can be cut open with a knife and the patient can continue to breathe safely and spontaneously, but stabbing the chest means death in a very short time [14]. This then is one of the earliest descriptions of the so-called pneumothorax problem. In practical terms, this means that the opening in the chest wall results in the loss of the normal negative intrapleural pressure leading to the outside air rushing in and collapsing the exposed lung. The patient struggles to breathe while the lung paradoxically shrinks during inspiration and expands during expiration, as the air is transferred between the healthy lung and the exposed lung. The mediastinum moves from side to side ("mediastinal flapping"), compressing the contralateral lung and interfering with the circulation. Cyanosis ensues, and the tachypnoic patient struggles for breath.

Only the very briefest of intrathoracic operations were attempted, and mostly extra-thoracic procedures were done in the first third of the twentieth century. Thousands of years ago it was known that most wounds to the chest were fatal. Even the ancients were curious about the airway: Hippocrates (460–370 BC) advised that a suffocating patient could be helped to breathe by putting a pipe into the larynx. Paracelsus (1493–1541) aided a patient with asphyxia by inflating the lungs via a tube and bellows.

A well-known thoracic surgeon John W Streider, the 52nd president of the American Association for Thoracic Surgery, noted that in that era "the period of operation was, with dismaying frequency, a race between the surgeon and the impending asphyxia of the patient." [15]

The dramatic entrance of inhalational anesthesia in the surgical arena in the 1840s led to rapid advances in several areas of surgery. The methods employed for the delivery of inhalational anesthesia were face mask and open drop administration of ether or chloroform with or without nitrous oxide. Muscle relaxants had yet to make an appearance, and endotracheal intubation was considered invasive and used rarely and only by experts. However, the standard of care for thoracic anesthesia was the aspiration of the bronchial secretions, and in 1936, Magill described a T connection for the endotracheal tube that he had devised [16].

1.3 Bronchoscopy

A key role in thoracic surgery and anesthesia is that of bronchoscopy. Gustav Killian, a German otolaryngologist from Freiberg, coined the term "direct bronkoscopie." Killian had performed a therapeutic bronchoscopy in 1876 for the first time, to remove a foreign body lodged in the right bronchus of a farmer, employing an esophagoscope and long rigid forceps [17, 18]. Inspired by this action of Killian, Philadelphia's Chevalier Jackson, also an otolaryngologist, developed a rigid bronchoscope and popularized the procedure of bronchoscopy in 1904. He kept a record of the foreign bodies he recovered with the help of a rigid bronchoscope. These objects are on display at the Mütter Museum in Philadelphia [19].

In 1930, Magill divided thoracic surgery procedures into two parts from the point of view of anesthesiologists. The first part covered surgeries that he termed "superficial," such as thoracoplasty, decortication, bronchial fistula repair, simple pulmonary abscess drainage, and exploratory thoracotomy. The second part of thoracic surgery procedures listed by Magill, such as lobectomies and pneumonectomies, were less common at that time. For these, he employed an endotracheal tube and nitrous oxide/oxygen and ether at low pressure for insufflation, with the patient breathing spontaneously. Provision for the assistance of ventilation, if required, was always made [20]. He proposed that "superficial" surgeries be handled using intercostal nerve blocks, supplemented with nitrous oxide in oxygen delivered via a face mask, noting that the mixture usually resulted in a degree of suboxygenation. Magill later used ether or chloroform along with the nitrous oxide and oxygen mixture [21].

However, both types of thoracic procedures led to one major problem: contamination of the healthy lung from pus or secretions emanating or trickling down from the operative site. This led researchers to evolve ways of isolating the diseased lung from the healthy one.

1.4 The Problem of Cross-Contamination

Gale and Waters, in 1931, tackled the problem of cross-contamination of the lungs by using endobronchial intubation of the healthy lung. For this, they employed a cuffed red rubber tube and dipped it in hot water to mold it into a curve. Using the bevel to direct the tube, it was advanced blindly into the appropriate bronchus. The endotracheal tube cuff was shaped and positioned in such a way that it sat on the carina occluding the entry to the bronchus on the side to be operated and thereby preventing infected secretions from trickling into the healthy lung [22].

The following year an endoscope was used by Coryllos, so that placement of the endotracheal tube was more accurate and regular suction of secretions via catheter was also carried out [23].

The bronchial blocker was another piece of airway equipment, evolved to better control the spread of secretions into the healthy lung. In 1935, a rubber balloon-tipped catheter was used by the Canadian surgeon Edward Archibald to occlude a bronchus which was supplying an infected pulmonary lobe. Once the balloon was inflated, it confined the secretions and slowly the lung to be operated collapsed. This occlusion of the particular bronchus was carried out just before a lobectomy. The angled or "Coude" tip helped maneuver the catheter into the target bronchus, and to be sure about the catheter location, radiographic check of position was done. The healthy lung in the meantime was ventilated via an endotracheal tube, which lay alongside the catheter which was being used as a bronchial blocker [24].

In 1936, Magill developed endobronchial tubes by using fine metal spiral tubing, coated with thin rubber, and featuring a cuff.

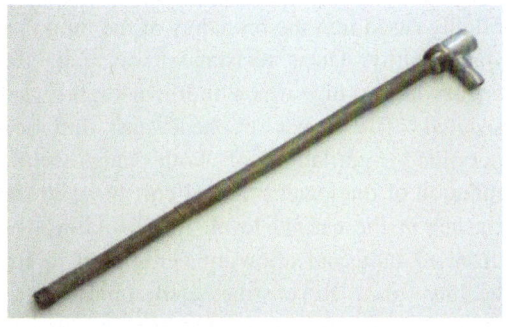

Magill's endobronchial tube. Image courtesy of the Geoffrey Kaye Museum of Anaesthetic History, VGKM1075

The spiral tubing acted as an air channel and was used to inflate the cuff. Initially, Magill used an endoscope like Coryllos did, for placing the endobronchial tube but abandoned it when he found that this dislodged the cuff and/or obstructed the upper lobe. So he decided on a lengthier cuff and combined its usage with regular suction of secretions. Another modification was made to endobronchial tubes taking into consideration the different angles the two main bronchi made at the carina. This led to the concept of the right and left endobronchial tubes, where the metal spiral of the tube was extended for better placement within the bronchus. The right endobronchial tube's spiral was extended so that the upper lobe bronchus was not accidentally occluded. A modification by Magill to the bronchial blocker was the incorporation of the inflating tube into the wall of the suction tube; the cuff was smaller and not covered with gauze. As a result, this bronchial blocker could be inserted into smaller airways, but on the downside, the small size meant it could displace easily [25]. Later, Magill described a combination of the tracheal tube and cuffed bronchial suction to be situated in the bronchus of the lung or lobe to be operated [26].

Emery Rovenstine, in 1936, described an endobronchial tube he had designed. It had two cuffs and was made from woven silk. Hot water was used to mold the tube so that it could be blindly eased into the bronchus of the lung that was healthy. Once resistance was felt, the endobronchial tube was withdrawn slightly and secured. The upper tracheal cuff inflation permitted ventilation of both lungs while inflation of the lower tracheal cuff blocked the trachea at the carinal level, thus isolating the diseased lung and allowing ventilation in the healthy one. Rovenstine also opined that controlled respiration and apnea were needed, recommending the lung separation technique so that the operative lung could be collapsed, thus providing the thoracic surgeon with a quiet field, unlike the time when the fastest surgeon was probably the best [27].

Another method of blocking the bronchus was by means of a ribbon gauze tampon, described by Clarence Crafoord from Sweden. The tampon was endoscopically positioned through an endotracheal tube [27].

1.5 Patient Position and Lung Contamination

The risk of contamination was always present since the patient was in the lateral position during surgery with the diseased lung superior and the normal or healthy lung dependent. At the time, most of the thoracic operations were done for infective diseases like pulmonary tuberculosis. This was because most patients were breathing spontaneously with some assistance by the anesthetist. So the research question was how to isolate the healthy lung? At first, a light depth of anesthesia was tried so that a patient's intact cough reflex would be sufficient for expectorating infective secretions.

Henry Beecher, in 1940, was of the opinion that a steep head-down position and an uncuffed endotracheal tube passed through a face mask would prevent contamination of the healthy lung as the secretions or pus would flow out with the help of gravity down the trachea and into the mask where they could be removed [28]. Other individuals tried patient positioning as a means of avoiding the soiling of the dependent lung. Overholt in 1946 advised the semi-prone position as a way to retain the secretions, whereas Parry Brown like Beecher allowed the pus to safely drain away from the non-operative lung [29, 30].

In 1943, one of the most popular bronchial blockers was introduced by Vernon Thompson, a British anesthetist. The components of this device were a long suction catheter and a rubber inflatable cuff. A bronchoscope was used to place the blocker in the diseased lung. The cuff was inflated, and there was a stylet in the lumen of the suction tube. On removal of the bronchoscope, the device was held in place with the help of gauze over the balloon which stuck to the bronchial mucosa. Another innovation in 1947 by Moody, Trent, and Newton had metal claws around the balloon to keep the blocker in place [27].

The insertion of the device by a bronchoscope with a longitudinal slot was devised by Solomon Albert in 1952 [31].

William Macewen, a Scottish scientist, practiced passing flexible metal tubes blindly into the larynx of cadavers. Later, in 1878, he did this in an awake patient with an oral tumor. With the correct positioning of the tube, an air chloroform mixture was delivered to the patient, who stopped coughing and gagging. However, Macewen abandoned this practice when he lost a patient [32].

It is interesting to note that a procedure done frequently by the thoracic surgeons, video-assisted thoracoscopy (VATS), owes its origins to the cystoscope in 1806, which went through many improvements and was finally used by Jacobaeus in 1910 for thoracoscopy.

In the same year, Jacobaeus wrote in the *Munich Journal*, suggesting that the cystoscope could be used to investigate serous cavities. This landmark article mentions three points which are significant even today: trocar introduction in such a way that no internal organ is injured or causes too much pain, the introduction of a transparent medium into the cavity such as filtered air, and employing a cystoscope that can fit inside a trocar. He writes about a two-cannula technique for looking into the abdomen (laparaskopie) and the pleurae (thorakoskopi) [33].

This pioneering paper had cited Forlanini's technique, which entailed blowing nitrogen or air into the pleural cavity and collapsing the lung, known as the pneumothorax treatment of tuberculosis. Jacobaeus made a second port for the introduction of cautery for lysing the adhesions formed by tuberculosis [34].

Jacobaeus operation as the technique came to be known was used for the treatment of tubercular pleural effusion for the next 45 years [35].

Even though Jacobaeus is considered the father of thoracoscopy, someone else had carried out the first thoracoscopy. In an article about the history of endoscopy and endoscopic equipment published in 1879, Josef Grunfeld talks about FR Cruise who carried out an endoscopic examination on a chest fistula using "a binocular device that made his instrument more perfect" [36]. The *Concise Dictionary of Irish Biography* states that Sir Francis Richard Cruise was born in Dublin in 1834 and died in 1912 around the time that Jacobaeus was getting famous for the technique of thoracoscopy. Even as a student Cruise devoted much of his time to the "light guide technique" as endoscopy was known at that time [37, 38].

In 1865, he published a paper titled "Endoscope as an aid to the diagnosis and treatment of disease." He had examined the interior of the pleura in an 11-year-old girl with empyema utilizing the pleurocutaneous fistula that had developed following pleural drainage. This was published in the *Dublin Quarterly Journal of Medical Science* in 1866 [39]. The appearance on the scene of anti-tubercular drugs closed the era of using pneumothorax for the treatment of pulmonary tuberculosis [35].

1.6 Chest Tubes

The concept and practice of chest tubes for draining empyema have been around for a long time; Hippocrates was probably the first individual to do so, and he even described the procedure, the incision, the cautery, and the metal tube he used [40]. Hundreds of years later, in 1860 a hypodermic for drainage of the empyema was developed by Hunter [41], while Playfair in the 1870s created an underwater seal for continuous drainage of empyema in a patient whose pus collection in the pleural space continued despite multiple aspirations [42].

The 1940s were important for the progress of anesthesia and the progress of thoracic surgery as a result of the introduction of curare for muscle relaxation and Alexander Fleming's discovery of penicillin. Curare allowed the anesthesiologist to have control over the airway without deep general anesthesia so that the problem of pneumothorax due to an opening in the pleura was largely solved. The drug was introduced into anesthesia practice by Griffith in 1942 [43], and Harroun wrote about its application in thoracic surgery in 1946 [44]. More complex pulmonary surgery and on sicker patients became possible with penicillin.

1.7 Role of Physiologists

Many of the advances in thoracic anesthesia were due to the airway equipment, which had been used elsewhere and then found its way into the anesthetist's armamentarium. This is true of the double-lumen tube (DLT) developed by Carlens for bronchospirometry. The use of this tube led to a crucial milestone in the evolution of thoracic anesthesia for it could bypass many difficulties in the process of one-lung ventilation and prevent cross-contamination. Endobronchial blockers also made an appearance at this time and were used for a variety of conditions. As with the DLTs, the bronchial blockers had many problems associated with them regarding correct placement, a small channel for suctioning, loss of seal, and intraoperative dislodgement [45, 46].

The physiologists were the pioneers responsible for the concept of one-lung anesthesia as early as 1871. They were carrying out experiments on animals in the laboratory while investigating bronchospirometry. The list of the researchers who used techniques to separate the airways to the two lungs includes renowned physiologist Eduard Pfluger (June 1829–March

1910) and the Frenchman Claude Bernard (July 1813–February 1878). The physiologists' purpose was to study gas exchange. Pfluger, Professor at the University of Bonn, was researching how gases from the lung reached the blood. He did this by using a catheter to sample the air in various parts of a dog's lungs [47]. A similar technique was used by Wolffberg in 1871. In 1905, Loewy and von Schrotter carried out 35 experiments on human volunteers to work out the cardiac output by using the Bohr equation and the Fick principle [48].

Head, Wolffberg, and Werigo continued to look into the respiratory physiology of dogs, but took an interest in independent lung spirometry, using separate tubes to intubate the right and left bronchi [48–50].

In 1889, Head designed a precursor to the double-lumen tube: a combination of a short tracheal cannula and a long cannula and a balloon, using it in dogs, turtles, and rabbits. Werigo's co-axial double-lumen tracheostomy cannula for dogs formed the basis for the first double-lumen bronchoscope used in man [50]. In 1912, Walter Hess used a variant of Head's device for physiologic experiments in rabbits. He added a carinal hook to stop the endobronchial tube from being advanced too far into the unilateral bronchus.

The development of anesthetic techniques has gone hand in hand with surgical advances and the late nineteenth century and early twentieth century saw many technical innovations, leading to the development of new equipment that has made life easier for the thoracic surgeon. The most important new equipment without which we cannot imagine anesthesia practice today is the endotracheal tube.

Ivan Magill and Stanley Rowbotham, both of whom served as medical officers during the First World War, created this tube. When the war was over, they worked at the Queen's Hospital for Facial and Jaw Injuries in Sidcup, Kent, England [51]. Here, the duo anesthetized patients who had received facial injuries in battle and needed plastic surgery.

The new science and practice of plastic surgery posed formidable challenges for the existing anesthesia techniques. The two innovators created wide bore single-lumen tracheal tubes (which allowed inspiration and expiration) that they used with throat packs, thus facilitating unhindered ventilation and also preventing aspiration of blood or debris entering the airway during the course of surgery. In addition, the two introduced other vital airway equipment, such as pharyngeal airways, insufflation catheters, and laryngoscopes [52].

The prevention of aspiration was dealt with by various techniques, such as the insertion of tampons. The cuff on the endotracheal tube was an improvement on these techniques. The cuff was first used at the Langenbeck's clinic in Berlin by Friedrich Trendelenburg, who was an assistant surgeon at that time [53].

A major obstacle in the way of a successful outcome of thoracic surgery was cross-contamination of the healthy lung by infected secretions and lack of control on the respiration. The operating conditions improved dramatically after the introduction of antibiotics and muscle relaxants in the 1940s, which allowed the further development of thoracic surgery. Pneumonectomy and lobectomy became commonplace in thoracic surgery operation theaters, and, slowly, complex procedures, such as tracheobronchial reconstructions, also started. Other major factors in improving surgical outcome were the lateral positioning of the patient to provide optimal access to the diseased lung and isolation of the lung by the use of new equipment.

Much of the equipment in use in thoracic anesthesia today originated as part of physiologists' experiments. The rigid double-lumen bronchoscope was used by Bjorkman, Jacobaeus, and Frenckner in their quest for determining lung volumes and the function of each lung, although the procedure was technically difficult and the conscious volunteer was extremely uncomfortable [54].

To overcome this drawback, Gebauer in 1939 [55] and Zavod in 1940 [56] constructed left-sided double-lumen catheters fashioned from soft rubber and made bronchospirometry more comfortable for volunteers. But even these catheters had disadvantages such as high resistance to airflow, small internal diameters, and required fluoroscopic positioning.

To improve on these shortcomings, a double-lumen catheter made of rubber, intended to be used for bronchospirometry, was developed by the Swedish physiologist Eric Carlens in 1949. With rigidity similar to that of a rubber urethral catheter, this was a left-sided double-lumen tube with a carinal hook to prevent the tube from descending too far into the bronchus [57].

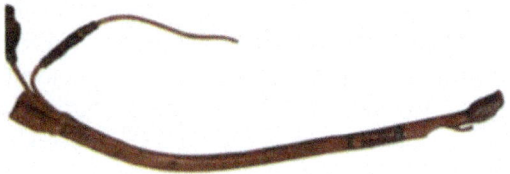

Carlens tube—Image courtesy Dr. Usha Saha

Carlens was also in favor of using atropine or scopolamine together with morphine, followed by a 2% tetracaine spray, to anesthetize the airway. To facilitate the easy navigation of the device past the vocal cords, a curved metal stylet was inserted into the tube and the carinal hook was tied down to the tube (to make the intubation easier). Carlens claimed to have carried out the procedure of bronchospirometry 100 times, using this equipment without any adverse outcome.

Later, Carlens and Viking Olov Bjork described the use of this equipment for delivering anesthesia on 20 patients undergoing pulmonary resection from November 1949 to February 1950 in the Sabbatsberg Hospital, Stockholm [58]. By 1952, the DLTs were being used routinely in this hospital and an article describing the benefits of this equipment on approximately 500 patients was published in the journal *Anesthesiology* [59].

1.8 DLT in Clinical Use

During this time, right lung surgery was done using a left-sided endobronchial tube for one-lung anesthesia. Surgery for the left lung was dangerous and this was because the right and left bronchial tree anatomy was unique to the two lungs. The distinctive anatomy of the right tracheobronchial tree meant that whenever the right main bronchus was intubated, the right upper lobe bronchus was prone to obstruction, thus leading to hypoxia or an incomplete collapse of the left lung because of herniation of the endobronchial cuff into the trachea, following which the left main bronchus was at risk of being partly blocked. This happens because in the adult the right upper lobe bronchus lies about 15 mm from the carina in women and 19 mm in men, while the left upper lobe emerges from the main left bronchus at 44 mm and 49 mm in women and men, respectively, thus the need for the cuff of right-sided endobronchial tubes to incorporate a slot and proper alignment, to ventilate the right upper lobe.

Despite its many advantages, the Carlens tube had shortcomings: difficult insertion associated with the carinal hook, trauma to airway structures, and the narrow lumens on the DLT which increased the expiratory resistance to the fresh gas flow. The last, according to Jenkins and Clarke, would probably preclude its use in patients with emphysema. In the case of left pneumonectomy, the DLT would need to be withdrawn into the trachea before the bronchus was clamped, and if the left main bronchus is blocked by tumor, then the Carlens DLT cannot be employed. Some modifications in the design of the DLT were clearly called for, the first one being constructed in 1959 by Bryce-Smith [60]. A year later, Bryce-Smith, and Salt, both from Oxford [61], and Malcolm White, from Middlesbrough [62], developed right-sided DLTs.

These modified DLT designs varied in the endobronchial sections, the position of the cuff, and the length of the endobronchial tube. The one designed by Bryce Smith curved posteriorly and to the left and had no carinal hook; the endobronchial tube continued for 7 cm as a single tube and had a cuff that on inflation stopped short of the opening of the upper lobe of the left main bronchus. The other difference being that in the Carlens DLT the two lumens were placed side by side or laterally, while in the Bryce-Smith and Salt design the lumens were placed anteroposteriorly.

The design of the DLT developed by White was like a Carlens tube which had been constructed for the right side. It had a carinal hook and an endobronchial cuff with a slit. The hook ensured that the slit in the endobronchial cuff faced the opening of the right upper lobe bronchus. Taking the DLT design a step further was Frank Robertshaw, from Manchester, who in 1962 designed DLTs for both right and left main bronchi in three sizes. These tubes had wider lumens than the earlier DLT designs, thus lessening the resistance to airflow. The left-sided Robertshaw DLT had the endobronchial tube angled at 45 degrees, while the right had the tube at an angle of 20 degrees and there was a slotted endobronchial cuff for right upper lobe aeration. There was no carinal hook [63].

1.9 Bronchial Blockers

One of the most famous thoracotomies took place on 23rd September 1951, where a left pneumonectomy for bronchogenic carcinoma was performed on King George VI. The anesthesiologists were Robert Machray and Cyril Scurr and the surgeon was Clement Price Thomas. The anesthesiologists avoided using an endobronchial tube and opted for a Thompson blocker and an endotracheal tube for the surgery, which was uneventful [64].

The German anesthetist Sturzbecher designed a unique endotracheal tube which incorporated two apparatuses into one: a bronchial blocker within an endotracheal tube; the blocker extended 7 cm or 9 cm beyond the distal end of the endotracheal tube (the shorter blocker intended for a main bronchus and the longer one for blocking a lobar bronchus). After endotracheal intubation, the blocker was directed into its desired position with the help of a stylet and a final check of the position was done by x-ray (a tiny metal tip was present in the blocker) [65, 66].

Robert Macintosh and Robert Leatherdale, in 1955, also described a combined endotracheal tube and bronchial blocker for left lung surgery and a left endobronchial tube for operations on the right lung [67]. The advantage of the combination, especially to the anesthetist, who serves as a thoracic surgery anesthetist occasionally, is that the equipment shape conforms to the shape of the left bronchus, making it easier to position and less prone to displacement during surgery.

William Vellacott, in 1954, described a right-sided endobronchial tube made of latex and wire for the express purpose of preventing the trickling down of purulent secretions from the right upper lobe bronchus to the healthy lung. For patients who had empyema and bronchopleural fistula, two cuffs were incorporated in the tube: a proximal one for the tracheal portion of the tube and a distal one for the bronchial portion. The bronchial cuff, when inflated, occluded the right upper lobe bronchus. A 2.5 cm opening between the two cuffs directed the anesthetic gases toward the left bronchus. The device is placed using a bronchoscope [68].

A radiological study by Wally Gordon and Ronald Green was carried out on 40 men and 40 women. This was done to find out the distance between the right upper lobe bronchus and the origin of the right main bronchus, which was found to be a centimeter or more (average 1.8 cm) in all the 80 patients. Based on their findings, the physicians developed a right endobronchial tube, made of rubber. Their unique design had the last 4 cm of the tube angulated at 15 degrees and a 2 × 3 mm lateral opening to which the endobronchial cuff was attached. When inflated, the tube directed the fresh gas flow to the right upper lobe bronchus. There was a hook akin to the one on a Carlens DLT, about a centimeter above this opening. A second endobronchial cuff with its lower margin 2 cm above the hook was also present. A stylet was used during the placement of this tube [69].

This tube was used in carcinoma bronchus, bronchial stenosis, and bronchoplastic procedures involving the left main bronchus [70].

William Pallister further modified this tube, which was normally blindly placed in position, so that it could be introduced into the appropriate position using a Magill bronchoscope [71].

1.10 Modification and Further Advancements

Several other modifications were made to endobronchial tubes and bronchial blockers, and though they were used successfully in thoracic cavity surgery, they had many drawbacks. The incomplete collapse of the lung to be operated and subsequent difficulty in carrying out the surgery, intraoperative displacement, and ventilation-perfusion mismatch leading to hypoxemia were common problems.

Slowly, the use of double-lumen tubes increased not only in Scandinavia but in other regions as well. The stage was set for a new era in the airway management of patients undergoing thoracic surgery as the red rubber DLTs gained recognition for it became apparent that the DLTs had all the advantages of the endobronchial tubes and bronchial tubes combined [72–74].

1.11 Evolution of Lung Isolating Devices

The evolution of lung isolating devices, however, did not stop here for it was soon realized that the red rubber DLTs too had significant shortcomings, such as problems with device insertion, intubation of the wrong bronchus, mucosal damage, malposition, hypoxemia, and even tracheobronchial rupture, which was attributed to over or asymmetrical inflation of the high-pressure, low-volume cuffs. In addition, the use of nitrous oxide during long surgery led to cuff distension [75].

Mucosal damage was also seen as a result of the reaction to the red rubber tubes and their rigidity. The search was on for a solution, and July 1977 saw Mallinckrodt conducting trials on a left-sided DLT made of polyvinyl chloride (PVC). The Broncho-Cath™ was the result of this trial [76]. Though it resembled the Robertshaw DLT it differed from it in that the high-volume, low-pressure cuffs inflated concentrically and the bronchial curvature of the DLT was less acute. The chemically inert PVC used for the Broncho was less of an irritant than red rubber to the airway. Other manufacturers like Sheridan, Portex, and Rusch also developed polyvinyl chloride DLTs. The shapes and properties of the cuffs in the bronchial and tracheal portions of the DLTs made by each of these companies were different [77, 78].

Another advantage of the PVC double-lumen tubes was that compared with the red rubber tubes these new tubes had thinner walls but approximately the same cross-sectional area as that of a red rubber tube [79].

Initial accounts detailing the superiority of the PVC tubes over the earlier red rubber ones appeared, but they were short-lived and malpositions and tracheobronchial rupture were also reported [80, 81].

1.12 Arrival of Fiberoptics

From the time that DLTs were first used, their positions were checked via visual means and by auscultation done after inflating the bronchial and tracheal cuffs and by consecutive clamping of the lumens. The efficacy of the above methods of tube placement was assessed in the mid-1980s by using a fiberoptic bronchoscope, and surprisingly 48% of the DLTs that were thought to be sited correctly were actually malpositioned [82].

Further research in DLT positioning by using fiberoptic bronchoscopes revealed that there was a narrow margin between correct placement and malposition and that flexion and extension of the neck also played a major role in dislodging the DLT from its proper position [83].

This research notwithstanding, the incorporation of bronchoscopy in ensuring optimal DLT placement remained an issue of dispute for 20 years [84, 85].

A national confidential inquiry into perioperative deaths (NCEPOD) in 1998 in patients who had esophago-gastrectomy mentioned that 30% of deaths reported were due to problems with the DLT: these ranged from multiple changes of the DLT, hypoxia, and hypoventilation. The most disturbing part of the report states that "no anesthetist reported using a fibreoptic bronchoscope to confirm the position of the tube, either before or during surgery, even when the tube was evidently incorrectly placed." [86]

Newer DLTs, such as the Silbronco tube, have been designed using medical-grade silicone to reduce trauma during insertion and ensuring shape retention even during prolonged surgery. An additional plus point for this tube is the wire reinforcement at the distal end that prevents kinking and obstruction [87].

The double-lumen tube serves to isolate the lungs during thoracic and thoracoscopic surgery. They are difficult to position in the appropriate position and even when they are they could shift when the patient is turned from supine to lateral or during surgery. This would lead to the improper collapse of the lung to be operated, airway trauma, and hypoxia among other risks. The position of the DLT requires checking by using endoscopy. The VivaSight DLT (ETView Ltd, M P Misgav 20174, Israel) use obviates the need to use a flexible bronchoscope to check the position of the DLT. This DLT is for single use and has a high-resolution camera incorporated in the distal end of the tracheal lumen. The camera provides continuous real-time images of the intubation using the VivaSight DLT as well as during position change and surgery, allowing the necessary adjustments to be made as soon as a malposition is diagnosed on the camera image. The device also has an in-built channel for removing secretions [88].

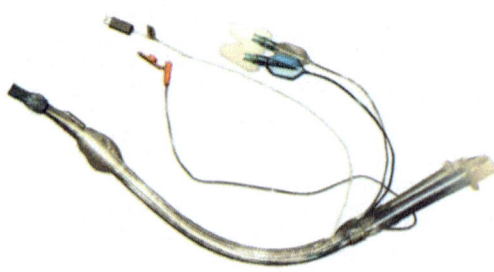

VivaSight DLT image: Author

The DLT cannot be used in all cases of thoracic surgery airway management, for example, in infants and small children. In 1969, Verlie Lines, from Sydney, Australia, and Raymond Vale, from London, UK, wrote about the use of 5 Fr Fogarty arterial embolectomy catheters for the selective bronchial blockade in this pediatric population [89, 90]. An example of the double-lumen tube meant for infants and children is the Marraro Paediatric Bilumen Tube [91].

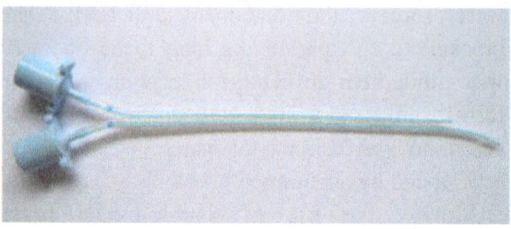

Marraro Paediatric Bilumen tube with permission of G. Marraro

A study of 200 patients in Canada by Robert Ginsberg of the Toronto Western Hospital described the use of the 8–14 Fogarty occlusion catheter for the bronchial blockade in adults undergoing thoracic surgery and concluded that the procedure was shorter and safer as compared to the one undertaken with the DLT [92].

Hiroshi Inoue and colleagues from Tokai University, Japan, in 1982, described a variation of the Fogarty catheter. The variation was the Univent tube, which is a single-lumen endotracheal tube manufactured from inert silicone. The anterior internal wall of the endotracheal had a small channel running its length, and a 2 mm torque-controlled bronchial blocker could be passed through it. After intubation, the endotracheal tube was rotated 90 degrees toward the side to be occluded and then the blocker was advanced out of the endotracheal tube, about 8 cm beyond the tip. Finer adjustment of the bronchial blocker was done via a bronchoscope or x-ray imaging [93].

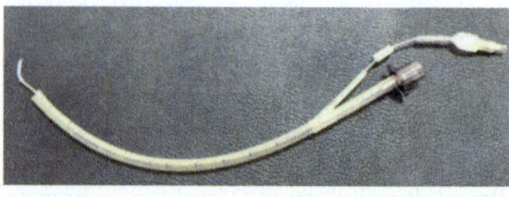

Univent tube® with movable bronchial blocker. Image: Author

The Univent tube appears to be akin to the combination of the endotracheal tube and endobronchial blocker devised by Magill almost half a century earlier before Inoue came up with his design of a method of isolating the lung [94].

The Fogarty catheter and the Univent tube were proof of the renewed interest in bronchial blockers, and 1999 saw the emergence of a new wire-guided BB developed by George Arndt and team from the University of Wisconsin. The BB could be placed coaxially via an endotracheal tube, aided by a pediatric bronchoscope [95].

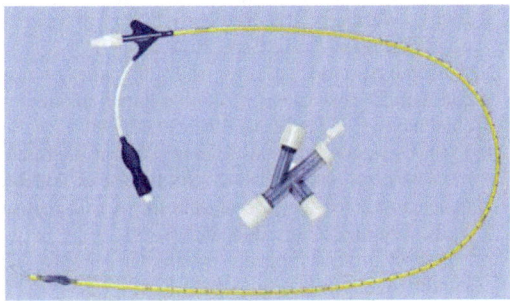

Arndt bronchial blocker. Image: Author

In 2005, Edmund Cohen from New York described another new BB with a soft nylon-deflecting tip controlled by a wheel located at the proximal end. After the BB was passed through an endotracheal tube, it was positioned with the help of a fiberoptic bronchoscope [96].

Even with varied equipment available for lung isolation, it may be difficult for the occasional thoracic anesthesiologist to achieve OLV with this BB. The DLT with its size and endobronchial limb proves more difficult to place than an SLT, and most BBs require endoscopy for optimal positioning and also take longer and need more intra-operative repositioning than a DLT.

A new DLT was designed to solve the problem of placement of BBs because even the Arndt and Cohen BB proved to be challenging in terms of fiberoptic placement. Known as the Papworth BiVent tube P3 Medical Ltd, Bristol, UK, it was designed by Ghosh and his colleagues from Bristol. It was designed to allow the reliable and safe use of any BB and to position it in the appropriate bronchus without the use of bronchoscopy. Made of dry natural rubber, it had two lumens that were D-shaped and placed longitudinally with a single inflatable, high-volume, low-pressure tracheal cuff. The distal part of the tube ended in two, pliable crescent-shaped flanges, which would rest on the carina, with the opening of the two lumens situated at the beginning of the main bronchi. When passed through the tube, the BB could be directed into the desired bronchus. Ghosh et al. carried out a study on manikins first [97] and then undertook a cadaveric study [98] on the Papworth BiVent tube before publishing their clinical experience in 2011 [99].

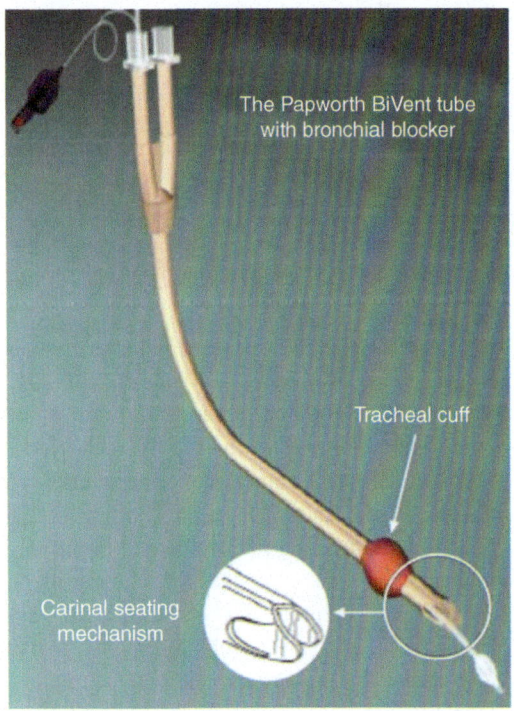

From P3 Medical, with permission

The search for an ideal BB continued, to overcome the problems associated with the BBs like difficulty in positioning and displacement during patient positioning or surgery [100]. The EZ-Blocker (Teleflex Life Sciences Ltd., Athlone, Ireland) developed by an anesthesiologist is easy to use for the occasional thoracic anesthesiologist. The EZ blocker is unique in that it has a Y-shaped distal end that fits on the bifurcation of the trachea. This permits placement of cuff in the main bronchi once the EZ blocker is inserted. The blocker cuff can be inflated just prior to lung isolation so there is less chance at misplacement or dislodging of the blocker [101]. One size can be used for most adult patients, whereas choosing an appropriate sized DLT is not so easy [102, 103].

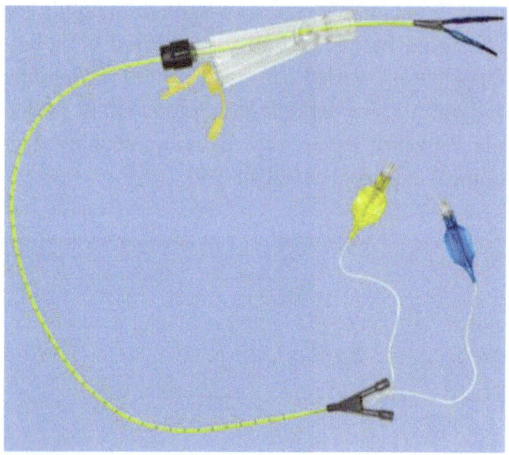

Rusch® EZ-Blocker™ Endobronchial blocker. Image: Author

Thoracic surgery has posed unique challenges for both the surgeon and anesthesiologist. Recognition of the problems and finding the appropriate solutions involved a slow and jerky progression and innumerable experiments on animals, lessons learned from the conflicts on the battlefield and training personnel, and improving monitoring and upgrading equipment. Endoscopes, monitors for real-time imagery apart from lung isolation techniques, gave rise to video-assisted thoracoscopies and tracheal reconstruction, among others. Concurrent developments in the areas of immunology and transplantation gave impetus to lung transplantation. These have been dealt with elsewhere in this book.

Thoracic surgery could reach the heights it has attained today only because of the development of endotracheal tubes, muscle relaxants, and the means to isolate lungs to contain infection to the operative site. A greater and detailed understanding of the anatomy and physiology of the thoracic cavity and the organs contained has enabled anesthesiologists to successfully tackle cases that would have been refused for surgery a mere 50 years ago.

"The more extensive a man's knowledge of what has been done, the greater will be the power of knowing what to do"—Benjamin Disraeli

References

1. Molnar TF, Hasse J, Jeyasingham K, et al. Changing dogmas: history of development in treatment modalities of traumatic pneumothorax, hemothorax, and posttraumatic empyema thoracis. Ann Thorac Surg. 2004;77:372–8.
2. Ball C, Westhorpe RN. The early history of ventilation. Anaesth Intensive Care. 2012;40:3–4.
3. Alliaume B, Coddens J, Deloof T. Reliability of auscultation in positioning of double-lumen endobronchial tubes. Can J Anaesth. 1992;39:687–90.
4. Klein U, Karzai W, Bloos F, et al. Role of fiberoptic bronchoscopy in conjunction with the use of double-lumen tubes for thoracic anesthesia: A prospective study. Anesthesiology. 1998;88:346–50.
5. Matas R. Intralaryngeal insufflation. Matas R. Intralaryngeal insufflation. JAMA. 1900;XXIV(22):1371–5.
6. Matas R. On the management of acute traumatic pneumothorax. Ann Surg. 1899;29(4):409–34.
7. Fell GE. Forced respiration in opium poisoning—its possibilities, and the apparatus best adapted to produce it. Buffalo Med Surg J. 1887;28(4):145–57.
8. O'Dwyer J. An improved method of performing artificial forcible respiration. Arch Pediatr. 1892;9:30–4.
9. Matas R. Artificial respiration by direct intralaryngeal intubation with a modified O'Dwyer tube and a new graduated air-pump, in its application to medical and surgical practice. Am Med. 1902;3:97–103.
10. Hutson LR, Vachon CA, Rudolph M. Innovator and pioneer in anesthesiology. Anesthesiology. 2005;103(4):885–9.
11. Cherian SM, Nicks R, Lord RS. Ernst Ferdinand Sauerbruch: rise and fall of the pioneer of thoracic surgery. World J Surg. 2001;25:1012–20.
12. Sauerbruch F. Present status of surgery of the thorax. JAMA. 1908;51:808.
13. Conacher I. History of thoracic anesthesiology. In: Slinger P, editor. Principles and practice of anesthesia for thoracic surgery. 2nd ed. New York: Springer; 2011. p. 1.
14. Celsus A. De Medicina. Loeb Classical Library 1938. http://penelope.uchicago.edu/Thayer/e/roman/texts/Celsus/home.html.
15. Streider JW. Anesthesia from the viewpoint of the thoracic surgeon. Anesthesiology. 1950;11:60–4.
16. Magill IW. Anaesthesia in thoracic surgery, with special reference to lobectomy: (Section of Anaesthetics). Proc R Soc Med. 1936;29:643–53.
17. Becker HD, Marsh BR. History of the rigid bronchoscope. In: Bolliger CT, Mathur PN, editors. Progress

in respiration research, Interventional bronchoscopy, vol. 30. Basel, Switzerland: Karger; 2000. p. 2–15.
18. Kollofrath O. Entfernungeines Knochenstücks aus dem rechten Bronchus auf natürlichem Wege und unter Anwendungder directen Laryngoscopie. Münchener Medizinische Wochenschrift. 1897;38:1038–9.
19. Mütter Museum, College of physicians of Philadelphia. Exhibition: Chevalier Jackson collection. Available from: http://muttermuseum.org/exhibitions/chevalier-jackson-collection
20. Magill IW. Discussion on anaesthesia in thoracic surgery, section of anaesthetics. Proc Roy Soc Med. 1930;23:771–82.
21. Magill IW. Anaesthesia in thoracic surgery, with special reference to lobectomy. Section of anaesthetics. Proc Roy Soc Med. 1936;29:643–53.
22. Gale JW, Waters RM. Closed endobronchial anesthesia in thoracic surgery: preliminary report. Anesth Analg. 1932;11:283–7.
23. Coryllos PN. A method of combined endotracheal anesthesia and suction in thoracoplasty for pulmonary tuberculosis: results in 41 cases (79 operations). Anesth Analg. 1932;11:138–44.
24. Archibald E. A consideration of the dangers of lobectomy. J Thorac Surg. 1935;4:335–51.
25. Westhorpe R. Magill's endobronchial tubes. Anaesth Intensive Care. 1992;20:409.
26. Cover note. Anaesthesia and Intensive Care, Vol. 30. No. 4. November, 1992
27. Mushin WW, Rendell-Baker L. The principles of thoracic anaesthesia past and present. Oxford: Blackwell Scientific Publications; 1953.
28. Beecher HKJ. Some controversial matters problems of anesthesia for intrathoracic surgery. J Thorac Surg. 1940;8:125.
29. Overholt RH, Langer L. The technique of pulmonary resection. Springfield: Charles C Thomas; 1949.
30. Parry Brown AI. Posture in thoracic surgery. Thorax. 1948;3:161–5.
31. Albert SN. A slotted bronchoscope for the introduction of bronchial blockers. Br J Anaesth. 1952;24:145.
32. Macewen W. Clinical observations on the introduction of tracheal tubes by the mouth, instead of performing tracheotomy or laryngotomy. Br Med J. 1880;2(1022):163–5.
33. Jacobaeus HC. Über die Möglichkeit, die Zystoskopie bei Untersuchung seröser Höhlungen anzuwenden. Münch Übermed Wschr. 1910;57:2090–2.
34. Jacobaeus HC. The cauterization of adhesions in artificial pneumothorax therapy of tuberculosis. Am Rev Tuberc. 1922;6:871–97.
35. Brandt HJ, Loddenkemper R, Mai J. Atlas of diagnostic thoracoscopy. Indications—technique. New York: Thieme Inc; 1985.
36. Grünfeld J. Zur Geschichte der Endoskopie und der endoskopischen Apparate. Medizinische Jahrbücher, K.K. Gesellschaft der Ärzte. Wien: Wilhelm Braumüller; 1879. p. 278.
37. Crone JS. A concise dictionary of Irish biography. Dublin 1937. Nendeln, Liechtenstein: Kraus Reprint; 1970. p. 44.
38. Anonymous. Sir Francis Cruise M.D. Br Med J. 1912;9:586.
39. Gordon S. Clinical reports of rare cases, occurring in the Whitworth and Hartwicke Hospitals: most extensive pleuritic effusion rapidly becoming purulent, paracentesis, introduction of a drainage tube, recovery, examination of interior of pleura by the endoscope. Dublin Q J Med Sci. 1866;41:83–90.
40. Hutchins RA. Hippocrates, writings. In: Great books of the Western world, vol. 29. Chicago: Encyclopedia Britannica; 1952. p. 142.
41. Hochberg LA. Thoracic surgery before the twentieth century. New York: Vantage Press; 1960. p. 255.
42. Playfair GE. Case of empyema treated by aspiration and subsequently by drainage: recovery. Br Med J. 1875;1:45.
43. Griffith HR, Johnson G. The use of curare in general anesthesia. Anesthesiology. 1942;3:418–20.
44. Harroun P, Hathaway HR. The use of curare in anesthesia for thoracic surgery; preliminary report. Surg Gynecol Obstet. 1946;82:229–31.
45. Campos JH, Kernstine KH. A comparison of a left-sided Broncho-Cath with the torque control blocker univent and the wire-guided blocker. Anesth Analg. 2003;96:283–9.
46. Narayanaswamy M, McRae K, Slinger P, et al. Choosing a lung isolation device for thoracic surgery: a randomized trial of three bronchial blockers versus double-lumen tubes. Anesth Analg. 2009;108:1097–101.
47. Wolffberg S. Über die Spannung der Blutgase in die Lungencapillaren. Pflügers Arch. 1871;4:465–92.
48. Loewy A, von Schrötter H. Untersuchungen über die Blutzirkulation beim Menschen. Z Exp Pathol. 1905;1:197–310. [Article in German].
49. Head H. On the regulation of respiration theoretical and experimental. J Physiol. 1889;10(1):279–90.
50. Werigo B. Zur Frageüber die Wirkung des Sauerstoffs auf die Kohlensäure ausscheidung in den Lungen. Pflügers Arch Ges Physiol. 1892;51:191–3. [Article in German].
51. Condon HA, Gilchrist E. Stanley Rowbotham: Twentieth century pioneer anaesthetist. Anaesthesia. 1986;41:46–52.
52. Bowes JB, Zorab JSM. Sir Ivan Magill's contribution to anaesthesia. In: Rupreht J, van Lieburg MJ, Lee JA, Erdmann W, editors. Anaesthesia. Berlin, Heidelberg: Springer; 1985. https://www.rcoa.ac.uk/lives-of-the-fellows/dr-edgar-stanley-rowbotham.
53. Trendelenburg F. Beiträge zu den operationen auf den Luftwegen. Arch Klin Chir. 1871;12:321–61.
54. Jacobaeus HC, Frenckner P, Björkman S. Some attempts at determining the volume and function of each lung separately. Acta Med Scandinav. 1932;79:174–215.
55. Gebauer PW. A catheter for bronchospirometry. J Thorac Surg. 1939;8:674–84.

56. Zavod WA. Bronchspirography: description of catheter and technique of intubation. J Thorac Surg. 1940;10:27–31.
57. Carlens E. A new flexible double-lumen catheter for bronchospirometry. J Thorac Surg. 1949;18:742–6.
58. Björk VO, Carlens E. The prevention of spread during pulmonary resection by the use of a double-lumen catheter. J Thorac Surg. 1950;20:157.
59. Bjork VO, Carlens E, Friberg O. Endobronchial anesthesia. Anesthesiology. 1953;14:60–72.
60. Bryce-Smith R. A double-lumen endobronchial tube. Br J Anaesth. 1959;31:274–5.
61. Bryce-Smith R, Salt R. A right-sided double lumen tube. Br J Anaesth. 1960;32:230–1.
62. White GM. A new double lumen tube. Br J Anaesth. 1960;32:232–4.
63. Robertshaw FL. Low resistance double-lumen endobronchial tubes. Br J Anaesth. 1962;34:576–9.
64. Ellis H. The pneumonectomy of George VI. In: Operations that Made History. London: Greenwich Medical Media; 1996. p. 123–30.
65. Stüertzbecher F. Die Blockade feuchter Lungen mit einem Spezialkatheter. Der Anaesthesist. 1953;2:151–2.
66. Oech SR. A cuffed endotracheal tube with an incorporated endobronchial blocker. Anesthesiology. 1955;16:468–9.
67. Macintosh R, Leatherdale RA. Bronchus tube and bronchus blocker. Br J Anaesth. 1955;27:556–7.
68. Vellacott WN. A new endobronchial tube for broncho-pleural fistula repair. Br J Anaesth. 1954;26:442–4.
69. Gordon W, Green RA. A new right endobronchial tube. Lancet. 1955;268:185.
70. Gordon W, Green RA. Right lung anaesthesia; anaesthesia for left lung surgery using a new right endobronchial tube. Anaesthesia. 1957;12:86–93.
71. Pallister WK. A new endobronchial tube for left lung anaesthesia, with specific reference to reconstructive pulmonary surgery. Thorax. 1959;14:55–7.
72. Zeitlin GL, Short DH, Ryder GH. An assessment of the Robertshaw double-lumen tube. Br J Anaesth. 1965;37:858–60.
73. Wood RE, Campbell D, Razzuk MA, et al. Surgical advantages of selective unilateral ventilation. Ann Thorac Surg. 1972;14:173–80.
74. Read RC, Friday CD, Eason CN. Prospective study of the Robertshaw endobronchial catheter in thoracic surgery. Ann Thorac Surg. 1977;24:156–61.
75. Borm D. Tracheo-bronchial ruptures during intubation anesthesias using the Carlens tube. Chirurg. 1977;48:793–5.
76. Burton N, Watson DC, Brodsky JB, et al. Advantages of a new polyvinyl chloride double-lumen tube in thoracic surgery. Ann Thorac Surg. 1983;36:78–84.
77. Fitzmaurice BG, Brodsky JB. Airway rupture from double-lumen tubes. J Cardiothorac Vasc Anesth. 1999;13:322–9.
78. Hannallah MS, Benumof JL, Bachenheimer LC, et al. The resting volume and compliance characteristics of the bronchial cuff of left polyvinylchloride double-lumen endobronchial tubes. Anesth Analg. 1993;77:1222–6.
79. Clapham MC, Vaughan RS. Bronchial intubation. A comparison between polyvinyl chloride and red rubber double lumen tubes. Anaesthesia. 1985;40:1111–4.
80. Burton NA, Fall SM, Lyons T, et al. Rupture of the left main- stem bronchus with a polyvinylchloride double-lumen tube. Chest. 1983;83:928–9.
81. Wagner DL, Gammage GW, Wong ML. Tracheal rupture following the insertion of a disposable double-lumen endotracheal tube. Anesthesiology. 1985;63:698–700.
82. Smith G, Hirsch N, Ehrenwerth J. Placement of double-lumen endobronchial tubes. Br J Anaesth. 1986;58:1317–20.
83. Benumof JL, Partridge BL, Salvatierra C, et al. Margin of safety in positioning modern double-lumen endotracheal tubes. Anesthesiology. 1987;67:729–38.
84. Brodsky JB, Shulman MS, Mark JB. Malposition of left-sided double lumen endobronchial tubes. Anesthesiology. 1985;62:667–9.
85. Pennefather SH, Russell GN. Placement of double lumen tubes—time to shed light on an old problem. Br J Anaesth. 2000;84:308–10.
86. Sherry K. Management of patients undergoing oesophagectomy. In: Gray AJG, Hoile RW, Ingram GS, Sherry KM, editors. The Report of the National Confidential Enquiry into Perioperative Deaths 1996/1997. London: The National Confidential Enquiry into Perioperative Deaths; 1998. p. 57–61.
87. Lohser J, Brodsky JB. Silbronco double-lumen tube. J Cardiothorac Vasc Anesth. 2006;20:129–31.
88. Dean C, Dragnea D, Anwar S, et al. The VivaSight-DL double-lumen tube with integrated camera. Eur J Anaesthesiol. 2016;33(4):305–8.
89. Vale R. Selective bronchial blocking in a small child. Case report. Br J Anaesth. 1969;41:453–4.
90. Lines V. Selective bronchial blocking in a small child. Br J Anaesth. 1969;41:893.
91. Marraro G. Selective endobronchial intubation: The Marraro Pediatric Bilumen Tube. Paediatr Anaesthesia. 1994;4:255–8.
92. Ginsberg RJ. New technique for one-lung anesthesia using an endobronchial blocker. J Thorac Cardiovasc Surg. 1981;82:542–6.
93. Inoue H, Shohtsu A, Ogawa J, et al. New device for one-lung anesthesia: endotracheal tube with movable blocker. J Thorac Cardiovasc Surg. 1982;83:940–1.
94. Magill IW. Anesthesia in thoracic surgery, with special reference to lobectomy. Proc Roy Soc Med. 1936;29:643–53.
95. Arndt GA, DeLessio ST, Kranner PW, et al. One-lung ventilation when intubation is difficult—presentation of a new endobronchial blocker. Acta Anaesthesiol Scand. 1999;43:356–8.

96. Cohen E. The Cohen flexitip endobronchial blocker: an alternative to a double lumen tube. Anesth Analg. 2005;101:1877–9.
97. Ghosh S, Falter F, Goldsmith K, et al. The Papworth BiVent tube: a new device for lung isolation. Anaesthesia. 2008;63:996–1000.
98. Ghosh S, Klein AA, Prabhu M, et al. The Papworth BiVent tube: A feasibility study of a novel double-lumen endotracheal tube and bronchial blocker in human cadavers. Br J Anaesth. 2008;101:424–8.
99. Ghosh S, Falter F, Klein AA, et al. The Papworth BiVent tube: initial clinical experience. J Cardiothoracic Vasc Anesth. 2011;25(3):505–8.
100. Narayanaswamy M, McRae K, Slinger P, et al. Choosing a lung isolation device for thoracic surgery: A randomized trial of three bronchial blockers versus double-lumen tubes. Anesth Analg. 2009;108:1097–101.
101. Mungroop HE, Wai PT, Morei MN, et al. Lung isolation with a new Y-shaped endobronchial blocking device, the EZ-Blocker. Br J Anaesth. 2010;104:119–20.
102. Brodsky JB, Lemmensh J. Tracheal width and left double-lumen tube size: a formula to estimate left-bronchial width. J Clin Anesth. 2005;17:267–70.
103. Hannallah MS, Benumof JL, Ruttimann UE. The relationship between left mainstem bronchial diameter and patient size. J Cardiothorac Vasc Anesth. 1995;9:119–21.

Ethical and Philosophical Considerations in Thoracic Anesthesia

2

Amitabh Dutta

2.1 Introduction

Thoracic anesthesia is a rapidly evolving subspecialty and has witnessed unprecedented advancement in recent years for keeping pace with surgery on and inside the chest cavity [1]. Powered by social media dissemination platforms, the growing awareness among the afflicted masses that their difficult-to-treat infectious (e.g., empyema thoracis, tubercular lung consolidations/masses) and non-infectious (e.g., lung malignancy, mass, thyroid enlargement, thymoma) lung problems can be approached safely with minimal access (thoracic video-endoscopy) or open surgery (thoracotomy, lung transplant) intervention has led to a quantum jump in thoracic surgery turnover in the last decade. Further, recent advances in thorax-specific radio diagnostics (HR-computed tomography, MRI, CT angiograms) and laboratory studies (markers, gene expert) have greatly facilitated decisive selectivity in approach to thoracic surgery, thereby ensuring lesser postsurgery morbidity and improved surgical outcome. Combined together, the above-stated elements of current-day thoracic surgery have propelled a proactive transit of orthodox conservatism and dogma-driven [2] management options to clear reasoned indications to surgery.

Despite significant advancements in thoracic surgery, dedicated thoracic surgery facilities are still difficult to find by, mainly because of the limited infrastructure (ORs, ICU, rehabilitation units) and for want of a seasoned and proficient team of experts (surgeons, anesthesiologists, intensivists, intervention chest physicians, transfusion specialists, and physiotherapists). Over and above the perceived inability to come around capacity and capability building issues in thoracic surgery, the patients continue to suffer with diminished respiratory reserves and deranged lung function because of the delay in reporting and reaching out to the tertiary care institution with requisite facilities. Additional reason for the protracted delay has to do with lack of courage in going for surgery, difficulty in arranging financial and backup human resources, and the fear of a futile surgery followed by prolonged rehabilitation. Current developments in thoracic surgery and anesthesia notwithstanding, the patients with significant thoracic pathology/issues land up in the OR in the late stage and, consequently, continue to return with a high degree of morbidity and mortality [3]. Therefore, there is an overriding need of an oversight mechanism

A. Dutta (✉)
Institute of Anaesthesiology, Pain and Perioperative Medicine, Sir Ganga Ram Hospital (sgrh.com), New Delhi, India

Ganga Ram Institute for Medical Education and Research (GRIPMER), New Delhi, India

Ethics Committee, Ganga Ram Institute for Medical Education and Research (GRIPMER), New Delhi, India

© Springer Nature Singapore Pte Ltd. 2020
J. Sood, S. Sharma (eds.), *Clinical Thoracic Anesthesia*,
https://doi.org/10.1007/978-981-15-0746-5_2

that looks beyond specifics of thoracic anesthesia/surgery healthcare to ward off undue patient dissatisfaction, controversies, and medicolegal fallout that commonly accompanies high-risk thoracic interventions. In this regard, approaching thoracic anesthesia healthcare delivery with a wider perspective gained through deliberations involving philosophical considerations and ethical dimensions is the way to go.

Another important aspect of thoracic surgery is the way one looks at thoracic healthcare delivery scope in entirety. This exercise lends significant advantage to the attending experts and the institution in planning anesthesia delivery along with the interventions therein, hospitalization, enhanced recovery [4–6], and following up the patient in the post-discharge period. In view of the intricate and contentious practice points of thoracic anesthesia, pre-evaluation of philosophical insights and attendant ethical burdens would proffer continuous refinement of the efficient planning, effective execution, and a safe patient.

2.2 Philosophical Considerations of Thoracic Anesthesia

The practice of anesthesia for thoracic surgery patients is a far departure from routine administration of standardized general anesthesia (GA) which involves ventilation of two healthy functional lungs. The many facets of problems which a thoracic anesthesiologist affronts warrant a proactive and continuously evolving thought process with a wider scope, deeper insight, and greater consistency to initiate and sustain an effective anesthesia healthcare delivery. There is a greater need for invoking one's philosophical domain to gain parity with anticipated/expected outcomes in thoracic anesthesia. The philosophical insights into thoracic anesthesia can be divided into four main elements: *first*, asking questions (why, how, when, etc.) concerning the job at hand, i.e., assessing the patient and preparing him/her for the surgery; *second*, arranging everything to ensure a safe anesthesia sojourn for the patient despite the anticipated rough surgical course; *third*, participating as a team to facilitate a positive outcome; and *fourth*, sustaining a transparent, clear, and multi-way communication between the anesthesiologist, surgery team, and the patient party (the patient, attendants, family members). The approach to thoracic anesthesia care therefore involves, apart from expert-specific deliverables (surgery, anesthesia), a continuous risk–benefit analysis and balancing. The core analytics and understanding of the case can be percolated to the relevant stakeholders to preempt shared decision-making and documentation, wherever necessary. The ability to stop for a while at every step of anesthesia care that empowers one to put a question on the veracity and benefit of an action before moving forward is likely to improve "benefit" and preclude "harm" in high-risk vulnerable patients.

Importantly, since almost all thoracic anesthesia interventions have greater element of invasiveness, they add up to iatrogenic surgical stress to the preexistent pulmonary and systemic comorbidities that the patients may already be harboring at the time of initial presentation. The active systemic disharmony secondary to anesthesia actions invites greater probability of complications than mere side effects that ensue otherwise. With an eye on ensuring patient safety, philosophical insights into thoracic anesthesia present two major areas that require to be dealt with (1) iatrogenic injury and (2) identifying and responding to the harm. To achieve the above, it calls for heightened elements of professionalism among expert anesthesiologists: namely, proficiency, dedication, and responsibility.

Since improving the quality of *decision and actions* in thoracic anesthesia has a significant direct bearing on patient's safety and surgical outcome, a practice aligned with the "DRIFT" (do-it-right-the-first-time) concept, as proposed by theorist Phil Crosby (1926–2001), is the way to go. Crosby defined the *four absolutes of quality management* [7]:

1. The **definition** of quality is *conformance to requirements*.
2. The **system** of quality is *prevention*.
3. The **performance** standard is *zero defects*.
4. The **measurement** of quality is the price of nonconformance.

Combining Crosby's DRIFT concept with Juran's "Quality Trilogy" [quality (planning, improvement, and control)] (Fig. 2.1) is probably the best way forward for safe practice of thoracic anesthesia [8]. The need for being careful in thoracic anesthesia stems from the fact that different patients with a similar set of problems behave variably after uniform application of standardized protocol-based conventions may surprisingly have contrasting outcomes. Therefore, each thoracic anesthesia patient is unique and requires exclusivity in approach. There seems to be great merit in dividing thoracic anesthesia delivery procedures into micro-processes; especially those having specific end-points, e.g., induction of anesthesia (absence of eyelash reflex) and intubation ($EtCO_2$ tracing on the monitor) (Table 2.1), should undergo continuous refinement, planning, and execution while they are being made to run in a particular sequence, each time.

2.3 Ethical Considerations

There are a multitude of extraordinary ethical implications of thoracic anesthesia for managing a major system surgery in the "vulnerable" compromised patients, for a thoracic surgery intervention not only aims at correcting the anatomical problem (e.g., excision of lung consolidation/mass lesion), but also looks to gain physiologic optimization and functional recovery; the anesthesia delivery warrants fine diligence in totality supporting the surgery cause. Therefore, there is a greater need for closely considering extraordinary surgical issues than what is routinely encountered. Also, the wider scope and depth of thoracic anesthesia presents us with new ethical challenges which are unlikely to get settled without dedicated deliberations around them. Despite a higher degree of expertise and professionalism, there are bound to be gaps because of new clinical

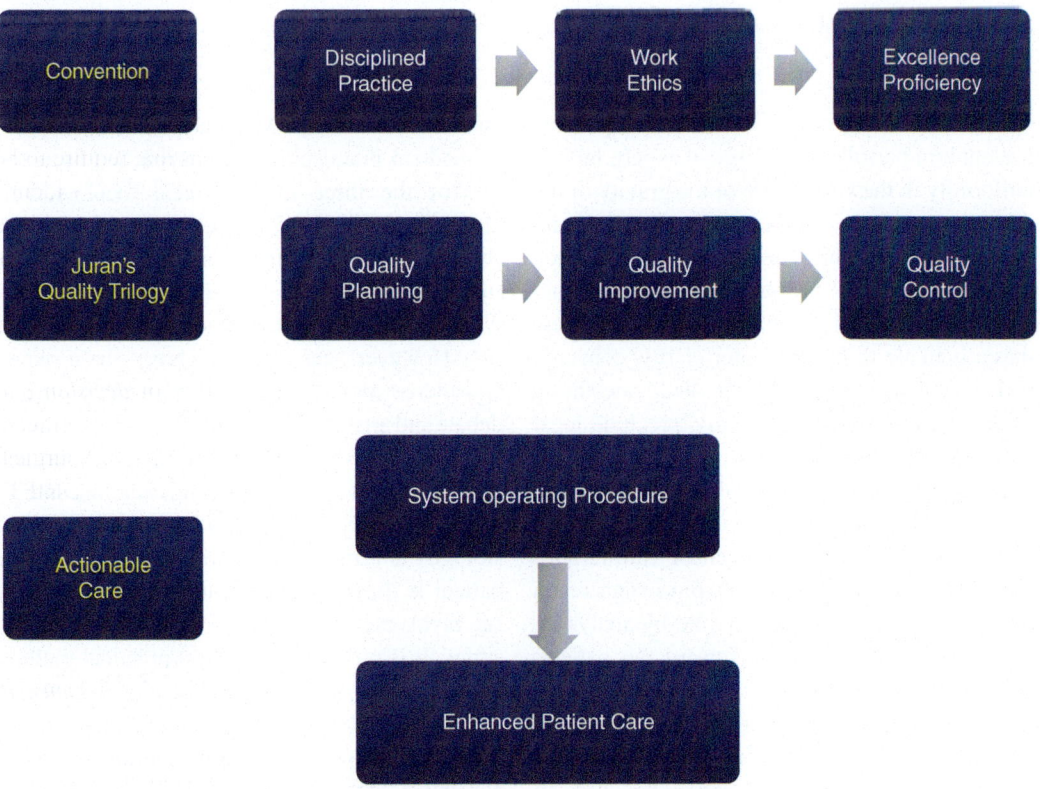

Fig. 2.1 Quality management in healthcare delivery

Table 2.1 Deconstructing micro-processes in thoracic anesthesia

Anesthesia Procedures and Processes	Reflective End-point (s)
Aerosolized nebulisation (salbutamol, pratropium)	FEV1 ↑ by 15%
Pre-oxygenation of lungs	$EtCO_2$ concentration > 90%
Induction of anesthesia (propofol, thiopental)	Loss of verbal contact/ eye lash reflex, BIS < 50
Tracheal Intubation	$EtCO_2$ tracing on monitor
Bronchial Intubation	Application of lung isolation assessment protocol
Depth-of-anesthesia	BIS< 50 (Inhalation, intravenous) MAC > 0.7 (Inhalation)
Muscle relaxation	Train-of-four = 0
Fluid administration	SVV > 10%-trigger for infusion
Coagulation status	TEG specifics
Blood loss	Onsite Haemoglobin assessment
Metabolic, Oxygenation, Ventilation status	Arterial blood gases profile
Reversal of muscle relaxant	TOF > 3
Retrieval from anesthesia	MAC < 0.1, BIS > 85

BIS Bispectral index, *MAC* Minimum alveolar concentration, *SVV* Stroke volume variation, *TEG* Thrombo-elastogram, *TOF* Train-of-four

situations and the stage at which the patients present him/herself to the surgical expert, lack of uniformity in the knowledge of the gravity of the problem among the team members, and for want of a controlled and comprehensive approach to the surgery and anesthesia. Assessment and addressing the ethical issues in thoracic anesthesia is likely to bring greater clarity, converge and channelize the surgical and anesthesia responses, and most importantly, preclude legal ramifications as a consequence. As an exception, evaluation of the ethical burdens of a thoracic anesthesia case needs to be both patient oriented (deontological) and society centric (utilitarian). In clinical practice of medicine, physicians reach a decision for the best patient care by analyzing their own moral obligation toward the patient, professionalism, and the nature of patient–physician relationship. Clinical ethics, i.e., the application of ethical theories, principles, rules, and guidelines in medical practice, becomes an aspect central to decision-making and should be handled sensitively. Medical ethics as applied to medical practice can be approached by using one of the three major ethical theories, i.e., *consequentialism* (where consequences of an action determine whether it is ethical), *deontology* (to be ethical is to do one's duty adequately), and *virtue* (ethics is a matter of streamlining virtues) [9]. However, any of the above three when considered alone or in a mix consumes time to debate and arrive at a decision. Therefore, the most common, practical, and time-efficient approach [10] to ethical analysis of a thoracic anesthesia case is principlism [11, 12], in which the anesthesiologist is a moral agent with duty obligations, patient is the central interest, and ethical analysis revolves around the golden four-principle ethics. It is purported to offer a practical method of dealing with real-world ethical dilemma. These principles supported by other individual principles allow one to consider the standard, normative, regulatory, and legalistic view of the ethics-related nuances, finally leading to a set of suggestions to move forward. A typical approach to ethical consideration in thoracic anesthesia involves (Table 2.2): *First*, the four golden principles of ethics [13] are applied in that order, followed by a normative analysis of inter-principle burdens and conflicts, if any. *Second*, the ethical principles are prioritized for application. *Lastly*, the aligned principles are applied in essence of *Principle of Totality of Responsibility* (ICMR 2006) [14].

Table 2.2 Ethical overview-analysis template for thoracic anesthesia

Levels of analysis	Applied imperative(s)
Level-one analysis: *Analyzing principle ethics*	
• Principle of respect for patient autonomy • Principle of beneficence • Principle of non-maleficence • Principle of justice	• Communication, shared decision-making, informed consent document • Patient benefit by CQI & TQM in anesthesia action • Enhance patient safety by identifying risk, preventing harm, and managing complication • Ensuring distributive justice by quality, equity, and fairness
Level-two analysis	
• Prioritizing ethical principles • Enhance communication clarity	• Align safety with risk : benefit analysis and informed consent • Primary communication to relate to anesthesia event
	Secondary communication (outcome, surgical courses) as a part of team Disseminate communication key points to stakeholder (inform surgery team, support staff)
• Resolving inter-principle burden • Balancing conflicts of interest	• Undertake normative analyses • Toe the line of *refusal, reversal,* and *referral*
	Proficiency and expertise-matched allocation
	Consultant involvement: *Difficult cases* **Supervised handling:** *Routine cases* **Training of student:** *Simulator-based*
Level-three analysis	
• Special situation consideration and response • Jehovah's Witnesses • High-risk surgery in a vulnerable patient	• Additional consent, restrategize plan • High-risk consent • Advance directives/"living will" – DNR/DNI/DNV decision – Organ donation
Level-four analysis	
• Principle of Totality of Responsibly	• Attending anesthesiologist to lead from the front

2.3.1 Ethical Principles Governing Medical Ethics

2.3.1.1 The Golden Four Principles of Ethics: [13]

Principle of Respect for Patient Autonomy

The *Principle of Respect for Patient Autonomy*, which subserves the ethos of shared decision-making in clinical practice, has a profound role to play in thoracic anesthesia. It entails detailed communication (with disclosure imperatives) with the patient and the family members and allows them to ask questions on the course of surgical intervention and the expected outcome, participate in decision-making, help them express their wishes and needs and how they look to prioritize them, and finally transfer one's responsibility to the attending anesthesiologists to sustain their free will when in anesthetized state. Importantly, during surgery, the deliberation on the "way to go" should always involve a family member, a close relative, or a legally appointed representative who has to be consistently available in and around the vicinity of the OR for discussing any emergent issues that may arise during surgery. A written informed consent is required to be co-signed by the patient stakeholders, anesthesiologist (both assessor and attending anesthesiologist), and the operating surgeon to be enshrined into a legal document called the informed consent form (ICF). The nature of ICF may vary depending upon patient vulnerability, incumbent risk, anticipated surgery course, and specific requirement of anesthesia (GA, local anesthesia, monitored anesthesia care). An additional high-risk consent has to be secured from the patient and attendants beforehand if the risk involved with anesthesia and surgery is high and the clinical threshold of the possibility of "harm" is low. In thoracic anesthesia practice, attention to detail and prudence are needed to get a dedicated ICF signed for transfusion of blood and blood products.

It is also very important how one stratifies the informed consent document depending upon the quantum of anticipated risk due to various factors, including patient vulnerability (general health and age), type of surgery (the extent of resection, blood loss, and depreciation of function of the operated/healthy lungs), and expected postsurgery outcome (ventilator dependence, need for tracheostomy, ventilator-associated pneumonia), among many. Not uncommonly, additional informed consent documents may have to be obtained for special requirements of the patients (e.g., Jehovah's Witnesses), anesthesiologists (high-risk consent for enhanced risks), surgeons (consent for decision on extension, modification, and abandonment of surgery in addition to the proposed surgery), and the institution [advance directives (do-not-intubate/ventilate/resuscitate orders), organ donation, end-of-life decisions].

Principle of Beneficence

Principle of Beneficence signifies that any patient coming to a healthcare delivery setup must get some benefit out of prescription and/or intervention exercise. In thoracic anesthesia, for anesthesiologist to understand the quantum and quality of benefits that the patient may get, there is a need to outline relevant details on a case-to-case basis and the possible imperatives arising out of anesthesia healthcare delivery. *First*, the safety of the patient is of paramount importance; administration of anesthesia and taking the patient through a contentious and difficult thoracic surgery is in itself a primary benefit. The use of invasive monitoring, albeit with a pinch of iatrogenic complication and associated cost implications, brings benefit to the patient in terms of facilitating a safe GA sojourn. Similarly, employing one-lung ventilation (OLV) that requires experience and proficiency forms a secondary benefit as it saves the normal dependent lung from contaminating spillage from the morbid lung and allows seamless surgery on the affected lung. In case of significant lung function deterioration following lung reduction surgery, the provision of postoperative intensive care and mechanical ventilation is reassuring and benefits the patient in terms of maintaining vital physiology, normalizing pulmonary function, and attaining independent respiration.

Overall, thoracic anesthesia promises benefits to the patient in terms of ensuring safety, complementing surgery, promoting pulmonary rehabilitation, and improving short-term surgical outcome. Conveying the details of benefits of thoracic anesthesia should form the basis of information sharing exercise at the time of securing a written informed consent document from the patients.

Principle of Non-maleficence

In thoracic anesthesia settings, *Principle of Non-maleficence* (Primum non Nocere) meaning "do no harm" subsumes central importance as there exists danger of patient getting harmed during the course of GA and surgical intervention. The assessor and the attending anesthesiologist are required to invest extraordinary focus in identifying different risk types (Fig. 2.2), communicate overall risk to members of surgical team, anticipate per-surgery events, and prepare the patient to undergo a well-planned GA. The essence of do-no-harm dictum dictates anesthesiologist to ensure safety by mitigating preventable (e.g., iatrogenic) and emergent (e.g., blood loss, bacteremia) harms during and after thoracic surgery.

Principle of Justice

Ethical *Principle of Justice* is the most unique aspect of medical ethics which not only looks at a patient as an individual but also as a unit of the community he/she belongs to. The Principle of Justice is described as the moral obligation to act on the basis of fair adjudication between competing claims and primarily ensures equality, equity, entitlement, non-discrimination, and fairness. Of the three categories of Principle of Justice, namely, fair distribution of scarce resources (distributive justice), respect for people's rights (rights based justice), and respect for morally acceptable laws (legal justice) [15], the first reflects more with the requirements and rigor of thoracic anesthesia. Thoracic surgery and anesthesia being a part of a highly specialized

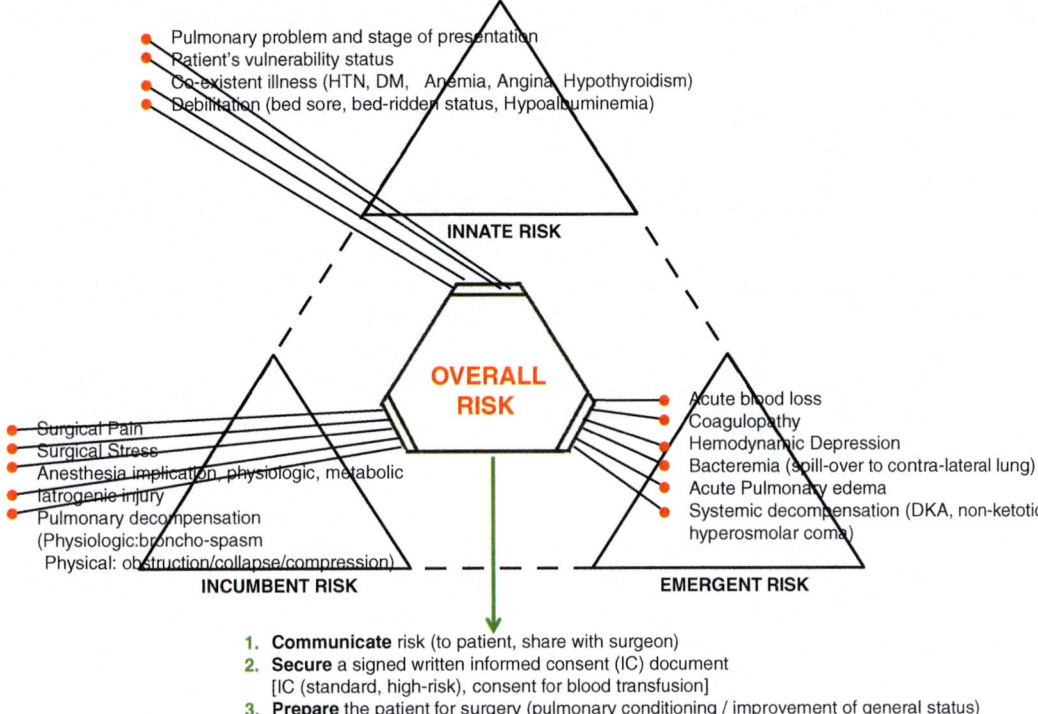

Fig. 2.2 Risk profiling and action in thoracic anesthesia

and scarcely available healthcare system tend to have a long list of patients awaiting surgery. Not uncommonly, when a thoracic anesthesia referral center is not able to cater to the needy patients along a consistent line of action, there may be long delays, labile priority allocation, and at times, increased costs. Therefore, sometimes, thoracic healthcare delivery setups are forced into a situation which undermines social justice, especially when viewed through utilitarian lens (utilitarianism: "maximum benefit to maximum no. of persons") [16, 17] or the society-centric approach to healthcare. Although the right to be treated equally and have equal access to thoracic healthcare facility may be the fundamental ideal for thoracic anesthesia practice, but on the ground, there are a multitude of factors (age, ethnic background, disability, financial position, level of insurance cover, and prognosis, among many) which adversely influence access to surgery, especially those having economic reason (Swiss Academy of Medical Sciences 2008) [18]. Therefore, at all times possible, consensus decisions on prioritizing thoracic surgery list should align with patients' need (severity of lung disease, life-threatening emergency) than other reasons.

At the time when tuberculosis, lung cancers, and incapacitating lung problems (severe COPD, large consolidation) are on the rise at an alarming rate, and the epidemic of smoking and air pollution not going to give any respite, there remains a dire need for the state health system to undertake capacity and capability building measures and situate additional thoracic surgery centers for the community at large. In this regard, at the institution level, policy changes to respond to the immediate patient load would be worthwhile, as would be the intent of the expert stakeholders (thoracic anesthesia team, operating surgeons, OR staff, intensive care personnel) to uphold the policy decisions to ensure equality, equity, and the objective veracity of arriving at surgical list movement.

2.3.2 The ICMR Twelve Principles of Ethics

The Indian Council of Medical Research (ICMR) [14], in its ethical guidelines for biomedical research in humans, offered an expansive 12-principle list of ethics to oversee planning, conduct, and reporting of medical research to safeguard human participants from any "harm" during the study. Although the implications of all the principles apply to the patients participating in research, the *Principle of Totality of Responsibility* relates somewhat directly to clinical care. The essence of this principle is that the attending anesthesiologist takes total responsibility of the standard four principles of ethics, resolve inter-principle conflicts, and apply them to the clinical case for deriving maximum benefit of anesthesia actions, procedures, and processes while being cognizant throughout of avoiding any harm to the patient.

2.4 Special Considerations in Thoracic Anesthesia

2.4.1 The Communication Challenge

In a typical thoracic anesthesia communication, the attending anesthesiologist is expected to review a thoracic surgery patient along the lines of ethical principles, strategize a plan for execution of anesthesia delivery, and communicate the patient party about the expected course of GA. However, while it is but obvious that conveying the "risk" component to the patient is always difficult, talking about the "benefits" is easy and reassuring, though it is primarily surgeon's privilege. Still, interactive deliberation with patients should carefully tread on two major lines: *First*, because the likelihood of the risk sublimating into significant adversity dominates the perioperative scene, any discussion in this regard should be initiated after careful "risk" profiling (Fig. 2.2). *Second*, though the expected benefits of a successful thoracic surgery may be magical and positively impact patient's quality of life, they become evident only after a protracted and focused postoperative recovery period and need not be overemphasized lest it would raise false expectations.

As a routine, it is necessary for the anesthesiologist to explain clearly to the patient and his/her family members the benefit of any extraordinary/invasive actions during administration of anesthesia. At all times, the anesthesiologists need to limit themselves and refrain from cross-communication of surgery details unless directed by the attending surgeon. The communication between the anesthesiologist and the patient party while the patient is anesthetized or on ventilatory support, as far as possible, should rivet around anesthesia care. In an exceptional situation only, when the surgeon is busy operating, at his behest and request, should communicating significant/emergent events be done and that too should toe a team-based approach.

2.4.2 Managing Conflicts of Interest (COI)

The nature of contentions and complicities of COI in medical practice has clouded thoracic anesthesia delivery too. COI, defined as "a set of circumstances that create a risk that professional judgment or action regarding a primary interest will be unduly influenced by a secondary interest" [19, 20], is omnipresent in clinical situations in one form or the other. COI in thoracic anesthesia is primarily *financial*, such as overuse of invasive monitoring, using costly selective anesthetic agents without the validated evidence, and disturbingly without giving due information/explanation to the patients and surgeon. Though the non-financial COIs, such as convenience-oriented practice (e.g., controlling case prioritization, selective availability only for elective day time cases, recusing oneself from emergency cases), glory/fame seeking behavior, and favoring your kin, among many. Therefore, it is important in major thoracic surgery cases where stakes are high or where risk profile is low or the patient is a candidate for recruitment into a study; the for identifying COI situations and balancing/obviating them is much required. If applicable, attending anesthesiologists should always tender COI declaration before starting the case lest there may be legal ramifications. The requirement of COI declaration becomes more pertinent in clinical practice of thoracic anesthesia, even more than that in clinical drug/device trial, because the indiscriminate use (without evidence/validation) of newer anesthetic agents *(desflurane, dexmedetomidine)*, hemodynamic drugs *(vasopressin analogues)*, monitoring gadgets *(invasive cardiac output monitoring)*, and equipment *(new double-lumen tube,* disposable fiberoptic scopes) ducks the obvious eyes and goes unnoticed most of the times. The COI declaration is an attempt to balance one's own interest with patient's interest and align with institutional norms and regulatory compliance specifics with the sole aim to identify and preclude any "harm" (physical, psychological, financial) to the patient arising out of the act of commission or omission.

The simplest way to approach the problems of COI situations is to consider as a routine, (1) whether one of the "3Rs," i.e., recuse, refuse, and refer, is applicable for a case; (2) submission of COI declaration; (3) undertaking reflective practice; and (4) refraining from introducing a costly new/selective drug or device without taking the patient and surgical team into confidence.

2.4.3 Research in Thoracic Anesthesia

The difficult nature of procedures in thoracic anesthesia calls for research of high scientific rigor. In order to advance understanding for the benefit of overall patient safety, the empirical and hypothetical research into thoracic anesthesia requires to identify and select the residual concerns that remain even after a structured reflective practice. To uphold patient safety during thoracic anesthesia, *first,* the administration of GA should be effective (no intraoperative awareness recall, no add-on hemodynamic stress, no iatrogenic procedure-related injury), efficient (minimum anesthetic agent utilization, quick recovery), and safe (continuous monitoring and pharmacovigilance, intensive care); *second,* to further the safety mandate, all the technical procedure should be facilitated by use of appropriate aids, such as Doppler ultrasound for nerve blocks and invasive limes, airway access using FOB guidance, and fluid administration based on hemodynamic parameters (e.g., stroke volume administration), to name a few; and *third*, the residual concern should be identified and researched upon. Though research in thoracic anesthesia patients can be difficult due to the difficult combination of patient vulnerability and major surgery, the potential for undertaking research should always be identified and converted. In view of the above, careful selection of patients and methods greatly subsumes critical importance. Since a prospective randomized study, which has the ability to generate robust clinical evidence, may not be feasible each time, every opportunity to report a case/a case series or undertake a retrospective analysis should not be missed, as the pilot data can form a strong ground for conducting a prospective study. For research in thoracic anesthesia, the patient and family members need to be taken into confidence by explaining the details, and a signed written informed consent is to be secured if they agree to participate in research of their own free will. Interestingly, a natural advantage to patient may be that in a clinical research situation, the attending anesthesia scientists become overly conscious toward the patient's well-being and avoidance of harm. A verified and validated patient information document and investigator COI declaration must accompany the signed informed consent form before the patient enters the recruitment phase of a prospective (empirical/randomized) study. Since funded clinical trials may be difficult to substantiate in thoracic anesthesia settings, at the policy level, investigator-initiated research should be supported by the institution with requisite infrastructure, a regulatory compliant system, and financial support (e.g., intramural funding).

2.4.4 Blood Transfusion Practices in Thoracic Anesthesia

The heightened possibility of blood loss during thoracic surgery makes it one of the most difficult surgical subspecialties for the attending anesthesiologist to manage. Since the chest wall, bronchial tree, and the pulmones are richly perfused, not uncommonly, blood loss during thoracic surgery can be significant necessitating transfusion of blood (RBC, whole blood) and blood products (fresh frozen plasma, platelet-rich plasma, cryoprecipitate). Since blood transfusion during surgery is fraught with risk, for the patient safety, a multispecialty approach with anesthesiologist, surgeon, physiologist, and transfusion expert is essential to address any adversity. Attending anesthesiologist needs to actively pursue this issue and place a plan cover for the anticipated blood loss during thoracic surgery. If blood loss during surgery is expected to be significant, it should be communicated to the patient party as is the risks (metabolic acidosis, coagulation abnormality, oxygen carrying capacity depreciation) and benefits (maintenance of adequate cardiac output) of the responsive transfusion during and after the surgery. An exclusive written documentation of informed consent for blood and blood product transfusion is absolutely necessary, both for the patient safety and for legal security of the responsible thoracic healthcare personnel. Further, the informed consent document should emphasize conveying to the patients the probable need for uncrossed blood transfusion in acute circumstances (emergency surgery, massive-continuous losses, unavailability of rare blood) and the attendant grave consequences [21].

A rare yet special situation regarding practice of blood transfusion in medicine is *Jehovah's Witnesses*. As a matter of belief-based principle, Jehovah's Witness patients refuse transfusion of blood and its selective products, and even the natural/recombinant hemoglobin irrespective of surgery indication or life-threatening emergency. The ethico-legal ramifications of refusing to accept blood transfusion may be dramatic and amount to life-threatening adversity [22]. Queerly, though the refusal to accept blood transfusion during thoracic surgery upholds Principle of Respect for Patient Autonomy, it works against moral obligation of the anesthesiologist's responsibility of avoiding harm and saving lives. The resultant inter-principle conflict is a matter of debate even among Jehovah's Witnesses, and there is a possibility that in the future, the legal position would change positively in favor of physicians, especially for the hapless anesthesiologist who has an added responsibility of caring for a non-communicative anesthetized patient [23].

Advance Directives in Thoracic Anesthesia

The thoracic surgery patients are likely to be more vulnerable and affected at the time of presenting to the referral tertiary care center. Also, a thoracic intervention involves the possibility of greater risk of surgical injury than that in other's surgery. The combination of patient vulnerability with difficult anesthesia care delivery which directly relates to surgical outcome has to be responded to by a careful plan, preparation, and conduct of thoracic anesthesia. The patients who have their own share of suffering even before they reach a veritable advanced thoracic center are likely to hoard their own opinion about outlook toward life and definition of suffering. They commonly prefer continuing walking toward greater safety, and most of the times, they do not want additional suffering because of the difficult surgery and protracted recovery course. Therefore, it is essential that a psychologist be part of the team to talk the patients out and help them overcoming their meaningless dogmas that hamper quality of care. Further, while exploring frantically for an appropriate high-end medical center for want of adequate treatment, many of the thoracic surgery patients would already have consumed their finances. These very patients participate actively in the decision-making about the prospective intervention and, not uncommonly, put forward their strong opinions. Legally, it is the duty of the thoracic anesthesia team to look into them and reach a fair balance before moving forward. This makes an interesting point as it activates another vital facet of present-day medicine practice, i.e., advance directives. An *advance directive*, also called a "living will" or a "personal directive," represents a legal document wherein a person specifies what actions should be taken during the course of their medical treatment health in case they are no longer able to make decisions for themselves for the reasons thereof (incapacitating illness, head injury, etc.). While advance directives have gained legal status in the USA, in other countries, it continues to be a legally persuasive exercise without the legal mandate.

A "living will" comprises specific directives on the course of medical treatment lines the providers and caregivers are expected to follow. Ethically, sometimes, advance directives, which may forbid the use of various kinds of medical treatment, can cut across the sanctity of *Principle of Beneficence*, by precluding actions beneficial to the patients. Of the many distressing examples of advance directives hampering treatment can be blocking administration of food through a gastric tube, withholding analgesia, not giving antibiotics, and in extreme circumstances, not employing the artificial airway access (tracheal tubes, tracheostomy), not using the supportive mechanical ventilation, and so on. Also a person, through the directives enshrined in his/her living will, may opt for not receiving any resuscitative efforts to prolong life. The decision to activate do-not-resuscitate (DNR) orders, which are being viewed in terms of do not ventilate, do not intubate, do not resuscitate, are contentious and difficult to reach at and requires careful deliberation along the lines of legal requirements of the respective state [24]. Interestingly, the patient self-determination act of the USA (PSDA, effective December 1991) requires healthcare providers (hospitals, nursing homes, etc.) to preempt their patients of their rights to document advance directives under state law [18]. Under the rights to a dignified life and dignified death, the Indian *Supreme Court* very recently (March 2018) allowed individuals for signing "living wills" and opting for passive euthanasia [25].

Thoracic anesthesiologists are likely to confront varied ethical intricacies burdening them with difficult-to-take decisions for the practice of anesthesia in thoracic surgery patients. In this regard, careful compliance with the existent legal statute of the land is a much required additional responsibility for them to shoulder. Recently, Rolnick, Asch, and Halpern, while commenting on the legal formalities that impose barriers to creating advance directives, recommended eliminating specific legal requirements to facilitate integration of advance directives with healthcare systems to improve the likelihood of their being used to achieve their intended goals [26].

2.5 Conclusions

Ethical and philosophical imperatives in thoracic anesthesia remain as relevant as they were before, only that creation of wider awareness around ethical principles governing medical practice and the ability of scientific evidence to question longstanding dogmas [2] have changed considerably. In medicine, since philosophical consideration and ethical analysis has potential to ease up translation of advancing scientific evidence into clinical practice realm, it is high time that thoracic anesthesia with its special set of intricacies (different airway access control modalities, one-lung ventilation, postoperative lung function rehabilitation, significant blood loss, cardiac and pulmonary function synchronization) be also subserved by guidelines/rules gleaned from such an exercise. This is likely to enhance patient safety in terms of preventing avoidable morbidities, identifying otherwise unforeseen harms, and planning better for every next case. The specifics related to the *direct* (patient autonomy and shared decision-making, risk–benefit analysis, decreasing iatrogenic harm, balancing conflicts of interest, etc.) and *indirect* (decision on postoperative intensive observation/ventilation, blood transfusion, DNR, advance directives, end-of-life decisions, organ donation) ethical implications of thoracic anesthesia need to be further explored in order to reach at and proffer a simple-to-communicate, easy-to-understand-and-apply, structured system of precision anesthesia practice.

References

1. Brodsky JB. The evolution of thoracic anesthesia. Thorac Surg Clin. 2005;15:1–10.
2. Kritek PA, Luks AM. Preventing dogma from driving practice. New Engl J Med. 2019;380:870–1. https://doi.org/10.1056/NEJMe1900708.

3. Berhard Z. Thoracic anesthesia. Curr Opin Anaesthesiol. 2001;14:47–9.
4. Dinic VD, Stojanovic MD, Markovic D, et al. Enhanced recovery in thoracic surgery: a review. Front Med (Lausanne). 2018;5:14. https://doi.org/10.3389/fmed.2018.00014.
5. Batchelor TJP, Rasburn NJ, Abdelnour-Berchtold E, et al. Guidelines for enhanced recovery after lung surgery: recommendations of the enhanced recovery after surgery (ERAS®) Society and the European Society of Thoracic Surgeons (ESTS). Eur J Cardio-Thorac Surg. 2018;55:91–115. https://doi.org/10.1093/ejcts/ezy301.2.
6. Batchelor TJP, Ljungqvist O. A surgical perspective of ERAS guidelines in thoracic surgery. Curr Opin Anaesthesiol. 2019;32:17–22.
7. Bill C. A TQM path to tomorrow: new ways for new days. In: Bill C, editor. The five pillars of TQM: how to make total quality management work for you. New York: Truman Talley Books; 1994. p. 478.
8. Juran J. The quality trilogy: a universal approach to managing for quality. Presented at the ASQC 40th Annual Quality Congress, Anaheim, California, 1986: pp. 1–9.
9. Taylor RM. Ethical Principles and concepts in Medicine. Bernat JL, Beresford HR, eds. Handb Clin Neurol. 2013;118:1–9. https://doi.org/10.1016/B978-0-444-53501-6.00001-9.
10. Pieterse AH, Stiggelbout AM, Montori VM. Shared decision making and importance of time. JAMA. 2019;322:25–6.
11. Hain R, Saad T. Foundations of practical ethics. Medicine. 2016;44:578–82.
12. Beauchamp TL, DeGrazia D. Principles and principlism. In: Khushf G, editor. Handbook of bioethics, philosophy and medicine. Dordrecht: Springer; 2004. p. 78.
13. Beauchamp TL, Childress JF. Principles of biomedical ethics. 5th ed. New York, NY: Oxford University Press; 2001.
14. Mathur M, editor. National ethical guidelines for biomedical and health research involving human participants. New Delhi: Indian Council of Medical Research; 2018. p. 2.
15. Gillon R. Medical ethics: four principles plus attention to scope. BMJ. 1994;309:184–8.
16. Zalta EN, Nodelman U, Allen C, et al. editors. The history of utilitarianism. Stanford Encyclopedia of Philosophy. Winter ed. Stanford, CA: Metaphysics Research Lab, Center for the Study of Language and Information, Stanford University; 2014. p. 94305.
17. Mandal J, Ponnambath DK, Parija SC. Utilitarian and deontological ethics in medicine. Tropical Parasitol. 2016;6:5–7.
18. Docker C. Advance directives/living wills. In: McLean SAM, editor. Contemporary issues in law, medicine and ethics. Aldershot: Dartmouth; 1996. p. 182.
19. Thompson DF. Understanding conflicts of interest. N Engl J Med. 1993;329:573–6.
20. Waisel DB. Ethics and conflicts of interest in anesthesia practice. In: Longnecker DE, Brown DL, Newman MF, et al. editors. Anesthesiology. 2nd ed. New York: McGraw Hill; 2012.
21. Miraflor E, Yeung L, Strumwasser A, et al. Emergency uncrossmatched transfusion effect on blood type alloantibodies. J Trauma Acute Care Surg. 2012;72:48–52.
22. Smith ML. Jehovah's Witness refusal of blood products. In: Post SG, editor. Encyclopedia of bioethics, vol. 3. 3rd ed. New York: Macmillan Reference-Thomson Gale; 2003. p. 1341–5.
23. Muramoto O. Medical confidentiality and the protection of Jehovah's Witnesses' autonomous refusal of blood. J Med Ethics. 2000;26:381–6.
24. American Medical Association. Guidelines for the appropriate use of do-not-resuscitate orders. Council on Ethical and Judicial Affairs. JAMA. 1991;265:1868–18.
25. Death with dignity: on SC's verdict on euthanasia and living wills. The Hindu. 10 March 2018 – via www.thehindu.com
26. Rolnick JA, Asch DA, Halpern SD. Delegalizing advance directives—facilitating advance care planning. N Engl J Med. 2017;376:2105–7.

Functional Anatomy of Thorax

Ajay Sirohi

The thorax is the region of the trunk that lies between the neck above and the abdomen inferiorly. The thoracic cavity contains the laterally placed pleura and lungs separated by a median partition, called the mediastinum.

Extent and boundaries of mediastinum are as follows: root of neck and thoracic outlet superiorly, diaphragm inferiorly, sternum anteriorly, and thoracic vertebrae posteriorly.

It contains heart and large blood vessels, thoracic duct and lymph nodes, vagus, phrenic nerves, sympathetic trunk, trachea and oesophagus.

A series of cross-sectional views through the thorax illustrate the relations of the structures that are contents of mediastinum and the rest of the thoracic cavity (Figs. 3.1, 3.2, 3.3, 3.4, 3.5 and 3.6).

An imaginary plane divides the mediastinum into a superior and an inferior part (Fig. 3.3). This plane passes anteriorly through the sternal angle and posteriorly to the inferior margin of fourth thoracic vertebra.

INFERIOR MEDIASTINUM is further divided into three parts:

1. Anterior mediastinum: Space between pericardium and sternum
2. Middle mediastinum: containing pericardium and heart
3. Posterior mediastinum: lying between pericardium and lower eight thoracic vertebrae

The arrangement of mediastinal structures from anterior to posterior is as follow:

Superior:	Inferior:
• Thymus	• Thymus
• Large veins	• Heart + pericardium + phrenic nerves
• Large arteries	
• Trachea	• Esophagus + thoracic duct
• Esophagus and thoracic duct	• Descending aorta
• Sympathetic trunk	• Sympathetic trunks

3.1 Upper Airway

The passage extending from the nostrils and lips to the lowest end of the larynx is referred to as the functional upper airway.

The nasal cavities are separated from each other by a septum (which is cartilaginous anteriorly and bony posteriorly). The cavities are bounded laterally by turbinate bones (upper, middle, and lower), with sinus openings in between. The soft and hard palate forms the floor of the nasal cavities.

The nasal cavities are internally lined by a richly innervated and vascular mucosa. During nasopharyngeal intubation and fiberoptic bronchoscopy, the anesthesiologist should be sensitive to the high vascularity of this mucosa.

A. Sirohi (✉)
Institute of Anaesthesiology, Pain and Perioperative Medicine, Sir Ganga Ram Hospital, New Delhi, India

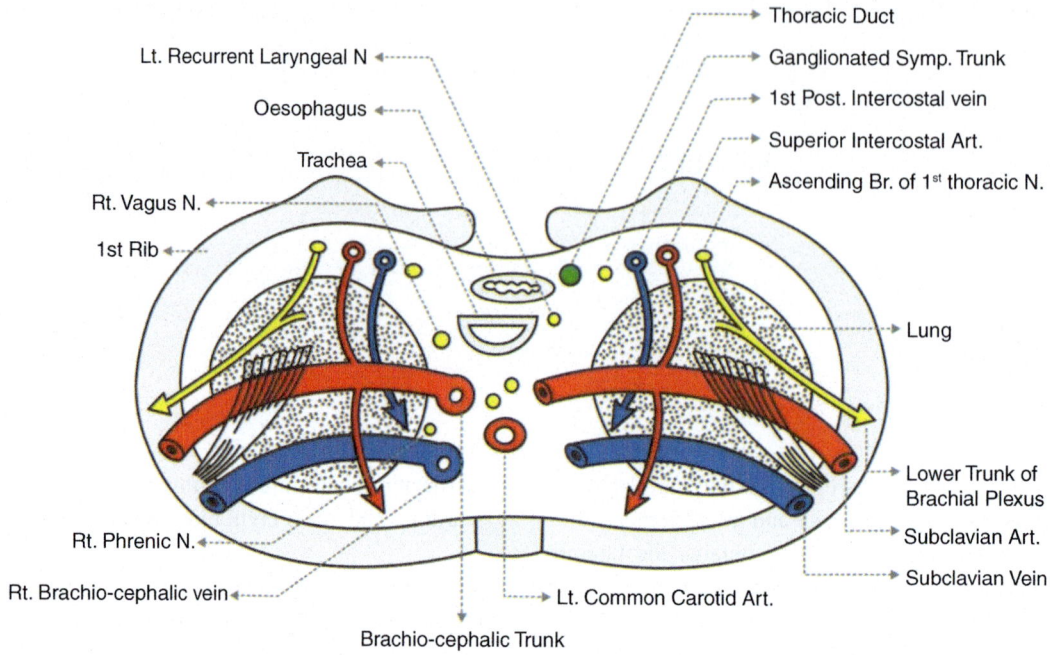

Fig. 3.1 Transverse section of thorax through the apices of both lungs

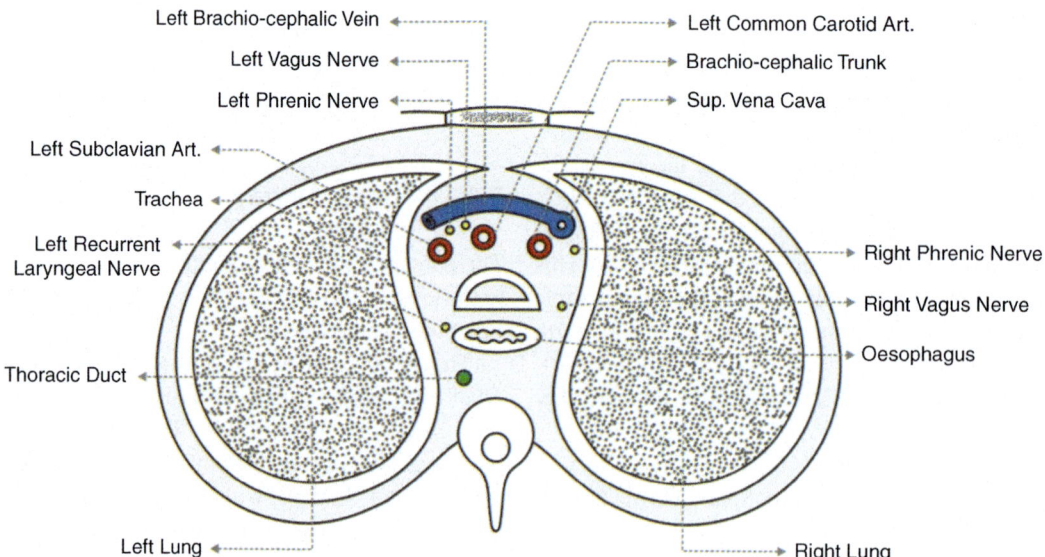

Fig. 3.2 Transverse section of thorax above the arch of aorta

3 Functional Anatomy of Thorax

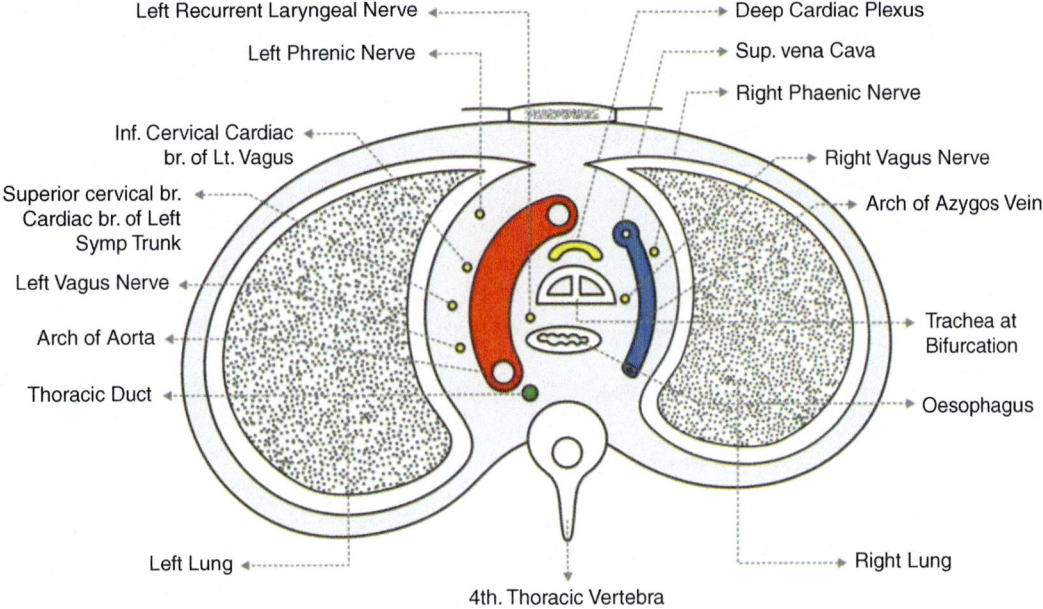

Fig. 3.3 Transverse section of thorax at the tracheal bifurcation

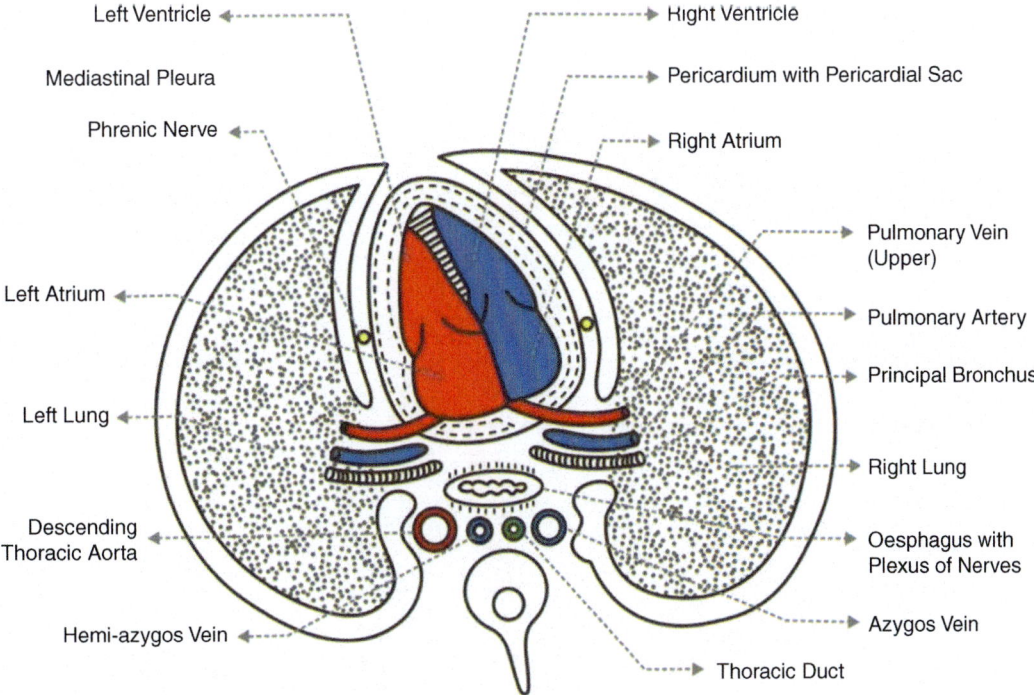

Fig. 3.4 Transverse section of thorax at the lung roots

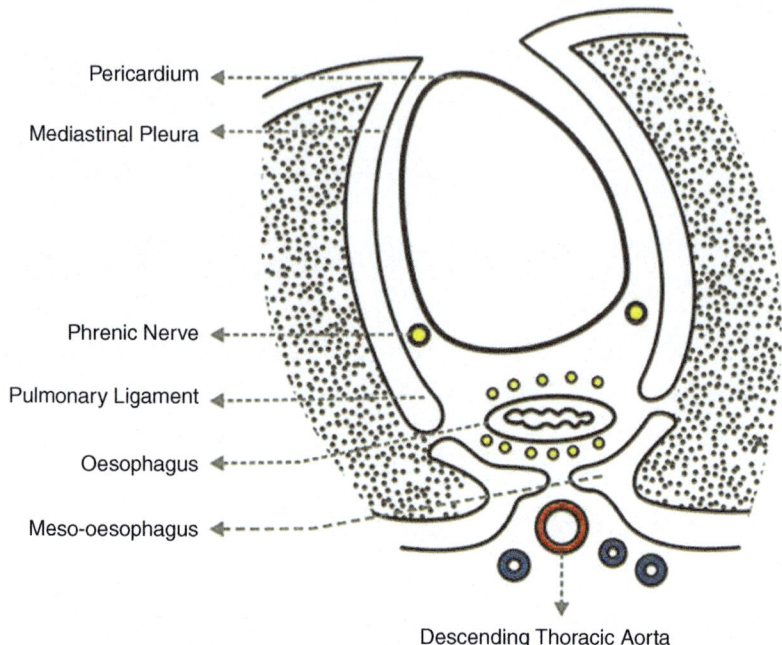

Fig. 3.5 Transverse section of thorax below the lung roots

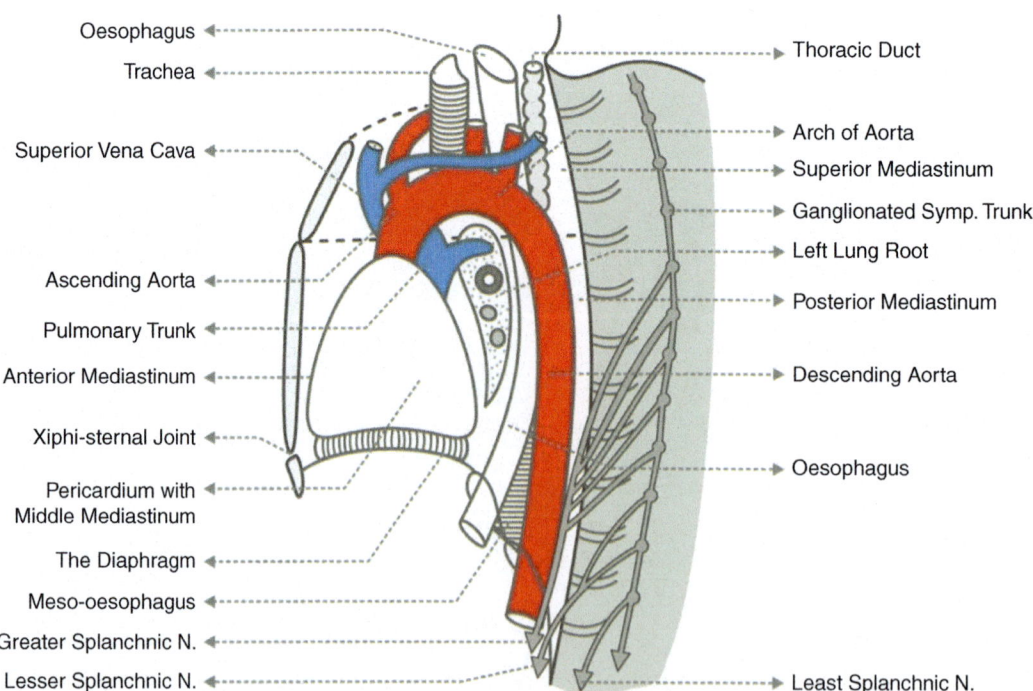

Fig. 3.6 Left lateral view of thoracic mediastinum

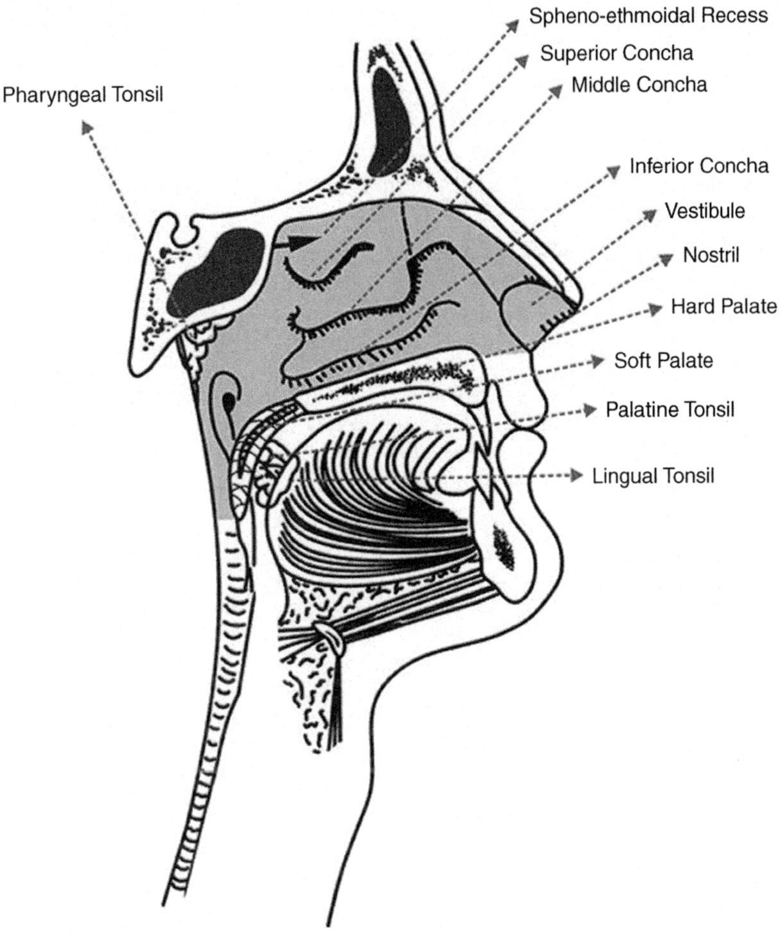

Fig. 3.7 Pharynx

- Pharyngeal Tonsil
- Spheno-ethmoidal Recess
- Superior Concha
- Middle Concha
- Inferior Concha
- Vestibule
- Nostril
- Hard Palate
- Soft Palate
- Palatine Tonsil
- Lingual Tonsil

3.2 Pharynx

It is a 12–15 cm long tube, with three regions: nasopharynx, oropharynx, and laryngopharynx (Fig. 3.7)

Nasopharynx is the part of the pharyngeal tube that lies between the base of skull and soft palate, behind the nasal cavities. It is lined by respiratory epithelium. It conditions the air entering during inspiration and propagates it ahead.

Oropharynx is the middle part of the pharyngeal tube that extends from the anterior tonsillar pillar to the superior border of epiglottis. It contains posterior one-third of tongue, lingual tonsils, palatine tonsils, and superior constrictor muscle. It helps in the voluntary and involuntary phases of swallowing.

Waldeyers' ring is a ring of lymphoid tissue in the naso- and oropharynx. It consists of two palatine tonsils, lingual tonsils and adenoid.

Laryngopharynx: is the distal part of pharynx. It is located between the epiglottis and cricoid cartilage, and continues into the esophagus below. It lies behind the larynx. Laryngopharynx contains two constrictor muscles, middle and inferior pharyngeal constrictors.

During general anesthesia, the tone of the tongue, hard palate, and pharyngeal musculature decreases, which may cause oropharynx to get obstructed [1, 2].

Airway resistance increases during hyperextension and hyperflexion of the cervical spine [3].

3.3 Larynx

The larynx is a tube that is located within the neck, anterior to the inferior portion of the pharynx and superior to the trachea. It extends from C4 to C6 vertebra, in adult, during normal respiration.

Its primary function is to form a passage of the airway, it prevents the entry of foreign body into the airway by closing the inlet immediately if there is a mechanical stimulus. Larynx also helps in voice production, coughing reflex, ventilatory functions, and also acts as a sense organ [4].

The larynx is made up of several cartilages: cricoid, thyroid, epiglottis (three unpaired cartilages), arytenoid, corniculate, cuneiform (three paired cartilages); and a number of intrinsic muscles. Laryngeal motion is helped by hyoid bone although technically it is not a part of larynx.

Laryngeal inlet is bounded by epiglottis, aryepiglottic folds, and arytenoids (Fig. 3.8).

Pyriform fossa: The larynx bulges into the pharynx posteriorly, creating a deep pharyngeal recess anteriorly on both sides. This fossa is laterally bound by thyroid cartilages. Sometimes foreign bodies tend to lodge in the pyriform fossa.

3.4 Trachea and Bronchial Tree

Trachea (a membrano-cartilaginous tube) is a continuation of larynx. It begins at the lower border of cricoid cartilage (opposite C6) and extends around 12 cm (in females)/14 cm (in males), through the neck and superior mediastinum and terminates in a bifurcation (called carina) into right and left principle bronchi, opposite the sternal angle (T4–T5 level). In the new born the trachea bifurcates at T3 vertebral level. In the standing position trachea bifurcation is at T6 level [5]. The tracheal diameter is approximately 22 ± 1.5 mm (in males) to 19 ± 1.5 mm (in females). The tracheal tube is made of 16–20 U-shaped cartilaginous rings. Posteriorly these rings are closed by fibrous tissue and trachealis muscle. The trachea is a midline tube except at its termination, where it deviates slightly to the right side due to the pressure of arch of aorta [6].

3.4.1 Relations of Trachea

- In the neck:
  - Anteriorly: Skin, superficial and deep cervical facia, overlapped by sternohyoid and sternothyroid muscle, crossed by isthmus of thyroid gland, opposite second, third and fourth

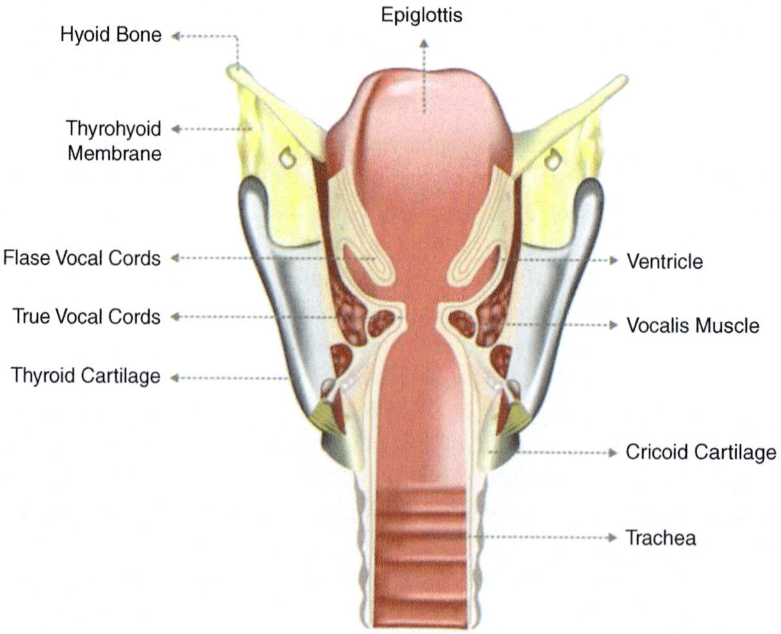

Fig. 3.8 Laryngeal inlet

tracheal rings, above, the isthmus is crossed by two Superior Thyroid arteries, below, the isthmus is related to Inferior Thyroid veins.
- Posteriorly: Oesophagus, which separates the trachea from the vertebral column and two Recurrent Laryngeal nerves or each side.
- Laterally: Lateral lobe of thyroid gland extending up to five to six rings of trachea, Common Carotid and Inferior Thyroid artery below the gland [7].
- In the thorax:
  - Anteriorly: Manubrium sterni, Inferior Thyroid veins, Left Brachiocephalic vein, Brachiocephalic Trunk, Left Common Carotid artery. At the bifurcation trachea is related with deep cardiac plexus and arch of aorta.
  - Posteriorly: left recurrent laryngeal nerve and Esophagus.
  - On right side: Right lung, Arch of Azygous vein, Right Vagus nerve.
  - On left side: Left Subclavian artery and Left common carotid, Arch of aorta and the left lung [8].

3.4.2 Bronchus

The two principle bronchi begin at the bifurcation of trachea and enter the hilum of the corresponding lung, where each bronchus subdivides into successive generations of smaller bronchi and finally end as terminal respiratory bronchioles. Each bronchus has an extrapulmonary and intrapulmonary component.

The right main bronchus is shorter (1.4–1.8 cm), wider (14–17.5 mm), and more vertical than the left bronchus. Hence, a foreign body in the trachea is usually aspirated into the right lung. Right bronchus passes downward and to the right from the bifurcation of trachea and makes an angle of 25 degrees from the median plane. It passes below the arch of azygous vein, enters the root of the right lungs, and reaches the hilum at the level of T5. In the lung, the right bronchus is crossed in front by the right pulmonary artery. Within the lung, the right principal bronchus divides into secondary or lobar bronchi. Each secondary bronchus subdivides into segmental or tertiary bronchi (Fig. 3.9) [9].

The area of the lung supplied by one tertiary bronchus is known as *bronchopulmonary segment*. The branches of pulmonary artery follow the tertiary bronchi and are segmental in distribution, whereas tributaries of pulmonary veins are intersegmental in drainage. A segmental bronchus may branch 6–18 times to produce 50–70 respiratory bronchioles which merge with the alveolar sac.

The left principle bronchus is longer, narrower, and more oblique then the right bronchus. It is on

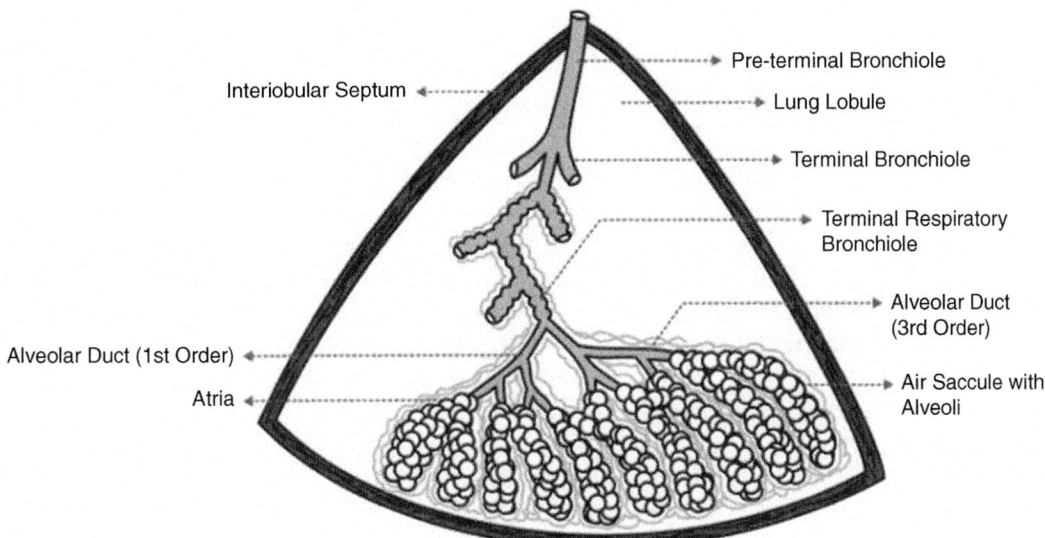

Fig. 3.9 Divisions of the bronchioles

an average 4.4–4.9 cm in length, and around 13–16.5 mm in diameter.

Left bronchus makes an angle of 45 degrees away from the median plane at the tracheal bifurcation and passes downward and to the left below the arch of the aorta. It enters the lung root and reaches the hilum at the level of T6. The left bronchus divides into upper and lower lobar bronchi to supply the respective lobe of the left lung.

However, all these dimensions can be quite variable among individuals and relationships of these structures can drastically change with chest pathologies [6].

Bronchopulmonary segments of the lungs (Fig. 3.10)

Right lung		Left lung	
Upper lobe	Apical	Upper lobe	Apical
	Anterior		Posterior
	Posterior		Anterior
			Upper lingular
Middle lobe	Medial		Lower lingular
	Lateral		
Lower lobe	Apical	Lower lobe	Apical
	Medial basal		Anteromedial basal
	Anterior basal		Lateral basal
	Lateral basal		Posterior basal
	Posterior basal		

3.4.3 Innervation

Tracheobronchial tree is innervated by anterior and posterior pulmonary plexus [8].

3.4.4 Circulation of the Tracheobronchial Tree

Tracheal and bronchial blood supply is from several sources [10].

The cervical trachea is supplied by Inferior Thyroid artery. The carina and distal trachea are supplied by bronchial arteries (internal thoracic artery) and also branches from innominate artery and descending Aorta. The segmental branches of bronchial arteries form a longitudinal network over the trachea and supplies it [11].

Though there is lot of variation in this blood supply, generally the left main bronchus is supplied by inferior bronchial artery, and the right main bronchus by posterior intercostal arteries (Fig. 3.11) [12].

3.5 Pleura and Lungs

The pleura is a thin closed serous sac into which each lung invaginates from the medial side. Each pleural cavity consists of two layers, an inner visceral and an outer parietal layer, and both layers are continuous around the lung root.

Parietal pleura is named according to the structures it lines: costal, diaphragmatic, cervical, and mediastinal.

Costodiaphragmatic recess:

It is a potential gap that is present between the parietal layer of pleura and the inferior border of the lung (Fig. 3.12).

3.5.1 Clinical Implication

Pleural tap is usually performed posterior to mid axillary line at one or more intercostal spaces below the fluid level with the patient in sitting position but not below the ninth intercostal space, lest it may injure the liver on the right side and spleen on the left side.

Entry of air in pleural cavity is called pneumothorax, which may lead to collapse of the lung. When the pleural cavity is exposed to the atmosphere it forms an *open pneumothorax*. When the opening of visceral pleura is valvular, it permits air entry into the pleural sac during inspiration but prevents air exit during expiration. This is known as *tension pneumothorax*, leading to lung collapse. It is a surgical emergency and managed by inserting chest tubes into the pleural cavity through the anterior part of the second intercostal space.

3.6 Lungs

Lungs are a pair of porous, elastic, and spongy essential organs of respiration. Each lung is covered by pleura except at the hilum.

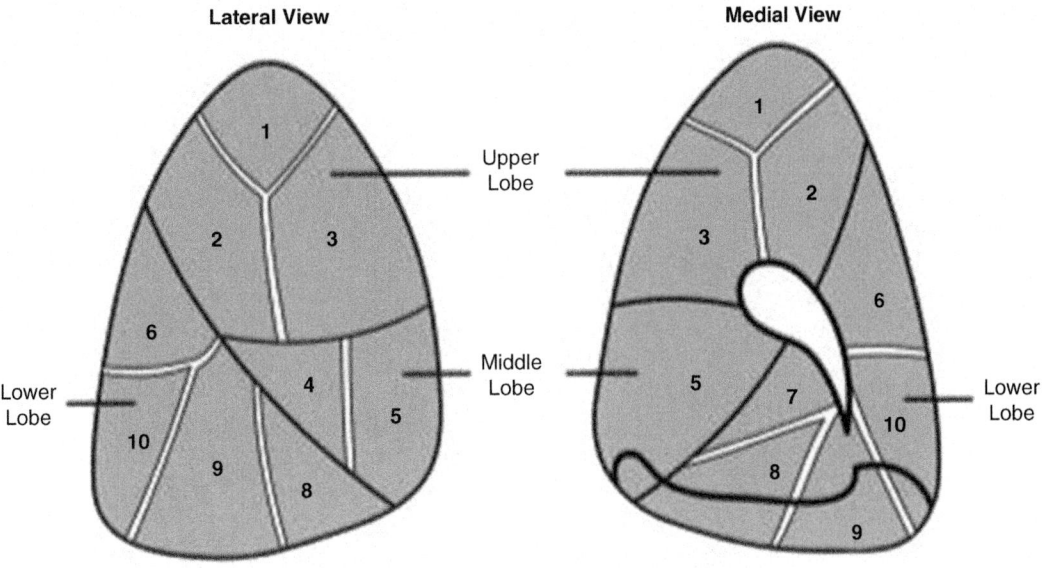

01 = Apical Segment of Upper Lobe; 02 = Posterior;
03 = Anterior; 04 = Lateral;
05 = Medial; 06 = Apical Segment of Lower Lobe;
07 = Medial Basal (Cardiac); 08 = Anterior Basal;
09 = Lateral Basal; 10 = Posterior Basal;

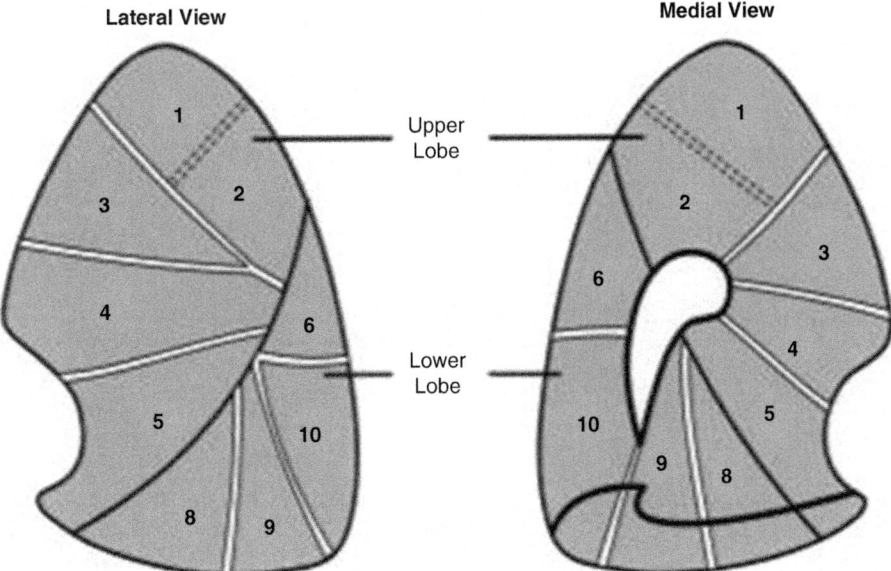

01 = Apical Segment of Upper Lobe; 02 = Posterior;
03 = Anterior; 04 = Superior Lingular;
05 = Inferior Lingular; 06 = Apical Segment of Lower Lobe;
09 = Lateral Basal; 08 = Anterior Basal;
  10 = Posterior Basal;

Fig. 3.10 Bronchopulmonary segments of right and left lungs

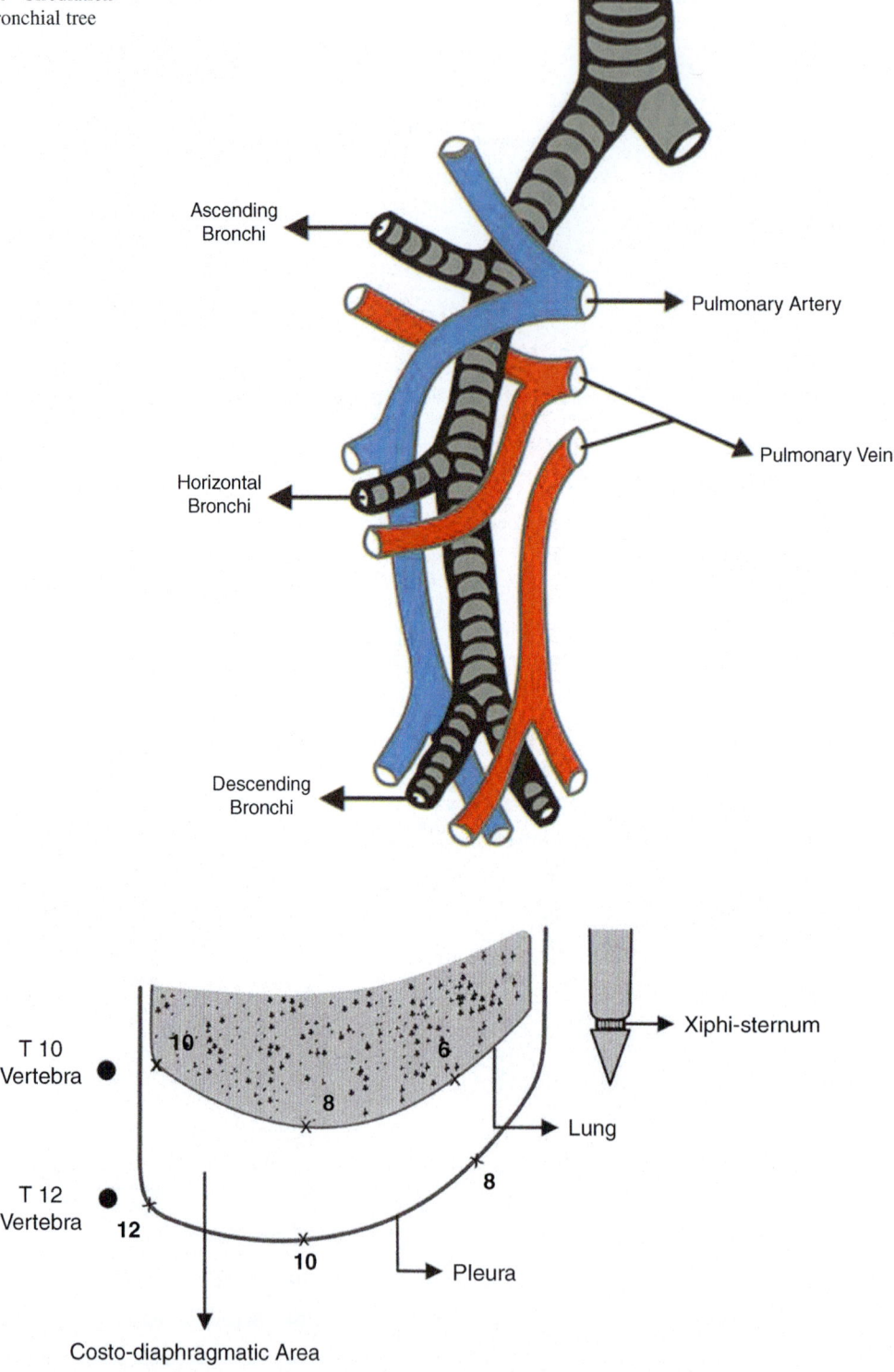

Fig. 3.11 Circulation of the bronchial tree

Fig. 3.12 Costodiaphragmatic recess

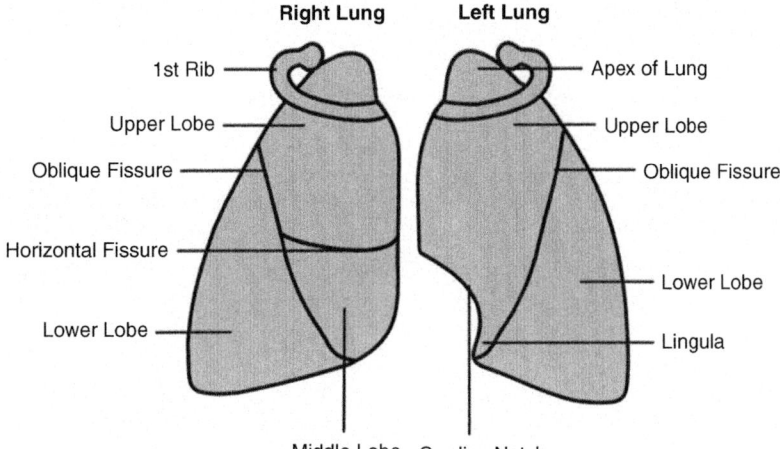

Fig. 3.13 Anatomy of lung (right and left)

Each lung is half conical in shape and presents an apex, base, costal, and medial surfaces and three borders anterior, posterior, and inferior (Fig. 3.13).

Apex of the lung is related to subclavian artery anteriorly, neck of the first rib posteriorly, trachea (right lung) and esophagus and thoracic duct (left lung) medially. Bases of the lung are related to the liver on the right side and stomach and spleen on the left side, separated by the diaphragm.

Costal surface: of the lung is smooth and is related to lateral thoracic wall separated by costal pleura. It has impressions for ribs and costal cartilages. The ribs coming in relation to the costal surface of the lung are: upper six ribs in the mid clavicular line, upper eight ribs in mid axillary line, and upper ten ribs in scapular line.

Medial surface: the posterior/Vertebral part is flat and related to the upper ten thoracic vertebrae.

The impressions and relations of mediastinal/anterior part are different on the right and left side (Fig. 3.14).

3.6.1 Lung Border

Anterior border is thin and occupies the costomediastinal recess of pleura. The anterior border of left lung follows the costo-mediastinal reflection up to the fourth costal cartilage and then it deviates laterally for 3.5 cm. It then it turns downwards and medially to forms a *cardiac notch* and reaches the sixth costal cartilage.

Posterior border is thick and rounded and occupies the paravertebral gutter. Inferior border is thin and occupies costodiaphragmatic recess of pleura.

3.6.2 Innervation of the Lungs

The autonomic nervous system is the main nervous system of the lungs that provides innervation through the pulmonary plexus, which surrounds the hila of the lungs [13].

3.6.3 Nutrition to the Lungs

The lung gets its nutrition from two sources:

- The conducting part, up to the beginning of respiratory bronchioles is supplied by bronchial arteries.
- Respiratory part is supplied by pulmonary artery via the pulmonary capillary plexus.

Venous drainage: the lungs are drained partly into pulmonary and partly into bronchial veins (Figs. 3.15 and 3.16).

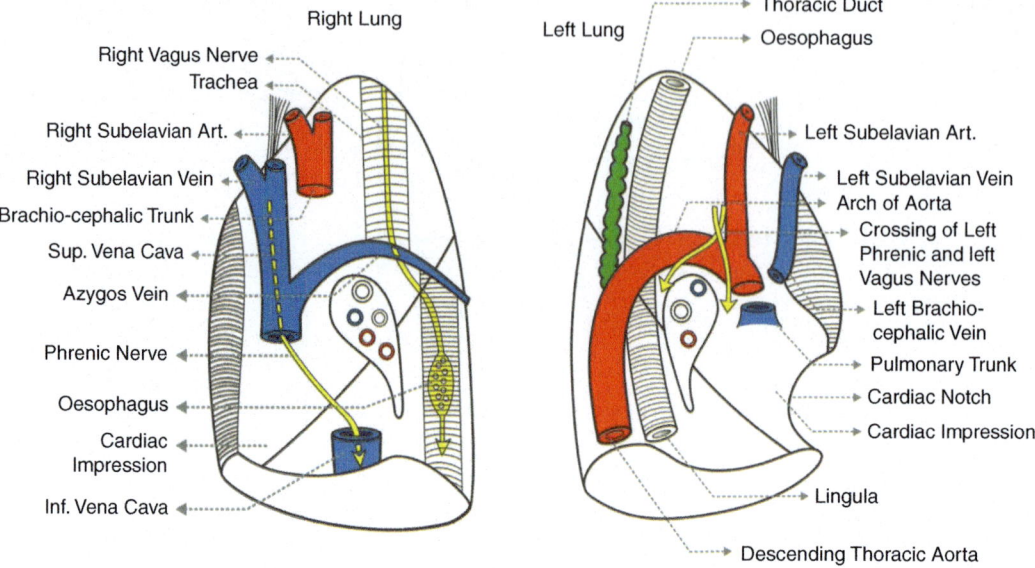

Fig. 3.14 Relations of the lungs

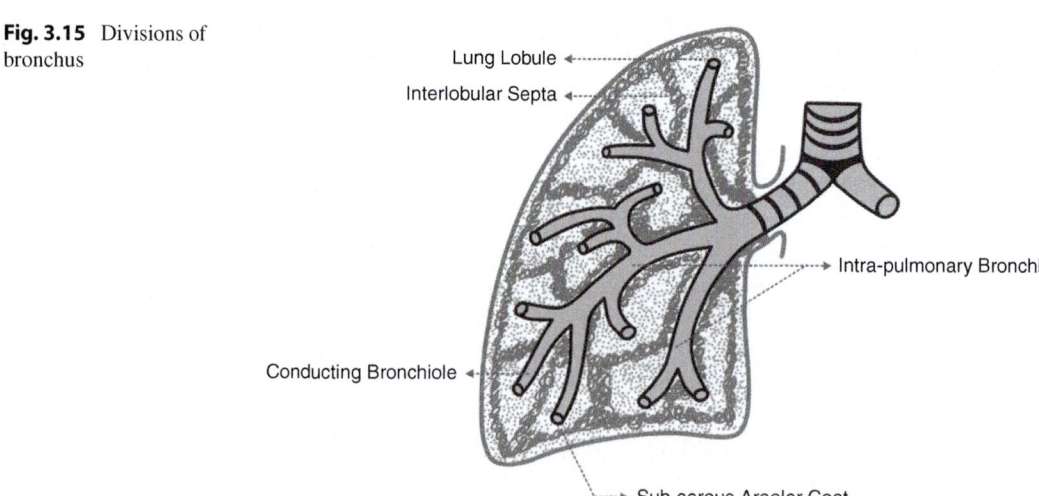

Fig. 3.15 Divisions of bronchus

3.7 Conclusion

Getting an in-depth understanding of the anatomy of thorax is an important prerequisite for a better understanding of thoracic pathology and surgical procedures. The better we understand the anatomical details of the thoracic region, the more errorless and accurate can be our surgical, anaesthetic and physiological approaches, leading to far lesser complications.

Therefore, the anatomy of the thoracic region could sometimes determine the very basis of a particular condition and the prognosis too, thus establishing the importance of understanding anatomy in great details, for better patient outcomes.

Fig. 3.16 Nutrition of the lung

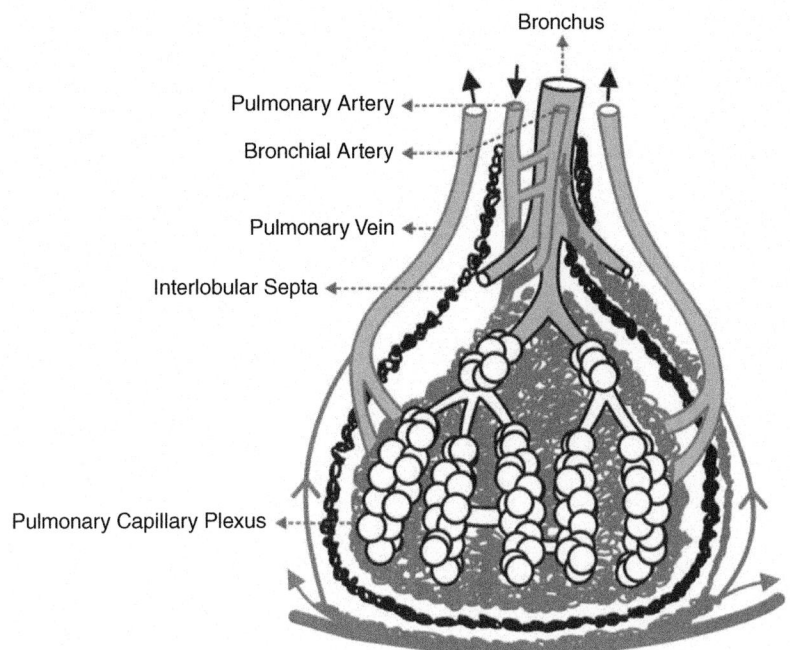

References

1. Hudgel DW, Hendricks C. Palate and hypopharynx—sites of inspiratory narrowing of the upper airway during sleep. Am Rev Respir Dis. 1988;138(6):1542–7.
2. Wheatley JR, Kelly WT, Tully A, et al. Pressure-diameter relationships of the upper airway in awake supine subjects. J Appl Physiol. 1991;70(5):2242–51.
3. Spann RW, Hyatt RE. Factors affecting upper airway resistance in conscious man. J Appl Physiol. 1971;31(5):708–12.
4. Bartlett D Jr. Respiratory functions of the larynx. Physiol Rev. 1989;69(1):33–57.
5. Gal TJ. Anatomy and physiology of the respiratory system and the pulmonary circulation. In: Kaplan JA, Slinger PD, editors. Thoracic anaesthesia. 3rd ed. Philadelphia: Churchill Livingstone; 2003. p. 57–70.
6. Sealy WC, Connally SR, Dalton ML. Naming the bronchopulmonary segments and the development of pulmonary surgery. Ann Thorac Surg. 1993;55(1):184–8.
7. Drake RL, Vogl W, Tibbitts A, et al. Illustration by Richard; Richardson, Paul. Gray's anatomy for students. 2nd ed. (PBK. ED). Philadelphia: Elsevier/Churchill Livingstone; 2005. p. 240.
8. Susan Standring Gray's Anatomy for Students. 40th Edn. Elsevier Churchill Livingstone Philadelphia 2008
9. Jackson CL, Huber JF. Correlated applied anatomy of the bronchial tree and lungs with a system of nomenclature. Chest. 1943;9:319–26.
10. Baile EM. The anatomy and physiology of the bronchial circulation. J Aerosol Med. 1996;9(1):1–6.
11. Minnich DJ, Mathisen DJ. Anatomy of the trachea, carina, and bronchi. Thorac Surg Clin. 2007;17(4):571–85.
12. Riquet M. Bronchial arteries and lymphatics of the lung. Thorac Surg Clin. 2007;17(4):619–38.
13. Belvisi MG. Overview of the innervation of the lung. Curr Opin Pharmacol. 2002;2(3):211–5.

Lung Physiology Relevant to Thoracic Anesthesia

Anil Kumar Jain

In health, lung function effortlessly and subconsciously producing adequate gas exchange, providing oxygen and removing carbon dioxide. Conscious respiratory action is noticed during exercise and also when diseases afflict the respiratory system. How does the respiratory system maintain normal function, what are the mechanisms available to maintain adequate gas exchange during abnormal situations, and how does anesthesia and surgery affect these functions should be understood by the anesthesia personnel. Patients subjected to thoracic surgery for various diseases already have a compromised function and may decompensate, if not properly prepared and handled during anesthesia and one lung ventilation. An in-depth knowledge of the normal respiratory physiology, various reflexes and mechanisms which come in play when the respiratory system is stressed, is mandatory.

Let us first see how lungs are ventilated.

4.1 Ventilation

Ventilation is ingress and egress of air in the lungs. On inspiration air enters and mixes with the air already present in the lung. Volume of air in the lungs depends on many factors such as size, sex and posture of the individual. The volume of air left in the lungs after normal exhalation, is the functional residual volume.

The functional residual volume or capacity (FRC) helps in preventing collapse of alveoli (Fig. 4.1) and enables uninterrupted oxygenation of blood [1].

The amount of tidal volume which takes part in gas exchange is alveolar ventilation. Ventilation of lungs depends on development of transpulmonary pressure (P_{TP}), which is the difference between alveolar pressure P_{alv} and pleural pressure (P_{PL}). For a given P_{TP}, volume-exchange will be determined by elastic and resistive properties of the lung.

4.2 Compliance

The lungs behave like elastic tissue and distend when pressure is applied and regain their shape on release of pressure. Compliance is reciprocal of the elastance and is the amount of volume change per unit of pressure change. Normal value is 0.2–0.3 L/cm H_2O [2]. It can be calculated by:

$$C = (V1 - V2)(P1 - P2) - 1$$

Relationship between pressure and volume is not linear, but curvilinear [2]. At extremes of lung volume, it is minimal. Compliance is low in

---

A. K. Jain (✉)
Institute of Anaesthesiology, Pain and Perioperative Medicine, Sir Ganga Ram Hospital, New Delhi, India

© Springer Nature Singapore Pte Ltd. 2020
J. Sood, S. Sharma (eds.), *Clinical Thoracic Anesthesia*,
https://doi.org/10.1007/978-981-15-0746-5_4

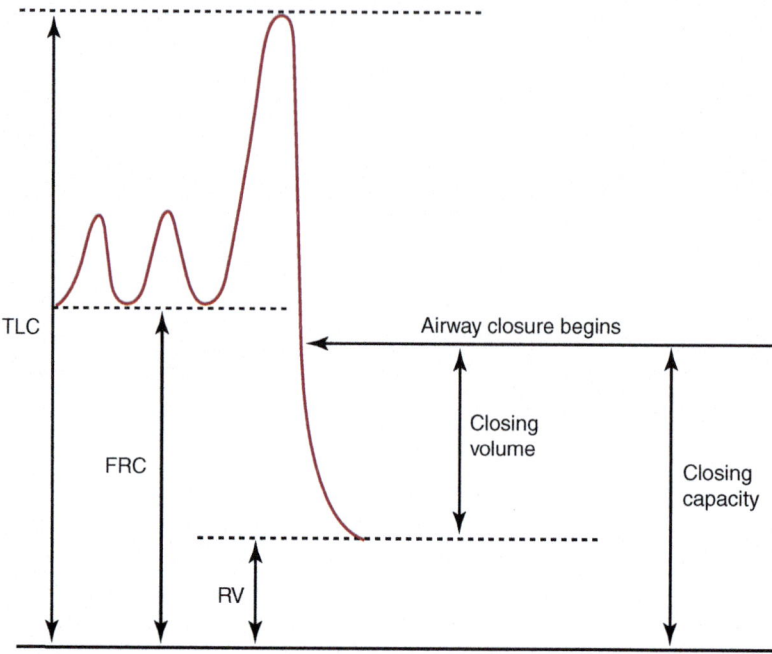

Fig. 4.1 Lung capacity and volume Lung capacity and volume (Source: Chap. 3. Respiratory system resistance permission. In: Nunn's Applied Respiratory Physiology. Fig 3.6)

diseases such as pulmonary fibrosis, sarcoidosis, COPD, alveolar edema and atelectasis, whereas it increases in emphysema and ageing. Anesthesia also produces fall in compliance.

4.3 Resistance of the Respiratory System

There are forces which oppose expansion of lung, of which airway resistance is a major component [3]. Pressure usually overcomes resistance, as resistance increases, more P_{TP} is required for same volume change. During positive pressure ventilation, driving pressure is applied to the endotracheal tube. Airway resistance is about 1 cm H_2O/L/s. Direct measurement of pressure drop along bronchial tree has proved that medium size bronchi are the major site of resistance. Resistance increases in intubated patients, COPD, asthma and also with turbulent air flow [4].

Resistance is inversely proportional to lung volume and increases sharply during forced exhalation. Small airways have no cartilage and are compressed on forced exhalation [3]. This compression produces flow limitation and may lead to dynamic hyperinflation of lung during tachypnea [5]. Equal pressure point (EPP) is a point in airway where intramural pressure is equal to extramural pressure and beyond this point airway collapse occurs [6].

Twenty per cent of total respiratory resistance is due to tissue resistance which may increase manyfold in respiratory diseases such as COPD and pulmonary fibromatosis [7]. Resistance offered by chest wall also increases in respiratory distress syndrome [8].

4.4 Distribution of Inhaled Air

In a spontaneously breathing patient, pleural pressure is the distending pressure for the lungs. Compliance of the lung and patient posture determine how air or gas will distribute in the lungs. Airway pressure is uniform all over the lung but in the upright posture, pleural pressure changes from apex to base of the lung. It increases 0.2 cm H_2O per centimetre of distance as we go from top of lung to bottom, so at the top pleural pressure is −8 cm H_2O while at the bottom of lung it is approximately −1.5 cm H_2O. Transthoracic pressure which produces distention of lung is higher at the top, so alveoli are more open at apex compared to the alveoli at bottom of the lung (Fig. 4.2). This gradient of pleural pressure is more in the diseased lung, such as in pulmonary edema [9].

Distribution of ventilation as assessed by radioactive xenon gas inhalation has shown that ventilation per unit volume of lung is greatest near bottom of lung. It decreases as we move towards apex. The dependent lung has good ventilation in lateral position.

P_{PL} is lowered by inspiratory effort of diaphragm to an equal amount all over the intrapleural space [10]. Alveoli at the base are more compliant, they lie on the steep portion of compliance curve, they expand more and air is preferentially distributed to basal areas.

At low lung volume (residual volume), intrapleural pressure is less negative, but the apex and base difference of pressure persists. The base of lung is compressed and its pressure exceed atmospheric pressure, so ventilation is poor at bases; whereas at the apex, ventilation is better as it is at steep portion of compliance curve.

The distribution of air is more uniform in prone when compared to supine position, even when vertical height is same in both positions. In prone position P_{PL} is more uniform [11]. Uniform distribution of gas in prone position is

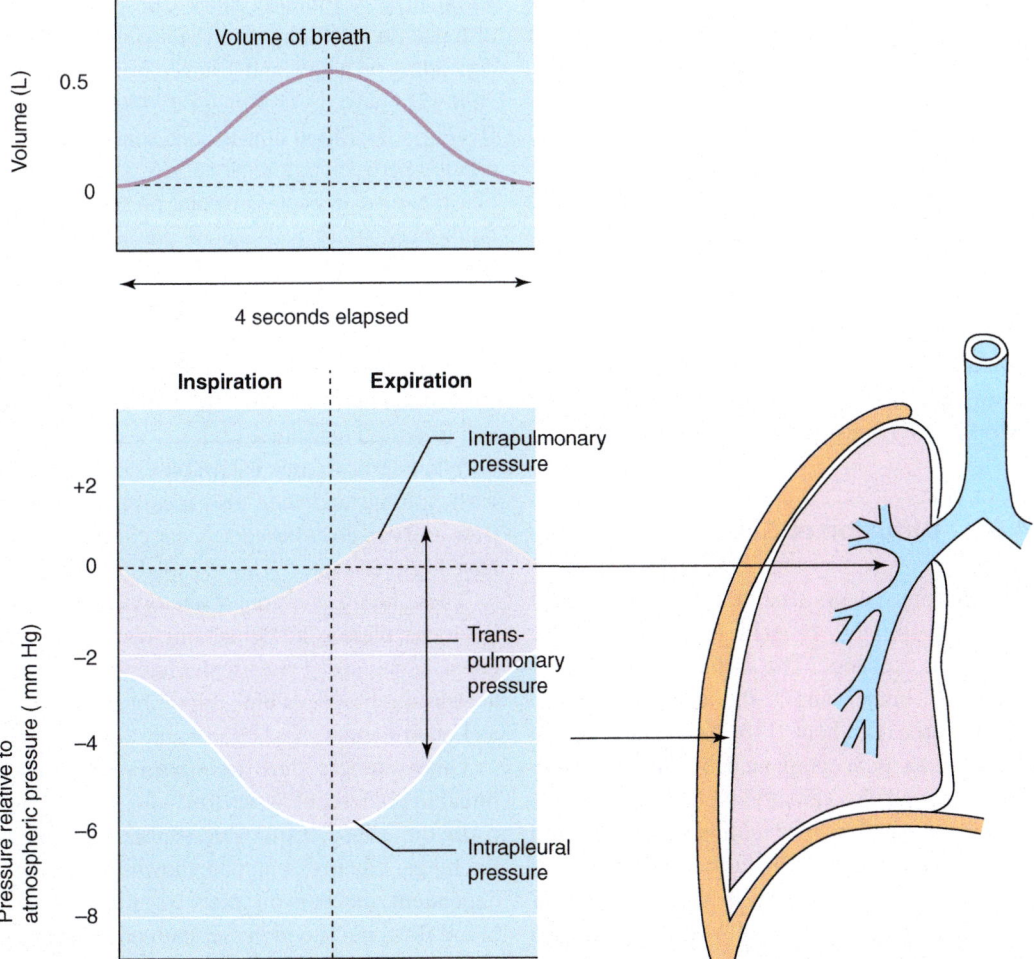

Fig. 4.2 Compliance curve and intrapleural pressure and regional ventilation. Source: https://owlcation.com/stem/Lung-Pressures-and-Lung-Compliance

also experimentally proven [12, 13]. Distribution is also affected by speed of gas flow. With low flows compliance is determinant, but at high flows resistance is the determinant of gas distribution [14, 15]. As the upper lung region has low resistance, it gets more ventilation and so at high flows gas distribution is more uniform; this is also revealed by xenon gas study in humans [14, 15].

4.5 Closure of Airways

Airway narrowing occurs during exhalation and forceful expiration. Volume at which small airways start closing is closing volume (CV), this is the volume of air which remains in lung above residual volume. Closing capacity is the sum of residual volume and closing volume [16]. Whenever P_{PL} increases excessively and exceeds PAW, it can produce collapse of airway. As basal P_{PL} is more, closure occurs at base (Fig. 4.3).

Factors like age, posture and anesthesia can affect CV. Ageing produces airway closure early during exhalation [17]. The supine position and anesthesia both reduce FRC such that CV encroaches it, leading to atelectasis (Fig. 4.4). Chronic obstructive lung disease also produces airway closure at higher lung volume, again increasing V/Q mismatch and hypoxia [16].

4.6 Diffusion of Gas

Gas exchange occurs after the 14th generation of airway. Respiratory bronchioles and alveoli are sites of air exchange. The surface area increases as bronchi branch and at the alveolar level the surface area is about 140 sq.m. Increase in surface area is accompanied by fall in airway resistance and also velocity of gas flow [18]. The velocity of gas flow in alveoli is very low, about 0.001 mm/s and it falls further and becomes stationary or zero when it touches alveolar membrane, now the rate of flow is even less than diffusion rate of O_2 and CO_2.

Complete gas mixing occurs in alveolus but in some conditions, such as emphysema, incomplete mixing may occur leading to layering of oxygen or CO_2 rich gases. CO_2-rich layer may be adjacent to alveolar membrane and oxygen may away from it and produce hypoxia [19].

4.7 Distribution of Blood Flow

Distribution of blood in pulmonary circulation depends on many factors of which gravity is the most important [20]. Gravity affects blood pressure in pulmonary vessels, which is modulated by posture of patients. In erect posture pressure at apex of lung is lower than at bases and so is blood flow which is least at apex. In lateral position blood flow is similarly altered, in erect posture different areas of lung receive unequal blood flow depending on height and distance from base. West et al. [21] have divided lung into three zones I to III (Fig. 4.5). Blood flow in each zone depends on relation between pulmonary artery, vein and alveolar pressure; in zone I alveolar pressure exceeds pulmonary artery and venous pressure so blood flow is minimal. In Zone III P_{PA}, P_{PV} always exceed P_{aLV} and blood flow is continuous during systolic and diastolic period. A zone IV has also been described in which blood is low because of gravity and induced compression of blood vessels and increased resistance [22].

When lung volume is low, bases of lungs have least volume and they also receive least blood flow as extra alveolar vessels are constricted and have high resistance. This is called zone 4.

These lung zones are not anatomical but physiological; there is no delineating border between zones. Zone size varies with change in posture, anesthesia, blood volume, blood pressure, IPPV and other factors.

Other authors have questioned the gravitational hypothesis of West [23].

In the 1990s, using microsphere studies of the lungs, Glenny et al. had shown that gravity-dependent mechanism plays a minor role in blood flow, but blood vessel path and branching have a major role in it [24]. Hilar regions have higher blood flow compared to the peripheral parts of lung. Recent research also highlights

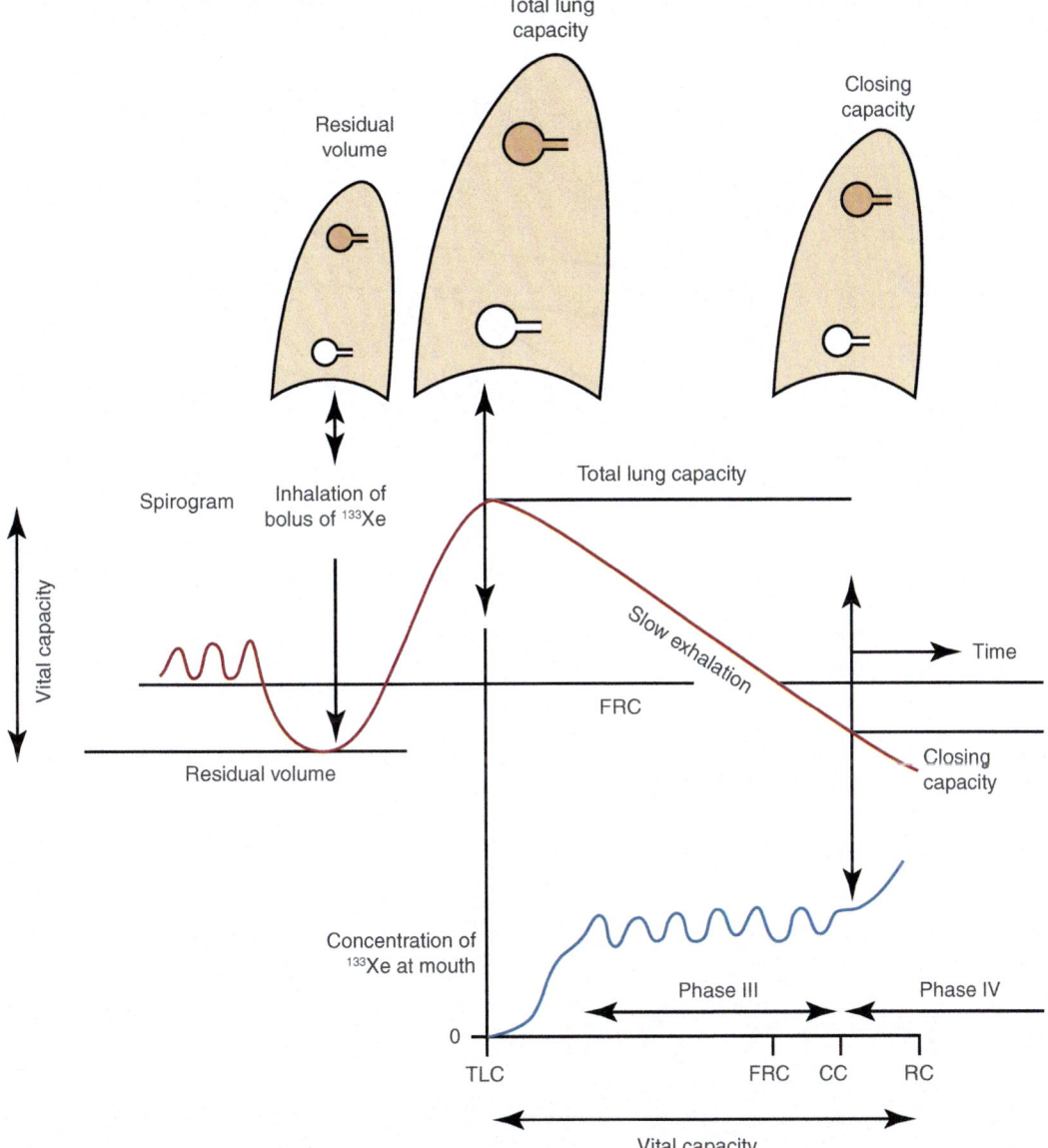

Fig. 4.3 Airway closing during breathing (Source: Chap 3. Respiratory system resistance permission. In: Nunn's Applied Respiratory Physiology. Fig. 3.14.)

that there is no recruitment of apical lung during exercise and when there are other causes of increased cardiac output [25].

Gravity influenced distribution of blood flow is seen in well expanded lungs with low pulmonary vascular pressures and well dilated vessels and may be absent in the lungs with high vascular pressure and low volume, as in lateral position.

4.8 Perfusion

Pulmonary blood vessels are wider and shorter and have low resistance and produce a pulsatile capillary [26]. Low pressure permits thin capillary which produces leakage of vascular content when exposed to sudden high pressure [27]. Vessel remodelling occurs when they are exposed to chronic elevated

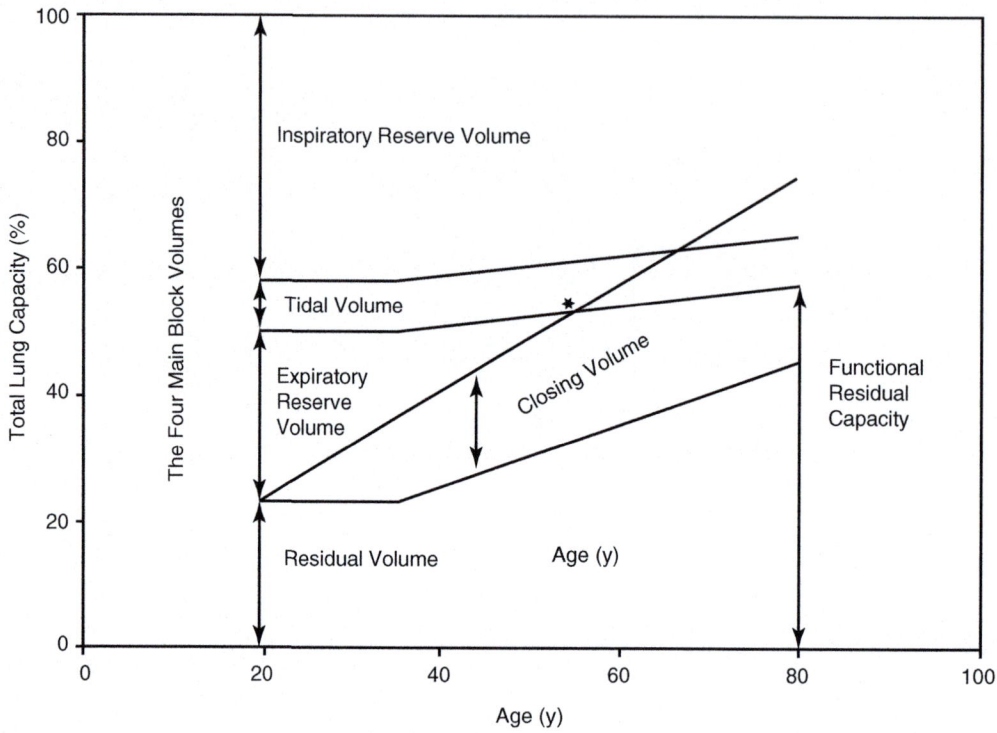

Fig. 4.4 Relationship between age and closing capacity (Source: Zaugg M, Lucchinetti E. Respiratory function in the elderly. *Anesthesiol Clin North Am.* 2000 Mar;18(1):47–58)

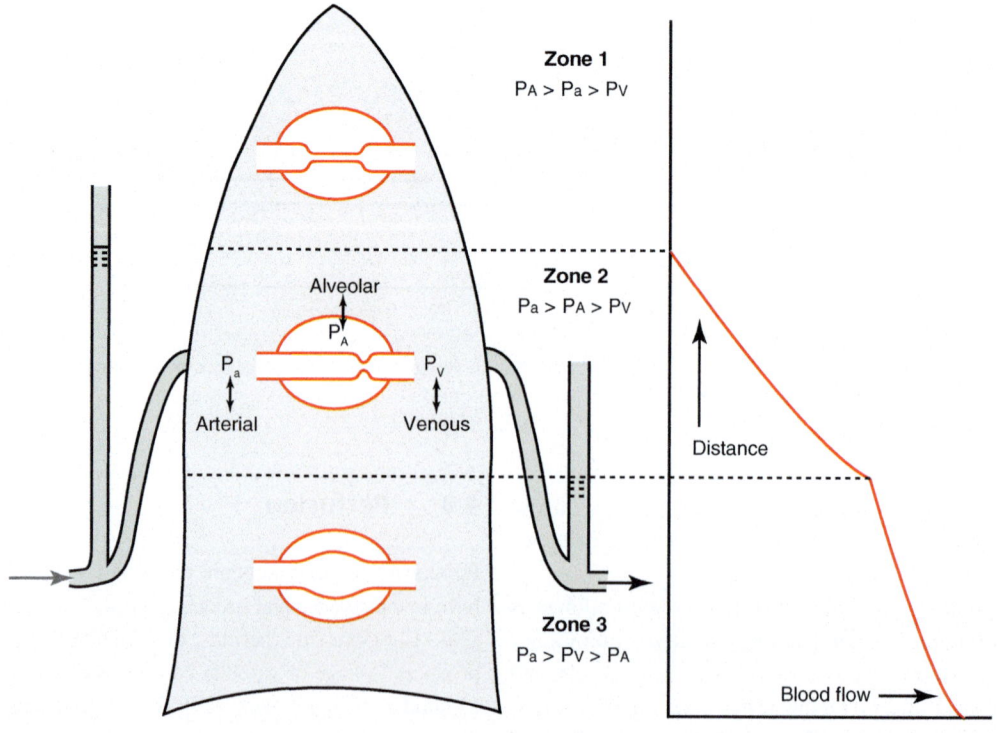

Fig. 4.5 Different zones in lung (Source: Respiratory physiology: the essentials. John B. West. 9th ed. Chap. 4 Fig. 4.8)

pressure at the expense of impaired diffusion [28, 29], and this prevents occurrence of pulmonary edema.

4.9 Hypoxic Pulmonary Vasoconstriction (HPV)

In response to fall in oxygen partial pressure in tissues, systemic vessels dilate to supply more blood and thereby more oxygen, but pulmonary vessels constrict when oxygen tension falls; this response is beneficial as it tries to match perfusion to low ventilation [30]. Mechanisms for HPV are not completely known, but many channels play a role in HPV, which include KV channels, L-type calcium channel, non-specific cation channels and also HPV endothelin receptor activation which produces a vasoconstrictor, endothelin [31–36]. During low alveolar oxygen tension HPV is initiated, which improves V/Q matching. Vasodilators and drugs which produce hypotension such as nitroprusside, nitrates, trinitroglycerin, nifedipine and other calcium channel blockers have inhibitory action on HPV and may increase V/Q mismatch [37]. These drugs by causing hypotension increase zone I of lung which also increases V/Q mismatch. Most volatile anesthetic agents suppress HPV [37]. Newer anesthetics sevoflurane and desflurane have minimal effect on HPV at less than 1MAC anesthesia. This suppression of HPV increases V/Q mismatch and thus may decrease PaO_2.

Intravenous anesthetic agents generally do not affect HPV but given in an inappropriate dose to a patient may lead to fall in blood pressure and increase the zone 1 of lung which may affect V/Q matching [1].

4.10 Anesthesia and Lung Function

Induction of general anesthesia (GA) whether IV or inhalational produces decrease in FRC; which promotes airway closure in the basal region (or dependent area) thereby producing atelectasis and hypoxia. Hypoxia is usually mild but some patients may have a severe fall in PaO_2 [38, 39]. About 15–20% of lung may collapse under anesthesia; this atelectasis is more in dependent area as compared to non-dependent [40].

During thoracic surgery and cardiopulmonary bypass, severe collapse of lung occurs, which may be more than 50% of lung volume [41]. This atelectasis may persist for days together after abdominal surgery and for several hours after thoracic surgery and a significant relation exists between amount of atelectasis and pulmonary shunt [42].

Atelectasis can be taken care of by several interventions such as use of positive end expiratory pressure [43, 44], recruitment manoeuvers, use of insoluble gas (nitrogen) [45] and maintenance of muscle tone [46].

4.11 Gas Exchange and Ventilation–Perfusion Inequality

Gas exchange difficulty occurs whenever there is ventilation–perfusion mismatch. The PaO_2 at apex of lung is 40 mm Hg more than at bases. As the total blood coming from base is more, it has more impact on PaO_2, as its PO_2 is low. The difference in ventilation is much less as compared to perfusion. Similarly the arterial $PaCO_2$ is higher at bases, when compared to apex of lung.

Segments of apical and basal region have threefold variation for ventilation and tenfold for blood perfusion. So V/Q ratio ranges from 5.0 approximately at apex and 0.5 at bases of lung, while V/Q is near 1 in the middle portion of lung (Fig. 4.6). The area of low ventilation–perfusion is slightly hypercapnic and hypoxic, area with high V/Q compensates for CO_2, but due to shape of oxygen dissociation curve it cannot compensate for oxygen. This results in significant difference in alveolar–arterial (A-a) gradient for oxygen wherever V/Q mismatch is significant (Fig. 4.7).

4.12 Ventilation–Perfusion During One Lung Ventilation (OLV) and Anesthesia

Gas exchange is impaired by anesthesia as there is development of atelectasis, which increases shunt and V/Q mismatch and produces fall in

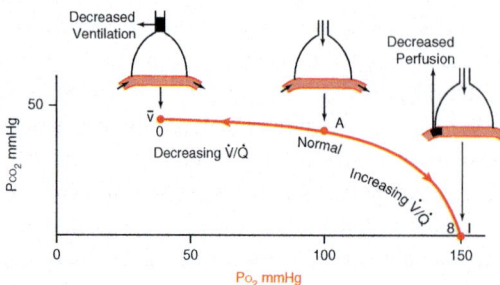

Fig. 4.6 V/Q ration effect on PO₂ and PCO₂ (Source: Respiratory physiology: the essentials. John B. West. 9th ed. Chap. 5 Fig. 5.7)

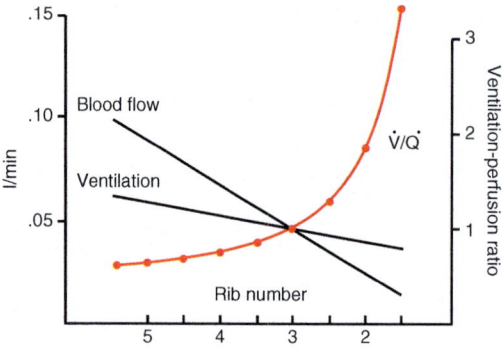

Fig. 4.7 Ventilation and perfusion distribution (Source: Respiratory physiology: the essentials. John B. West. 9th ed. Chap. 5 Fig. 5.8)

oxygenation. CO_2 elimination is usually preserved as compensatory increase in ventilation is sufficient to correct CO_2 elimination.

The arterial oxygenation is further impacted by obesity, smoking and ageing [47, 48]. Venous admixture, which is the amount of venous blood that mixes with arterial blood, without oxygenation, is also more during anesthesia, producing fall in PaO_2.

4.13 Lateral Position V/Q Mismatch

4.13.1 Conscious Awake Patient

Perfusion of blood is more in the dependent lung. Sixty-five per cent of cardiac output goes to the dependent right lung, whereas left lung when dependent receives 55% of cardiac output. Ventilation of dependent lung also is better as compliance curve of alveoli in dependent region is steep. So in the awake, lateral position ventilation and perfusion is better in the dependent lung. Lateral position V/Q match is similar to upright position.

Induction of anesthesia in a spontaneously breathing patient, results in decrease in FRC by 15–20% and the position of each lung on compliance curve also changes. The dependent lung slips to the flat portion and the non-dependent to steeper portion of compliance curve, so mismatch of ventilation–perfusion occurs more in dependent lung.

Institution of skeletal muscle paralysis and IPPV leads to better compliance of non-dependent lung, perfusion remains as before, so there is increase in mismatching of ventilation and perfusion. Loss of negative intrapleural pressure on opening the chest, leads to further decrease in compliance of dependent lung, as the weight of mediastinum compresses the dependent lung. The non-dependent lung compliance increases as it becomes free and not limited by chest wall; its perfusion is not altered, but V/Q mismatch increases, Zone I increases in the non-dependent lung, when TLV is being applied. Ventilation is diverted to the dependent lung on institution of OLV, and this improves V/Q matching as perfusion is already better there, but this increases true shunt in the operated or non-dependent lung.

During thoracic surgery as patient is in lateral decubitus position, atelectasis increases. On initiation of one lung ventilation, lung which is not ventilated continues to get perfusion with blood and acts as shunt. This shunt fraction can be decrease by accelerating collapse of the lung, since collapse of lung would decrease its blood supply due to HPV. Collapse of lung is hastened by using soluble gas for ventilation before blocking the ventilation.

It has been shown experimentally that collapse is faster when using N_2O–O_2 for lung ventilation compared to air. Surgical retraction and the HPV decreases blood flow in the non-ventilated lung [49].

The degree of shunt can be measured by shunt equation:

$$\frac{Qs}{QT} = \frac{CcO_2 - CaO_2}{CcO_2 - CvO_2}$$

which can be further simplified, when ($CcO_2 = PaO_2$)

$$\frac{Qs}{QT} = \frac{(1 - SaO_2)}{1 - SvO_2}$$

Thus changes in SvO_2 and SaO_2 could be used to see effect on shunt of any intervention.

Occurrence of shunt or venous admixture plays a major role in blood oxygenation when OLV is employed. PaO_2 during OLV is influenced by amount of blood flow through the non-ventilated lung and oxygen content of mixed venous blood. Mixed venous oxygen is predicted by oxygen delivery and oxygen consumption (VO_2). Usually it is shown that oxygen delivery, oxygen consumption and haemoglobin are constant during a short time period (Fig. 4.8).

When right to left shunt or venous admixture is present, any change in delivery of oxygen will impact mixed oxygen saturation. Increasing oxygen delivery by raising cardiac output and increasing Hb will improve mixed venous oxygen tension and also increase PaO_2. Low mixed venous oxygen tension will lead to fall in arterial oxygenation at any given shunt fraction. A drop in cardiac output and haemoglobin level also produces reduction in PaO_2.

The lateral position improves perfusion and ventilation in dependent lung and so improves oxygenation as shunt fraction also is reduced (Fig. 4.9). The arterial oxygen tension improves with head up tilting of patient which is due to reduction in shunt fraction (Fig. 4.10).

One lung ventilation can affect gas exchange as blood continues to flow in lung which is not

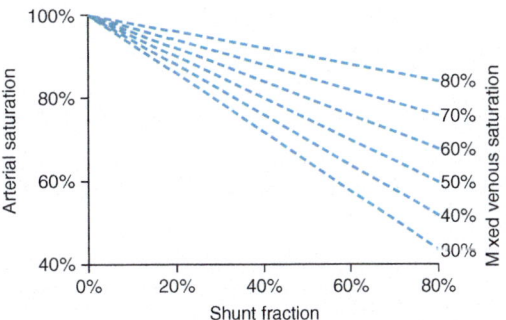

Fig. 4.8 Effect of shunt fraction on oxygen saturation (Source: Barbeito A, Shaw AD, Grichnik K: Thoracic Anesthesia: www.accessanesthesiology.com)

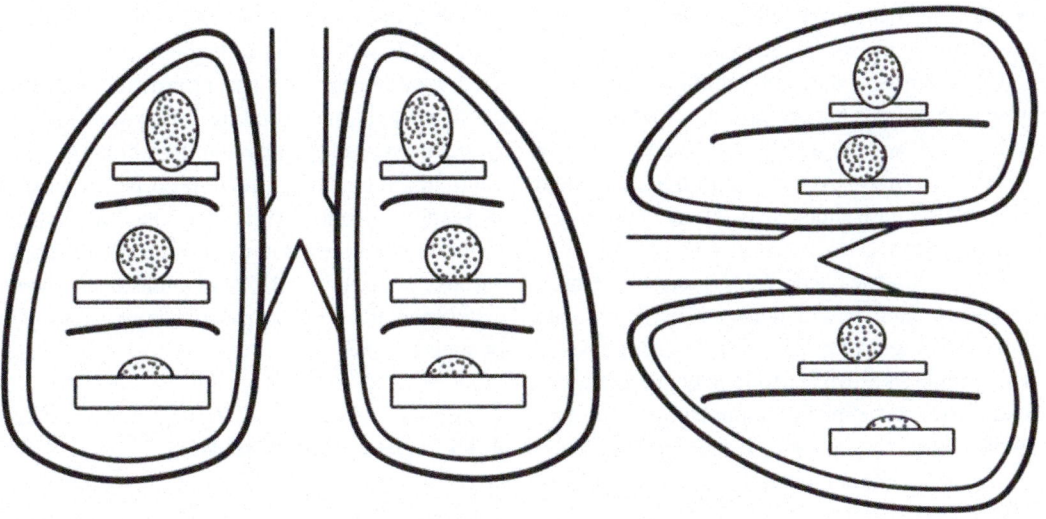

Fig. 4.9 Body positions and *V/Q* (Source: Barbeito A, Shaw AD, Grichnik K: Thoracic Anesthesia: www.accessanesthesiology.com)

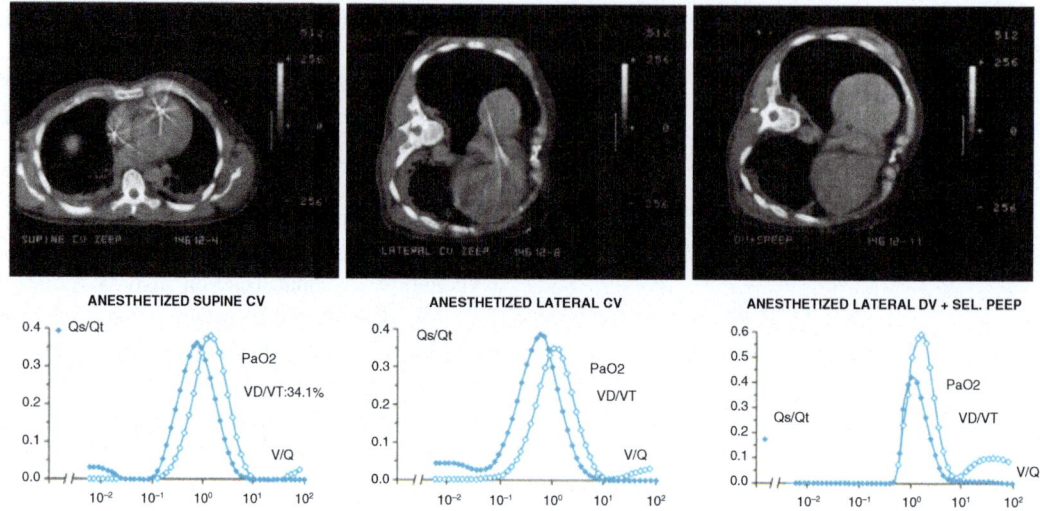

Fig. 4.10 Body position and ventilation–perfusion (Source: Barbeito A, Shaw AD, Grichnik K: Thoracic Anesthesia: www.accessanesthesiology.com)

ventilated and contributes to shunt or venous admixture and lower PaO_2 and may produce hypoxia. Regaining pre-OLV conditions in the lung will take time, which results in poor oxygen tension in post-operative period [50]. Reducing blood flow to non-dependent lung can improve oxygenation [51, 52].

Causes of poor oxygenation during OLV are increased shunt fraction from non-ventilated lung and venous admixture or low V/Q region development in dependent lung [53]. PEEP and recruitment manoeuvre (RM) to dependent lung may improve gas exchange [54].

Uniform distribution of ventilation and dead space reduction is the mechanism of RM maneuver [55]. Positive pressure also has negative impact, as it may divert blood to non-dependent lung and increase shunt, so cautious PEEP use is necessary [56].

Total collapse and compression of non-dependent lung would decrease perfusion and improve oxygenation [57, 58]. Other measures which could improve PaO_2 are inhalation of nitric oxide (NO) and almitrine administration intravenously. Whereas NO has meagre effect when used alone, combining it with almitrine results in better oxygenation [59, 60].

Almitrine when used in the proper doses, does not affect cardiac output, but impacts the oxygenation positively [59]. HPV is potentiated by almitrine thereby reducing shunt. HPV is not the only factor but an important contributor to moving blood away from non-ventilated area of lung.

4.14 Effect of Ventilation

Improperly applied IPPV could result in auto-PEEP generation during OLV, especially in diseased lung. Low auto-PEEP may improve oxygenation by decreasing lung collapse but high auto-PEEP will produce hemodynamic effects such as impairing venous return and reducing cardiac output and resulting in hypotension and reducing oxygenation by shunting blood to non-ventilated lung. This effect could be minimized by identifying auto-PEEP and reducing it and by proper ventilation strategy of lung. Biologically variable ventilation (BVV) also has been shown experimentally to improve oxygenation in animals [61–63].

4.15 pH Manipulation

Pulmonary vasodilatation is produced by alkalosis and vasoconstriction by acidosis. HPV is affected by $PaCO_2$ in animals and is minimal at $PaCO_2$ of 20 mm Hg. Effect of alkalosis or acute respiratory acidosis on HPV is minimal in humans [64–67].

4.16 Supine Position

The dependent areas receive more perfusion and V/Q mismatch increases as the dependent area receives less ventilation. During OLV the V/Q mismatch further increases as shunt in the non-ventilated lung increases [68].

4.17 Prone Position

V/Q matching matching, compliance improves and lung volumes are preserved leading to better PaO_2. Gas exchange is better than supine position but lateral posture is best for oxygenation [69, 70].

4.18 Conclusion

Understanding respiratory physiology along with mechanics of respiration and gas exchange is essential for correcting V/Q mismatch perioperatively.

Anesthesia and surgery can produce collapse of lung which is enhanced by improper ventilation of lung. Per-operatively this could manifest as fall in partial pressure of oxygen and produce difficulty in maintaining oxygen saturation. During one lung anesthesia, perfusion of non-ventilated lung produces venous admixture or shunt. This shunt fraction could be minimized by accelerating collapse of lung. Improper ventilation and position of patient would add to the venous admixture by producing collapse in the ventilated lung.

References

1. Kavanach B, Hedenstierna G. Respiratory physiology and pathophysiology. In: Miller RS, editor. Miller's anaesthesia. 8th ed. Philadelphia: Elsevier; 2015. p. 444–72.
2. Grassino AE, Rpissos G. Static properties of the lung and chest wall. In: Crystal RG, West JB, Weibel ER, et al. editors. The lung: scientific foundations. 2nd ed. Philadelphia: Lippincott-Raven; 1997. p. 1187.
3. Pedley TJ, Kamm RD. Dynamics of gas flow and pressure flow relationship. In: Crystal RG, West JB, Weibel, Barnes PJ, editors. The lung: scientific foundations. 2nd ed. Philadelphia: Lippincott Raven; 1997. p. 1365.
4. Slats AM, Janssen K, van Schadewijk A, et al. Bronchial inflammation and airway responses to deep inspiration in asthma and chronic obstructive pulmonary disease. Am J Respir Crit Care Med. 2007;176(2):121–8.
5. Calverley PM, Koulouris NG. Flow limitation and dynamic hyperinflation: key concepts in modern respiratory physiology. Eur Respir J. 2005;25(1):186–99.
6. Mead J, Turner JM, Macklem PT, et al. Significance of the relationship between lung recoil and maximum expiratory flow. J Appl Physiol. 1967;22(1):95–108.
7. Verbeken EK, Cauberghs M, Mertens I, et al. Tissue and airway impedance of excised normal, senile, and emphysematous lungs. J Appl Physiol (1985). 1992;72(6):2343–53.
8. Bachofen H, Scherrer M. Lung tissue resistance in diffuse interstitial pulmonary fibrosis. J Clin Invest. 1967;46(1):133–40.
9. Hubmayr RD. Perspective on lung injury and recruitment: a skeptical look at the opening and collapse story. Am J Respir Crit Care Med. 2002;165(12):1647–53.
10. Milic-Emile J. Ventilation distribution. In: Hammid Q, Shannon J, Martin J, editors. Physiologic bases of respiratory disease. Hamilton, ON: BC Decker; 2005.
11. Ganesan S, Lai-Fook SJ, Schürch S. Alveolar liquid pressures in nonedematous and kerosene-washed rabbit lung by micropuncture. Respir Physiol. 1989;78(3):281–95.
12. Mayo JR, MacKay AL, Whittall KP, et al. Measurement of lung water content and pleural pressure gradient with magnetic resonance imaging. J Thorac Imaging. 1995;10(1):73–81.
13. Petersson J, Sánchez-Crespo A, Rohdin M, et al. Physiological evaluation of a new quantitative SPECT method measuring regional ventilation and perfusion. J Appl Physiol (1985). 2004;96(3):1127–36.
14. Bryan AC, Bentivoglio LG, Beerel F, et al. Factors affecting regional distribution of ventilation and perfusion in the lung. J Appl Physiol. 1964;19:395–402.
15. Bake B, Wood L, Murphy B, et al. Effect of inspiratory flow rate on regional distribution of inspired gas. J Appl Physiol. 1974;37(1):8–17.
16. Milic-Emili J, Torchio R, D'Angelo E. Closing volume: a reappraisal (1967–2007). Eur J Appl Physiol. 2007;99(6):567–83.
17. Teculescu DB, Damel MC, Costantino E, et al. Computerized single-breath nitrogen washout: predicted values in a rural French community. Lung. 1996;174(1):43–55.

18. Haefeli-Bleuer B, Weibel ER. Morphometry of the human pulmonary acinus. Anat Rec. 1988;220(4):401–14.
19. Adaro F. Limiting role of stratification in alveolar exchange of oxygen. Respir Physiol. 1976;26(2):195–206.
20. Hughes JMB. Distribution of pulmonary blood flow. In: Crystal RG, West JB, Weibel ER, Barnes PJ, editors. The lung: scientific foundations. 2nd ed. Philadelphia: Lippincott-Raven; 1997. p. 1523–36.
21. West JB, Dollery CT, Naimark A. Distribution of blood flow in isolated lung; relation to vascular and alveolar pressures. J Appl Physiol. 1964;19:713–24.
22. Hughes JM, Glazier JB, Maloney JE, et al. Effect of lung volume on the distribution of pulmonary blood flow in man. Respir Physiol. 1968;4:58–72.
23. West JB. Studies of pulmonary and cardiac function using short-lived isotopes oxygen-15, nitrogen-13 and carbon-11. Prog At Med. 1968;2:39–64.
24. Glenny RW. Blood flow distribution in the lung. Chest. 1998;114(1 Suppl):8S–16S.
25. Robertson HT, Hlastala MP. Microsphere maps of regional blood flow and regional ventilation. J Appl Physiol (1985). 2007;102(3):1265–72.
26. Dawson CA, Linehan JH. Dynamics of blood flow and pressure flow relationships. In: Crystal RG, West JB, Weibel ER, Barnes PJ, editors. The lung: scientific foundations. 2nd ed. Philadelphia: Lippincott-Raven; 1997. p. 1503–22.
27. Bachofen H, Schurch S, Weibel ER. Experimental hydrostatic pulmonary edema in rabbit lungs. Barrier lesions. Am Rev Respir Dis. 1993;147:997–1004.
28. Jeffery PK. Remodeling and inflammation of bronchi in asthma and chronic obstructive pulmonary disease. Proc Am Thorac Soc. 2004;1:176–83.
29. Townsley MI, Fu Z, Mathieu-Costello O, et al. Pulmonary microvascular permeability. Responses to high vascular pressure after induction of pacing induced heart failure in dogs. Circ Res. 1995;77:317–25.
30. Sommer N, Dietrich A, Schermuly RT, et al. Regulation of hypoxic pulmonary vasoconstriction: basic mechanisms. Eur Respir J. 2008;32(6):1639–51.
31. Archer SL, Weir EK, Reeve HL, et al. Molecular identification of O2 sensors and O2-sensitive potassium channels in the pulmonary circulation. Adv Exp Med Biol. 2000;475:219–40.
32. Sham JS, Crenshaw BR Jr, Deng LH, et al. Effects of hypoxia in porcine pulmonary arterial myocytes: roles of K(V) channel and endothelin-1. Am J Physiol Lung Cell Mol Physiol. 2000;279(2):L262–72.
33. McMahon TJ, Moon RE, Luschinger BP, et al. Nitric oxide in the human respiratory cycle. Nat Med. 2002;8(7):711–7.
34. O'Brien RF, Robbins RJ, McMurtry IF. Endothelial cells in culture produce a vasoconstrictor substance. J Cell Physiol. 1987;132(2):263–70.
35. Hieda HS, Gomez-Sanchez CE. Hypoxia increases endothelin release in bovine endothelial cells in culture, but epinephrine, norepinephrine, serotonin, histamine and angiotensin II do not. Life Sci. 1990;47(3):247–51.
36. Rakugi H, Tabuchi Y, Nakamaru M, et al. Evidence for endothelin-1 release from resistance vessels of rats in response to hypoxia. Biochem Biophys Res Commun. 1990;169(3):973–7.
37. Bjertnaes LJ, Hauge A, Nakken KF, et al. Hypoxic pulmonary vasoconstriction: inhibition due to anesthesia. Acta Physiol Scand. 1976;96(2):283–5.
38. Hedenstierna G. Contribution of multiple inert gas elimination technique to pulmonary medicine. Ventilation-perfusion relationships during anaesthesia. Thorax. 1995;50(1):85–91.
39. Moller JT, Cluitmans P, Rasmussen LS, Houx P, et al. Long-term postoperative cognitive dysfunction in the elderly ISPOCD1 study. ISPOCD investigators. International study of post-operative cognitive dysfunction. Lancet. 1998;351(9106):857–61.
40. Hedenstierna G. Effects of body position on ventilation/perfusion matching. In: Gulio A, editor. Anaestheisa, pain, intensive carfe and emergency medicine—APICE. Milan: Springer; 2005. p. 3–15.
41. Tenling A, Hachenberg T, Tydén H, et al. Hedenstierna G. Atelectasis and gas exchange after cardiac surgery. Anesthesiology. 1998;89(2):371–8.
42. Lindberg P, Gunnarsson L, Tokics L, et al. Atelectasis and lung function in the postoperative period. Acta Anaesthesiol Scand. 1992;36(6):546–53.
43. Hedenstierna G, Edmark L. The effects of anesthesia and muscle paralysis on the respiratory system. Intensive Care Med. 2005;31(10):1327–35.
44. Musch G, Harris RS, Vidal Melo MF, et al. Mechanism by which a sustained inflation can worsen oxygenation in acute lung injury. Anesthesiology. 2004;100(2):323–30.
45. Rothen HU, Sporre B, Engberg G, et al. Influence of gas composition on recurrence of atelectasis after a reexpansion maneuver during general anesthesia. Anesthesiology. 1995;82(4):832–42.
46. Hedenstierna G, Tokics L, Lundquist H, et al. Phrenic nerve stimulation during halothane anesthesia. Effects of atelectasis. Anesthesiology. 1994;80(4):751–60.
47. Pelosi P, Ravagnan I, Giurati G, et al. Positive end-expiratory pressure improves respiratory function in obese but not in normal subjects during anesthesia and paralysis. Anesthesiology. 1999;91(5):1221–31.
48. Coussa M, Proietti S, Schnyder P, et al. Prevention of atelectasis formation during the induction of general anesthesia in morbidly obese patients. Anesth Analg. 2004;98(5):1491–5.
49. Ishikawa S, Nakazata K, Makita K. Progressive changes in arterial oxygenation during one-lung anaesthesia are related to the response to com-

pression of the non dependent lung. Br J Anaesth. 2003;90:21–6.
50. Benumof JL. One-lung ventilation and hypoxic pulmonary vasoconstriction: implications for anesthetic management. Anesth Analg. 1985;64(8): 821–33.
51. Karzai W, Schwarzkopf K. Hypoxemia during one-lung ventilation: prediction, prevention, and treatment. Anesthesiology. 2009;110(6):1402–11.
52. Hedenstierna G, Reber A. Manipulating pulmonary blood flow during one-lung anaesthsia. Acta Anaesthesiol Scand. 1996;40(1):2–4.
53. Klingstedt C, Hedenstierna G, Baehrendtz S, et al. Ventilation-perfusion relationships and atelectasis formation in the supine and lateral positions during conventional mechanical and differential ventilation. Acta Anaesthesiol Scand. 1990;34:421–9.
54. Tusman G, Böhm SH, Melkun F, et al. Alveolar recruitment strategy increases arterial oxygenation during one-lung ventilation. Ann Thorac Surg. 2002;73:1204–9.
55. Tusman G, Böhm SH, Sipmann FS, et al. Lung recruitment improves the efficiency of ventilation and gas exchange during one-lung ventilation anesthesia. Anesth Analg. 2004;98:1604–9.
56. Slinger PD, Kruger M, McRae K, et al. Relation of the static compliance curve and positive end-expiratory pressure to oxygenation during one-lung ventilation. Anesthesiology. 2001;95:1096–102.
57. Ishikawa S, Nakazawa K, Makita K. Progressive changes in arterial oxygenation during one-lung anaesthesia are related to the response to compression of the non-dependent lung. Br J Anaesth. 2003;90:21–6.
58. Pfitzer J. Acute lung injury following one-lung anaesthesia. Br J Anaesth. 2003author reply;91:153–4.
59. Moutafis M, Liu N, Dalibon N, et al. The effects of inhaled nitric oxide and its combination with intravenous almitrine on Pao2 during one-lung ventilation in patients undergoing thoracoscopic procedures. Anesth Analg. 1997;85:1130–5.
60. Silva-Costa-Gomes T, L. Gallart, J. Vallès, et al. Low- vs high-dose almitrine combined with nitric oxide to prevent hypoxia during open-chest one-lung ventilation. Br J Anaesth. 2005;95:410–6.
61. Lefevre GR, Kowalski SE, Girling LG, et al. Improved arterial oxygenation after oleic acid lung injury in the pig using a computer-controlled mechanical ventilator. Am J Respir Crit Care Med. 1996;154(5):1567–72.
62. Boker A, Graham MR, Walley KR, et al. Improved arterial oxygenation with biologically variable or fractal ventilation using low tidal volumes in a porcine model of acute respiratory distress syndrome. Am J Respir Crit Care Med. 2002;165(4):456–62.
63. Boker A, Haberman CJ, Girling L, et al. Variable ventilation improves perioperative lung function in patients undergoing abdominal aortic aneurysmectomy. Anesthesiology. 2004;100(3):608–16.
64. Lloyd TC Jr. Influence of blood pH on hypoxic pulmonary vasoconstriction. J Appl Physiol. 1966;21(2):358–64.
65. Benumof JL, Mathers JM, Wahrenbrock EA. Cyclic hypoxic pulmonary vasoconstriction induced by concomitant carbon dioxide changes. J Appl Physiol. 1976;41(4):466–9.
66. Benumof JL, Wahrenbrock EA. Blunted hypoxic pulmonary vasoconstriction by increased lung vascular pressures. J Appl Physiol. 1975;38(5):846–50.
67. Bergofsky EH, Lehr DE, Fishman AP. The effect of changes in hydrogen ion concentration on the pulmonary circulation. J Clin Invest. 1962;41:1492–502.
68. Bardoczky GI, Szegedi LL, d'Hollander AA, et al. Two-lung and one-lung ventilation in patients with chronic obstructive pulmonary disease: the effects of position and FiO_2. Anesth Analg. 2000;90(1):35–41.
69. Albert RK. Prone ventilation. Clin Chest Med. 2000;21(3):511–7.
70. Pelosi P, Croci M, Calappi E, et al. The prone positioning during general anesthesia minimally affects respiratory mechanics while improving functional residual capacity and increasing oxygen tension. Anesth Analg. 1995;80(5):955–60.

Thoracic Anesthesia Equipment

Shvet Mahajan and Akhil Kumar

5.1 Introduction

A variety of lung isolation techniques are used for the purpose of one-lung ventilation, which is a prerequisite for many thoracic, cardiac, and esophageal surgical procedures. The equipment used to facilitate the lung isolation includes double lumen tubes, bronchial blockers, and the single-lumen endotracheal tubes. The bronchial blockers are used in two ways, attached to single-lumen tube Torque Controlled Blocker Univent® or with a standard single-lumen tube like the wire-guided endobronchial blocker Arndt® blocker [1], the Cohen® tip-deflecting endobronchial blocker [2], or the Fuji Uniblocker™ [3]. The recent development of newer lung isolation devices such as the Silbroncho DLT along with the use of different kinds of video laryngoscopy equipment like the Glidescope® [4] has greatly facilitated lung isolation in patients with difficult airways.

S. Mahajan (✉) · A. Kumar
Institute of Anaesthesiology, Pain and Perioperative Medicine, Sir Ganga Ram Hospital, New Delhi, India

5.2 Double-Lumen Endotracheal Tubes

A little more than half a century ago, Carlens and Bjork pioneered the first double-lumen tube, which was used for lung isolation [5]. Ever since then all the generations of DLT have been influenced by the Carlens DLT. The DLT is designed for both the left or the right side according to which mainstem bronchus is to be accommodated. The form of the different sides of the DLT is manufactured to conform to the unique anatomy of the left or right bronchus.

In essence, a DLT is the end result of bonding two single-lumen tubes one of a greater length than the other. The shorter tube in a DLT is meant for the trachea and has a high volume and low-pressure cuff and is placed just above the carina. The longer tube is smaller low-volume, high-pressure bronchial cuff is ideally positioned below the tracheal carina but before the takeoff of any lobar bronchi. A transverse section of the two tubes is in the shape of a "D" with the straight line of the Ds facing each other in the midline. The cuffs, their pilot balloons, and the connection site at the top of each of the two tubes are all color coded (white for tracheal and blue for endobronchial tube). Once the DLT is properly placed both tracheal and bronchial cuffs are inflated. To achieve selective OLV, the lumen of the contralateral lung is clamped.

DLTs are available from different manufacturers: Mallinckrodt Broncho-Cath® (St. Louis, MO), the Sheridan® Sher-I-Bronch®(Argyle, NY), Rusch®(Duluth, GA), and Portex®(Keene, NH) the smallest available is 26 French (Fr) followed by 28, 32, 35, 37, 39, and 41 Fr. The size 6 to 7 mm internal diameter single-lumen tracheal tubes have resistance that is comparable to that in each of the lumens of DLTs ranging from 35 to 41 Fr [6].

5.3 Selection of the Proper Size of DLT (Refer Chap. 10 for Further Details)

5.3.1 Margin of Safety (Fig. 5.1)

The key to safety is the correct positioning of the DLT. This is dependent on the span of the tracheabronchial tree linking the most distal and the proximal acceptable positions for placement of the DLT [7, 8]. The other factors are the length of the DLT cuff and the bronchial segment into which the DLT is placed. A long mainstem bronchus or short DLT cuff increases the margin of safety.

Each side DLT has its own set of problems, relating to anatomical structure and DLT movement with extension and flexion of the neck.

5.3.1.1 Left-Sided Tube
The average length of the left bronchus lying between the carina and origin of the upper lobe bronchus is 5.6 cm. The most proximal acceptable position for the bronchial cuff of the left-sided DLT is just below the carina while the acceptable most distal position is the bronchial lumen tip at the proximal edge of the secondary carinal orifice. Intraoperatively the surgical manipulation can lead to neck movement of up to 3.5 cm [9], so the safety margin is small. Position the bronchial cuff too proximally and there could be obstruction of the trachea or even the contralateral right mainstem bronchus, while a more distal placement could lead to upper or lower bronchus obstruction.

5.3.1.2 Right-Sided Tube
The safety margin for right-sided tubes is significantly less than left-sided tubes. This is due to the shorter right mainstem bronchus that originates at 1.5–2 cm beyond the carina. The ventilation of the right upper lobe is the key factor in the correct position of a right-sided DLT. The opening for the right upper lobe in the DLT (which is placed beyond the bronchial cuff) has to be aligned with the right upper lobe orifice. The margin of safety for right-sided tube is dependent on the length of the ventilation opening and the diameter of the right upper lobe orifice, thus malposition when using the right DLT is a distinct possibility.

5.3.2 Specific Tubes

5.3.2.1 Carlens Double-Lumen Tube (Fig. 5.2)
The Carlens tube is a left-sided DLT with a carinal hook. This hook or spur aids in the proper placement of the DLT and minimizes movement after placement. It was the earliest DLT used for lung isolation [5]. It is available in size 41, 39, 37, and 35 Fr. The Carlens DLT has oval lumens, hence passing of suction catheter was occasionally difficult. The presence of hook increases difficulty and laryngeal trauma during intubation, more malpositions, and interference during pneumonectomies [10]. When the verification of the DLT placement is complicated as in cases with massive hemoptysis the Carlens tube may be especially useful [11].

5.3.2.2 White Double-Lumen Tube
This DLT like the Carlens tube has a carinal hook, but is designed to be placed in the right mainstem bronchus. It has a slit in the bronchial cuff that allows ventilation of the right upper lobe bronchus.

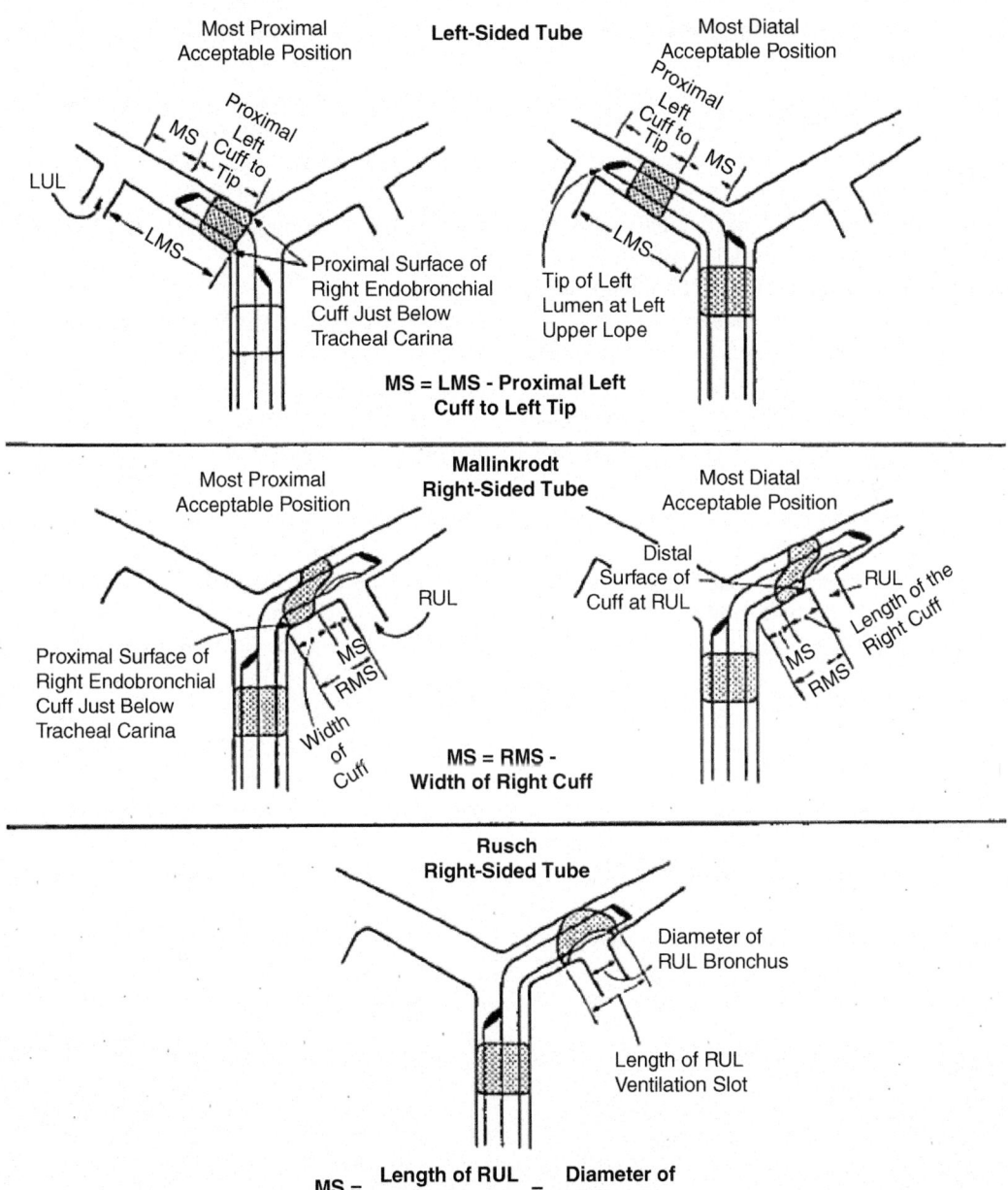

Fig. 5.1 The margin of safety (MS) in positioning double-lumen endotracheal tubes

5.3.2.3 Robertshaw Double-Lumen Tube (Figs. 5.3 and 5.4)

This DLT made an appearance in the field of lung isolation devices in 1962. The first Robertshaw DLTs were constructed from reusable red rubber but later, newer generations are made of clear, nontoxic plastic, and are disposable. Unlike the Carlens DLT, the Robertshaw DLTs may be used for both right and left mainstem bronchi and the absence of the carinal hook means that optimal positioning and easy intubation are possible. The tubes are available in sizes 41, 39, 37, 35, 28, and 26 Fr. This DLT with its design of providing a large lumen meant a decrease in airway resistance and easy removal of secretions. Like the Carlens tube, the lumens are D-shaped placed side by side, but are larger in size. Like other DLTs, the Robertshaw DLTs also have two curves (in planes approximately 90-degrees apart).

The right-sided Robertshaw DLTs the bronchial portion of is angled at 20 degrees [12]. Like other right-sided DLTs, there is an opening on the lateral aspect of the bronchial cuff. This opening is distal to the bronchial cuff and extends tangentially toward the medial surface. The bronchial segment is 23 mm for sizes 35/37 and 25 mm for sizes 39/41 Fr [13].

5.3.2.4 Broncho-Cath Double Lumen

This DLT may or may not have a carinal hook. In the right-sided version of this DLT the bronchial cuff has a unique shape, like a skewed doughnut or S shaped with its upper lateral tip that is closer to the upper right lobe opening being nearer the trachea, while the lower edge of the cuff is near the medial bronchial wall. The slot in the DLT for ventilation of the upper lobe bronchus is just distal to the bronchial cuff. The recent version of this DLT has no bevel on the bronchial segment.

In the left-sided version of this DLT which is also available with or without the carinal hook, the bronchial section is angled at approximately 45 degrees [14–16]. The average length of this segment is 30 to 31 mm and has a curved tip [13].

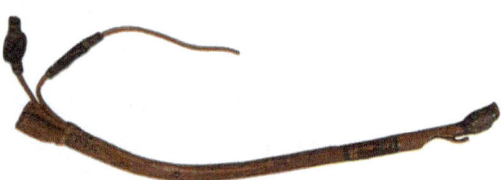

Fig. 5.2 Carlens DLT. Carlens tube—image courtesy Dr. Usha Saha

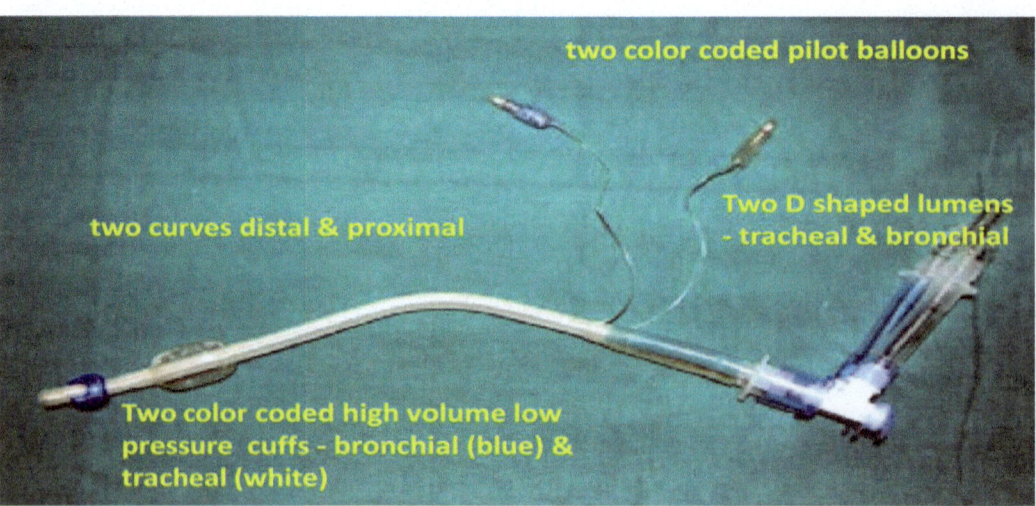

Fig. 5.3 Robertshaw DLT

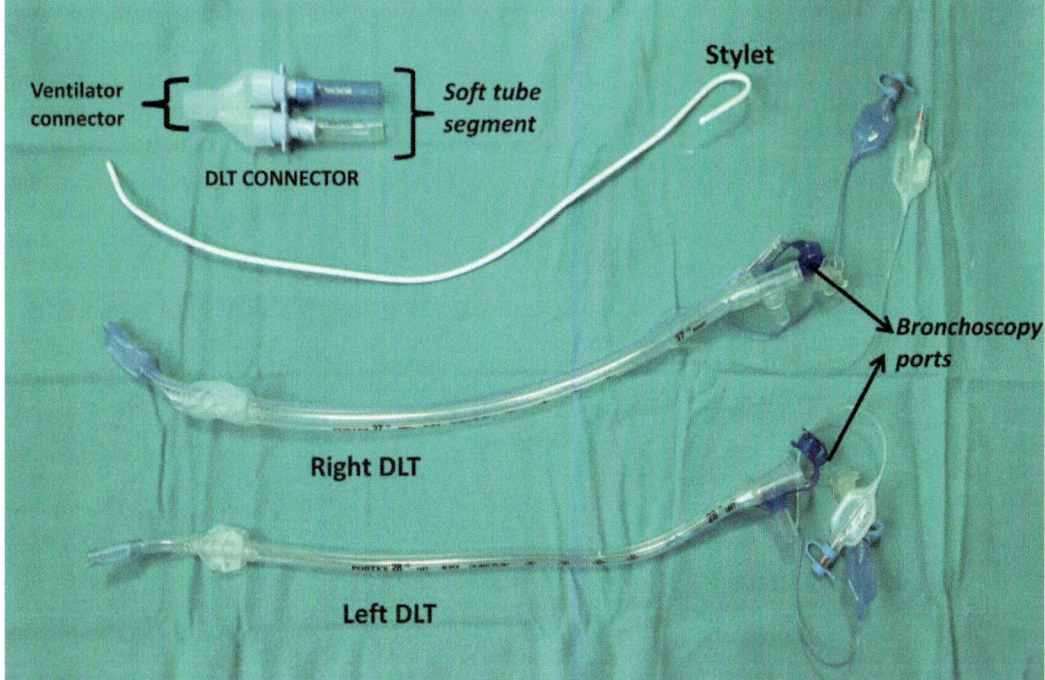

Fig. 5.4 Robertshaw DLT

5.3.2.5 Sher-I-Bronch Double Lumen Tube

The right-sided version of this DLT has two bronchial cuffs, one above and one below the slot (13 to 14 mm long) for ventilation of the right upper lobe bronchus.

The bronchial section of the left-sided Sher-I-Bronch double-lumen tube has a bevel, an average length of 34 mm and is at an angle of 34 degree from the main tube [13].

1. Methods of Insertion (refer chap. 10 for further details)
2. Placement Techniques (refer chap. 10 for further details)

5.3.2.6 Silbroncho DLT (Fig. 5.5)

It is a 100% silicone double-lumen tube for one-lung ventilation developed by Fuji Systems

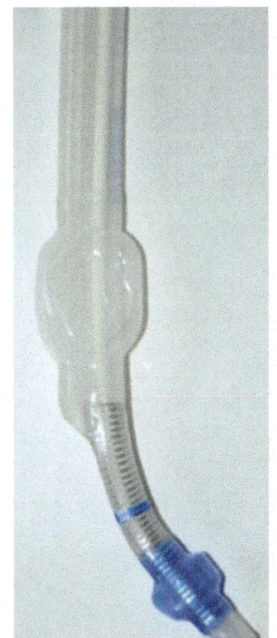

Fig. 5.5 Silbroncho DLT

in Tokyo, Japan. Its unique characteristic is the soft, flexible wire-reinforced endobronchial tip. This feature decreases kinking and allows X-ray verification of the DLT placement. In addition, the safety margin is increased by the short bronchial tip reduced bronchial size. In a study by Lee et al. Silbroncho® [17] was found to be superior to a polyvinyl chloride tube (Broncho-Cath®). It has a beveled tip that makes it easier for the tube to pass through the vocal cords. It is available in sizes 33, 35, 37, and 39 Fr.

5.3.2.7 Cliny Right-Sided DLT (Fig. 5.6)

Create Medic Co., Ltd., Yokohama, Japan developed a right-sided DLT. Useful for patients with very short-right mainstem bronchus. The unique features of this DLT are a long oblique bronchial cuff with its proximal section facing the tracheal orifice and two ventilation slots for the right-upper lobe [18].

5.3.2.8 Papworth Bivent Tube (Fig. 5.7)

This DLT was designed for the anesthesiologists who occasionally handle cases where lung

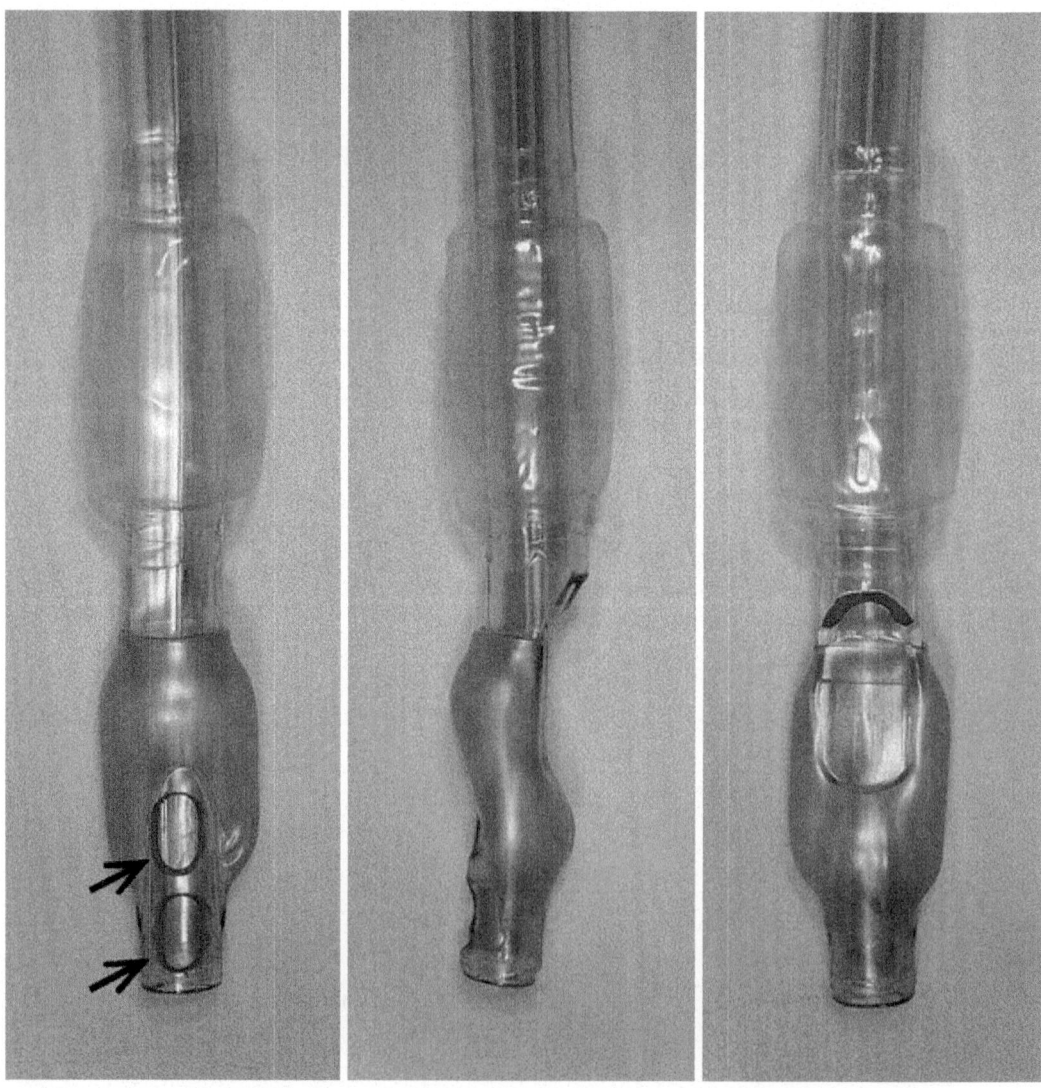

Fig. 5.6 Cliny® Right-sided, double-lumen endobronchial tube (Arrows: Indicate two ventilation shots)

5 Thoracic Anesthesia Equipment

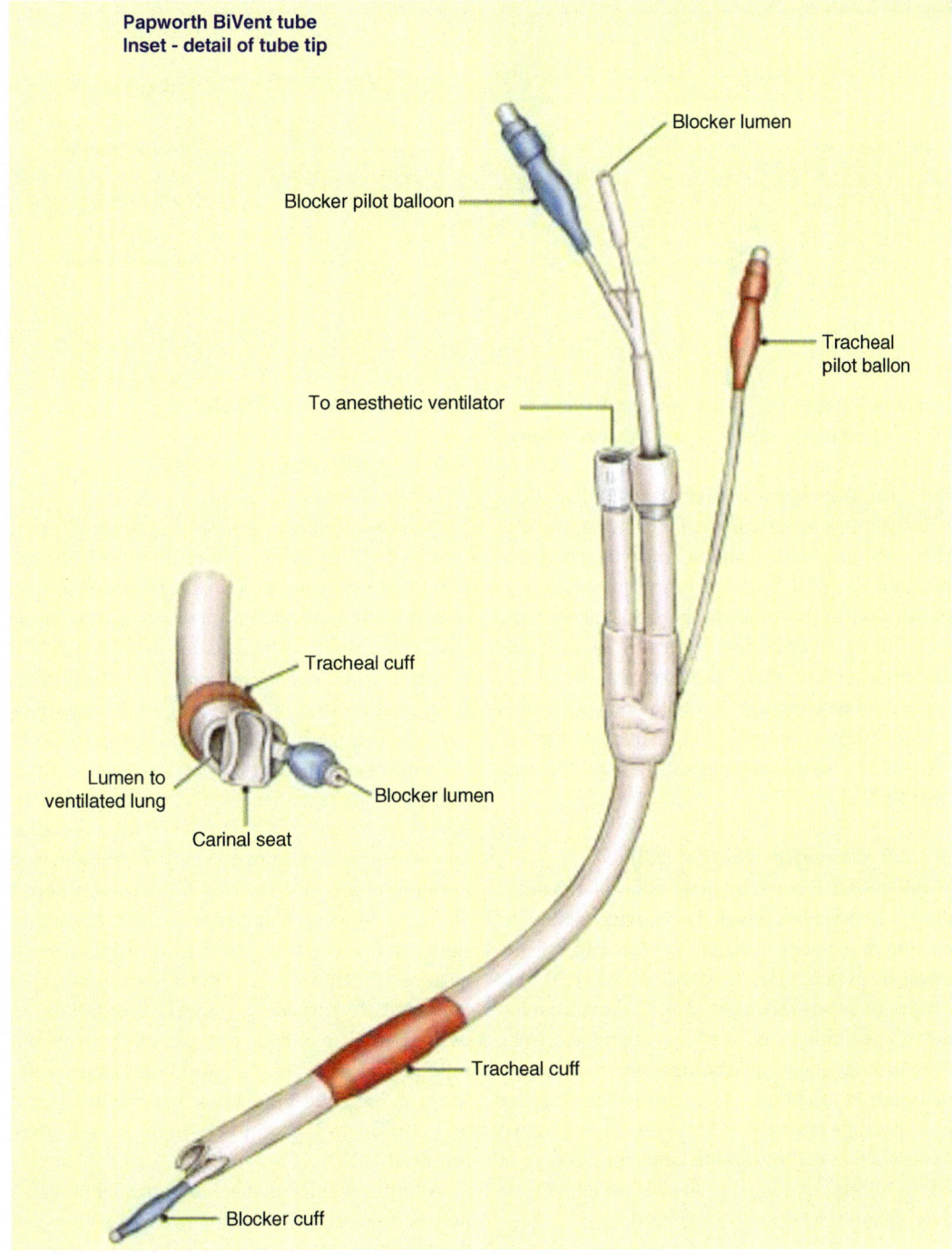

Fig. 5.7 Papworth BiVENT tube

Fig. 5.8 Viva Sight DLT

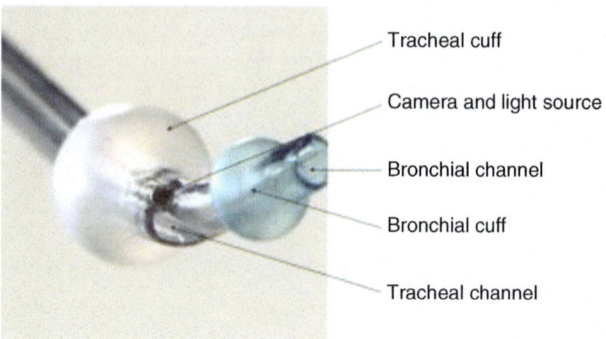

isolation is required. The Papworth BiVent tube [19, 20] is made up of two D-shaped lumens which are centrally positioned side by side, and has a distal end that is pliable and splits into a fork that fits onto the carina. The tube has a posterior curvature and a single low volume, high-pressure tracheal cuff. A bronchial blocker is inserted down the lumen to the lung that has to be isolated. At present only 43 Fr size is available. No endoscopic guidance is necessary. The advantage is that it can be used for both open and closed thoracic surgery as rapid lung isolation is possible and a satisfactory operating field is soon obtained [21].

5.3.2.9 Vivasight-DLT (Fig. 5.8)

VivaSight-DLT is a new generation of left-sided double-lumen tube, which has an integrated high-resolution camera situated at the end of the tracheal lumen. The camera allows real-time images of the airway to be viewed during intubation, positioning as well as perioperatively. Malpositions and dislocations are thus easily detected. In addition, for clearing the imaging lens, the tube has an injection port leading to two lumens along the wall of the tube, which opens at the distal end of imaging lens. VivaSight–DL is available in sizes 35, 37, 39, and 41 Fr.

5.3.2.10 Complications of DLT Placement (Refer Chap. 10 for Further Details)

5.4 Bronchial Blockers

5.4.1 Indications and Use

Bronchial blockers may be used as an alternative to DLT to achieve lung isolation. Proper placement of bronchial blocker balloon within the mainstem bronchus restricts gas flow to that entire lung. When using a DLT it is not possible as in a small patient, difficult intubation, nasal intubation, subglottic stenosis, tracheostomized patient, or if postoperatively the endotracheal intubation has to be continued [22]. In rare situations, bronchial blockers may be used for isolation of a smaller specific lung segment [22]. If a patient is on anticoagulants a bronchial blocker is a better choice since its placement is less traumatic than the insertion of a DLT [23]. Reduction of carbon dioxide in the dead space may be achieved by using a modified blocker to deliver fresh gas near the end of the tracheal tube [24]. Lastly, if sequential blockage of the lungs is required then a blocker may be useful and shifted to the opposite lung as and when required [25].

A hollow center channel in bronchial blockers may be used to apply suction to assist collapse of the lung or to apply continuous positive airway pressure.

5.4.2 Types of Blockers

Bronchial blockers are of two types: where they form an integral part of a combination with a standard single-lumen endotracheal tube, such as the Torque Controlled Blocker Univent® [26]; or independent bronchial blockers which are used with a customary single-lumen endotracheal tube, e.g., the wire-guided endobronchial blocker Arndt® [1] blocker, the Cohen® tip-deflecting endobronchial blocker [2], the Fuji Uniblocker™ [3, 27] or the Rusch® EZ blocker™.

5.4.3 Torque Controlled Blocker Univent® (Fig. 5.9)

This is a later version of the Univent (a single-lumen tube combined with a bronchial blocker) that was introduced by Inoue et al. [28] in 1982. The Torque Controlled Blocker Univent® (TCBU) was introduced in 2001. The Univent®resembles a single-lumen endotracheal tube with channel enclosing a movable bronchial blocker along its concave side. The device can be maneuvered into the desired main bronchus or specific bronchi. Manufactured from non-latex material, the TCBU has a malleable shaft allowing easier maneuverability into the chosen bronchus. For complete blockage, 4–8 ml of air is the volume needed to inflate the TCBU's high-pressure, low-volume cuff [29, 30], while 2 ml is required for a selective lobar blockade [31–33]. There is a small lumen for suctioning that needs to be closed before inserting the tube. The internal diameter (ID) of the Univent® in adults ranges from 6.0 to 9.0 mm; however, the 2-mm diameter of the enfolded channel for the bronchial blocker, means that the OD is larger than that of a regular single-lumen endotracheal tube, plus the ovoid cross section of the device requires two measurements of the outer diameter. The inner lumen is reduced by allowing space for the blocker. The blocker can be moved >10 cm beyond the main body.

An advantage of the Univent® is that CPAP application is possible by attaching a small 4.5-mm connector from a single-lumen endotracheal tube to the enclosed bronchial blocker, which is then fixed to a standard CPAP system [34, 35]. High-frequency jet ventilation (HFJV) has also been used successfully with the Univent® tube in a patient with tracheal carina resection [36, 37].

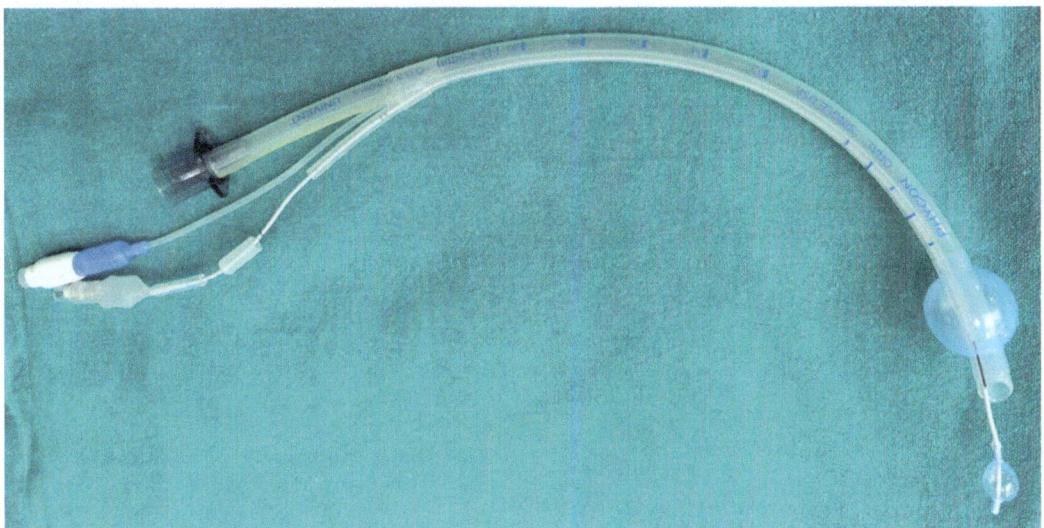

Fig. 5.9 Univent blocker

5.4.3.1 Placement, Position, and Confirmation of Univent® Tubes

Certain steps are imperative prior to using bronchial blockers. Check for leaks in the bronchial blocker and tube cuffs. Lubricate the blocker and the tube. Following cuff deflation ensure free movement of blocker by pushing it back and forth. Endotracheal tube intubation is carried out once the bronchial blocker is fully retracted, this is followed by tube cuff inflation and patient ventilation. Next, the bronchial blocker is directed into the desired bronchus with the aid of a fiberoptic scope. Twisting the shaft can direct the blocker tip into the desired bronchus [38]. There is another technique for bronchial blocker insertion. Following endotracheal intubation, use a fiberscope to direct the tube into the desired bronchus. Next, the bronchial blocker is inserted into the bronchus and the endotracheal tube withdrawn into the trachea. However, this method can cause trauma to the airway [39]. The Univent® bronchial blocker's best position in either left- or right-sided bronchus is when there is no air leak with full cuff inflation. On fiberoptic bronchoscopy, the outer surface of the cuff lies just below the tracheal carina, typically ≥5 mm inside the desired bronchus and the terminal end of Univent® tube should be at least 1–2 cm above the tracheal carina.

5.4.3.2 Complications and Pitfalls

- Danger of bronchial blocker being incorporated into the stapling line [40].
- Inflation of bronchial blocker cuff near the tracheal lumen can result in respiratory arrest [41].
- Failure to achieve lung separation [42].
- Lack of seal within the bronchus [43].
- Structural complications like fracture of bronchial cap connector [44].
- Malpositions with surgical manipulations [45].

The preferred technique of optimal placing of the Univent® and correcting intraoperative malpositions, is by using fiberoptic bronchoscopy.

5.4.4 Wire-Guided Endobronchial Blocker (Arndt® Blocker) (Fig. 5.10)

This is an independent bronchial blocker [1] and is employed when a single-lumen endotracheal tube is already in situ. There are two parts to the Arndt® blocker: a blocking catheter and a special airway connector.

The catheter cuff is elliptical or spherical shaped, low pressure, and high volume. A flexible

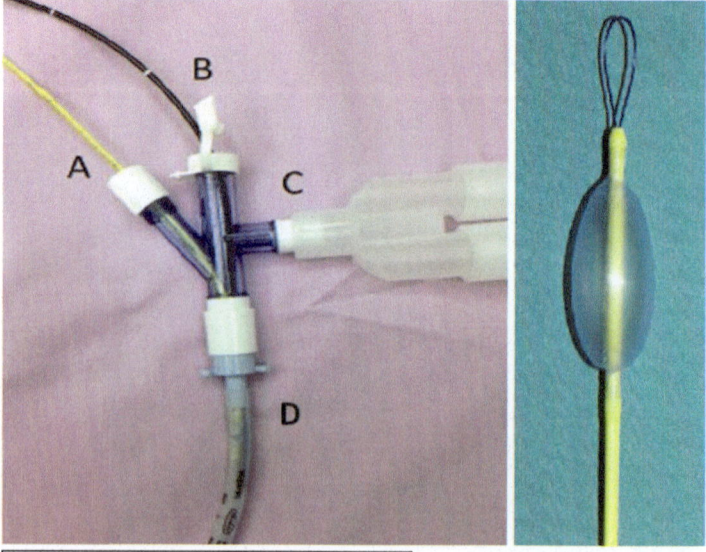

Fig. 5.10 Arndt blocker

- Port A : For bronchial blocker
- Port B: For FOB
- Port C: Anesthesia breathing system
- Port D: Attaches to the tracheal tube

nylon is passed from the proximal portion of the catheter to the distal end where it emerges as a loop the size of which can be adjusted by advancing or advancing the assembly. The inner lumen of the catheter measures 1.4 mm in diameter. There are side holes at the distal end of the catheter, which are present only in the 9 Fr Arndt® blocker. These openings aid in lung deflation.

The airway adapter has four parts:

1. 15 mm female connector for the tracheal tube.
2. 15 mm male connector for a side port that links to the anesthesia breathing system.
3. Roughly 30-degree angled port for the bronchial blocker.
4. A port for flexible endoscope.

5.4.4.1 Placement, Position, and Confirmation of Arndt® Blocker

It is imperative to follow these procedures to ease insertion of the bronchial blocker: inflate cuffs, check for leaks then deflate; lubricate both the blocker and the fiberoptic bronchoscope. For the right mainstem bronchus, the bronchial blocker with the spherical cuff is used whereas for the left mainstem bronchus elliptical or spherical cuff can be employed.

Following tracheal intubation and ventilation, a multiport adapter is attached between the breathing system and the tracheal tube. Prior to insertion of blocker, the cuff should be fully deflated and open the blocker port. The fiberoptic bronchoscope is used to place the Arndt® blocker through the endotracheal tube and the wire-guide loop is used to direct the blocker into the desired "mainstem" bronchus.

The wire-guide loop is used in two ways: [46] it is either closely wound around the tip of fiberscope which then directs the blocker into its desired location or [47] a track for the blocker is provided when the fiberscope is passed through the loop into the desired bronchus. Next, 2–3 ml of air is used to inflate the blocker balloon for selective lobar blockade or 5 to 8 ml if the total bronchial blockade is the target.

When switching patient position from supine to lateral decubitus, it is imperative that the blocker cuff be deflated and the device moved to 1 cm beyond the optimal position, this is done to prevent dislodgement. Reconfirm proper placement of device once the lateral decubitus position has been finalized. Removal of the wire loop converts the 1.4-mm channel into a suction port or for the application of a CPAP device.

The optimal blocker position in the desired bronchus is achieved under vision with the fiberoptic bronchoscope when the exterior of the blocker balloon is seen at least 5-mm below the tracheal carina on the targeted bronchus and the proper seal obtained.

5.4.4.2 Complications and Pitfalls
- More frequent incidence of malposition compared to the TCBU [48].
- Longer time to collapse the lung as compared to the Univent tube or DLT [49, 50].
- Potential for inclusion of guidewire or tip of bronchial blocker in stapling line [51].
- Shearing of balloon when removing through multiport connector [52].
- At the end of surgery, it is important to deflate the cuff of the Arndt blocker before withdrawing it and the multiport connector but not via the unlocked blocker port.

5.4.5 Cohen® Flexitip Endobronchial Blocker (Fig. 5.11)

Available only in size 9 Fr this device is 65 cm in length has an inner lumen 1.4 mm in diameter enables lung isolation via a conventional single-lumen endotracheal tube. The Cohen® endobronchial blocker has a special deflecting tip which aids in precision placement of the blocker under bronchoscopic guidance. The low-pressure, high-volume spherical shaped balloon at the tip requires a volume of 5 to 8 ml for optimal inflation. The proximal end of this blocker has a wheel

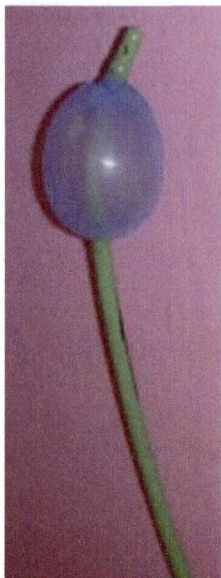

Fig. 5.11 The Cohen flexitip bronchial blocker with a multiport connector and proximal wheel control

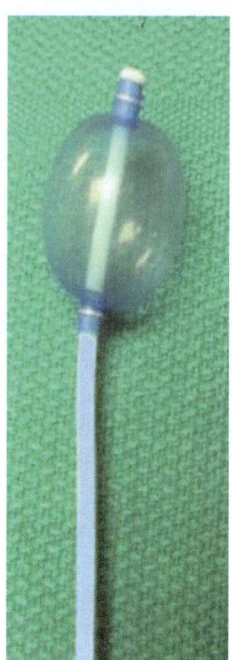

Fig. 5.12 Fuji Uniblocker™

that can be operated with thumb and forefinger to manipulate blocker tip movement. There are side holes built-in between the tip and the balloon of the blocker, which aid in lung deflation or oxygen insufflation. The device has distance markings and an indicator arrow at the proximal end that shows in which direction the tip deflects.

5.4.5.1 Placement, Position, and Confirmation of Cohen® Blocker

The Cohen® blocker is advanced through an 8.0-mm ID single-lumen endotracheal tube. A multiport airway adapter like the Arndt is placed on the endotracheal tube. Before insertion, the blocker is lubricated and the bronchial balloon tested and then fully deflated. The bronchoscope is advanced through the bronchoscopy port till the carina is visible. Cohen® endobronchial blocker is then passed through the blocker port and fiberoptic bronchoscope used to observe the direction of the blocker into the desired "mainstem" bronchus. The direction of tip deflection is confirmed by the black mark at the proximal end of the blocker. The black mark should face the main bronchus which is to be blocked. This is achieved by twisting the proximal end of the blocker. The deflection of the blocker tip should be done with the wheel under direct vision, while keeping the bronchoscope position stable. In most cases, a 10–45 degree deflection is sufficient to direct the blocker into "mainstem" bronchus to be blocked. The balloon is then inflated under bronchoscopic guidance with 5–8 ml of air. The optimal position is achieved when the outer surface of the blocker balloon is seen with a fiberoptic bronchoscope at least 5-mm below the tracheal carina inside the desired "mainstem" bronchus.

5.4.6 Fuji Uniblocker™ (Fig. 5.12)

Like the Arndt® and Cohen® bronchial blockers, the Fuji Uniblocker™ is an independent bronchial blocker that is placed through the standard endotracheal tube. It is available in 4.5 Fr and 9 Fr sizes and is 65 cm in length with a central channel of 2 mm internal diameter. It also has a soft silicon high-volume balloon that incorporates gas barrier technology which stabilizes the gas volume and pressure over time [53]. This blocker has torque-control, plus an integrated shaft that allows guidance through the appropriate bronchus. The Fuji Uniblocker™ with its swivel connector enables easy insertion of the fiberoptic bronchoscope.

5.4.6.1 Placement, Position, and Confirmation of Fuji Uniblocker™

Before insertion, lubrication of blocker ensures smooth passage through the single-lumen endotracheal tube. After testing the blocker balloon for leaks, it is fully deflated. A fiberoptic bronchoscope is used to place the Fuji Uniblocker™ into a single-lumen endotracheal. The torque control shaft on the blocker permits entry into the target bronchus. The correct position of the blocker is confirmed with the fiberoptic bronchoscope: the fully inflated blocker 4–8 ml of air and lies at least 5-mm below the tracheal carina inside the desired mainstem bronchus.

5.4.7 Rusch® EZ-Blocker™ (Fig. 5.13)

This blocker provides lung isolation by insertion through a standard single-lumen endotracheal tube. There are two distal extensions of the EZ® Blocker each having a central lumen and an inflatable cuff. Radio-opaque material is used for the two distal extensions, the tips and the shaft. The two distal extensions are in separate colors for the purpose of identification. The blue distal extension has additional blue pinstripes as symbols for CPAP purposes. These colored and symbolic identifications are repeated on each equivalent balloon assembly for cuff inflation. Printed depth markers indicate the distance to the distal tip of EZ™ Blocker. The EZ-Multiport Adapter is used for connection to ventilation devices and allows introduction of a fiberoptic bronchoscope for placement and proper positioning.

5.4.7.1 Placement, Position, and Confirmation of EZ-Blocker™

After intubation with a suitable-sized endotracheal tube, the EZ-Multiport adapter should be connected to the endotracheal tube, and ventilation initiated. Check both cuffs for leakage and asymmetric inflation. The cuffs are then deflated completely. The distal part of EZ-Blocker™ and bronchoscope are lubricated for smooth passage through endotracheal tube. The endotracheal tube should be positioned 4-cm above the carina to guarantee optimal functioning of EZ-Blocker™. The EZ-Blocker™ is introduced through a port of multiport adapter. The fiberoptic bronchoscope is then introduced through another port to view the airway and the EZ-Blocker™. The EZ-Blocker™ is then advanced under direct visual control until both extensions are just outside the endotracheal tube. The device is then further advanced under visual guidance until both distal extensions have been introduced in both mainstem bronchi. The appropriate distal extension cuff is inflated via the respective balloon; the blue striped proximal balloon corresponds to the distal cuff on blue extension. Isolate the target lung and auscultate the contralateral lung for sufficient ventilation. The fiberoptic bronchoscope is removed only after the final check of the position of the inflated cuff.

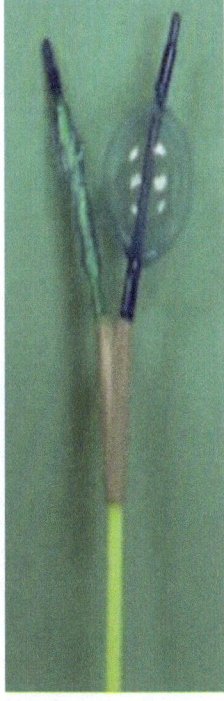

Fig. 5.13 EZ blocker

5.4.8 Fogarty Embolectomy Catheter as a Bronchial Blocker (Fig. 5.14)

The Fogarty is specifically designed as a vascular surgery tool, but may be used as a bronchial blocker to achieve lung isolation [54] if traditional bronchial blockers are not available. The occlusion balloon is high-pressure, low-volume cuff needing 0.5–10 ml of air to achieve lung isolation. The wire stylet with the Fogarty catheter can be molded at its distal end for guiding the catheter into the target bronchus. Common sizes used in adults include: number

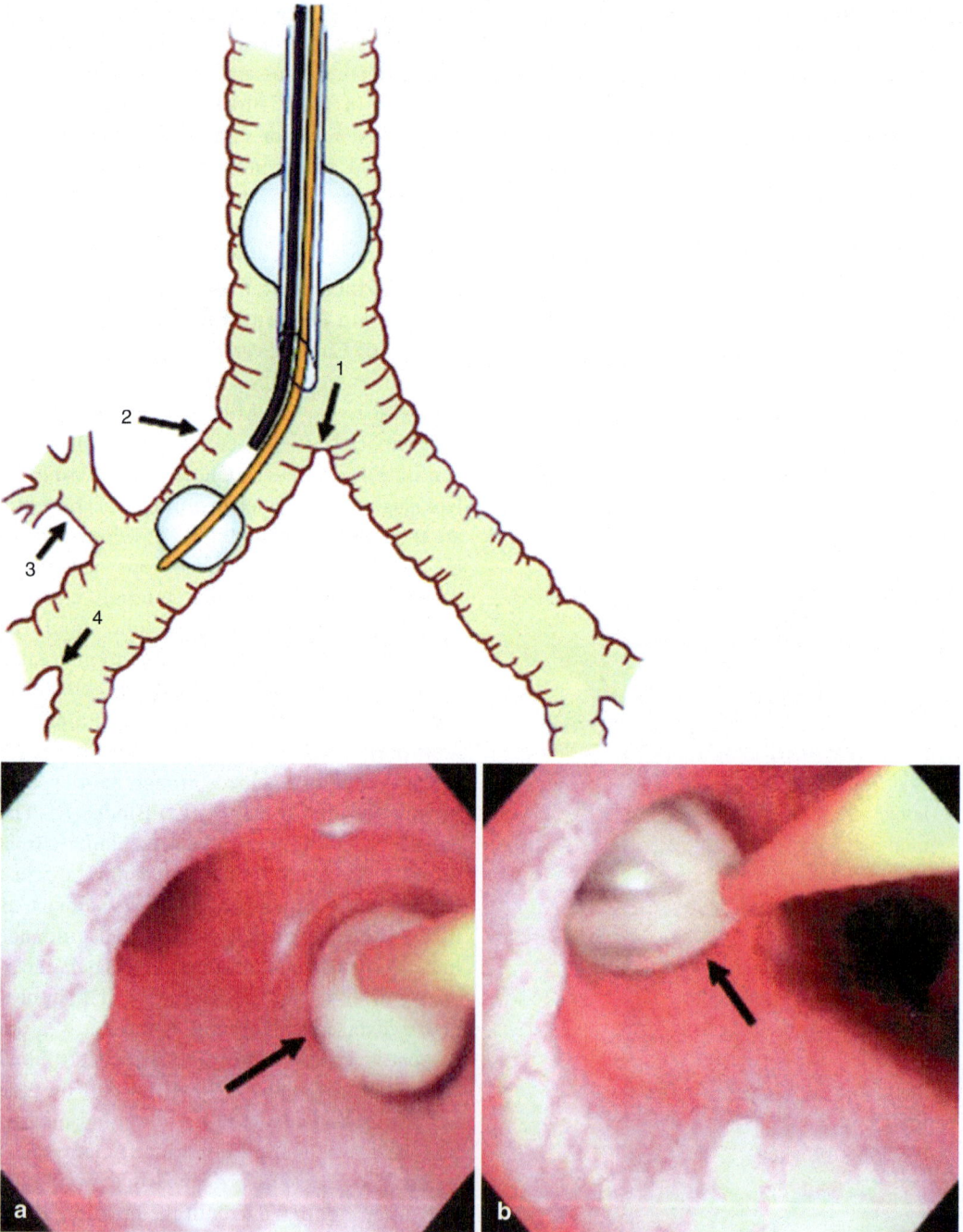

Fig. 5.14 Fogarty embolectomy catheter as a bronchial blocker

6.0, 8/14, or 8/22 F, which has a length of 80 cm. The figures marked on the catheter refer to device size followed by inflated balloon diameter (mm).

The Fogarty catheter has the advantage of being used in an already intubated patient without having to resort to tube exchange or during nasotracheal intubation and OLV. They can also be used in pediatric patients (refer Chap. 17) and for selective lobar bronchial blockade [55].

5.4.8.1 Placement, Position, and Confirmation of Fogarty Catheter

After lubrication of the blocker, check the balloon for leaks and then fully deflate it. The fiberscope is used to direct the catheter through the endotracheal tube. Under vision direct, the Fogarty catheter into the desired bronchus, inflate the catheter cuff then withdraw the fiberscope. Air leak prevention and making an airtight seal between the elbow connector of a breathing circuit and that of the single-lumen tube connector is done by using a customized 9 Fr arrow-Flex sheath and a twist-lock device used with the diaphragm of a Portex bronchoscope swivel connector [56]. The Arndt multiport adapter also allows the independent passage of any blocker and fiberoptic bronchoscope.

5.4.8.2 Complications and Pitfalls
- The device should not be used in those with latex allergy since the Fogarty catheter is manufactured from natural rubber latex.
- Suction or oxygen insufflation is not possible as it has a hollow blind center.
- No guide wire so pairing with fiberoptic bronchoscope not possible.
- Placing device outside the endotracheal tube can avoid air leak from the breathing circuit which is possible when a device placed within the single-lumen endotracheal tube.
- Inclusion in staple line, when used for selective lobar blockade, is a possibility.

5.5 Lung Isolation in Presence of a Tracheostomy

The shortened airway and the small and restrictive stoma pose a challenge for achieving OLV in the tracheostomized patients. Bronchial blockers can be placed either within or alongside a reinforced single-lumen ETT or a disposable cuffed tracheostomy cannula [57–61]. Alternatively, the bronchial blocker may be placed through the vocal cords and then alongside the tracheostomy tube [61, 62]. Use of small DLT placed via a tracheostomy tube has been reported, although positioning can be difficult [63, 64].

5.6 Lung Isolation in an Anticipated Difficult Airway

The key objective is to secure the airway [57]. If difficult bag-mask ventilation is also anticipated, awake intubation is necessary, which is best done with single-lumen ETT [65]. While awake fiberoptic intubation and placement of a DLT has been described, guiding a stiff, large-diameter DLT through the oropharynx over a short, pliable bronchoscope can be difficult [57, 66].

For those patients who cannot be intubated orally, awake nasotracheal intubation with a single lumen ETT is an option [58, 65, 67].

If mask ventilation is possible, either awake intubation, or intubation after induction of general anesthesia with a SLT or a DLT can be done [63]. A video laryngoscope may be used post-induction to guide placement of a DLT [63, 68–70].

Bronchial blockers are the easiest and safest means for lung isolation when an SLT is used to secure a difficult airway [57]. Alternatively, airway exchange catheter can be used to replace SLT with DLT once general anesthesia is established. To minimize the risk of exchange failure and airway trauma, the AEC should have the hollow center as well as a universal adapter to facilitate oxygenation as needed, and should be at least 83-cm long [65]. The catheter should not be inserted more than 24-cm at the lip to avoid airway injury during exchange. The use of fiberoptic bronchoscope to exchange a nasotracheal SLT for an oral DLT has also been described [71].

5.7 Need for Postoperative Ventilation

Once the surgery is over in patients who will need extended postoperative ventilation, the DLT should be replaced by an SLT.

In case of limited period of postoperative ventilation, a left DLT may be left in place, while right DLT should be replaced because of more chances of malposition with patient movement. A Univent tube <7.5-mm ID should be changed to standard ETT for postoperative ventilation as soon as possible [72]. For bronchial blockers inserted via a large (≥8-mm ID) SLT to achieve lung isolation, the blocker balloon should be deflated and blocker removed.

5.8 Single-Lumen Tubes

Lung isolation can also be accomplished by placing a single-lumen endotracheal tube within the right or left mainstem bronchus, resulting in ventilation of only the intubated lung. They are sometimes used in pediatric patients (refer Chap. 14 on pediatric lung isolation) and may also be useful in selected patients with abnormal tracheobronchial anatomy, as well as in emergency situations, like unilateral pulmonary hemorrhage or copious purulent material, when immediate isolation of healthy lung is necessary [57], especially when DLTs or blockers are not available.

5.8.1 Standard Single-Lumen Tube

If the length of the cuff and the tube beyond it (>4 cm) is longer than the DLT, obstruction of the upper lobe bronchus is a possibility. To prevent this mishap, distance from the tip of the tube to the cephaloid border of the cuff must be less than the length of the "mainstem" bronchus [73]. The recommendations for single-lumen tube is one half to one size smaller than usual in adults [74] and 0.5 mm to 2 mm smaller in children [75, 76].

5.8.2 Special Single-Lumen Endobronchial Tubes (Fig. 5.15)

Specialized long single-lumen endotracheal tubes are preferred if endobronchial placement of the single-lumen tube is necessary. These specifi-

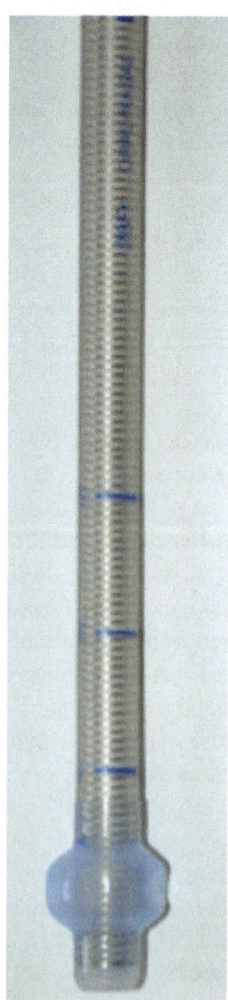

Fig. 5.15 Special single-lumen endobronchial tubes

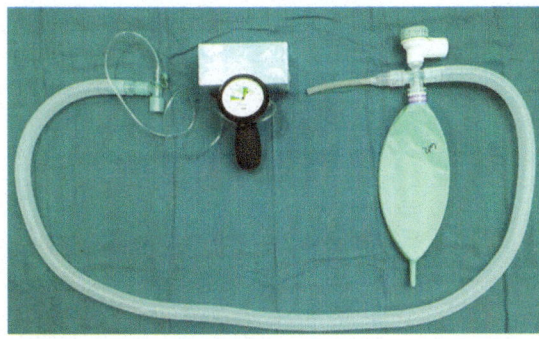 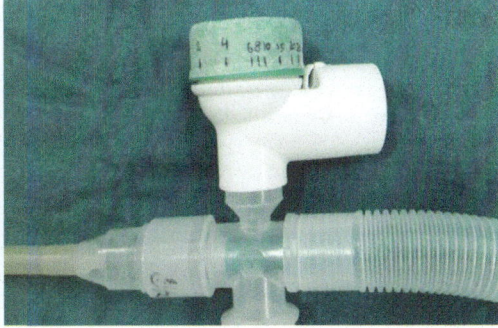

Fig. 5.16 CPAP devices. Indigenous continuous positive airway pressure (CPAP) device for mitigation of hypoxemia during One-Lung Ventilation (OLV)

cally designed tubes are placed in endotracheal position, then passed into the mainstem bronchus using fiberoptic guidance [57]. Fuji Systems in Tokyo, Japan has developed a Phycon single-lumen tube that is longer (40 cm), has a short cuff. and does not have a Murphy eye, thus increasing the margin of safety when placed in "mainstem" bronchus for one-lung ventilation.

5.9 CPAP Devices (Fig. 5.16)

Hypoxemia, resulting from ventilation–perfusion mismatch and intrapulmonary shunt, is one of the major complications of OLV [77]. A variety of approaches to prevent hypoxemia have been developed. Application of continuous positive airway pressure (CPAP) to the non-ventilated lung is one way to avoid hypoxia. Easy application of CPAP can be achieved using commercial devices with a CPAP adaptor, which can be attached to either the open lumen of the DLT or the suction port of a bronchial blocker. The oxygen flow rate for generating the CPAP is 5 l/min from the wall outlet. CPAP pressure can be adjusted from 1 to 10 cm H_2O as per requirement. If commercial CPAP is not available then an AMBU bag with a PEEP valve can be used to deliver CPAP.

An indigenously created CPAP device for the alleviation of hypoxemia during one-lung ventilation was assembled from Bain's modification of the Mapleson D circuit [78]. A flow of 5 l/min of oxygen flow was used with the standard Bain's circuit. A cuff pressure monitor is attached to the CO_2-sampling site and the patient end of the circuit is blocked. Next is the calibration of the adjustable pressure-limiting (APL) valve. Start with the APL valve in the open position then gradually close it: the pressure in the circuit will increase, as seen in the cuff pressure monitor. The APL valve is then marked according to the pressure displayed. Intraoperatively the patient end of the circuit is attached to the DLT lumen leading to the non-ventilated lung while the machine end is attached to an oxygen source, which is delivering 5 l/min. So, now the CPAP can be delivered by rotating the calibrated APL valve to the required amount.

5.10 Airway Exchange Catheters (AEC) (Fig. 5.17)

Airway Exchange Catheters (AEC) are essential to the armamentarium of thoracic anesthesiologists. They are used not only in patients with difficult laryngoscopic view but also facilitate exchanging from SLT to DLT prior to surgery or DLT to SLT in case postoperative ventilation is required.

While gum elastic bougie [79], an Aintree® catheter [80] (Cook Critical Care) has been used with an SLT, the Frova® intubating catheter [81] (Cook Critical Care) has been used for DLTs. Various lengths and sizes of AEC are available. An AEC must be >70 cms in length to ensure successful tracheal introduction of DLT. Before attempting tube exchange, the AEC should be lubricated and

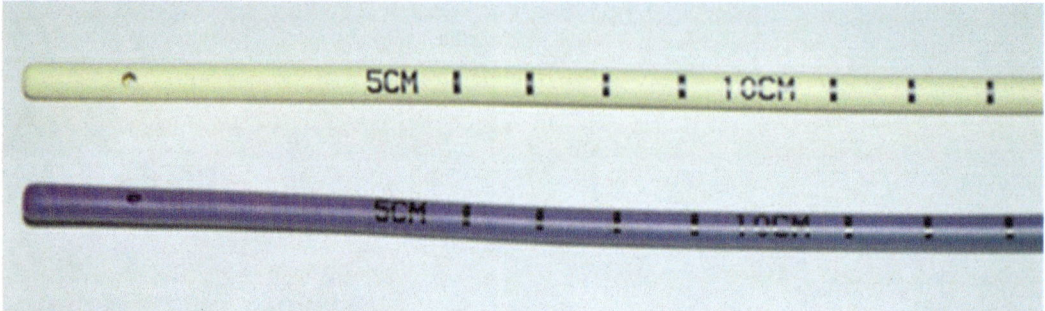

Fig. 5.17 Airway exchange catheters (AEC)

must be tested whether AEC fits in the DLT. AEC should never be advanced against resistance. Lifting the supraglottic tissue with a laryngoscope and rotating the tube counterclockwise by 90° provides a smooth passage through glottis and prevents impingement at vocal cords and arytenoids, respectively. Depth markings of AEC and tube should be noted. AEC should never be more than 25–26 cms into the airway. A system for jet ventilation should be available, in case the tube cannot be advanced. Tube impingement can occur during DLT to SLT exchange, the incidence of which can be reduced by placing an AEC in each lumen of DLT.

5.11 Fiberoptic Bronchoscope

This is the preferred way of achieving optimal positioning of lung isolation devices in supine, lateral decubitus, or when a malposition takes place.

The components of the flexible fiberscope system are: (1) Eyepiece, (2) Control section, (3) Insertion cord, (4) Universal cord for light transmission, and (5) Light source.

The main component of the fiberscope is the insertion cord which contains a collection of approximately 10,000 glass fibers, 25 μ each in diameter. To keep the light from being lost during transmission, each fiber is coated with a 1-μ layer of glass having different optical density. This helps in the total internal reflection of light entering the fiber. Individual fibers cannot provide a good resolution and hence the need for a collection of approximately 10,000 fibers in a bundle. The fiberscope contains another set of fiberoptic bundles to serve as a cable for transmitting light from a light source to the end of the insertion cord. However, these bundles need not be coherent as those in the insertion cord as they do not transmit any image.

The size of flexible fiberscope recommended for 26, 28, and 32 Fr DLT is 2.2-mm outer diameter whereas the sizes of 3.5 or 4.2 mm is preferred for 35, 37, 39, and 41 Fr DLT.

5.12 Videolaryngoscopes

Videolaryngoscopes are known to improve glottic view [82], (Cormack and Lehane grade as well as percentage of glottic opening scale) over the Macintosh blade laryngoscope. They can be especially useful in difficult airway scenarios. D blade videolaryngoscopes are beneficial substitutes to the standard Macintosh laryngoscope for routine DLT insertion [83]. Glidescope® has been successfully used in patients with a difficult airway [4, 84]. Intubation facilitated by bending the stylet of DLT so that the DLT curve follows the curve of glidescope. The McGrath™ [85], Airtraq™ [86], Pentax® airwayscope [87, 88], have also been used for insertion of DLT.

5.13 Conclusion

Right- and left-sided DLTs are most commonly used to provide lung isolation. They are the best choice in cases requiring lung isolation.

With the development of fiberoptic bronchoscopic techniques, the use of bronchial blockers has increased. They are a superior option for patients with difficult airways, for selective lobar ventilation, or wherever postoperative mechanical ventilation is required.

AEC can also be used in cases of difficult laryngoscopic view as well as for exchanging SLT to DLT or vice versa.

Various types of videolaryngoscopes are now available that can be used to achieve lung isolation in difficult airway scenarios.

References

1. Arndt GA, Kranner PW, Rusy DA, et al. Single-lung ventilation in a critically ill patient using a fiberoptically directed wire-guided endobronchial blocker. Anesthesiology. 1999;90:1484–6.
2. Cohen E. The Cohen flexitip endobronchial blocker: an alternative to a double lumen tube. Anesth Analg. 2005;101:1877–9.
3. Narayanaswamy M, McRae K, Slinger P, et al. Choosing a lung isolation device for thoracic surgery: a randomized trial of three bronchial blockers versus double-lumen tubes. Anesth Analg. 2009;108:1097–101.
4. Chen A, Lai HY, Lin PC, et al. Glide Scopeassisted double-lumen endobronchial tube placement in a patient with an unanticipated difficult airway. J Cardiothorac Vasc Anesth. 2008;22:170–2.
5. Bjork VO, Carlens E. The prevention of spread during pulmonary resection by the use of a double-lumen catheter. J Thorac Surg. 1950;20:151–7.
6. Hannallah MS, Miller SC, Kurzer SI, et al. The effective diameter and airflow resistance of the individual lumens of left polyvinyl chloride double-lumen endobronchial tubes. Anesth Analg. 1996;82:867–9.
7. Benumof JL. Improving the design and function of double–lumen tubes. J Cardiothorac Vasc Anesth. 1988;2:729–33.
8. Benumof JL, Partridge BL, Salvatierra C, et al. Margin of safety in positioning modern double-lumen endotracheal tubes. Anesthesiology. 1987;67:729–38.
9. Saito S, Dohi S, Naito H. Alteration of double-lumen endobronchial tube position by flexion and extension of the neck. Anesthesiology. 1985;62:696–7.
10. Newman RW, Finer GE, Downs JE. Routine use of Carlens double-lumen endobronchial catheter: an experimental and clinical study. J Thorac Cardiovasc Surg. 1961;42:327.
11. Thangathurai D, Roessler P, Milhail M. Is there a role for the Carlen's double–lumen tube in cardiothoracic anesthesia? J Cardiothorac Vasc Anesth. 1996;10:693.
12. Conacher ID, Herrema IH, Batchelor AM. Robertshaw double lumen tubes: a reappraisal thirty years on. Anaesth Intensive Care. 1994;22:179–83.
13. Watterson LM, Harrison GA. A comparison of the endobronchial segment of modern left–sided double-lumen tubes in anesthesia for bilateral sequential lung transplantation. J Cardiothorac Vasc Anesth. 1996;10:583–5.
14. Brodsky JB, Macario A. Modified Broncho Cath double–lumen tube. J Cardiothorac Vasc Anesth. 1995;9:784–5.
15. Fortier G, Bergeron C, Bussieres JS. New landmarks improve the positioning of the left Broncho-Cath double-lumen tube-comparison with the classic technique. Can J Anesth. 2001;48:790–4.
16. Yahagi N, Furuya H, Matsui J, et al. Improvements of the left Broncho-Cath double-lumentube. Anesthesiology. 1994;81:781–2.
17. Lee JS, Kil TY, Chung JY. Comparison of a silicon double-lumen Endobronchial tube (Silbroncho (R)) with a polyvinyl chloride tube (Broncho-Cath (R)) in right-side thoracic surgery. Korean J Anesthesiology. 2005;48(5):509–13.
18. Hagihira S, Takashina M, Mashimo T. Application of a newly designed right-sided, double-lumen endobronchial tube in patients with a very short right mainstem bronchus. Anesthesiology. 2008;109:565–8.
19. Ghosh S, Falter F, Goldsmith K, et al. The Papworth BiVent tube: a new device for lung isolation. Anaesthesia. 2008;63:996–1000.
20. Ghosh S, Klein AA, Prabhu M, et al. The Papworth BiVent tube: a feasibility study of a novel double-lumen endotracheal tube and bronchial blocker in human cadavers. Br J Anaesth. 2008;101:424–8.
21. Ghosh S, Falter F, Klein AA, et al. The Papworth BiVent tube: initial clinical experience. J Cardioth Vascular Anesth. 2011;25:505–8.
22. Campos JH. An update on bronchial blockers during lung separation techniques in adults. Anesth Analg. 2003;97:1266–74.
23. Herenstein R, Russo JR, Mooka N, et al. Management of one–lung anesthesia in an anticoagulated patient. Anesth Analg. 1988;67:1120–2.
24. Frolich MA. Postoperative atelectasis after one–lung ventilation with a Univent tube in a child. J Clin Anesth. 2003;15:159–63.
25. Capdeville M, Hall D, Koch CG. Practical use of a bronchial blocker in combination with a double-lumen endotracheal tube. Anesth Analg. 1998;87:1239–41.
26. Campos JH, Kernstine KH. A comparison of a left-sided Broncho-Cath with the torque control blocker univent and the wireguided blocker. Anesth Analg. 2003;96:283–9.
27. Campos JH. Which device should be considered the best for lung isolation: double-lumen endotracheal tube versus bronchial blockers. Curr Opin Anaesthesiol. 2007;20:27–31.
28. Inoue H, Shohtsu A, Ogawa J, et al. New device for one-lung anesthesia: endotracheal tube with movable blocker. J Thorac Cardiovasc Surg. 1982;83:940–1.
29. Benumof JL, Gaughan SD, Ozaki G. The relationship among bronchial blocker cuff inflation volume, proximal airway pressure, and seal of the bronchial blocker cuff. J Cardiothorac Vasc Anesth. 1992;6:404–8.

30. Hannallah SM, Benumof JL. Comparison of two techniques to inflate the bronchial cuff of the Univent® tube. Anesth Analg. 1992;75:784–7.
31. Campos JH. Effects on oxygenation during selective lobar versus total lung collapse with or without continuous positive airway pressure. Anesth Analg. 1997;85:583–6.
32. Campos JH, Ledet C, Moyers JR. Improvement of arterial oxygen saturation with selective lobar bronchial block during hemorrhage in a patient with previous contralateral lobectomy. Anesth Analg. 1995;81:1095–6.
33. Hagihira S, Maki N, Kawaguchi M, Slinger P. Selective bronchial blockade in patients with previous contralateral lung surgery. J Cardiothorac Vasc Anesth. 2002;16:638–42.
34. Benumof JL, Gaughan S, Ozaki GT. Operative lung constant positive airway pressure with the Univent® bronchial blocker tube. Anesth Analg. 1992;74:406–10.
35. Baraka A, Sibai AN, Nawfal M, et al. Underwater seal for CPAP oxygenation during one-lung ventilation by a Univent ® tube. Middle East J Anesthesiol. 1996;13:581–3.
36. Ransom E, Detterbeck F, Klein JI, et al. Univent® tube provides a new technique for jet ventilation. Anesthesiology. 1996;84:724–6.
37. Williams H, Gothard J. Jet ventilation in a Univent® tube for sleeve pneumonectomy. Eur J Anaesthesiol. 2000;18:407–9.
38. Baraka A. The Univent tube can facilitate difficult intubation in a patient undergoing thoracoscopy. J Cardiothorac Vasc Anesth. 1996;10(5):693–4.
39. Doyle DJ. A simple technique for placement of the Univent bronchial blocker. Anesthesiology. 1993;79:399.
40. Thielmeier KA, Anwar M. Complication of the Univent tube. Anesthesiology. 1996;84:491.
41. Dougherty P, Hannallah M. A potentially serious complication that resulted from improper use of the Univent tube. Anesthesiology. 1992;77:835.
42. Peragallo RA, Swenson JD. Congenital tracheal bronchus: the inability to isolate the right lung with a univent bronchial blocker tube. Anesth Analg. 2000;91:300–1.
43. Asai T. Failure of the Univent bronchial blocker in sealing the bronchus. Anaesthesia. 1999;54:97.
44. Campos JH, Kernstine KH. A structural complication in the torque control blocker Univent: fracture of the blocker cap connector. Anesth Analg. 2003;96:630–1.
45. Campos JH, Reasoner DK, Moyers JR. Comparison of a modified double-lumen endotracheal tube with a single-lumen tube with enclosed bronchial blocker. Anesth Analg. 1996;83:1268–72.
46. Campos JH. Progress in lung separation. Thorac Surg Clin. 2008;15:71–83.
47. Campos JH. Current techniques for perioperative lung isolation in adults. Anesthesiology. 2002;97:1295–301.
48. Campos JH, Kernstine KH. A comparison of a left-sided Broncho-Cath, with the torque control blocker Univent® and the wire-guided blocker. Anesth Analg. 2003;96:283–9.
49. Karzai W. Alternative method to deflate the operated lung when using wire –guided endobronchial blockade. Anesthesiology. 2003;99:239–40.
50. Arndt GA. Endobronchial blocker response. Anesthesiology. 2003;99:240.
51. Soto RG, Oleszak SP. Resection of the Arndt bronchial blocker during stapler resection of the left lower lobe. J Cardiothorac Vasc Anesth. 2006;20:131–2.
52. Prabhu MR, Smith JH. Use of the Arndt wire-guided endobronchial blocker. Anesthesiology. 2002;97:1325.
53. Roscoe A, Kanellakos GW, McRae K, et al. Pressures exerted by endobronchial devices. Anesth Analg. 2007;104:655–8.
54. Ginsberg RJ. New technique for one-lung anesthesia using an endobronchial blocker. J Thorac Cardiovasc Surg. 1981;82:542–6.
55. Otruba Z, Oxorn D. Lobar bronchial blockade in bronchopleural fistula. Can J Anaesth. 1992;39:176–8.
56. Rajan GRC. An improved technique of placing a coaxial endobronchial blocker for one-lung ventilation. Anesthesiology. 2000;93:1563–4.
57. Collins SR, Titus BJ, Campos JH, et al. Lung isolation in the patient with a difficult airway. Anesth Analg. 2018;126:1968.
58. Campos JH, Kernstine KH. Use of the wire-guided endobronchial blocker for one-lung anesthesia in patients with airway abnormalities. J Cardiothorac Vasc Anesth. 2003;17:352.
59. Bellver J, García-Aguado R, De Andrés J, et al. Selective bronchial intubation with the univent system in patients with a tracheostomy. Anesthesiology. 1993;79:1453.
60. Dhamee MS. One-lung ventilation in a patient with a fresh tracheostomy using the tracheostomy tube and a Univent endobronchial blocker. J Cardiothorac Vasc Anesth. 1997;11:124.
61. Tobias JD. Variations on one-lung ventilation. J Clin Anesth. 2001;13:35.
62. Robinson AR 3rd, Gravenstein N, Alomar-Melero E, et al. Lung isolation using a laryngeal mask airway and a bronchial blocker in a patient with a recent tracheostomy. J Cardiothorac Vasc Anesth. 2008;22:883.
63. Coe VL, Brodsky JB, Mark JB. Double-lumen endobronchial tubes for patients with tracheostomies. Anesth Analg. 1984;63:882.
64. Brodsky JB, Tobler HG, Mark JB. A double-lumen endobronchial tube for tracheostomies. Anesthesiology. 1991;74:387.
65. Campos JH. Lung isolation techniques for patients with difficult airway. Curr Opin Anaesthesiol. 2010;23:12.
66. Patane PS, Sell BA, Mahla ME. Awake fiberoptic endobronchial intubation. J Cardiothorac Anesth. 1990;4:229.

67. Angie Ho CY, Chen CY, Yang MW, et al. Use of the Arndt wire-guided endobronchial blocker via nasal for one-lung ventilation in patient with anticipated restricted mouth opening for esophagectomy. Eur J Cardiothorac Surg. 2005;28:174.
68. Chen A, Lai HY, Lin PC, et al. GlideScope-assisted double-lumen endobronchial tube placement in a patient with an unanticipated difficult airway. J Cardiothorac Vasc Anesth. 2008;22:170.
69. Hernandez AA, Wong DH. Using a Glidescope for intubation with a double lumen endotracheal tube. Can J Anaesth. 2005;52:658.
70. Liu TT, Li L, Wan L, et al. Videolaryngoscopy vs. Macintosh laryngoscopy for double-lumen tube intubation in thoracic surgery: a systematic review and meta-analysis. Anaesthesia. 2018;73:997.
71. Satya-Krishna R, Popat M. Insertion of the double lumen tube in the difficult airway. Anaesthesia. 2006;61:896.
72. Slinger PD, Lesiuk L. Flow resistances of disposable double-lumen, single-lumen, and Univent tubes. J Cardiothorac Vasc Anesth. 1998;12:142.
73. Oh AY, Kwon WK, Kim KO, et al. Single-lung ventilation with a cuffed endotracheal tube in a child with a left mainstem bronchus disruption. Anesth Analg. 2003;96:696–7.
74. Hammer GB. Single-lung ventilation in infants and children. Paediatr Anaesth. 2004;14:98–102.
75. Baraka A. Right bevelled tube for selective left bronchial intubation in a child undergoing right thoracotomy. Pediatr Anaesth. 1996;6:487–9.
76. Heidegger T, Heim C. Esophageal detector device: not always reliable (letter). Ann Emerg Med. 1996;28:582.
77. Han JI. One lung anesthesia. Korean J Anesthesiol. 2005;48:449–58.
78. Kumar A, Pappu A, Sharma S, et al. Indigenous continuous positive airway pressure device for mitigation of hypoxemia during one lung ventilation. Anesth Analg. 2016;123(6):1636.
79. Latto IP, Stacey M, Mecklenburgh J, et al. Survey of the use of the gum elastic bougie in clinical practice. Anaesthesia. 2002;57:379–84.
80. Higgs A, Clark E, Premraj K. Low-skill fibreoptic intubation: use of the Aintree catheter with the classic LMA. Anaesthesia. 2005;60:915–20.
81. Vlachtsis H, Veltman M. Shearing of a Frova intubating introducer by a Bronchocath double lumen tube. Anaesthesia. 2006;61:197–8.
82. Lin W, Li H, Liu W, et al. A randomized trial comparing the CEL-100 videolaryngoscope (TM) with the Macintosh laryngoscope blade for insertion of double-lumen tubes. Anaesthesia. 2012;67:771–6.
83. Shah SB, Bhargava AK, Hariharan U, et al. A randomized clinical trial comparing the standard Mcintosh laryngoscope and the c-mac d blade video laryngoscope™ for double lumen tube insertion for one lung ventilation in Onco surgical patients. Indian J Anaesth. 2016;60:312–8.
84. Ueshima H, Kitamura A. Combination of Parker flex-IT™ Stylet and McGRATH MAC for effective double lumen tube intubation. Saudi J Anaesth. 2014;8:574.
85. Hirabayashi Y, Seo N. The Airtraq laryngoscope for placement of double-lumen endobronchial tube. Can J Anaesth. 2007;54:955–7.
86. Poon KH, Liu EH. The airway scope for difficult double-lumen tube intubation. J Clin Anesth. 2008;20:319.
87. Suzuki A, Kunisawa T, Iwasaki H. Double lumen tube placement with the Pentax-airway scope. Can J Anaesth. 2007;54:853–4.
88. Lewis JW Jr, Serwin JP, Gabriel FS, et al. The utility of a double-lumen tube for one-lung ventilation in a variety of noncardiac thoracic surgical procedures. J Cardiothorac Vasc Anesth. 1992;6:705–10.

Preoperative Assessment of Thoracic Surgery Patient

Jayashree Sood and Nitin Sethi

6.1 Introduction

The goals of preoperative assessment of a patient presenting for thoracic surgery are primarily to identify patients at high risk for developing perioperative morbidity and secondarily to institute appropriate management protocols to reduce the risk.

The underlying etiology for thoracic disease can be divided into two broad categories: infections and cancers. Infective etiology is commonly seen in the south Asian population with tuberculosis being the most common infection [1]. Lung infection can manifest as empyema, lung abscess, and bronchiectasis [2]. Thoracic cancers can either involve the mediastinum (thymomas, lymphomas) or the lung parenchyma (primary or metastatic) [3, 4]. A few percentage of patients may also present with noninfective and nonmalignant lung lesions such as bullous lung disease [5] and cysts [6].

An important point to remember during preoperative evaluation is that cancer surgeries are never completely elective and unnecessarily delaying cancer surgery pending certain investigations carries the risk of inadvertent tumor progression [7]. Even after appropriate preoperative optimization there will be certain patients with compromised lung function. Such patients may be candidates for limited lung resection surgeries [8]. The most common cause of postoperative morbidity after thoracic surgery is either respiratory (atelectasis, pneumonia, and respiratory failure) occurring in 15–20% of patients [9] or cardiovascular (arrhythmias, ischemia) occurring in 10–15% of patients [10].

6.2 Preoperative Evaluation

Preoperative evaluation primarily focuses on evaluation of two major organ systems: respiratory and cardiovascular.

6.2.1 Respiratory System

6.2.1.1 Clinical History
Eliciting a good clinical history is the initial step in arriving at a diagnosis. The symptoms of respiratory ailments can be categorized as in the following subsections.

Bronchopulmonary Symptoms
Bronchopulmonary symptoms occur due to the involvement of lung parenchyma resulting in cough, sputum, dyspnea, and wheezing. Cough is the most common presenting symptom. In areas which are endemic for tuberculosis, any patient with history of cough lasting for more than 3

J. Sood (✉) · N. Sethi
Institute of Anaesthesiology, Pain and Perioperative Medicine, Sir Ganga Ram Hospital, New Delhi, India

© Springer Nature Singapore Pte Ltd. 2020
J. Sood, S. Sharma (eds.), *Clinical Thoracic Anesthesia*,
https://doi.org/10.1007/978-981-15-0746-5_6

weeks, associated with low grade fever, malaise, and weight loss should raise the suspicion of tuberculosis. Cough, along with purulent sputum, indicates presence of underlying infection. Production of copious amount of sputum along with hemoptysis and cough is suggestive of bronchiectasis. Chronic smokers usually present with chronic dry cough initially, but may be associated with sputum production later. Presence of hemoptysis along with cough or failure of change in quality and quantity of sputum despite antibiotic therapy in chronic smokers raises a high suspicion of lung carcinoma [11, 12]. The presence of dyspnea indicates diminished respiratory reserve due to impaired lung parenchyma function. Wheezing occurs mainly due to the presence of air flow limitation in the small airways of the lung [13].

Chest pain can occur due to the presence of pleural effusion secondary to infection mainly tuberculosis or progression of lung tumor into the pleura. The pain can be mild, dull aching in nature or can be pleuritic which worsens on coughing and breathing [14].

Extrapulmonary Intrathoracic Symptoms
These symptoms occur due to the invasion of the tumor to the surrounding structures such as the pleura, chest wall (pain), superior vena cava (SVC syndrome), pericardium (pericarditis), brachial plexus, and recurrent laryngeal nerve (hoarseness) [15].

Extra-thoracic Metastatic Symptoms
These symptoms result from the metastases of the tumor cells outside the thoracic cavity. Lung tumor metastasis can occur to the following organs: brain, skeleton, liver, adrenals, gastrointestinal tract, kidneys, and pancreas [15].

Extra-thoracic Nonmetastatic Symptoms
Extra-thoracic nonmetastatic symptoms or paraneoplastic syndrome is due to the secretion of endocrine- or endocrine-like substances by the tumor cells. These commonly include Cushing's syndrome, carcinoid syndrome, excessive antidiuretic hormone secretion, hypocalcemia and myopathy (Eaton–Lambert Syndrome) [16].

Nonspecific Symptoms
Patient with chronic infective lung pathology or tumor may also manifest with weight loss, anorexia, malaise, and lethargy. They may be severely nutritionally depleted leading to muscle wasting subsequently resulting in wasting of the respiratory muscles [16].

In patients with lung carcinoma, a detailed history of chemotherapy should also be obtained due to their systemic side effects (bleomycin, mitomycin: pulmonary toxicity; doxorubicin: cardiac toxicity; cisplatin: renal toxicity) [17].

6.2.1.2 Investigations
Investigations required for patients undergoing thoracic surgery can be categorized as:

1. Laboratory
2. Radiology
3. Pulmonary function assessment

Laboratory Investigations
Those essential for a patient undergoing thoracic surgery include complete blood count, renal and liver function tests, Gram stain, sputum cytology, and sputum/blood cultures (Table 6.1) [18].

Radiology Investigations
Preoperative assessment of X-ray chest and CT scan is essential for qualitative evaluation of pulmonary or extrapulmonary lesions and detection of any airway compromise. A large pleural

Table 6.1 Laboratory investigation

Investigation	Significance
Complete blood count	Polycythemia: Seen in smokers indicates hemoglobin desaturation Leucocytosis: presence of underlying infection
Gram stain	Indicates types of infective microorganisms
Sputum cytology	Aids in diagnosis of cancer
Sputum and blood	Isolation of causative microorganism and determination of antibiotic sensitivity
Liver function tests	Deranged in patient on antitubercular drugs and in tumor metastasis
Renal function test	Indicated in elderly patients and in tumor metastasis

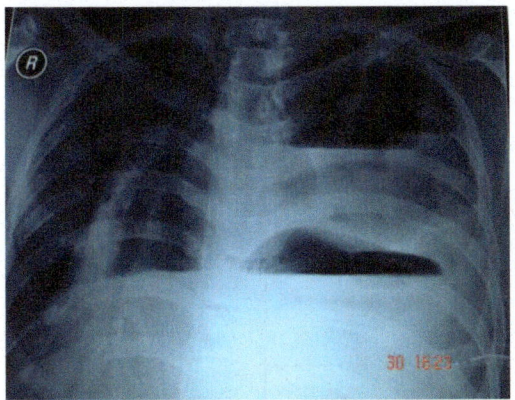

Fig. 6.1 Left-sided hydropneumothorax causing right-sided tracheal deviation

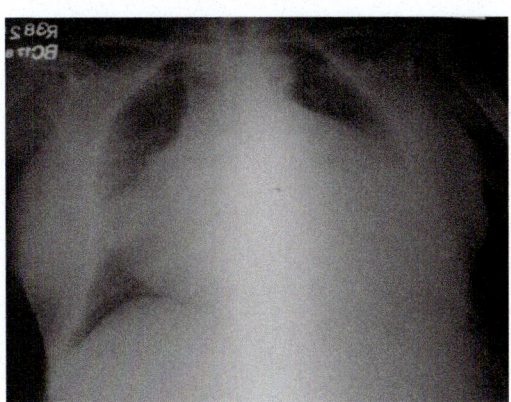

Fig. 6.2 Large anterior mediastinal mass

effusion can lead to deviation of mediastinum including the trachea to the opposite side (Fig. 6.1). Mediastinal masses such as thymomas can result in direct tracheal compression (Fig. 6.2). Lung parenchymal tumors can cause compression of the distal bronchus. Endobronchial tumors can result in obstruction of bronchial lumen which can make placement of double lumen tubes difficult. All cancer patients should undergo a repeat radiological evaluation prior to surgery if there has been a delay of several weeks between the initial evaluation and planned surgery, because tumors can grow in the intervening period resulting in airway compression which may not have been evident earlier. A thorough radiological evaluation done preoperatively helps the anesthesiologist in formulating an airway management protocol prior to anesthesia induction [19].

Pulmonary Function Assessment

Pulmonary function assessment evaluates three aspects of lung function: respiratory mechanics: the process of inhaling oxygen and exhaling carbon dioxide; lung parenchyma function: the process involving gas exchange (oxygen and carbon dioxide) across the alveolar–capillary membrane; and cardiopulmonary function: the process of carrying oxygen from lungs to the tissues and carbon dioxide from tissues to the lungs [20].

Respiratory Mechanics

The important determinants of lung mechanical function are the assessment of various lung volumes using spirometry (Fig. 6.3). Lung volumes routinely measured for patients undergoing thoracic surgery are forced expiratory volume in the 1st second (FEV_1), forced vital capacity (FVC), maximal voluntary ventilation (MVV), and residual volume/total lung capacity ratio (RV/TLC) [21].

Predicted postoperative FEV1% (Ppo FEV1 %) is a validated test for predicting postoperative respiratory complications in patients undergoing lung resection. Its calculation is based on the % of functional lung tissue removed. The whole lung is divided into 42 subsegments; 22 subsegments are in the right lung (6 segments in the upper lobe, 4 in the middle lobe, and 12 in the lower lobe) and 20 subsegments are in the left lung (10 in the upper lobe and 10 in the lower lobe) [22].

$$\text{Ppo FEV}_1\% = \text{preoperative FEV}_1\% \times \left(1 - \%\text{functional lung tissue removed}/100\right)$$

If a patient is planned for left upper lobectomy, then the % functional lung tissue removal will be 23.8% (10/42 × 100). Assuming a preoperative FEV_1 of 60%, the Ppo FEV_1% will be 45.7%.

Another formula for determining PpoFEV_1% is based on the quantitative radionuclide perfusion scar, wherein the fraction of total perfusion for the resected lung is measured [23].

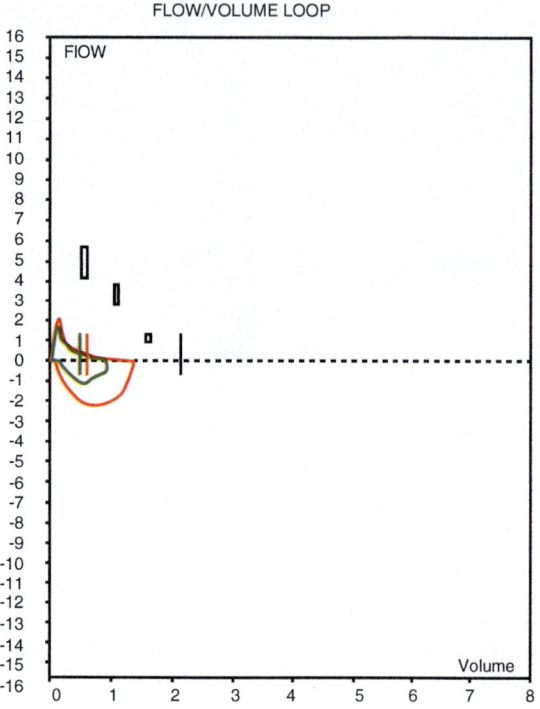

DYNAMIC LUNG VOLUMES & FLOW RATES

		PRE		POST		
	PREDICTED	OBSERVED	% PRED	OBSERVED	% PRED	% CHANGE
FVC(L)	2.15	0.94	44	1.37	63	46
FEV1(L)	1.78	0.54	30	0.63	35	16
FEV 3s(L)	----	0.80	----	0.98	----	23
FEV1/FVC(%)	76.83	57.55	75	45.82	60	-20
PEF(L/S)	5.29	1.73	33	2.14	40	24
MEF(L/S)	2.66	0.30	11	0.23	9	-22
MEF75(L/S)	4.88	0.83	17	0.67	14	-19
MEF50(L/S)	3.27	0.35	11	0.27	8	-23
MEF25(L/S)	1.11	0.13	11	0.11	10	-13
FVC ins(L)	----	0.80	----	1.29	----	62
PIF(L/S)	----	1.14	----	2.18	----	92
FI50(L/S)	----	1.14	----	2.16	----	90
Texp(Sec)	----	4.69	----	9.83	----	110

Fig. 6.3 Spirometry

$$PpoFEV_1\% = \text{preoperative } FEV_1 \times (1 - \text{fraction of total fraction for the resected lung})$$

The risk of developing a postoperative complication increases if the Ppo $FEV_1 < 40\%$, in the elderly population the risk is found to increase if the Ppo $FEV_1 < 45\%$ [24].

A better predictor of postoperative complication is the actual postoperative FEV_1, because it takes around 6 months for the postoperative FEV_1 values to reach the levels as determined by Ppo

FEV_1. However, the actual postoperative FEV_1 cannot be determined preoperatively, therefore the reliance on PpoFEV$_1$ [25].

Patients with Ppo $FEV_1 < 40\%$, who are at an increased risk of developing postoperative complication should undergo a thorough assessment of pulmonary function, i.e., assessment of lung volumes and airway resistance in a pulmonary function laboratory using whole-body plethysmography [20].

Pulmonary Parenchymal Function

The preliminary assessment of pulmonary parenchymal function is done by arterial blood gas analysis. Room air $PaO_2 < 60$ mmHg and a $PaCO_2 > 45$ mmHg are indicators of risk of developing postoperative complications.

A more precise assessment of the lung parenchymal function is the determination of diffusion capacity for carbon monoxide (DLCO), an indicator of total functional surface area of the alveolar capillary interface. Like Ppo FEV_1, Ppo DLCO can also be determined using the similar calculation. A Ppo DLCO < 40% correlates with increased risk of developing respiratory and cardiac complications postoperatively [23].

The two most valid preoperative tests for predicting perioperative risk are Ppo FEV_1 and Ppo DLCO.

Cardiopulmonary Function

Cardiopulmonary function assessment is carried out in cardiopulmonary function exercise test (CPET) laboratory wherein a patient is made to exercise in a bicycle ergometer or treadmill. The most important parameter assessed in a CPET laboratory is the maximal oxygen consumption (VO_2 max), considered to be a relevant predictor of outcome post thoracic surgery. Patients with VO_2 max < 15 ml/kg/min are at increased risk of developing postoperative morbidity [26]. CPET is quite expensive and is not routinely available at all centers, especially in the developing nations. Various surrogate tests for assessment of cardiopulmonary function have been developed which can be easily performed in the preoperative period. These include stair climbing test, 6-min walk test and the shuttle-walk test.

Stair Climbing Test (SCT)

Patients ability to climb three flights of stairs (12–14 m) is considered an acceptable risk for lobectomy (FEV1 > 1.7 l; VO_2 max: 12 ml/kg/min), whereas an ability to climb five flights of stair (22 m) is considered an acceptable risk for pneumonectomy (FEV1 > 2 l; VO_2 max > 20 ml/kg/min) [27].

6-Minute Walk Test

Patients are asked to walk as far as possible in 6 min along a flat corridor. Ability to walk 2000 ft correlates with VO_2 max 15 ml/kg/min. VO_2 max can also be determined using the formula VO_2 max = distance in meter/30 [28].

Shuttle-Walk Test (SWT)

Patients are asked to walk back and forth between two markers kept 10 m apart. The walking speed is increased each minute in a graded pattern as per protocol. Ability to complete 25 shuttles without interruption correlates with a VO_2 max > 15/ml/kg/min [29].

Patients who develop > 4% desaturation during exercise testing are at increased risk of developing complications [23].

Further refinement in assessment of pulmonary function post lung resection is the use of regional lung function tests using imaging diagnostics. The commonly used imaging modalities for assessment of regional lung function are:

1. *Radionuclide V/Q lung scan*: This test is the gold standard for assessment of ventilation perfusion abnormalities. Regional ventilation is estimated by scanning with radio labelled xenon-133 whereas for regional perfusion technetium -99m macroaggregated albumin is used. This test is more precise for determining postoperative lung function after pneumonectomy as compared to lobectomy [30].
2. *Pulmonary Quantitative CT-scanning:* This test quantifies areas of ventilation as normal parenchyma, atelectasis, and emphysema. It is a more precise determinant of post lobectomy lung function in comparison to post pneumonectomy lung function [31].

3. *Three-dimensional dynamic perfusion MRI:* It is used for assessment of regional pulmonary blood flow and exhibits good correlation with postoperative FEV_1 values [32].

The suitability for pulmonary resection can be summarized as per the American College of Chest Physicians (ACCP) evidence-based clinical practice guidelines (Fig. 6.4) [33].

For patients with low or absent cardiac risk factors, the Ppo FEV_1 % and Ppo DLCO % is determined. If the Ppo FEV_1 and Ppo VLCO are > 60% then the patients are categorized as low risk (mortality < 1%). If the Ppo FEV_1 and Ppo DLCO are 30–60% then the patients are subjected to SCT or SWT. If the SCR distance is > 22 m or the SWT distance is > 400 m, then the patients are at low risk for developing complications post surgery. However, if the distance covered in SCT or SMT is less than the prescribed limit then the patients are subjected to CPET. CPET is also done in patients with Ppo FEV_1 or Ppo DLCO < 30%. CPET results are interpreted as follows: low risk (mortality <1%) if VO_2 Max > 20 ml/kg/min, moderate risk (morbidity/mortality risk 1–10%) if VO_2 Max 10–20 ml/kg/min, and high risk (morbidity/mortality risk > 10%) if VO_2 Max < 10 ml/kg/min.

6.2.2 Cardiovascular System Evaluation

Patients undergoing pulmonary resection are at an intermediate risk of developing postoperative cardiac complications such as myocardial infarction, arrhythmias, and cardiac arrest, having an incidence of 2–3% [33]. Many of the patients undergoing thoracic surgery have history of smoking and advanced age putting them at risk of developing coronary artery disease (CAD) and LV dysfunction. The presence of underlying long standing COPD can lead to pulmonary hypertension resulting in chronic cor pulmonale. Patients with elevated pulmonary vascular resistance (PVR) cannot accommodate increased pulmonary blood flow post lung resection or pneumonectomy due to the non-distensible vasculature resulting in post lung resection pulmonary edema [34]. Patients with history of CAD, long standing hypoxemia and or ECG changes suggestive of pulmonary hypertension/right heart enlargement (right axis deviation, ↑R, ↑S wave in V2-V6, ↓T wave, ↓ST in V2-V6, V2-V6, ↑P in II, III) or coronary ischemia (Q waves, left bundle branch block, diaphasic P wave in V1, ↑ST, ↓ST, ↓T, U wave) should undergo a baseline echocardiogra-

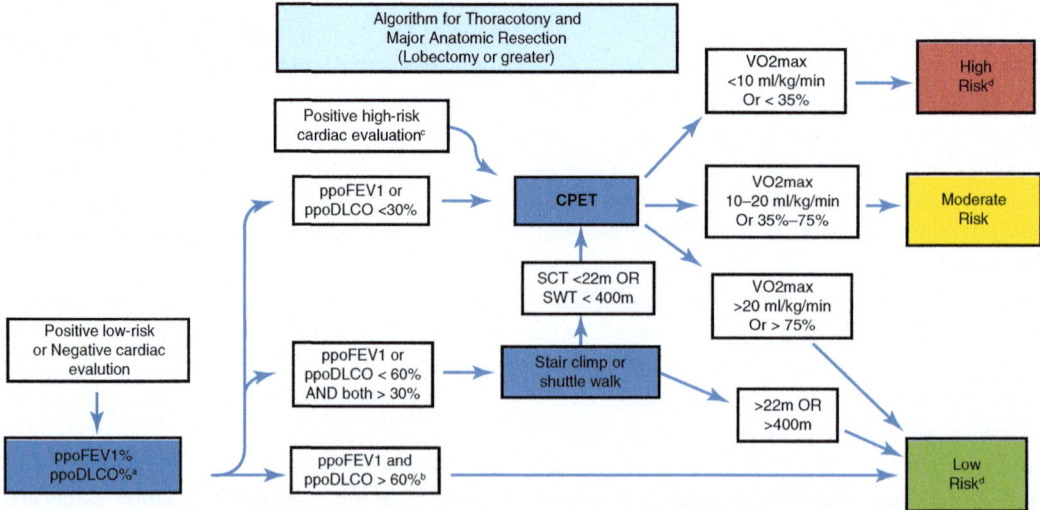

Fig. 6.4 Physiologic evaluation resection algorithm. Reproduced with permission from Elsevier Inc., License Number: 4460121260316. License date: Nov 01, 2018. From: Brunelli A, et al. Physiologic evaluation of the patient with lung cancer being considered for resectional surgery: Diagnosis and management of lung cancer, 3rd ed: American College of Chest Physicians evidence-based clinical practice guidelines. Chest 2013;143:e166S-e190S

phy followed by noninvasive exercise testing which includes exercise ECG and thallium scan (Fig. 6.5). Patients with normal exercise ECG can proceed for surgery; however, if it is suggestive of ischemia then thallium exercise test should be done. If thallium exercise test is normal then the thoracic surgery can be performed; if however; it is positive for ischemia then a coronary angiography should be planned [35]. An alternative to thallium exercise test is the stress transthoracic echocardiography (dipyridamole or dobutamine). If coronary angiography is indicative of significant CAD then a coronary artery bypass grafting may be required prior to or at time of thoracic surgery. If the patient undergoes CABG or coronary stenting prior to thoracic surgery then a delay of at least 6 weeks is needed before the thoracic surgical procedure can be performed [36]. If the patient in need of CABG requires a limited pulmonary resection for the control of tumor then both the procedures can be performed simultaneously. The lung resection should be performed after CABG during a combined procedure after ensuring adequate myocardial function and hemostasis [37].

Another way of cardiovascular risk assessment in patients undergoing thoracic surgery is by applying the thoracic revised cardiac risk index (ThRCRI) (Fig. 6.6) [38]. In ThRCRI, 1.5 points each are given for patients undergoing pneumonectomy, history of previous ischemic heart disease, history of previous stroke or

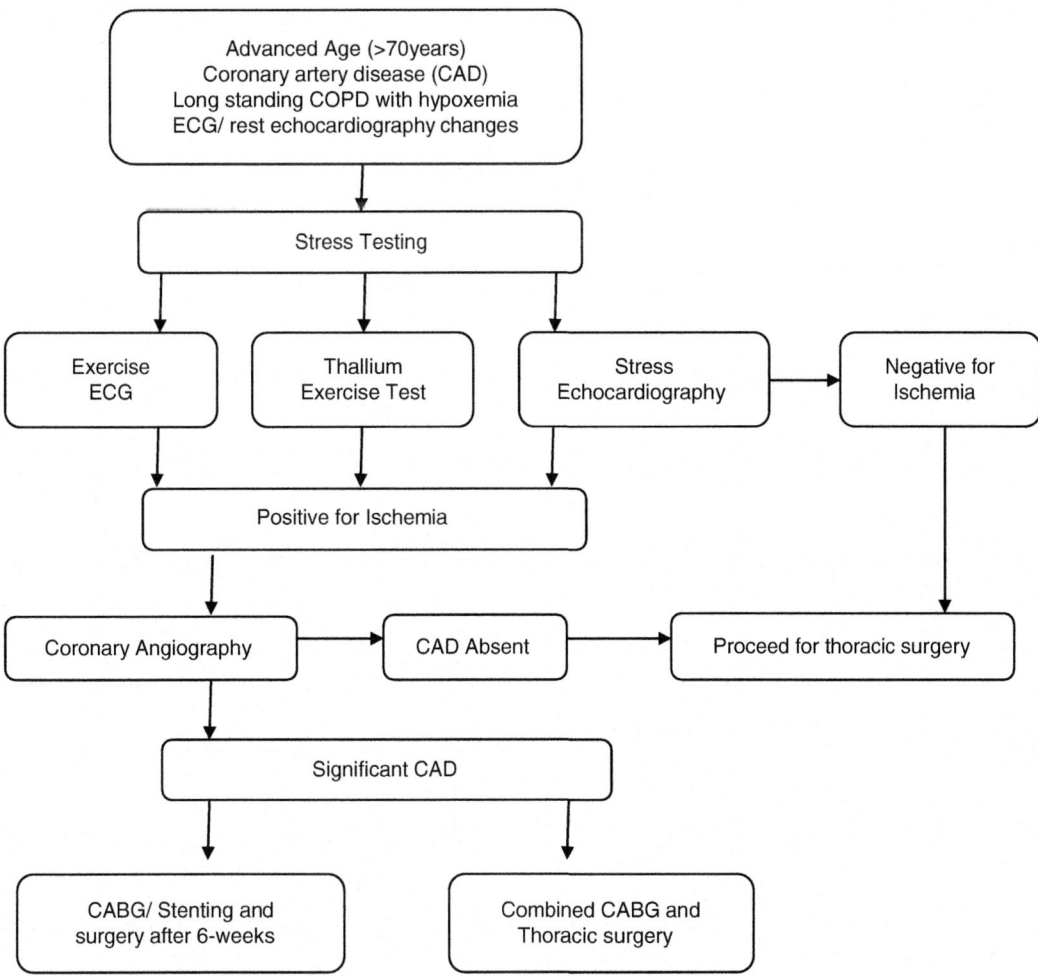

Fig. 6.5 Preoperative cardiovascular function evaluation

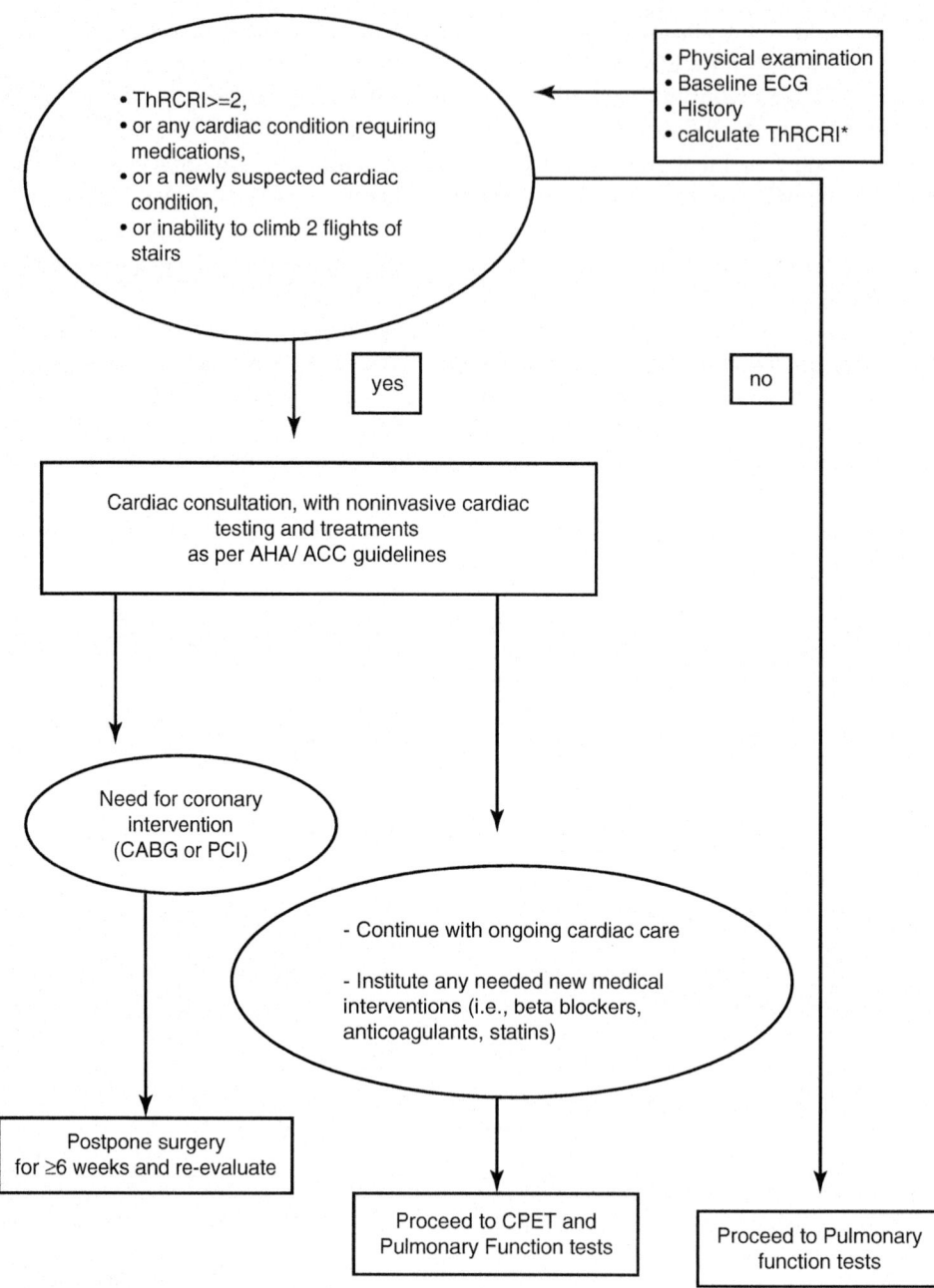

*ThRCRI *(Thoracic revised Cardioc Risk Index).*
- Pnemonectomy: 1.5 points
- Previous ischemic heat disease: 1.5 points
- Previous stroke or TIA: 1.5 points
- Creatinine > 2mg/dl: 1 point

Fig. 6.6 Thoracic revised cardiac risk index (ThRCRI). Reproduced with permission from Elsevier Inc., License Number: 4460121260316. License date: Nov 01, 2018. From: Brunelli A, et al. Physiologic evaluation of the patient with lung cancer being considered for resectional surgery: Diagnosis and management of lung cancer, 3rd ed: American College of Chest Physicians evidence-based clinical practice guidelines. Chest 2013;143:e166S-e190S

transient ischemic attack and 1 point is given for serum creatinine value >2 mg/dl. If the patient has ThRCRI score >2, or any one of the following: any cardiac ailment requiring treatment, a newly diagnosed cardiac condition and inability to climb at least 2 flight of stairs then a thorough cardiac work-up as per the American Heart Association/American College of Cardiologists Guidelines is essential [39].

Perioperative/postoperative atrial fibrillation and flutter (POAF) is one of the most common dysrhythmia occurring in patients undergoing thoracic surgery, especially pulmonary resection and esophageal surgery with an incidence of 13–26% [40]. POAF can result in ventricular dysfunction and sustained hemodynamic instability. Risk of POAF can be categorized from low risk to high risk as per the surgical procedure being performed. Low risk procedures (<5% incidence) include decortication, tracheal stenting, mediastinoscopy, thoracoscopy, wedge resection; intermediate risk procedures (5–15% incidence) include segmentectomy, thoracoscopic sympathectomy; and high risk procedures (>15% incidence) include anterior mediastinal mass resection, open or thoracoscopic lobectomy, tracheal resection and reconstruction, esophagectomy, and lung transplantation [40]. Apart from the surgical risk factors there are various patient-related risk factors for POAF which include history of hypertension, coronary artery disease, obesity, smoking, advanced age, genetic abnormalities, and male sex [41].

Apart from assessment of the respiratory and cardiovascular systems, evaluation of renal parameters is also essential. Patient having a serum creatinine >2 mg/dl or those undergoing hemodialysis may have a prolonged postoperative stay [20].

6.2.3 Airway Evaluation

Patients with previous history of radiotherapy, infection, pulmonary or airway surgery may have a difficult endobronchial intubation. Prior to surgery recent bronchoscopy, X-ray, and CT scan reports should be reviewed to rule out any recent changes in the airway anatomy in comparison to baseline evaluation, as tumors may progressively increase in size and cause airway distortion if there is a significant time lag between initial evaluation and surgery [20].

6.3 Preoperative Preparation

6.3.1 Respiratory System

Patients undergoing thoracic surgery are prone to develop various complications such as atelectasis, bronchospasm, respiratory tract infection, and pulmonary edema. Preoperative pulmonary rehabilitation therapy can help prevent these complications. The most commonly followed rehabilitation therapy is the "five-pronged" regimen [34]. The components of the "five-pronged" regimen are explained below.

6.3.1.1 Cessation of Smoking
Cessation of smoking preoperatively results in a significant reduction in postoperative respiratory morbidity. Benefits of smoking cessation are best accrued if it is stopped for more than 4–8 weeks as it results in improvement in ciliary action, macrophage activity, diminished sputum production, and an overall reduction in postoperative respiratory complications. Even a short duration of cessation up to 12–48 h results in reduction in carboxyhemoglobin levels [42].

6.3.1.2 Bronchodilator Therapy
Patients with COPD, asthma, or history of smoking are prone to have hyperreactive airways resulting in bronchospasm. These patients benefit from preoperative bronchodilator therapy. Drugs used for bronchodilator therapy include sympathomimetics, methylxanthines, and steroids. Sympathomimetics include β_2-agonists such as salmeterol, albuterol, formoterol, and anticholinergics such as ipratropium given mainly via the inhalation route. These drugs increase adenylyl cyclase activity thereby increasing cyclic adenosine monophosphate (CAMP) levels, which relaxes the bronchial smooth muscle. Methylxanthines include theophylline and

aminophylline which increase CAMP levels by preventing its degradation by inhibiting the enzymatic activity of phosphodiesterase. Steroids are per se not bronchodilators but due to their anti-inflammatory action, they help in reducing mucosal edema and release of bronchoconstrictors. They can be administered by inhalation, oral, or intravenous route [43].

6.3.1.3 Loosening of Secretions

Persistent accumulation of secretions in the respiratory tract can result in atelectasis and pulmonary infection. Hydration of the respiratory tract helps in loosening and thinning of secretions which allows their easy removal. Jet humidification or an ultrasonic nebulizer generates water aerosols which are delivered into the respiratory tract by a mask in a spontaneously breathing patient and helps in effectively mobilizing the secretions. In addition, adequate oral or intravenous fluid intake should be there to maintain hydration [44].

Broad spectrum antibiotics should be prescribed to treat pulmonary infection. This will reduce the viscosity and volume of secretions.

6.3.1.4 Removal of Secretions

Various maneuvers such as postural drainage, coughing, chest physiotherapy, and forced expiratory technique (FET) help in effectively mobilizing the secretions. Chest physiotherapy, which involves percussion, and postural drainage help in moving the secretions from peripheral to the central airways, whereas coughing helps in clearing the secretions from the central airways. An effective alternative to coughing is the use of FET wherein forced expiration its initiated from 50% of the inspiratory reserve lung volume to residual volume [45].

6.3.1.5 Patient Motivation and Preoperative Stabilization

Last but not the least it is very important to educate the patient regarding the nature of surgery and postoperative management strategy which includes pain management and respiratory physiotherapy. In addition to psychological preparation, any preexisting comorbidities should be stabilized. Initiation of preoperative physical rehabilitation and ensuring adequate nutrition can result in an improvement in postoperative outcome [34].

6.3.2 Cardiovascular System

Due to the high incidence of POAF in patients undergoing thoracic surgery, prophylactic use of various drugs including antiarrythmics, β-blockers, magnesium, and statins have been evaluated for prevention of arrhythmias [40].

Beta blockers in patients undergoing thoracic surgery, should be continued and not be stopped. Prophylactic use of β-blockers in patients who previously are not on treatment with β-blockers is not recommended [46]. Patients with hypomagnesaemia should be administered intravenous magnesium to replete their body stores, as low magnesium levels are precursors for arrhythmias [40]. Currently there is no role of digoxin in prevention of POAF. In patients at intermediate to high risk for developing POAF intravenous amiodarone administered via infusion either during surgery or during the first 24–48 h after surgery has been shown to reduce the incidence of POAF [47]. Diltiazem given prophylactically in patients undergoing lobectomy or pneumonectomy has shown a reduction in the incidence of atrial fibrillation and supraventricular tachycardia [48].

6.4 Conclusion

A good preoperative evaluation and preparation of a patient scheduled for thoracic surgery is essential for a successful postoperative outcome. Clinical history and examination done meticulously are essential for a diagnosis to be made. Pulmonary function tests performed preoperatively help in assessing the risk of perioperative morbidity and mortality. A fine pronged strategy for preoperative optimization is recommended.

References

1. Chakraborty AK. Epidemiology of tuberculosis: current status in India. Indian J Med Res. 2004;120(4):248–76.
2. Yazbeck MF, Dahdel M, Kalra A, Browne AS, et al. Lung abscess: update on microbiology and management. Am J Ther. 2014;21(3):217–21.
3. Herbst RS, Heymach JV, Lippman SM. Lung cancer. N Engl J Med. 2008;359(13):1367–80.
4. Dubashi B, Cyriac S, Tenali SG. Clinicopathological analysis and outcome of primary mediastinal malignancies—A report of 91 cases from a single institute. Ann Thorac Med. 2009;4(3):140–2.
5. Tulay CM, Özsoy IE. Spontaneous pneumothorax recurrence and surgery. Indian J Surg. 2015;77(Suppl 2):463–5.
6. Trotman-Dickenson B. Cystic lung disease: achieving a radiologic diagnosis. Eur J Radiol. 2014;83(1):39–46.
7. Colice GL, Shafazand S, Griftin JP, et al. Physiologic evaluation of the patient with lung considered for resectional surgery. ACCP evidenced based clinical prochiegindelunes (2nd Edition). Chest 2017; 132:161S–775.
8. Burke JR, Duarte IG, Thourani VH, et al. Preoperative risk assessment for marginal patients requiring pulmonary resection. Ann Thorac Surg. 2003;76(5);1767–73.
9. Licker MJ, Widikker I, Robert J, et al. Operative mortality and respiratory complications after lung resection for cancer: impact of chronic obstructive pulmonary disease and time trends. Ann Thorac Surg. 2006;81(5):1830–7.
10. Wright CD, Gaissert HA, Grab JD, et al. Predictors of prolonged length of stay after lobectomy for lung cancer: a Society of Thoracic Surgeons General Thoracic Surgery Database risk-adjustment model. Ann Thorac Surg. 2008;85(6):1857–65.
11. Terasaki G, Paauw DS. Evaluation and treatment of chronic cough. Med Clin North Am. 2014;98(3):391–403.
12. Irwin RS, Baumann MH, Bolser DC, et al. Diagnosis and management of cough executive summary: ACCP evidence-based clinical practice guidelines. Chest. 2006;129(1 Suppl):1S–23S.
13. Rabe KF, Watz H. Chronic obstructive pulmonary disease. Lancet. 2017;389(10082):1931–40.
14. Lee RW, Hodgson LE, Jackson MB, et al. Problem based review: pleuritic chest pain. Acute Med. 2012;11(3):172–82.
15. Hammerschmidt S, Wirtz H. Lung cancer: current diagnosis and treatment. Dtsch Arztebl Int. 2009;106(49):809–18.
16. Walter FM, Rubin G, Bankhead C, et al. Symptoms and other factors associated with time to diagnosis and stage of lung cancer: a prospective cohort study. Br J Cancer. 2015;112(Suppl 1):S6–13.
17. Allan N, Siller C, Breen A. Anaesthetic implications of chemotherapy. Continuing education in anaesthesia. Crit Care Pain 2012; 12:52–6.
18. O'Neill F, Carter E, Pink N, et al. Routine preoperative tests for elective surgery: summary of updated NICE guidance. BMJ. 2016;354:i3292.
19. Whitten CR, Khan S, Munneke GJ, et al. A diagnostic approach to mediastinal abnormalities. Radiographics. 2007;27(3):657–71.
20. Slmger O, Darling G. Preanesthetic assessment to thoracic surgery. In: Slinger P, editor. Principles and practice of anesthesia for thoracic surgery. New York: Springer; 2011, p. 11–34.
21. Culver BH. Preoperative assessment of the thoracic surgery patient: pulmonary function testing. Semin Thorac Cardiovasc Surg. 2001;13(2):92–104.
22. British Thoracic Society; Society of Cardiothoracic Surgeons of Great Britain and Ireland Working Party. BTS guidelines: guidelines on the selection of patients with lung cancer for surgery. Thorax. 2001;56(2):89–108.
23. Colice GL, Shafazand S, Griffin JP, et al. American College of Chest Physicians. Physiologic evaluation of the patient with lung cancer being considered for resectional surgery: ACCP evidenced-based clinical practice guidelines (2nd edition). Chest. 2007;132(3 Suppl):161S–77S.
24. Win T, Jackson A, Sharples L, et al. Relationship between pulmonary function and lung cancer surgical outcome. Eur Respir J. 2005;25(4):594–9.
25. Brunelli A, Rocco G. Spirometry: predicting risk and outcome. Thorac Surg Clin. 2008;18(1):1–8.
26. Weisman IM. Cardiopulmonary exercise testing in the preoperative assessment for lung resection surgery. Semin Thorac Cardiovasc Surg. 2001;13(2):116–25.
27. Brunelli A, Al Refai M, Monteverde M, et al. Stair climbing test predicts cardiopulmonary complications after lung resection. Chest. 2002;121(4):1106–10.
28. ATS Committee on Proficiency Standards for Clinical Pulmonary Function Laboratories. ATS statement: guidelines for the six-minute walk test. Am J Respir Crit Care Med. 2002;166(1):111–7.
29. Win T, Jackson A, Groves AM, et al. Relationship of shuttle walk test and lung cancer surgical outcome. Eur J Cardiothorac Surg. 2004;26(6):1216–9.
30. Win T, Laroche CM, Groves AM, et al. Use of quantitative lung scintigraphy to predict postoperative pulmonary function in lung cancer patients undergoing lobectomy. Ann Thorac Surg. 2004;78(4):1215–8.
31. Wu MT, Pan HB, Chiang AA, et al. Prediction of postoperative lung function in patients with lung cancer: comparison of quantitative CT with perfusion scintigraphy. AJR Am J Roentgenol. 2002;178(3):667–72.
32. Ohno Y, Koyama H, Nogami M, et al. Postoperative lung function in lung cancer patients: comparative analysis of predictive capability of MRI, CT, and SPECT. AJR Am J Roentgenol. 2007;189(2):400–8.

33. Brunelli A, Kim AW, Berger KI, et al. Physiologic evaluation of the patient with lung cancer being considered for resectional surgery: Diagnosis and management of lung cancer, 3rd ed: American College of Chest Physicians evidence-based clinical practice guidelines. Chest. 2013;143(5 Suppl):e166S–90S.
34. Benumof Jl, Alfery DD. Anaesthesia for thoracic surgery. In: Miller RD, Cucbiara EF, Millar ED, et al. editors. Anaesthesia, 5th edn. Philadelphia, PA: Churchill Livingstone; 2000; p. 1665–752.
35. Peters RM. The role of limited resection in carcinoma of the lung. Am J Surg. 1982;143(6):706–10.
36. Daye J, Boatman D, Peters C, et al. Brilakis ES. Perioperative risk of patients undergoing noncardiac surgery after coronary artery bypass surgery. J Investig Med. 2008;56(6):878–81.
37. Prokakis C, Koletsis E, Apostolakis E, et al. Combined heart surgery and lung tumor resection. Med Sci Monit. 2008;14(3):CS17–21.
38. Brunelli A, Varela G, Salati M, et al. Recalibration of the revised cardiac risk index in lung resection candidates. Ann Thorac Surg. 2010;90(1):199–203.
39. Lee TH, Marcantonio ER, Mangione CM, et al. Derivation and prospective validation of a simple index for prediction of cardiac risk of major noncardiac surgery. Circulation. 1999;100(10):1043–9.
40. Frendl G, Sodickson AC, Chung MK, et al. American Association for Thoracic Surgery. 2014 AATS guidelines for the prevention and management of perioperative atrial fibrillation and flutter for thoracic surgical procedures. J Thorac Cardiovasc Surg. 2014;148(3):e153–93.
41. January CT, Wann LS, Alpert JS, et al. American College of Cardiology/American Heart Association Task Force on Practice Guidelines. 2014 AHA/ACC/HRS guideline for the management of patients with atrial fibrillation: a report of the American College of Cardiology/American Heart Association Task Force on Practice Guidelines and the Heart Rhythm Society. J Am Coll Cardiol. 2014;64(21):e1–76.
42. Lee SM, Landry J, Jones PM, et al. The effectiveness of a perioperative smoking cessation program: a randomized clinical trial. Anesth Analg. 2013;117(3):605–13.
43. Cazzola M, Page CP, Calzetta L, et al. Pharmacology and therapeutics of bronchodilators. Pharmacol Rev. 2012;64(3):450–504.
44. Chopra SK, Taplin GV, Simmons DH, et al. Effects of hydration and physical therapy on tracheal transport velocity. Am Rev Respir Dis. 1977;115(6):1009–14.
45. Varela G, Novoa NM, Agostini P, et al. Chest physiotherapy in lung resection patients: state of the art. Semin Thorac Cardiovasc Surg. 2011;23(4):297–306.
46. POISE Study Group, Devereaux PJ, Yang H, et al. Effects of extended-release metoprolol succinate in patients undergoing non-cardiac surgery (POISE trial): a randomised controlled trial. Lancet. 2008;371(9627):1839–47.
47. Riber LP, Christensen TD, Jensen HK, et al. Amiodarone significantly decreases atrial fibrillation in patients undergoing surgery for lung cancer. Ann Thorac Surg. 2012;94(2):339–44.
48. Amar D, Roistacher N, Burt ME, et al. Effects of diltiazem versus digoxin on dysrhythmias and cardiac function after pneumonectomy. Ann Thorac Surg. 1997;63(5):1374–81.

Patient Positioning in Thoracic Surgery

Bhuwan Chand Panday

7.1 Introduction

Positioning of a patient plays an important role in all surgical procedures. Good dissection and manipulation are possible only with adequate exposure of the surgical field. This in turn can be easily attained with appropriate adjustment of the operating table and use of accessories like a hand support. Various positions have been described for thoracic surgeries, but none of these positions are free of complications. The complications may vary from mild to life-threatening hemodynamic changes. The surgeon and anesthesiologist must be aware about the required body position for a specific type of surgery. Prior to final positioning, all the necessary precautions must be taken. Once the surgery has started, it is difficult to manipulate or change the patient position. Though most of the thoracic surgical procedures are conducted in the lateral position, some procedures are conducted in other positions as well. There are some universal precautions which must be practiced in all positions, e.g. eye care, padding of all bony prominences, avoidance of excessive abduction and extension of limbs, neck and spine. Prophylactic precautions for deep vein thrombosis is another important measure, which must be considered prior to the surgery. If needed, low molecular weight heparin may be administered prior to the surgical procedure. In addition to this, specific care is required for some specific positions. Various commonly used patient positions in thoracic surgery are described below.

Supine This position is the most commonly used position in general surgery, but unfortunately this is less commonly used in thoracic surgery. Abduction of arms produces pressure on the brachial plexus by the humerus. It becomes severe if the abduction is more than 90° and sustained for prolonged periods of time and so reducing abduction to less than 90° is recommended. It is mandatory to adequately support all the limbs and joints to avoid over-stretching related trauma. The forearm of the patient should preferably be kept in the supine position, because pronation may lead to pressure-dependent ulnar nerve lesion [1]. The eyelids should be taped to avoid exposure keratitis. There are only a few thoracic procedures conducted in supine position, e.g. thymectomy. A thick roll under the back is required to displace the thymus anteriorly (Fig. 7.1) for better exposure. The head is tilted to one side and the left upper limb is kept on a soft gel pad over the bean bag. Excessive turning of the head may lead to brachial plexus injury. Procedures with expected long duration are provided with adequate DVT prophylactic (Fig. 7.2) measures (e.g. DVT pump and safe use of perioperative low molecular weight heparin).

B. C. Panday (✉)
Institute of Anaesthesiology, Pain and Perioperative Medicine, Sir Ganga Ram Hospital, New Delhi, India

Semi-Fowler's position This is not a new position; it is a simple sitting position with some inclination at the back. This position is most commonly used in the ward/room where the patient is kept in a semi-sitting upright position (Fig. 7.3). The abdominal muscles are relaxed and oxygenation is better in this position. There are four types of Fowler's positions described, depending on the surgical need. Based on the angle of inclination, Fowler's positions are divided into four types, i.e. low, semi, standard and high. In thoracic surgery the semi-Fowler's is used; here the angle of inclination is 30–45° at the trunk. Surgeries which require diaphragm and abdominal structures to descend for better surgical exposure of thoracic structures are preferred to be done in this position. The Semi-Fowler's position is preferred over the lateral position, due to better exposure of the sympathetic chain and comfort of the surgeon [2]. In addition, this position is also beneficial in patients with acute respiratory distress syndrome (ARDS) in terms of improving oxygenation [3].

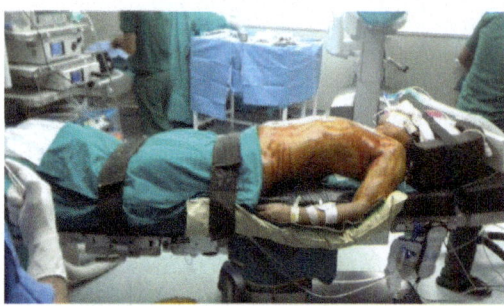

Fig. 7.1 Position for robotic thymectomy

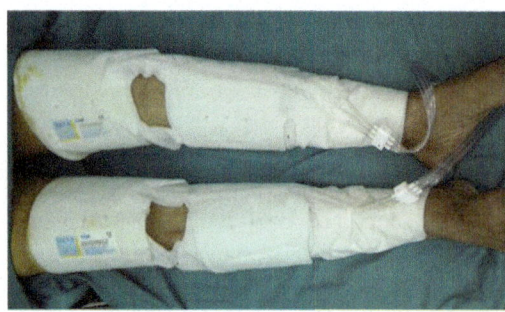

Fig. 7.2 DVT pump

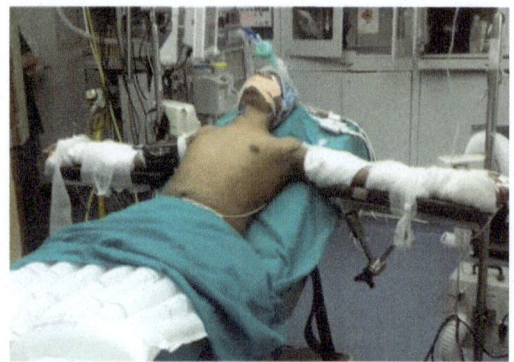

Fig. 7.3 Semi-Fowler's position

7.1.1 Lateral

This is one of the most commonly used positions in thoracic surgery. This position is associated with various changes in hemodynamics and position-related trauma. Since it shifts the mediastinum and abdominal viscera towards the dependent side, there will be ventilation–perfusion mismatch due to increase of blood flow and decrease of ventilation on the dependent side. Adequate knowledge of these changes and application of all precautionary measures could prevent the perturbations in physiology and position (Figs. 7.4 and 7.5) related trauma. The various preventive measures include: (a) adequate

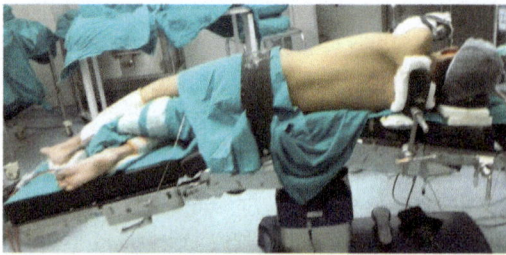

Fig. 7.4 Lateral position with adequate padding and strapping

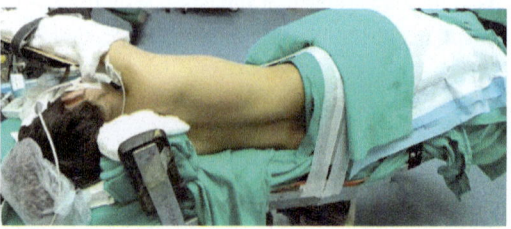

Fig. 7.5 Lateral position with lateral flexion of the spine

padding of all bony prominences (b) eye protection (c) optimum spine curvature with gentle handling during flexion and extension avoiding hyperextension in the upper limb to reduce stretching of nerves in the axillary area by keeping the axillary roll way from the arm pit to prevent brachial plexus injury. Even the peripheral nerves can be traumatized if the forearm is not kept properly [4]. Keeping the large bore intravenous line in the upper arm provides an easy access to administer drugs and fluid. Blood pressure measurement in the lower or dependent arm is advocated, though it may not provide accurate values. Displacement of the double lumen tube is not uncommon, but this can be averted with adequate fixation and assessment of the tube cuff position immediately after turning the patient to the lateral position. There are significant changes in various hemodynamic parameters as well (For details see Chap. 8).

7.1.2 Reverse Trendelenburg (rT) Position

This position is often used in thoracic surgical procedures (Fig. 7.6). Esophageal mobilization and esophagectomy is done preferably in this position. The surgeon mobilizes the esophagus from the left side and therefore one lung ventilation is required. Here the angle of inclination must be measured [5] and the surgeon informed in case of steep positioning. Oxygenation is improved due to better expansion of thoracic cavity and lungs as a result of the descent of abdominal contents. It has been shown that patient kept prone if given the rT position is beneficial in terms of reducing the intraocular pressure [6]. The rT position leads to stasis of venous blood in lower limbs with predisposition to deep vein thrombosis (DVT). Incidence of hypotension and venous air embolism is also common in this position. Adequate strapping and support will prevent slipping of the patient from the operating table. The beneficial effect of this position was studied in 70 patients who underwent angiography; these patients were given 30–45° head up position and reported less back pain with less vascular complications [7].

7.1.3 Prone

This position is less commonly used in thoracic surgery. A few decades ago surgeons preferred the prone position, especially in non-dry lung cases. Thoracotomy was regularly performed in prone and neck flexed positions [8]. Even in the present scenario, some surgeons prefer conducting esophageal mobilization in the prone rather than the supine position. It has also been noticed that this uncommon position results in decreased workload and procedure time and has better ergonomics than the supine decubitus position [9]. In another interesting study conducted in 58 patients, they compared the prone versus lateral position for esophagectomy and concluded that surgery in the prone position is less invasive and associated with less systemic inflammatory response and is safe for the patient [10]. But the prone position is not without complications, varying from minor haemodynamic changes to major cardiac events. There are some complications which are less troublesome and can be managed conservatively, e.g. pain in anterolateral thigh due to compression injury to the lateral femoral cutaneous nerve injury [11, 12]. While some may lead to permanent damage, e.g. postoperative vision loss due to increased orbital pressure [13] and nerve damage, pre-positioning preventive measures and proper planning may prevent these inadvertent position-related events.

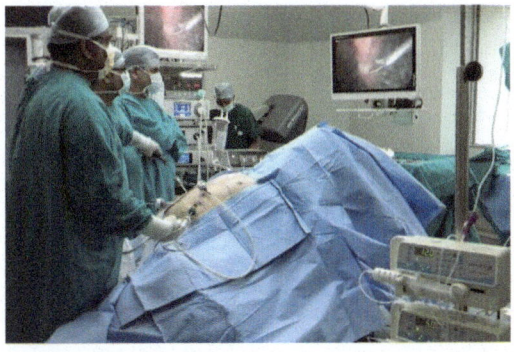

Fig. 7.6 VATS lobectomy in the reverse Trendelenburg position

7.1.4 Semi-prone

This is another less commonly used position in thoracic surgery. Esophagectomy, lobectomy and lymph node dissection are commonly done in the prone position [14–16]. A study conducted in this position reported that the surgeon was comfortable and conversion rate of VATS to open thoracotomy was less. Lifting of the upper arms of the patient is also not needed, there is less fatigue and better ergonomic conditions achieved [16].

7.2 Clinical Pearls

Appropriate positioning is essential not only for adequate surgical exposure but also greatly enhances the intraoperative comfort. Knowledge of various positions and their effect on physiology, combined with adequate preventive measures and agile response during emergent situations will lead to a smooth, and uneventful recovery.

References

1. Knight DJW, Mahajan RP. Patient positioning in anaesthesia. Continuing education in anaesthesia. Crit Care Pain. 2004;4:160–3.
2. Kuhajda I, Djuric D, Milos K, et al. Semi-Fowler vs. lateral decubitus position for thoracoscopic sympathectomy in treatment of primary focal hyperhidrosis. J Thorac Dis. 2015;7(Suppl 1):S5–S11.
3. Shah DS, Desai AR, Gohil N. A comparison of effect of semi fowler's vs side lying position on tidal volume & pulse oxymetry in ICU patients. Innovat J Med Health Sci. 2012;2:81–5.
4. Tuncali BE, Tuncali B, Kuvaki B, et al. Radial nerve injury after general anaesthesia in the lateral decubitus position. Anaesthesia. 2005;60(6):602–4.
5. Carey TW, Shaw KA, Weber ML, et al. Effect of the degree of reverse Trendelenburg position on intraocular pressure during prone spine surgery: a randomized controlled trial. Spine J. 2014;14(9):2118–26.
6. Kohli M, Panday BC, Sood J. Smart phones application for intraoperative patient care. Anesth Analg. 2017;124:1731–2.
7. Thangkratok P. The effect of reverse Trendelenburg position on back pain after cardiovascular angiography and interventions. BKK Med J. 2016;12:28–32.
8. Brown AI. Posture in thoracic surgery. Thorax. 1948;3(3):161–5.
9. Shen Y, Feng M, Tan L, et al. Thoracoscopic esophagectomy in prone versus decubitus position: ergonomic evaluation from a randomized and controlled study. Ann Thorac Surg. 2014;98(3):1072–8.
10. Kubo N, Ohira M, Yamashita Y, et al. Thoracoscopic esophagectomy in the prone position versus in the lateral position for patients with esophageal cancer: a comparison of short-term surgical results. Surg Laparosc Endosc Percutan Tech. 2014;24(2):158–63.
11. Juhl CS, Ballegaard M, Bestle MH, et al. Meralgia paresthetica after prone positioning ventilation in the intensive care unit. Case Rep Crit Care. 2016;2016:7263201.
12. Gupta A, Muzumdar D, Ramani PS. Meralgia paraesthetica following lumbar spine surgery: a study in 110 consecutive surgically treated cases. Neurol India. 2004;52(1):64–6.
13. Kumar N, Jivan S, Topping N, et al. Blindness and rectus muscle damage following spinal surgery. Am J Ophthalmol. 2004;138(5):889–91.
14. Lin J, Kang M, Chen C, et al. Thoracoscopic oesophageal mobilization during thoracolaparoscopy three-stage oesophagectomy: a comparison of lateral decubitus versus semiprone positions. Interact Cardiovasc Thorac Surg. 2013;17(5):829–34.
15. Lin Z, Xi J, Xu S, et al. Uniportal video-assisted thoracic surgery right mediastinal lymph node dissection in semiprone position. Asvide. 2015;2:170.
16. Lin Z, Xi J, Xu S, et al. Uniportal video-assisted thoracic surgery lobectomy in semiprone position: primary experience of 105 cases. J Thorac Dis. 2015;7(12):2389–95.

Monitoring in Thoracic Surgery

Bhuwan Chand Panday

8.1 Introduction

Monitoring is an integral part of our life, affecting it one way or the other; food, education, security and health. Even animals monitor the environment for their food and survival. Monitoring is so important that it affects almost all aspects of life, e.g. security, food, education, and health. Monitoring the patient is since antiquity. The ancient Indian surgical textbook 'Sushruta Samhita' described monitoring during pregnancy [1]. Monitoring of various parameters can guide the the health care worker regarding deviation from the normal path. Sensitive monitors can detect and warn even minimal changes in hemodynamics and other important parameters. Intervention at the initial stage can decrease morbidity and mortality. In the health care system, there has been a vast advancement in newer technology, various gadgets and tools of monitoring are evolving rapidly. Monitoring with recently developed devices has proved to be of utmost importance in improving the health care system.

B. C. Panday (✉)
Institute of Anaesthesiology, Pain and Perioperative Medicine, Sir Ganga Ram Hospital, New Delhi, India

8.2 Electrocardiogram

An electrocardiogram is amongst the basic parameters required for all procedures. These waveforms are encoded with wide range of information. An experienced or skillful physician can interpret different segments, wave morphology and arrhythmias, providing crucial information. In advanced monitoring systems, most of the calculations (ST elevation/depression, arrhythmias etc.) are done by computerized analysis and displayed on the monitor. Abnormal changes in ECG waveforms may be life threatening; these changes can be tall T waves, severe arrhythmias, heart blocks, ST depression/elevation etc. In addition, ST elevation with coving may also be present in cases of severe hyponatremia and mimics myocardial infarction [2]. Instant interpretation and quick intervention can surely convert an impending disaster to a fruitful outcome. They also warn you in case of any alarming change in the waveform.

Thoracic surgery requires great skill, where surgical manipulations are constantly being done. Vital organs are in close proximity to the surgical field; therefore, trauma to heart, lungs and diaphragm is not uncommon. During manipulation even the slight abnormal deviation may lead to major complications. Even a slight touch to the pericardium leads to instant changes in ECG morphology. Quick communication and agile response of surgeon (Fig. 8.1) and anesthesiologist decreases the morbidity. Abdominal manipulation close to the diaphragm may inadvertently produce a tear in the diaphragm which may lead to pneumothorax. This pneumothorax is instantly reflected in the ECG waveform. Right or left sided pneumothorax may reflect with different changes in these waves. Right sided pneumothorax is reflected as poor-R wave progression in V1–3 leads, q waves can be found in V4–6, II, III and aVF. Low QRS voltage and less commonly T wave inversion with right axis deviation is also detected [3]. There may also be some nonspecific changes in waveforms (Fig. 8.2). In case of left side pneumothorax, right axis deviation, decline in QRS amplitude and precordial T wave inversion are noted [4]. The electrocardiographic features are different from acute myocardial infarction as there is absence of significant Q waves and elevated ST-segment. Awareness about the occurrence of these ECG changes during left or right sided pneumothorax will help and guide the physician for the appropriate management.

Tension pneumothorax may also present with ECG changes similar to acute myocardial infarction [5]. A few studies have also tried to corelate hypovolemia with heart rate variation indices (based on ECG changes) [6] but further evaluation is required to establish a relationship.

8.3 Pulse Oximetry (Plethysmography)

Invention of plethysmography has revolutionized the monitoring of arterial oxygen saturation noninvasively. It instantly provides the real time percentage of arterial blood oxygen saturation. Though the probe is usually applied in the supine position, it is important to know that the value may differ when applied while sitting and standing. The best value of arterial oxygenation saturation reported is in the upright, sitting position [7]. Not only the patient position but the probe placement site (finger, ear lobe etc.) also affects the percentage saturation values, it has been noted that the best corelation with PaO_2 was found to be with finger plethysmography [8]. It has also been noted that even fingers have different SpO_2 values, and highest values were reported with middle finger and thumb [9].

Patient undergoing abdominal surgery close to the diaphragm may lead to inadvertent trauma to the diaphragm and sudden development of tension pneumothorax, which may be reflected in pulse oximeter. Instant interpretation and intervention could save the patient [10]. Patients with preexisting lung disease (carcinoma, bronchiectasis etc.) usually present with low SpO_2 values. Pleural effusion may also affect the arterial saturation. Interestingly, it has been noticed that a patient

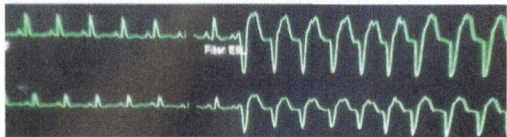

Fig. 8.1 Change in waveform during pericardium touch

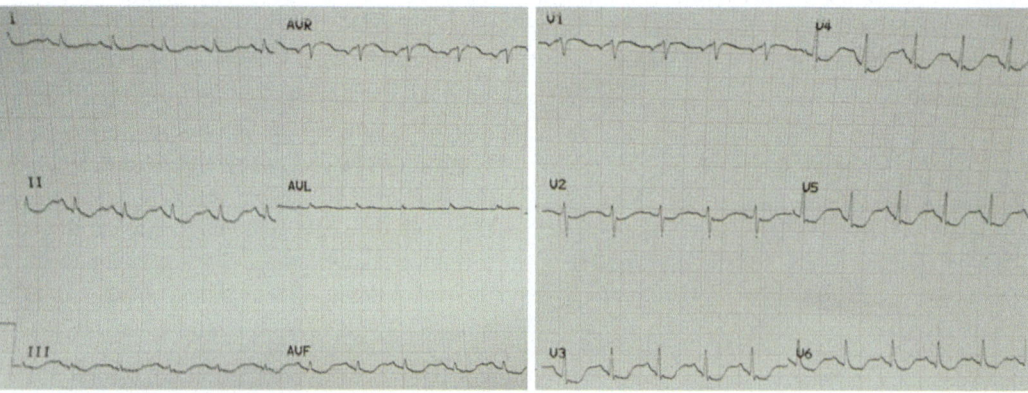

Fig. 8.2 Right sided pneumothorax

with a small unilateral pleural effusion, if kept in the lateral position with the effusion site dependent, produces decrease in arterial oxygen saturation. Contrary to this, if a large pleural effusion site is kept non-dependent in the lateral position, there is a decrease in the saturation level [11].

It would be prudent to have an adequate knowledge about the pulse oximeter's mechanism of working and the conditions where the numerical values or waveforms are not appropriate, e.g. intravascular dye, nail polish, methemoglobinemia, carbon-monoxide poisoning, motion artefact, cold peripheries, electrical interference and interference with ambient light.

8.3.1 Recent Advances in Pulse Oximetry

8.3.1.1 Oxygen Reserve Index (ORI)

Traditionally used plethysmograph is based on two wavelengths to detect the level of saturation but recently developed pulse co-oximetry using multiple wavelengths provides values which represent saturation in real time as well as oxygen reserve. Oxygen reserve index is a dimensionless index with a range of 0–1, reflecting a variation in PaO_2 (in the range of 100–200 mmHg) [12]. It provides early and impending information regarding decrease in oxygen status than the SpO_2 monitor [13]. Early warning of deteriorating values is of immense importance, especially in cases of one lung ventilation [14]. ORI values significantly corelate with PaO_2 values [14]. ORI can be monitored continuously, which may be beneficial to decrease the frequency of arterial blood sampling. This tool is useful to avoid any hypoxic or hyperoxic injury and also provides an instant value to guide oxygen therapy [12]. It has also been observed that the motion artefacts may also mask the values, to assess and overcome these problems, an interesting study was conducted which concluded with the superiority of Masimo co-oximeter over the simple pulse oximeter [15].

8.3.1.2 Pleth Variability Index (PVI)

This new generation co-oximeter, in addition to saturation and ORI values, also provides guidance about fluid administration. Optimum fluid requirement during the intraoperative period is reduced under its guidance. It is especially beneficial in critically ill patients where the volume of fluid administration is of vital importance. It might be advantageous to predict the fluid responsiveness for avoiding hypo- or hypervolemia. Administration of optimum fluids leads to better peripheral perfusion and lower lactate levels [16]. It is also a useful tool to predict the fluid responsiveness and a guiding tool to precisely administer fluids to avoid hypo- or hypervolemia, especially in critically ill patients [17], though large studies and further evaluation is required to establish the strong corelation between the PVI and fluid status.

8.4 Blood Pressure

8.4.1 Non-invasive Blood Pressure Monitoring

It is a basic yet an important measure to assess the cardiovascular status. Adequate perfusion pressure is required to maintain the functioning of all the organ systems. Non-invasive blood pressure monitoring is the most commonly used method to assess the hemodynamics. Prior to measuring the blood pressure one must have basic knowledge about its working, importance of appropriate cuff size and the site of application. The blood pressure values may vary with different body positions. Blood pressure is higher in the standing position in comparison to supine and systolic pressure is more affected than the diastolic pressure. Even in each of the lateral positions (right/left lateral) due to hydrostatic pressure, blood pressure in the upper arm is significantly lower than the lower arm. Accurate pressure can be obtained if the arm is at the heart level [18, 19].

8.4.2 Invasive Blood Pressure

Invasive arterial blood pressure monitoring is required in case of haemodynamically unstable, critically ill patients and for procedures where major blood loss is expected. An arterial catheter is placed inside an artery and connected to a transducer with a pressure line. It provides real time and beat to beat changes in blood pressure. Though it gives accurate values, there are certain precautions needed before deciphering any reading, e.g. appropriate transducer height, adequate flushing of the entire tubing (to avoid any bubble-related dampening), avoid over or under dampening, use pressure tubings to avoid kinking and compliance related artefacts and transducer zeroing. The radial artery is the most common artery used for pressure monitoring, due to the ease of access and presence of dual blood supply in the hand. The femoral artery is the second most commonly used site for arterial cannulations. In some medical institutes, brachial artery is preferred over radial artery due to a lower complication rate [20, 21]. Other less commonly used sites for continuous invasive arterial blood pressure are the ulnar, dorsalis pedis, and axillary arteries.

In thoracic surgical procedures, which are mostly done in the lateral decubitus position, we prefer the radial artery at the dependent limb and the transducer must remain at the level of the right atrium for precise blood pressure measurement.

8.5 Central Venous Pressure (CVP)

The CVP gives an idea about the intravascular fluid status. It is best measured in the supine position, but various procedures are conducted in the lateral, Trendelenburg, reverse Trendelenburg or prone positions where the values may change drastically. Position of the transducer plays an important role for an accurate reading. Knowledge about various positions and their effects on the venous pressure is important. There are some changes that take place in the lateral position, which may not provide the correct values. A unique study compared the lateral (30° left or right) with the supine position; they recommended supine phlebostatic axis position is more precise for CVP values [22]. Thoracic surgical patients require one lung ventilation with higher inspiratory pressure. On several occasions, PEEP is required to improve ventilation and oxygenation. It has been noticed that application of high PEEP (15 cm H_2O) during ventilation does not change the CVP significantly in the supine and lateral decubitus positions, while it alters the CVP values in the prone position [23, 24]. Most of the lung resection procedures (lobectomy, pneumonectomy, etc.) require a dry lung for better outcome. Minimal but adequate fluid administration is recommended to avoid bleeding but at the same time maintaining adequate perfusion. A fine balance between fluid administration and fluid loss is required to maintain adequate perfusion pressure. Hypovolemia may lead to AKI, inadequate cerebral perfusion; while hypervolemia may cause interstitial oedema, cardiac overload, wound dehiscence, etc. CVP monitoring plays a crucial role in patients with major fluid shifts, or wherever minimal fluid administration is recommended. But the value of CVP is not reliable in case of the lateral position. A unique study was conducted to assess the CT scan guided blood levels of both the atria in the lateral position. They reported significant difference in blood levels of both the atria, lower atria has higher blood levels in the lateral position. These changes in atria must be considered while keeping the transducer at an appropriate level [25].

8.6 End Tidal Carbon Dioxide Monitoring (EtCO$_2$)

Capnography is a mandatory monitoring for a patient undergoing any procedure under general anesthesia. It is also the gold standard to confirm the correct placement of an endotracheal tube. In addition it also provides information regarding adequacy of ventilation and displays the waveform as well as provides the digital value. The value gives an idea about the highest $EtCO_2$ level but there are many variations in the waveform morphology. Higher CO_2 values mean hypoventilation prompting a change in the ventilator strategy for adequacy of ventilation. Sudden drastic decrease in values may be due to pulmonary embolism or tube migration into the right main bronchus [26]. Similarly, there are many deviations of waveforms in cases of pulmonary disease, endotracheal tube migration and tube secretions. Laparoscopic surgery using CO_2 insufflation to distend abdomen, may alarmingly increase the $EtCO_2$ levels. Instant interpretation of an abnormal waveform may decrease the morbidity.

Thoracic surgical procedures are commonly done in the lateral position with bronchial blockers or double lumen tubes. Confirmation of lung isolation techniques with bronchial blocker can be achieved with capnography, although it is not a sensitive monitor to detect migration of double lumen tube [27].

In an interesting study, neonates were intubated with double lumen tubes and an air sample was taken from distal part of the tube, $EtCO_2$ values (distal portion of DLT) were measured and compared with the $PaCO_2$ values. Both the values were very close to each other, but further evaluation is required [28]. Another important way to assess the capnography in critically ill patients is dual lung capnography. This is rarely used, but plays an important role to detect critically low perfusion. In this technique, the sample gas is taken from both the lungs and evaluation is done to assess the perfusion [29].

8.6.1 Airway Pressure

Controlled ventilation under general anesthesia results in airway pressures whose determinants are airflow, airway resistance and alveolar compliance. These parameters can be calculated with the help of the following equation:

$$\text{Airway pressure} = \text{flow} \times \text{resistance} + \text{alveolar pressure}$$

In volume controlled ventilation (VCV), volume delivered is fixed while peak and plateau pressures vary. In case of pressure controlled ventilation (PCV) both the pressures (peak and plateau) are constant but there is change in the volume delivered. Peak and plateau pressures are important parameters to assess the airway system. Peak airway pressure is measured when there is airflow during inspiration, and is determined by lung resistance. An increase in isolated peak airway pressure (VCV) reflects elevation in airway resistance. Increase in peak airway pressure may be due to kinking or narrowing of airway tubings, secretions, high tidal volume, lung diseases or when the patient is emerging out of anesthesia. Plateau pressures are measured at the end of the inspiration (inspiratory pause) with no air flow in the circuit. Plateau pressure is important as a surrogate marker of alveolar pressure which reflects lung compliance. Increase in the plateau pressure indicates decrease in lung compliance.

During thoracic surgery, application of one lung ventilation leads to elevation of peak and plateau airway pressures with a safe upper limit of peak airway pressure of 35 cm H_2O.

In some instances it has been noticed that these airway resistances may also increase in case of ventilatory dysfunction or in cases of inappropriate ventilator setting. Prompt evaluation and instant intervention will lead to a favourable outcome.

8.6.2 Loops During Mechanical Ventilation (Figs. 8.3 and 8.4)

8.6.2.1 Flow–Volume (F–V) Loops/ Pressure–Volume (P–V) Loops

Flow–volume loops are graphical representations of inspiratory and expiratory cycles of respiratory volumes. The graphical representation of one cycle of inspiration and expiration, forms a unique circular shape. Each half of this circle is contributed to during inhalation and exhalation. A thorough evaluation of these loops provides information regarding peak flow rate, airway pressures, tidal volume, lung and airway pathology, leaks in the airway, air trapping and presence of secretions. It has also been noticed that during single lung ventilation development of auto-PEEP is also common during thoracic surgery [30].

8.6.3 Early Detection of Displaced Double Lumen Tube

1. **Bronchial cuff pressure monitoring**

    In one lung ventilation one of the most common complications of double lumen tube (DLT) is displacement of the bronchial cuff. Even after proper positioning and adequate fixation of the DLT, its displacement is common during positioning or during surgical manipulation at the hilar region. It has been seen that regular monitoring of the bronchial cuff pressure is helpful in diagnosing DLT

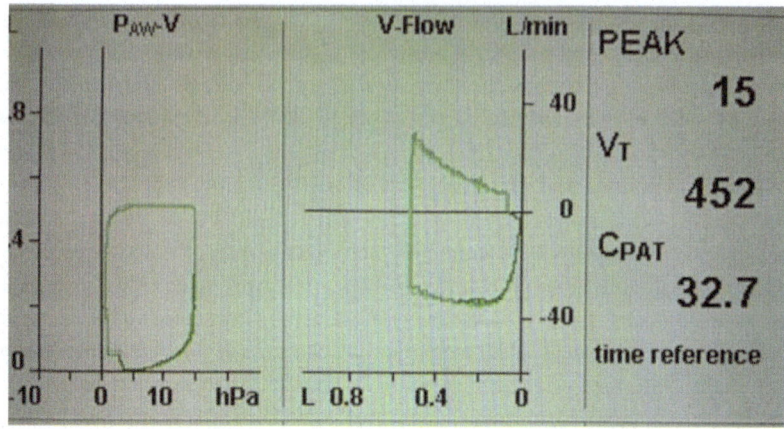

Fig. 8.3 Normal traces of P–V loops and F–V loops during both lung ventilation

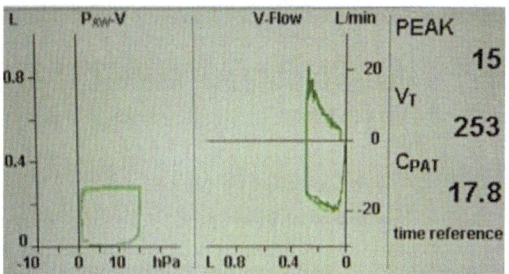

Fig. 8.4 Normal traces of P–V loops and F–V loops during one lung ventilation

displacement [31]. A sudden decrease in cuff pressure (bronchial cuff pressure) indicates that the cuff is displaced from the narrow part of bronchus to the bigger diameter of the trachea.

2. **Airwave monitor**

    This novel device is based on acoustic reflectometry to monitor the position and obstruction of the endotracheal tube [32]. It is developed to sense the obstruction and migration at the initial stages. Early diagnosis and prompt intervention decrease morbidity. However, further evaluation and larger studies are required to establish the relationship.

3. **Flow–volume/Pressure–volume loops**

    Displacement of the DLT leads to a sudden decrease in flow and increase in expiratory resistance with change in the morphology of the loop predicting displacement. An abnormally large area of pressure–volume loop can be detected during malpositioning of DLT (Fig. 8.5) [33, 34]. Corrective measures should be taken promptly, with fibre-optic bronchoscope to guide the readjustment of the tube.

8.7 Cardiac Status

8.7.1 Trans-thoracic Echocardiography (TTE)

Trans-thoracic echocardiography is a rapid, easy and non-invasive method to assess the cardiac status. Patient with suspected or known cardiac dysfunction must be evaluated thoroughly for risk assessment. Detailed evaluation of regional wall motion abnormality, valvular function, clot or vegetation and left ventricular ejection fraction is conducted with ease. Assessment of fluid and vascular systems add valuable information and guide the physician in precise management and optimization.

8.7.2 Trans-oesophageal Echocardiography (TEE)

TEE is an expensive diagnostic tool but provides real time cardiac status during the intraoperative period without affecting the surgical field. TEE is also easy to use in various positions due to its flexibility. Training with basic knowledge and orientation is required, since images displayed are different from

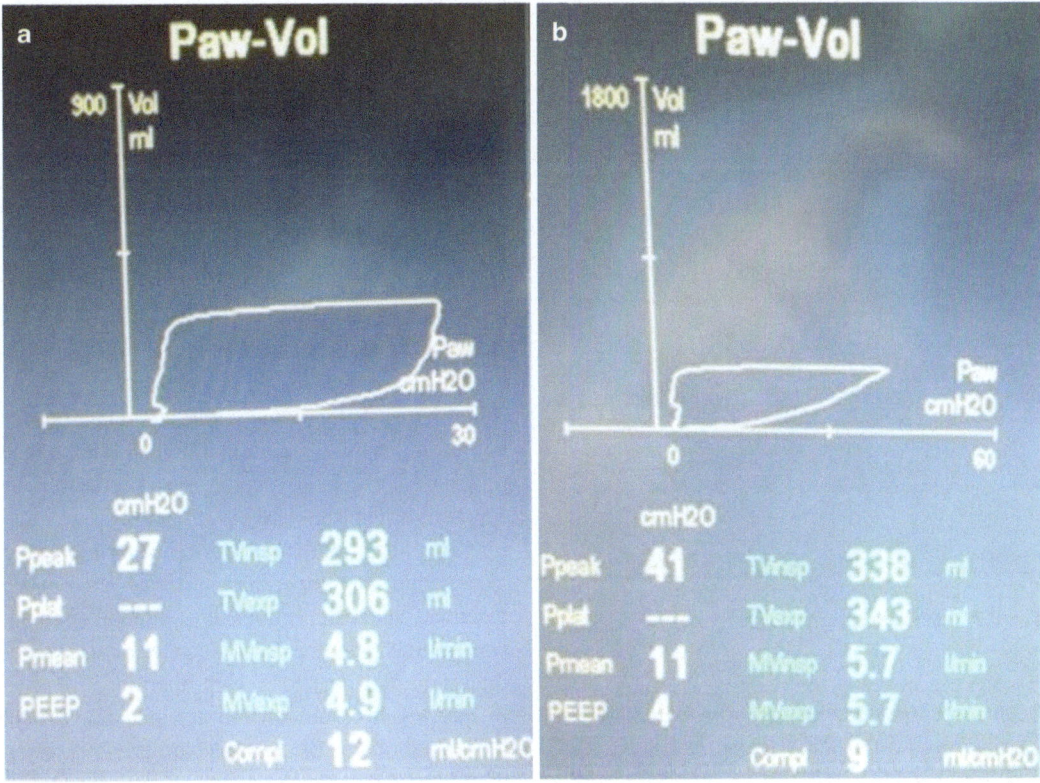

Fig. 8.5 (a) Area of the curve is enlarged (b) peak airway pressure is very high

trans-thoracic echocardiography. Apart from the cardiac status it has also proven to be a very sensitive tool to detect air embolism (bubbles of 0.2 ml). This would lead to rapid diagnosis, early intervention, and fruitful outcome. TEE is also playing an important role in localizing lesions present close to the heart. It also guides the surgeon during surgery to evaluate the extent of residual tumours.

8.8 Depth of Anesthesia

Various monitoring devices are available to measure the depth of anesthesia but the basic functioning is through the processing of various electrical signals generated in the brain. Commonly used monitors are entropy and Bispectral index (BIS). Both of them require electrode application on the forehead. BIS is the more commonly used monitor with a scale

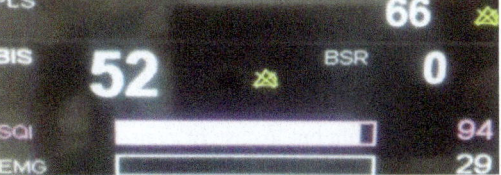

Fig. 8.6 Bispectral index

of 1–100, used with general anesthesia. It is recommended to keep BIS values in the range of 40–60 (Fig. 8.6) to avoid intraoperative awareness.

8.9 Analgesia

The most fearful factor to avoid in any surgical procedure is pain. But unfortunately there was no monitoring device available to assess 'pain' till the last few years. A few anesthesia monitors have

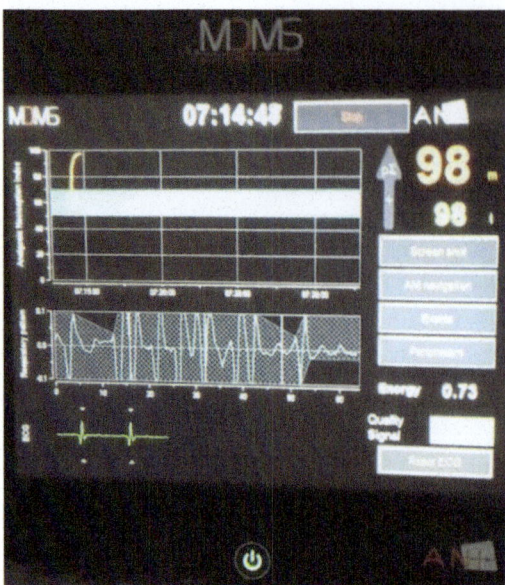

Fig. 8.7 Anti-nociceptive index

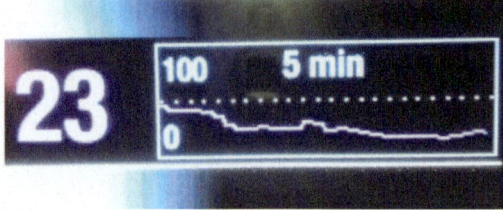

Fig. 8.8 Surgical plethysmography index

8.10 Temperature

The human body cannot tolerate temperatures below and above a certain range. Maintenance of temperature is advocated to continue proper functioning of the body. An awake individual may use warm clothes or warm air during winter to maintain the temperature and vice versa in hot weather. Under the influence of general anesthesia, he may become hypothermic, due to vasodilatation and heat loss. Hypothermia (Fig. 8.9) in long cases is not uncommon and may affect the metabolism of various drugs. Prevention of loss of heat may be achieved with warm air/mattress or warm fluid to maintain the body temperature. Nasal/oral or rectal probe may be used to measure the temperature, which provides basics to control temperature. Thoracic surgical procedures require special attention due to long cases and major fluid shifts. Temperature monitoring is mandatory in cases of sympathectomy, since early change in temperature will assure the surgeon of success.

been incorporated with recently validated nociceptive monitors. Anti-Nociceptive Index (ANI) and Surgical Pleth Index (Plethysmography) are two newer parameters developed to assess the analgesia in these patients.

The basic mechanism of ANI (Fig. 8.7) is based on measurement of parasympathetic activity, which is based on RR variation in the ECG, during the respiratory cycle. If the values are high it means predominance of parasympathetic tone and no pain but in case of pain, sympathetic activity predominates and so the ANI values decrease. Apart from the analgesia, it has also played a crucial role in cases where the surgical manipulation is close to the vagus nerve, since a stimulus close to the vagus instantly increases the ANI values and warns the surgeon, as it increases the parasympathetic activity.

Surgical pleth index (Fig. 8.8) is based on amplitude and heart rate of photoplethysmography. Various studies have been conducted to evaluate the correlation. Values below 50 are considered as adequate analgesia while higher values require further analgesic doses.

8.11 Fluid Status

Non-thoracic procedures tolerate sufficient fluid loss without affecting the surgical field. But, in cases of lung resection, it is mandatory to keep the lungs dry for better surgical conditions. Minimal fluid transfusion is advocated especially in cases where large lung resection or pneumonectomy is planned. There are various methods to assess the fluid status and gradual ongoing loss during the procedures, e.g. monitoring the output

Fig. 8.9 Monitoring parameters

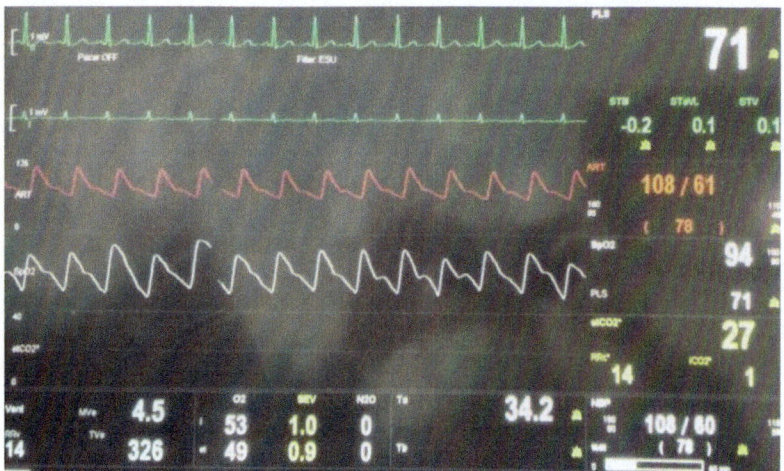

(urine output, blood loss, etc.) and replacing it as per the requirement. Tachycardia and hypotension are the surrogate indicators of hypovolemia. With increase in severity of blood loss, high blood lactate level in the ABG is an indicator of inadequacy of tissue perfusion.

Regular assessment of precise fluid status and transfusion of adequate volume to maintain optimum perfusion pressure is the mainstay of favourable outcome in thoracic cases. Lung resection cases require 'bone dry lung' to avoid bleeding and to provide better surgical conditions. Critically ill patients undergoing major lung resection need precise fluid balance, which can be achieved with advanced monitoring of stroke volume variation (SVV) and pulse pressure variation (PPV). These parameters can be derived from the arterial waveform analysis. Earlier, evaluation of these parameters (SVV) was advocated for closed chest, with both lungs under controlled ventilation. In these cases SVV less than 10%, correlate with adequate fluid status and values of more than 13% predicts fluid deficit. SVV guided fluid infusion predicts fluid responsiveness (Fig. 8.10) in gastro-surgical cases [35]. In a unique study in thoracic cases where patients were kept in the lateral decubitus position with one lung ventilation, they concluded that SVV guided fluid transfusion in these patients does not cause any hypervolemia [36]. Pulse pressure variation is another sensitive tool to evaluate the fluid responsiveness [37].

8.12 Monitoring of Neuromuscular Blockade

Intraoperative monitoring of neuromuscular blocking drugs helps in assessment of the residual effect of these drugs. Administration of neuromuscular blocker drugs under monitoring will avoid unnecessary delay in extubation. It is especially helpful in the elderly, critically ill patients and in patients suffering with myasthenia gravis. Myasthenic patients require a very low dose of non-depolarizing agents (atracurium) for adequate effect.

8.13 Clinical Pearls

Use of state-of-the-art monitoring devices facilitates in early detection, quick intervention at the initial stage in high risk cases, may lead to a favourable outcome.

Prophylactic care to avoid DVT, nerve injury, soft padding of all bony landmarks, adequate strapping to avoid falls will provide adequate surgical exposure without any complications.

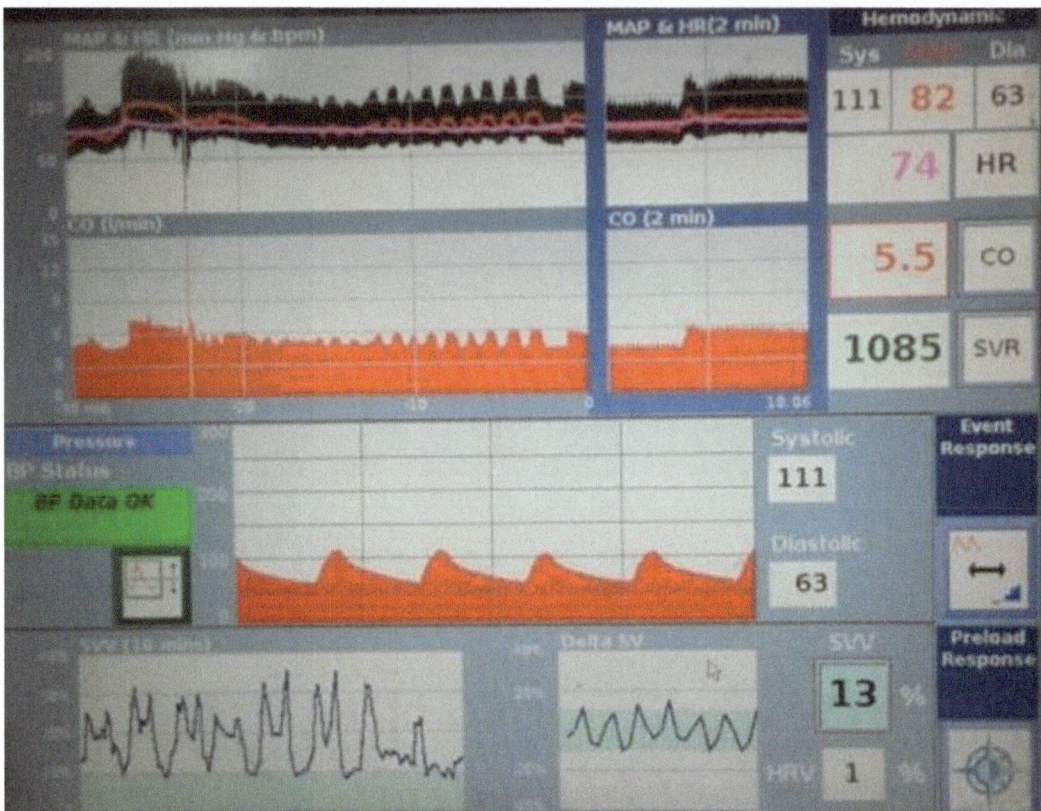

Fig. 8.10 LiDCO monitoring

References

1. Kaviraj doctor Ambikadutt Shastri. Sushruta Samhita: Sharira-Sthanam; Garbhavkrantishariram, vol 1. Publiisher-Chaukhmba Sanskrit Sansthan, Varanasi; Reprint 2014.
2. Tamene A, Sattiraju S, Wang K, et al. Brugada-like electrocardiography pattern induced by severe hyponatraemia. Europace. 2010;12(6):905–7.
3. Tsilakis D, Kranidis A, Koulouris S, et al. ECG changes associated with right-sided pneumothorax. Hosp Chron. 2007;2(3):108–10.
4. Walston A, Brewer DL, Kitchens CS, et al. The electrocardiographic manifestations of spontaneous left pneumothorax. Ann Intern Med. 1974;80(3):375–9.
5. Saks MA, Griswold-Theodorson S, Shinaishin F, et al. Subacute tension hemopneumothorax with novel electrocardiogram findings. West J Emerg Med. 2010;11(1):86–9.
6. Ryan KL, Rickards CA, Ludwig DA, et al. Tracking central hypovolemia with ecg in humans: cautions for the use of heart period variability in patient monitoring. Shock. 2010;33(6):583–9.
7. Ceylan B, Khorshid L, Güneş ÜY, et al. Evaluation of oxygen saturation values in different body positions in healthy individuals. J Clin Nurs. 2016;25(7-8):1095–100.
8. Laishley RS, Aps C. Tension pneumothorax and pulse oximetry. Br J Anaesth. 1991;66(2):250–2.
9. Neagley SR, Zwillich CW. The effect of positional changes on oxygenation in patients with pleural effusions. Chest. 1985;88(5):714–7.
10. Laishley RS, Aps C. Tension pneumothorax and pulse oximetry. Br J Anaesth. 1991;66(2):250–2.
11. Michaelides SA, Michailidis AR, Bablekos GD, et al. Does size matter concerning impact of position on oxygenation status in spontaneously breathing patients with unilateral effusion? Postgrad Med J. 2018;94(1108):81–6.
12. Scheeren TWL, Belda FJ, Perel A. The oxygen reserve index (ORI): a new tool to monitor oxygen therapy. J Clin Monit Comput. 2018;32(3):379–89.
13. Szmuk P, Steiner JW, Olomu PN, et al. Oxygen reserve index: A novel noninvasive measure of oxygen reserve—a pilot study. Anesthesiology. 2016;124(4):779–84.
14. Koishi W, Kumagai M, Ogawa S, et al. Monitoring the Oxygen Reserve Index can contribute to the

early detection of deterioration in blood oxygenation during one-lung ventilation. Minerva Anestesiol. 2018;84(9):1063–9.
15. Barker SJ. "Motion-resistant" pulse oximetry: a comparison of new and old models. Anesth Analg. 2002;95(4):967–72.
16. Forget P, Lois F, de Kock M. Goal-directed fluid management based on the pulse oximeter-derived pleth variability index reduces lactate levels and improves fluid management. Anesth Analg. 2010;111(4):910–4.
17. Cannesson M, Desebbe O, Rosamel P, et al. Pleth variability index to monitor the respiratory variations in the pulse oximeter plethysmographic waveform amplitude and predict fluid responsiveness in the operating theatre. Br J Anaesth. 2008;101(2):200–6.
18. Eşer I, Khorshid L, Güneş UY, et al. The effect of different body positions on blood pressure. J Clin Nurs. 2007;16(1):137–40.
19. Park HS, Park KY. Blood pressure variation on each measuring site in the right lateral position. J Korean Academy Nurs. 2002;32(7):986–91.
20. Lakhal K, Robert-Edan V. Invasive monitoring of blood pressure: a radiant future for brachial artery as an alternative to radial artery catheterisation? J Thorac Dis. 2017;9(12):4812–6.
21. Singh A, Wakefield BJ, Duncan AE. Complications from brachial arterial pressure monitoring are rare in patients having cardiac surgery. J Thorac Dis. 2018;10(2):E158–9.
22. Potger KC, Elliott D. Reproducibility of central venous pressures in supine and lateral positions: a pilot evaluation of the phlebostatic axis in critically ill patients. Heart Lung. 1994;23(4):285–99.
23. Hong SH, Choi JH, Lee J. The changes of central venous pressure by body posture and positive end-expiratory pressure. Korean J Anesthesiol. 2009;57(6):723–8.
24. Gandhi SK, Munshi CA, Coon R, et al. Capnography for detection of endobronchial migration of an endotracheal tube. J Clin Monit. 1991;7(1):35–8.
25. Song IK, Ro S, Lee JH, et al. Reference levels for central venous pressure and pulmonary artery occlusion pressure monitoring in the lateral position. J Cardiothorac Vasc Anesth. 2017;31(3):939–43.
26. Gandhi SK, Munshi CA, Coon R, et al. Capnography for detection of endobronchial migration of an endotracheal tube. J Clin Monit. 1991;7(1):35–8.
27. Fisicaro MD, Maguire DP, Armstead VE. Using the capnograph to confirm lung isolation when using a bronchial blocker. J Clin Anesth. 2010;22(7):557–9.
28. Kugelman A, Zeiger-Aginsky D, Bader D, et al. A novel method of distal end-tidal CO2 capnography in intubated infants: comparison with arterial CO2 and with proximal mainstream end-tidal CO2. Pediatrics. 2008;122(6):e1219–24.
29. Shankar KB, Russell R, Aklog L, et al. Dual capnography facilitates detection of a critical perfusion defect in an individual lung. Anesthesiology. 1999;90(1):302–4.
30. Bardoczky G, d'Hollander A, Yernault JC, et al. On-line expiratory flow-volume curves during thoracic surgery: occurrence of auto-PEEP. Br J Anaesth. 1994;72(1):25–8.
31. Araki K, Nomura R, Urushibara R, et al. Displacement of the double-lumen endobronchial tube can be detected by bronchial cuff pressure change. Anesth Analg. 1997;84(6):1349–53.
32. Nacheli GC, Sharma M, Wang X, et al. Novel device (AirWave) to assess endotracheal tube migration: a pilot study. J Crit Care. 2013;28(4):535.e1–8.
33. Bardoczry G, deFrancquen P, Rocmans P, et al. Monitoring of flow-volume and pressure-volume loops during one lung ventilation. J Cardiothoracic Vascular Anaesth 1994;8(3):59.
34. Bardoczky GI, Levarlet M, Engelman E, et al. Continuous spirometry for detection of double-lumen endobronchial tube displacement. Br J Anaesth. 1993;70(5):499–502.
35. Li C, Lin FQ, Fu SK, et al. Stroke volume variation for prediction of fluid responsiveness in patients undergoing gastrointestinal surgery. Int J Med Sci. 2013;10(2):148–55.
36. Haas S, Eichhorn V, Hasbach T, et al. Goal-directed fluid therapy using stroke volume variation does not result in pulmonary fluid overload in thoracic surgery requiring one-lung ventilation. Crit Care Res Pract. 2012;2012:687018.
37. Grassi P, Lo Nigro L, Battaglia K, et al. Pulse pressure variation as a predictor of fluid responsiveness in mechanically ventilated patients with spontaneous breathing activity: a pragmatic observational study. HSR Proc Intensive Care Cardiovasc Anesth. 2013;5(2):98–109.

Part II

Anesthesia for Operative Procedures

9.2 Glycocalyx

The endothelial surface layer (ESL) comprising of endothelial glycocalyx and plasma proteins helps in the mechanism of fluid transit across the vasculature (Fig. 9.1).

The glycocalyx is present on the luminal side of the vascular endothelium and comprises of proteoglycans, glycolipids and glycoproteins [7].

It absorbs the plasma proteins, e.g. albumin to form an endothelial surface (ESL) layer (1 mm) and traps around 700–1000 ml of plasma at the ESL [8]. This directs the oncotic pressure to retain the plasma which should have otherwise been forced into the interstitium, if Starling's principle was totally applicable.

It excludes erythrocytes and thus protein-rich plasma is predominant in this layer. The glycocalyx along with endothelial cells form the endothelial surface layer (ESL) [9]. This layer is 0.4–1.2 μg thick and in equilibrium with the plasma and requires normal levels of plasma albumin for its function.

Thus both endothelial cell layer and glycocalyx layer maintain a vascular barrier. Trans-endothelial pressure difference and plasma subglycocalyx colloid oncotic pressure are central to fluid filtration, with interstitial colloid oncotic pressure (COP) being nearly zero [10]. At subnormal capillary pressure transcapillary flow is zero. With increased capillary pressure, the COP increases and fluid movement occurs in relation to trans-endothelial pressure difference.

Therefore, when colloid is transfused it distributes in the plasma, maintains COP, decreases capillary pressure, thus decreasing fluid filtration [11]. A crystalloid infusion, on the other hand, increases COP, increases capillary pressure resulting is more fluid filtration.

There is also a small area below the glycocalyx (the subglycocalyx space). Plasma proteins diffuse into this space under conditions of low transcapillary fluid filtration. The protein in this area is cleared into the interstitium, thus maintaining low oncotic pressure in this area and favouring fluid retention in the vascular compartment.

Therefore, low vascular hydrostatic pressure allows more fluid filtration into the interstitium while increased hydrostatic pressure in the vessels increases fluid filtration in the

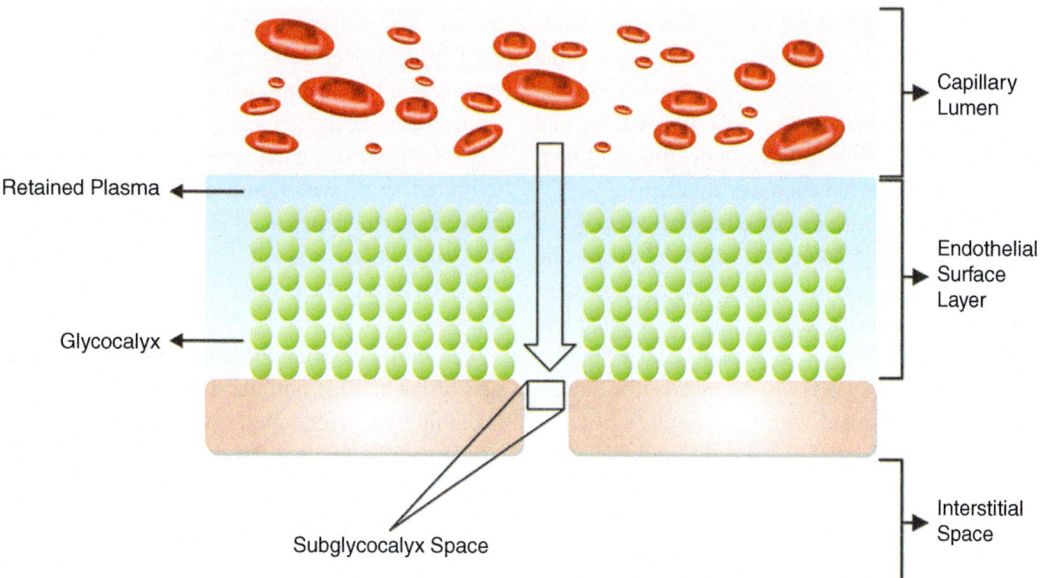

Fig. 9.1 The endothelial surface layer (ESL) is comprised of the endothelial glycocalyx and retained plasma proteins on the luminal surface of the capillary endothelium

Fluid Management

Shikha Sharma

9.1 Introduction

Any student of thoracic anesthesia embarks on the journey with the message of low fluid infusion for thoracic surgical cases. This message is not without reason as reports suggest that increased fluid infusion can lead to complications like acute kidney injury and acute lung injury.

There have been significant advances in the surgical technique from open surgery to video assisted surgery and now robotic surgery. In spite of these advances there is no significant change in the rate of pulmonary complications mortality rate or length of hospital stay [1, 2].

Volume of intravenous fluid administered is one of the main factors considered responsible for morbidity and mortality following lung resection with an incidence of 3–10% (morbidity) and mortality of 25–60% following pneumonectomy. Lesser resections have a lower incidence [3–6].

All major surgeries whether GI surgery or thoracic surgery recommend less IV fluid for the fear of tissue oedema and subsequent anastomotic leak. This factor is more pronounced in thoracic surgical cases, especially those involving parenchymal excision. To clarify this by an example, in a patient with cardiac output of 5 L and 60% of this perfuses the right lung (3 L) and 40% perfuses the left lung (2 L). If right sided pneumonectomy or bilobectomy is performed then this blood needs to be accommodated by the left lung or remaining part of right lung (2 lt + 3lt)—leading to a situation of autologous overload. This situation can be further complicated by generous IV fluid infusion. In reality does this really happen? No, not even in patients with carcinoma lung in whom the lung parenchyma is otherwise normal and the lung has to make sudden adjustment for the cardiac output it has to accommodate. In chronic destroyed lung, compensatory mechanisms are already in place and perfusion to this lung is already curtailed. Nature does not waste its resources, therefore, in case of destroyed lung, perfusion preferentially increases to the healthy lung.

This can be further explained with an everyday example. If a garden of a particular size is irrigated with water and this garden is now halved but the water used for irrigation remains the same, then does it get flooded? No, not necessarily because some water is taken up by the soil.

Similarly, to extend this example to the lung, part of the cardiac output, after lung resection, is taken up by a layer called glycocalyx, apart from adjustment in the vascular tree.

S. Sharma (✉)
Institute of Anaesthesiology, Pain and Perioperative Medicine, Sir Ganga Ram Hospital, New Delhi, India

subglycocalyx decreasing the oncotic pressure and retaining fluid in the vessels [9, 12].

Thus fluid flux is driven by the oncotic pressure difference between the ESL and capillary lumen with no role play by interstitial tissue oncotic pressure.

Fluid reuptake is through sympathetically mediated lymph return [13].

Perioperative fluid management is thus based on the concept of tissue oedema being the result of breakdown of ESL and glycocalyx.

It has been suggested that ischemia–reperfusion injury, inflammation and atrial natriuretic peptide [14–16], released in response to fluid overload can disrupt the endothelial glycocalyx.

In contrast, pretreatment with hydrocortisone, antithrombin [17] and use of sevoflurane [18] can protect the glycocalyx endothelium.

It is important to stress here that investigators have proposed that pulmonary capillary ESL is thicker than microcirculation of other organs [19].

Acute lung injury causes pulmonary capillary leakage [20–22]; there is presence of glycosaminoglycan fragments and glycocalyx components in lavage fluid suggesting the role of pulmonary glycocalyx layer in lung injury.

Table 9.1 Factors affecting endothelial layer

Protective	Non-protective
Glucocorticoids	Inflammation
Albumin	Sepsis
Sevoflurane	Ischemia–reperfusion
Fresh frozen plasma	Surgical trauma
Lung-protective ventilation	Hyperglycemia
Antithrombin III	Hypoxia
	Hypertension
	High tidal volumes
	Hypervolemia

9.3 Glycocalyx and Normovolemia

In cases of fluid overload, ANP is released from cardiac atria which causes destruction of endothelial glycocalyx and fluid shift into the interstitium by increased vascular permeability.

A study by Chappel studied the effect of volume loading with colloid on capillary permeability [16]. There was a significant increase in serum ANP levels and increased levels of hyaluronan and syndocan-1 which are components of endothelial glycocalyx.

9.4 Effect of Mechanical Ventilation of Glycocalyx

Glycocalyx also regulates endothelial integrity through nitric oxide and reactive oxygen [23]. Increased intravascular hydrostatic pressure and laminar shear stress in the vascular lumen change capillary barrier function and produce pulmonary oedema [24, 25].

Along with this, in a lung ventilated with tidal volumes of 6–8 ml/kg increases intravascular pressure increasing the lung endothelial permeability. This effect is less when tidal volumes of 4–6 ml/kg are used (lung protective strategy).

Also, when left atrial pressure is 17 cm H_2O, the increase in endothelial permeability is fivefold when low tidal volume is used and 15-fold when high tidal volume is used (Table 9.1).

Acute lung injury and increased capillary permeability

ALI and ARDS have been defined as a syndrome of increased permeability and inflammation with hypoxemia and bilateral lung infiltrates on chest X-ray, independent of PEEP used and pulmonary artery occlusion pressure of 18 mmHg or less.

9.5 Genesis of Pulmonary Oedema in Thoracic Surgery

The two main mechanisms responsible for pulmonary oedema following thoracic surgery are increase in capillary permeability and increase in pulmonary capillary hydrostatic pressure.

A special mention is needed for patients with interstitial lung disease and ARDS. In these patients, the actual lung tissue which is ventilated is 200–500 g (healthy lung) and thus the lung is more vulnerable to ventilator induced lung injury (VILI). This is because if tidal volume is calculated on the basis of body weight, the TV delivered can cause biotrauma to the remaining healthy lung, initiating local inflammatory process leading to increased permeability and pulmonary oedema [26–28].

9.6 Concept of Third Space

Classically, the third space is separate from the interstitial space and which does not participate in fluid exchange between interstitium and intravascular space [29]. Its location is still unknown but leads to fluid replacement regimens targeted towards this hypothetical space. The refrain for thoracic anesthesiologists is that there is no third space in the chest, implying the use of a restrictive fluid regimen.

9.7 Lymphatics and RV Dysfunction

ARDS, following thoracic surgery is caused not only by fluid overload but also occurs even when fluid restrictive strategy is applied [30].

Lung lymphatics play an important role in fluid clearance and when interstitial fluid resulting from capillary filtrate is in excess of the lymphatic drainage capacity, pulmonary oedema occurs [31].

Although lymph flow can increase sevenfold in response to increased interstitial pressure [32], this capacity can decrease in the perioperative period due to factors like surgical trauma [31].

Pulmonary lymphatic drainage is different for both lungs with >90% being ipsilateral for the right lung and 55% is contralateral or ipsilateral for the left lung [33].

Thus in the case of right pneumonectomy, there is an increased risk of pulmonary oedema as more than 90% of the lymphatic drainage is lost [34, 35], whereas left pneumonectomy has little effect due to contralateral lymphatics being present.

Right ventricular dysfunction also reduces drainage capacity of lymphatics [36]. Right ventricular dysfunction is common after lung resection surgery [37], due to increased afterload and tachycardia [38, 39].

9.8 Restrictive Fluid Therapy

Reducing the amount of intravenous fluid transfusion minimizes the hydrostatic pressure in thoracic surgical patients as they are prone to develop interstitial and pulmonary oedema due to pre-existing disease of the lung along with deleterious effects of one lung ventilation, surgical trauma, ischemia–reperfusion injury effect of transfusion of blood products and exposure to microbes as well as volutrauma and barotrauma due to mechanical ventilation. This trauma can damage the glycocalyx endothelial cells, epithelial alveolar cells and surfactant [40, 41].

A restrictive fluid regimen is recommended but can cause acute kidney injury specially in patients with chronic renal disease, hypertension or peripheral vascular disease. The patients require an adequate perfusion pressure for tissue perfusion which can be maintained by the use of vasopressors guided by the use of invasive haemodynamic monitors. These can give early warning signs [42].

Anesthesia per se also causes hypotension and vasodilatation and thus depth of anesthesia monitor can allow appropriate dose titration.

9.9 Goal Directed Therapy (GDT)

Thus the best course of action is to employ goal directed therapy (GDT) using measurement of stroke volume, pulse pressure variation and stroke volume variation (SVV).

Clinically, hourly urine output needs to be measured and a target of 0.5–1 ml/kg/h is unnecessary and there only needs to be some urine output per hour to be sure of tissue perfusion.

GDT can also result in positive fluid balance and use of "restrictive fluid therapy" can cause perioperative oliguria with increased risk of postoperative acute renal failure [43, 44].

Lymphatics can get disrupted due to preoperative chemotherapy or surgical dissection. This can hamper fluid drainage and increase the chances of lung oedema and thereby affect gas exchange.

With no consensus among the thoracic anesthesiologists regarding optimal fluid requirement and in the absence of any guidelines, there is great variation in the amount of fluid transfused. It ranges from 3–4 ml/kg/g to 10–12 ml/kg/h while others recommend GDT.

With GDT, it is easier to achieve a pre-specified goal [45]:

- If PPV or SPV are >10–15% then a fluid challenge of 250 ml is administered till the variation is <10%.
- Stroke volume should be maximum for optimal intravascular volume, thus when PPV or SPV is <10%, the stroke volume is taken as the new baseline.
- TEE can estimate volume status and guide fluid administration, based on LV cavity size.

9.10 Zero Balance Approach

In the absence of any RCTs, conservative fluid approach or zero balance approach is highly recommended. Stress of surgery releases the anti-diuretic hormone and also activates renin-angiotensin-aldosterone system. These lead to retention of salt and water.

The zero balance approach requires administration of 1–4 ml/kg/h of fluid to counteract the vasodilatory effects of anesthesia along with administration of vasopressors to maintain normal haemodynamics.

The zero balance strategy includes the following [46]:

1. Intraoperative administration of balanced crystalloid solution at 1–3 ml/kg/h.
2. Blood for blood should be the approach in case of blood loss.

To achieve this goal:

1. Preoperatively, patient should be encouraged to take a carbohydrate drink up to 2 hours before surgery (ERAS Chap. 24).
2. Intraoperatively, balanced crystalloid solution limited to 1–2 ml/kg/h and blood products for blood loss which should be separate from the calculation of maintenance fluid [47].
3. A restrictive approach is applied in patients with major lung resection and in those with moderate risk (zero balance). CVP or PCWP are not good measures of volume status, thus urine output/hr should be noted.
4. There should be a low threshold for administration of vasopressors to counter anesthesia-induced vasodilatation and convert hypovolemia to normovolemia.
5. The goal directed and restrictive approach should continue in the postoperative period for up to 8–12 h.
6. Oral hydration needs to be monitored specially in patients undergoing right pneumonectomy.

As heart rate, arterial pressure and central venous pressure are unreliable indicators of fluid status, cardiac output, stroke volume, extravascular lung water, cerebral oxygenation and central venous oximetry can be valuable adjuncts [48, 49].

Till the monitors of these parameters are more freely available, the anesthesiologist can rely on basics like ongoing blood and fluid losses, maintenance of vital signs and urine output as signs of adequate perfusion.

Recent data suggests that crystalloid administration should be < 2L intraoperatively. < 3L during first 24 h postoperatively, with a total fluid balance of less than 20 ml/kg during the first 24 h postoperatively. Fluid restriction not only prevents ALI, but helps in the resolution of ALI already developed, without the added risk of AKI [50, 51].

9.11 Causes of Fluid Overload

Lung lymphatics are responsible for transport of fluid from the interstitium. Pulmonary resection can impair this ability. The lymphatic drainage of right lung is mainly ipsilateral (>90%) but of left side is contralateral (>55%), so a right pneumonectomy can decrease capillary filtrate in the intestitium and result in pulmonary oedema and cause acute lung injury. Left pneumonectomy, on the other hand, has little effect on lymphatics [40, 41].

The other causes of ALI are [52–54]:

- Volume induced lung injury
- Ischemia–reperfusion injury
- Oxygen toxicity

Exposure of 100% O_2 is tolerated by the healthy lung for nearly 12 h, before demonstrating capillary leak and the duration is much less in patients with other risk factors.

9.12 Pitfalls of Restrictive Fluid Therapy

While hypovolemia can cause insufficient oxygen delivery and affect organ functions, hypervolemia can cause interstitial oedema with impaired diffusion of oxygen.

Clinical studies have shown that liberal fluid resuscitation in various surgical procedures leads to poor clinical outcome due to increased chances of wound dehiscence, anastomotic leaks and overload.

Apart from the quantity, the type of fluid is also important; crystalloids can cause hyperchloremic acidosis while colloids (HES) are incriminated in renal damage specially when transfused in patients with sepsis.

In thoracic surgery, fluid infusion in excess of 6–8 ml/kg/h is a risk factor for acute lung injury (ALI), acute respiratory distress syndrome (ARDS), pneumonia and atelectasis.

However, in complex surgeries and critical patients, the concomitant use of vasopressors can mask volume depletion and the need for fluid resuscitation.

Avoiding fluid overload appears to be important in preventing ALI. Historically, the incidence of renal injury has been regarded as very low (1.4%) by The Society of Thoacic Surgeons National Database.

Two recent studies have reported the incidence as 6.8 and 5.9% [55, 56].

The role of TEE, pulse pressure variation and SVV has been examined in lung resection surgery.

TEE measures the cardiac output even when heart rate and blood pressure remain unchanged.

Both the TEE and PPV or SVV use heart–lung interaction during mechanical ventilation to assess responsiveness to fluid.

During one lung ventilation and with the use of protective lung ventilation, it is suggested that blood shunted through the nonventilated lung does not contribute to the PPV and SVV value and thus a SVV > 8% and PPV > 6% correlates with fluid responsiveness compared with PPV of 13% and SVV > 12% otherwise (two lung ventilation).

Monitoring of extravascular lung water by pulse contour cardiac output (PiCCO) system offers prognostic and therapeutic information in patients with ALI. Its accuracy is however, affected by a decrease in pulmonary blood volume [57, 58].

Thus, TEE, PPV/SVV, PiCCO appear to be promising techniques to guide fluid therapy.

9.13 Key Points

1. Total positive fluid balance in the first 24 h should not exceed 10–20 ml/kg.
2. Intraoperatively crystalloid administration should be 1–2 ml/kg/h.
3. Colloids should only be used for replacement of blood loss if blood is not administrated.
4. There is no third space loss.
5. Urine output of >0.5 ml/kg/h is unnecessary; however, there should be some urine output per hour as a guide for adequate tissue perfusion.
6. Inotropes should be used to counter vasodilation due to anesthesia.

References

1. Gopaldas RR, Bakaeen FG, Dao TK, et al. Video-assisted thoracoscopic versus open thoracotomy lobectomy in a cohort of 13 619 patients. Ann Thorac Surg. 2010;89:1563–70.
2. Louie BE, Farivar AS, Aye RW, et al. Early experience with robotic lung resection results in similar operative outcomes and morbidity when compared with matched video-assisted thoracoscopic surgery cases. Ann Thorac Surg. 2012;93:1598–604.

3. Parquin F, Marchal M, Mehiri S, et al. Postpneumonectomy pulmonary edema: analysis and risk factors. Eur J Cardiothorac Surg. 1996;10:929–32.
4. Licker M, de Perrot M, Spiliopoulos A, et al. Risk factors for acute lung injury after thoracic surgery for lung cancer. Anesth Analg. 2003;97:1558–65.
5. Alam N, Park BJ, Wilton A, et al. Incidence and risk factors for lung injury after lung cancer resection. Ann Thorac Surg. 2007;84:1085–91.
6. Marret E, Miled F, Bazelly B, et al. Risk and protective factors for major complications after pneumonectomy for lung cancer. Inter Cardiovasc Thorac Surg. 2010;10:936–9.
7. Becker BF, Chappell D, Jacob M. Endothelial glycocalyx and coronary vascular permeability: the fringe benefit. Basic Res Cardiol. 2010;105:687–701.
8. Pries AR, Secomb TW, Gaehtgens P. The endothelial surface layer. Pflugers Arch. 2000;440:653–66.
9. Chappell D, Jacob M, Hofmann-Kiefer K, et al. A rational approach to perioperative fluid management. Anesthesiology. 2008;109:723–40.
10. Woodcock TE, Woodcock TM. Revised Starling equation and the glycocalyx model of transvascular fluid exchange: an improved paradigm for prescribing intravenous fluid therapy. Br J Anaesth. 2012;108:384–94.
11. Rehm M, Bruegger D, Christ F, et al. Shedding of the endothelial glycocalyx in patients undergoing major vascular surgery with global and regional ischemia. Circulation. 2007;116:1896–906.
12. Chappell D, Jacob M. Role of the glycocalyx in fluid management: small things matter. Best Pract Res Clin Anaesthesiol. 2014;28:227–34.
13. Woodcock TE, Woodcock TM. Revised Starling equation and the glycocalyx model of transvascular fluid exchange: an improved paradigm for prescribing intravenous fluid therapy. Br J Anaesth. 2012;108:384–94.
14. Rehm M, Haller M, Orth V, et al. Changes in blood volume and hematocrit during acute preoperative volume loading with 5% albumin or 6% hetastarch solutions in patients before radical hysterectomy. Anesthesiology. 2001;95:849–56.
15. Bruegger D, Schwartz L, Chappell D, et al. Release of atrial natriuretic peptide precedes shedding of the endothelial glycocalyx equally in patients undergoing on- and off-pump coronary artery bypass surgery. Basic Res Cardiol. 2011;106:1111–21.
16. Chappell D, Bruegger D, Potzel J, et al. Hypervolemia increases release of atrial natriuretic peptide and shedding of the endothelial glycocalyx. Crit Care. 2014;18:538.
17. Chappell D, Dorfler N, Jacob M, et al. Glycocalyx protection reduces leukocyte adhesion after ischemia/reperfusion. Shock. 2010;34:133–9.
18. Chappell D, Heindl B, Jacob M, et al. Sevoflurane reduces leukocyte and platelet adhesion after ischemia-reperfusion by protecting the endothelial glycocalyx. Anesthesiology. 2011;115:483–91.
19. Schmidt EP, Yang Y, Janssen WJ, et al. The pulmonary endothelial glycocalyx regulates neutrophil adhesion and lung injury during experimental sepsis. Nat Med. 2012;18:1217–23.
20. Constantinescu AA, Vink H, Spaan JA. Endothelial cell glycocalyx modulates immobilization of leukocytes at the endothelial surface. Arterioscler Thromb Vasc Biol. 2003;23:1541–7.
21. Vink H, Constantinescu AA, Spaan JA. Oxidized lipoproteins degrade the endothelial surface layer: implications for platelet-endothelial cell adhesion. Circulation. 2000;101:1500–2.
22. Huxley VH, Williams DA. Role of a glycocalyx on coronary arteriole permeability to proteins: evidence from enzyme treatments. Am J Physiol Heart Circ Physiol. 2000;278:1177–85.
23. Collins SR, Blank RS, Deatherage LS, et al. Special article: the endothelial glycocalyx: emerging concepts in pulmonary edema and acute lung injury. Anesth Analg. 2013;117:664–74.
24. Dull RO, Mecham I, McJames S. Heparan sulfates mediate pressure-induced increase in lung endothelial hydraulic conductivity via nitric oxide/reactive oxygen species. Am J Physiol Lung Cell Mol Physiol. 2007;292:1452–8.
25. Dull RO, Jo H, Sill H, et al. The effect of varying albumin concentration and hydrostatic pressure on hydraulic conductivity and albumin permeability of cultured endothelial monolayers. Microvasc Res. 1991;41:390–407.
26. Zeldin RA, Normandin D, Landtwing D, et al. Postpneumonectomy pulmonary edema. J Thorac Cardiovasc Surg. 1984;87:359–65.
27. Blank RS, Hucklenbruch C, Gurka KK, et al. Intraoperative factors and the risk of respiratory complications after pneumonectomy. Ann Thorac Surg. 2011;92:1188–94.
28. Kutlu CA, Williams EA, Evans TW, et al. Acute lung injury and acute respiratory distress syndrome after pulmonary resection. Ann Thorac Surg. 2000;69:376–80.
29. Jacob M, Chappell D, Rehm M. The 'third space'—fact or fiction? Best Pract Res Clin Anaesthesiol. 2009;23:145–57.
30. Slinger P. Fluid management during pulmonary resection surgery. Ann Card Anaesth. 2002;5:220–4.
31. Chau EH, Slinger P. Perioperative fluid management for pulmonary resection surgery and esophagectomy. Semin Cardiothorac Vasc Anesth. 2014;18:36–44.
32. Zarins CK, Rice CL, Peters RM, et al. Lymph and pulmonary response to isobaric reduction in plasma oncotic pressure in baboons. Circ Res. 1978;43:925–30.
33. Nohl-Oser HC. An investigation of the anatomy of the lymphatic drainage of the lungs as shown by the lymphatic spread of bronchial carcinoma. Ann R Coll Surg Engl. 1972;51:157–76.
34. Turnage WS, Lunn JJ. Postpneumonectomy pulmonary edema. A retrospective analysis of associated variables. Chest. 1993;103:1646–50.

35. Verheijen-Breemhaar L, Bogaard JM, van den Berg B, et al. Postpneumonectomy pulmonary oedema. Thorax. 1988;43:323–6.
36. Laine GA, Allen SJ, Katz J, et al. Effect of systemic venous pressure elevation on lymph flow and lung edema formation. J Appl Physiol. 1986;61:1634–8.
37. Pedoto A, Amar D. Right heart function in thoracic surgery: role of echocardiography. Curr Opin Anaesth. 2009;22:44–9.
38. Reed CE, Dorman BH, Spinale FG. Mechanisms of right ventricular dysfunction after pulmonary resection. Ann Thorac Surg. 1996;62:225–31.
39. Okada M, Ota T, Matsuda H, et al. Right ventricular dysfunction after major pulmonary resection. J Thorac Cardiovasc Surg. 1994;108:503–11.
40. Abbas SM, Hill AG. Systematic review of the literature for the use of oesophageal Doppler monitor for fluid replacement in major abdominal surgery. Anaesthesia. 2008;63:44–51.
41. Phan TD, Ismail H, Heriot AG, et al. Improving perioperative outcomes: fluid optimization with the esophageal Doppler monitor, a metaanalysis and review. J Am Coll Surg. 2008;207:935–41.
42. Brandstrup B. Fluid therapy for the surgical patient. Best Pract Res Clin Anaesthesiol. 2006;20:265–83.
43. Corcoran T, Rhodes JE, Clarke S, et al. Perioperative fluid management strategies in major surgery: a stratified meta-analysis. Anesth Analg. 2012;114:640–51.
44. Chong MA, Wang Y, Berbenetz NM, et al. Does goal-directed haemodynamic and fluid therapy improve peri-operative outcomes?: a systematic review and meta-analysis. Eur J Anaesthesiol. 2018;35:469–83.
45. Bundgaard-Nielsen M, Holte K, Secher NH, et al. Monitoring of peri-operative fluid administration by individualized goal-directed therapy. Acta Anaesthesiol Scand. 2007;51:331–40.
46. Cecconi M, Parsons AK, Rhodes A. What is a fluid challenge? Curr Opin Crit Care. 2011;17:290–5.
47. Ansari BM, Zochios V, Falter F, et al. Physiological controversies and methods used to determine fluid responsiveness: a qualitative systematic review. Anaesthesia. 2016;71:94–105.
48. Funk DJ, Moretti EW, Gan TJ. Minimally invasive cardiac output monitoring in the perioperative setting. Anesth Analg. 2009;108:887–97.
49. Thiele RH, Bartels K, Gan TJ. Inter-device differences in monitoring for goal-directed fluid therapy. Can J Anaesth. 2015;62:169–81.
50. Ahn HJ, Kim JA, Lee AR, et al. The risk of acute kidney injury from fluid restriction and hydroxyethyl starch in thoracic surgery. Anesth Analg. 2016;122:186–93.
51. National Heart, Lung, and Blood Institute Acute Respiratory Distress Syndrome (ARDS) Clinical Trials Network, Wiedemann HP, Wheeler AP, et al. Comparison of two fluid-management strategies in acute lung injury. N Engl J Med. 2006;354:2564-2575.
52. Licker M, Fauconnet P, Villiger Y, et al. Acute lung injury and outcomes after thoracic surgery. Curr Opin Anaesthesiol. 2009;22:61–7.
53. Staub N. Pulmonary edema due to increased microvascular permeability to fluid and protein. Circ Res. 1978;43:143–51.
54. Klein J. Normobaric pulmonary oxygen toxicity. Anesth Analg. 1990;70:195–207.
55. Kohl B, Deutschman CS. The inflammatory response to surgery and trauma. Curr Opin Crit Care. 2006;12:325–32.
56. Ray JF 3rd, Yost L, Moallem S, et al. Immobility, hypoxemia, and pulmonary arteriovenous shunting. Arch Surg. 1974;109:537–41.
57. Kobayashi M, Koh M, Irinoda T, et al. Stroke volume variation as a predictor of intravascular volume depression and possible hypotension during the early postoperative period after esophagectomy. Ann Surg Oncol. 2009;16:1371–7.
58. Michard F. Bedside assessment of extravascular lung water by dilution methods: temptations and pitfalls. Crit Care Med. 2007;35:1186–92.

Lung Isolation Techniques

10

Namrata Ranganath and Kavitha Lakshman

Keywords

One-lung ventilation · Double-lumen tubes
Single lumen tubes · Bronchial blockers
Lung separation

10.1 History of Lung Isolation

In 1931, Gale and Waters inserted a cuffed rubber endotracheal tube into the bronchus for the first time to achieve lung isolation in thoracic procedures [1, 2]. This was further modified by Archibald in 1935 who used rubber endobronchial blocker that was positioned by radiography. In the following year, Sir Ivan Magill further improved the positioning of rubber endobronchial blocker by passing a rigid endoscope though its lumen to achieve more precise positioning under direct vision. This was followed with the introduction of double-lumen bronchial tube by Gabauer and later Carlens and this marked the start of the era of lung isolation.

Lung isolation is usually achieved through three methods, namely, Double-Lumen Tubes (DLT), Bronchial Blockers, and Single Lumen Tubes (SLT). Among the various methods, DLTs are considered the gold standard for achieving lung isolation and are most commonly used. The DLT is a bifurcated tube having both an endotracheal and an endobronchial lumen and can be used to achieve either the right or the left lung isolation. In the second method, the bronchial blockers block the mainstem bronchus so that the lung distal to the occlusion is collapsed by air absorption. These bronchial blockers are inflatable devices that can be placed alongside the standard endotracheal tube or can be contained in the separate channel provided inside a modified SLT such as the Univent tube (outside the ETT or inside the ETT). In lung isolation through an SLT or an endobronchial tube, the contra-lateral lung is protected by advancing the SLT or an endobronchial tube into the contra-lateral main stem bronchus while simultaneously allowing for the collapse of lung on the side of surgery. Nowadays, an SLT is rarely used in adult practice because of the difficulty in positioning a standard SLT inside the bronchus. Also, there exists a limited access to the non-ventilated lung, when an SLT is used. However, an SLT is still used in some adult cases of difficult airways, carinal resection, or after a pneumonectomy and also in infants and small children. When used in infants and small children, a pediatric endotracheal tube which is uncuffed and uncut is advanced under direct vision into the main stem bronchus using an infant or pediatric bronchoscope.

N. Ranganath (✉) · K. Lakshman
Department of Anesthesiology and Pain Relief,
Kidwai Memorial Institute of Oncology,
Bengaluru, Karnataka, India

© Springer Nature Singapore Pte Ltd. 2020
J. Sood, S. Sharma (eds.), *Clinical Thoracic Anesthesia*,
https://doi.org/10.1007/978-981-15-0746-5_10

10.2 Double-Lumen Endotracheal Tubes

The DLT designed by Carlens for the purpose of lung surgery in the year 1950 was a huge leap in thoracic anesthesia as it allowed the anesthesiologist to attain and maintain lung isolation in the majority of patients through laryngoscopy and auscultation. The Carlens DLT had a high resistance to flow due to a narrow lumen and had a carinal hook that made it difficult to maneuver it through the glottis in some patients. To overcome these limitations, Robertshaw in the 1960s modified the Carlens DLT by using large-diameter D-shaped lumens to offer low flow resistance and by removing the carinal hook to facilitate the insertion. The large-diameter lumen offers additional advantage by allowing for easy passage of a suction catheter and the fixed curvature of the D-shaped lumen helps in facilitating proper positioning and in reducing the possibility of kinking. The Robertshaw design is available as separate left- and right-sided DLTs (Fig. 10.1). Based on the Robertshaw DLT, disposable DLTs made of polyvinyl chloride were introduced in the 1980s. These DLTs were provided with radiographic markers near the endotracheal cuff and endobronchial cuff and also around the ventilation slot for the right upper lobe bronchus in the right-sided DLT. Additionally, there was a bright blue colored, endobronchial cuff in which low-volume and low-pressure was incorporated for easy visualization during confirmation of tube placement during fiber-optic bronchoscopy. Though there are various types of DLT, all have similar design where two endotracheal tubes are "bonded" together lengthwise. One lumen reaches up to main stem bronchus, while the second lumen will reach up to the distal trachea distal. Lung separation is achieved by inflating both the proximal tracheal cuff and the distal bronchial cuff (see "Positioning of DLT"). In case of right-sided DLTs, the endobronchial cuff is slotted to facilitate right upper-lobe ventilation because the right main stem bronchus is shorter and has limited capacity to accommodate both the right-bronchial lumen tip and the cuff. The initial reusable DLTs were made of red rubber tubes having high-pressure cuffs which become stiffer and brittle with time thereby making the placement increasingly more difficult and traumatic. Then the disposable DLTs made of nontoxic plastic with Z-79 markings were used. These DLTs conformed to the anatomy of the patient when the plastics warmed up from the patient's body temperature. However, the repositioning of the same tube became more difficult due to this increased malleability. Presently, high-volume, low-pressure, and color-coded cuffs are used in the DLTs. The bronchial cuff along with the pilot balloon and connector are color coded blue while the tracheal cuff along with the pilot balloon and connector are transparent or white. To achieve and maintain a balance between an adequate seal and mucosal perfusion, cuff inflation pressure is maintained at 15–30 mmHg [3–7].

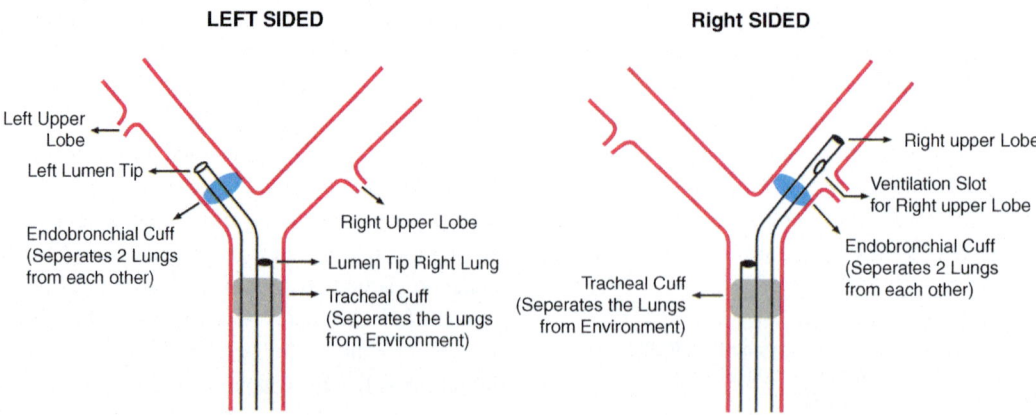

Fig. 10.1 Essential features and parts of right and left sided double lumen tubes

10.3 Indications for Use of Lung Separation Techniques

The indications for lung isolation are quite different from lung separation and it is important to distinguish the same.

10.3.1 Lung Isolation

Whenever the non-diseased lung is threatened with contamination by blood or pus from the diseased lung, the lungs must be isolated to prevent potentially life-threatening complications. Lung isolation is also indicated in broncho-pleural and bronchocutaneous fistulas, where there is inadequate ventilation because of the existence of a low-resistance pathway during positive-pressure ventilation for the delivered tidal volume. Finally, to prevent the contralateral lung from drowning, lung isolation is indicated during bronchopulmonary lavage for alveolar proteinosis or cystic fibrosis. However, in modern anesthesia practice, these situations are relatively uncommon and constitute about less than 10% of all thoracic procedures.

10.3.2 Lung Separation

Lung separation can be considered for all other indications of OLV where there is no potential risk of contaminating the dependent lung. All the relative indications for adequate surgical exposure, video-assisted thoracoscopic surgery (VATs) which requires a well collapsed lung for diagnostic and therapeutic procedures, are included in this category [8–10]. Lung separation is considered in the majority of the procedures where OLV is indicated while lung isolation is required only in a minority [11, 12].

10.3.3 Absolute Indications

1. To avoid spillage or contamination from one lung to the other:
   (a) Infection
   (b) Massive hemorrhage
2. To control the distribution of ventilation:
   (a) Broncho-pleural fistula
   (b) Broncho-pleural cutaneous fistula
   (c) Surgical opening of a major conducting airway
   (d) Giant unilateral lung cyst or bulla
   (e) Life-threatening hypoxemia related to unilateral lung disease
3. Unilateral broncho-pulmonary lavage—Pulmonary alveolar proteinosis

10.3.4 Relative Indications

1. Surgical exposure—high priority:
   (a) Thoracoscopy
   (b) Mediastinal exposure
   (c) Thoracic aortic aneurysm
   (d) Upper lobectomy
   (e) Pneumonectomy
2. Surgical exposure—medium or low priority:
   (a) Middle and lower lobectomies
   (b) Sub-segmental resections
   (c) Esophageal resection
   (d) Procedures on the thoracic spine
   (e) Pulmonary edema after cardio-pulmonary bypass
   (f) Hemorrhage following removal of pulmonary emboli
   (g) Severe hypoxemia due to lung disease involving one side

10.4 Selection of Double-Lumen Bronchial Tube

10.4.1 Right-Sided Versus Left-Sided Double-Lumen Tubes

It is recommended to intubate the non-operative bronchus to minimize tube displacement (i.e., a left-sided DLT used for right lung surgery), especially bronchial surgeries [13]. However, there exists a controversy for left-sided lung procedures due to the anatomic variability of the right upper lobe. There is potentially a greater risk of upper lobe obstruction whenever a right-sided DLT is used. This is because the right main bronchus is considerably shorter than the left bronchus, resulting in a narrow margin of safety for the right main bronchus. Also, the difficulty encountered in positioning of the bronchial portion of the right-sided DLT for maintaining adequate lung isolation and adequate ventilation of the right upper lobe bronchus can cause difficulties during surgery, like severe hypoxia that can occur during isolated ventilation of the right lung [14]

In practice, left-sided DLTs are preferred for all lung surgeries by most anesthesiologists due to perceived safety and this is despite the existence of inadequate evidence on actual increased safety, when intraoperative hypoxia, hypercapnia, and high airway pressures are used as criteria [15, 16]. Whenever there is a need for manipulation of the left main stem bronchus, the left-sided DLT is usually withdrawn and repositioned with the bronchial port above the carina. In general, left-sided DLT can be used for all surgeries of the lung except for the surgeries that involve the left main stem bronchus (including sleeve resection) where right-sided DLTs are preferred.

Contraindications for DLT use include anatomic barriers like carinal or bronchial lesions, strictures, vascular compression by aortic aneurysm, and aberrant bronchus that make positioning difficult or dangerous [17–19]. Right-sided DLTs may be indicated in cases where placement of a left-sided DLT becomes impossible due to tortuosity and compression of the trachea or left main stem bronchus. For patients with special conditions and unusual anatomic variability, newly designed DLTs are used [20].

10.4.2 Size of Double-Lumen Tube

The size that provides near-complete seal of the bronchial lumen without cuff inflation is the ideal size of a DLT. For a left-sided DLT, the proper size should have a bronchial tip that is 1–2 mm smaller than the patient's left bronchus diameter so as to allow space for the deflated bronchial cuff. The mucosal damage caused by the high inflation pressures of a smaller tube are nearly comparable to those caused by forcing a larger tube into a smaller bronchus [21]. Choosing the correct size of tube every time is nearly impossible even when using height- and weight-based DLT size estimates [22].

10.4.2.1 Based on Sex and Height of the Patient

SIZE 35 Fr is recommended for females of height less than 160 cm, 37Fr for females of height more than 160 cm, 39 Fr for males of height less than 170 cm, and a 41 Fr for males of height more than 170 cm [8].

One can also use a formula based on height to decide the optimal depth of insertion for left-sided DLTs. Depth of insertion in cm [at incisors] =12+patient height [cm]/10

Studies have shown that in an average Asian population, DLT size cannot be predicted from the height and hence alternative methods should be used. We use one size smaller than that calculated by the height of the patient.

Brodsky and Lemmens [10], based on their vast experience of 1170 left-sided DLT placements, found that the average depth of left-sided DLT placement in a 170 cm tall man or woman was 28–29 cm, with a change of approximately ±1.0 cm for each 10 cm change in height

10.4.2.2 Based on Radiological Studies

Tracheal and bronchial dimensions can also be measured directly from the chest radiograph or chest CT scan. Diameter of the left bronchus can be measured in almost 75% of the patients using a chest radiograph. In conditions where direct measurement of the left main bronchus is not possible or difficult, the left bronchial diameter can be estimated accurately by multiplying the tracheal width by 0.68 (direct proportional relationship between width of the left bronchus and trachea) [23].

10.4.2.3 A Flexible Fiberoptic Bronchoscope (FFB)

An FFB can be passed through the bronchial lumen to assess the appropriate placement of the DLT during insertion (Table 10.1). The common

Table 10.1 Table comparing ease of insertion of various sizes of flexible fibreoptic bronchoscope in DLT of various sizes

FFB OD size (mm)	DLT size (F)	Fit of FFB inside DLT
5.6	All sizes	Does not fit
	41	Passes easily
	39	Moderately easy to pass
4.9	37	Tight fitting, requiring lubricant
	35	Does not fit
3.6–4.2	All sizes	Easily passes in all except 26,28,32
Approximately 2.0–2.8	All sizes	Special arrangements are needed by most operating rooms to obtain this size FFB (only 2.0 passes through size 26)

practice of fiberoptic bronchoscopy has lessened the risk of undetected distal/proximal placement or migration of the bronchial tip/bronchial cuff.

10.5 Placement of Double-Lumen Tube

There are two ways of placing a double-lumen tube:

1. Blind Technique
2. Direct vision technique

The DLT should be checked and prepared before using. The tracheal cuff (high volume, low pressure) will accommodate approximately 20 ml of air, while the bronchial cuff can accommodate 3 ml of air. After checking cuff integrity, the cuffs should be completely deflated and the tube should be liberally coated with a water-soluble lubricant. The stylet should be lubricated and gently placed into the bronchial lumen and should be slightly withdrawn taking care not to disturb the tube's preformed curvature. Placing DLTs is more difficult as compared with SLTs because DLTs are larger in diameter and length when compared to SLTs. A Macintosh blade and preferably a large blade should be used for tracheal intubation because it provides the largest area for passing the tube. It is important that a DLT should never be forced into position.

10.5.1 Blind Technique

The distal concave curvature of the tube should face anteriorly during the tube insertion. Once the tip of the DLT crosses the vocal cords, the stylet is removed carefully and then the tube is rotated through an angle of 90° (left rotation for left-sided tube and right rotation for right-sided tube). Further advancement of the tube is stopped as soon as resistance is encountered. Resistance to further passage indicates the firm placement of the tube tip in the main stem bronchus. Rotation as well as further advancement of the tube needs to be performed gently and should be performed under direct laryngoscopy to prevent any interference and injury of hypopharyngeal structures. To avoid tracheal or bronchial laceration it is important to remove the stylet. The tracheal cuff is inflated on reaching the desired depth and the DLT is secured. The patient is then connected to the ventilator to commence mechanical ventilation. Care must be taken to ensure that there is no tear or puncture of both the tracheal cuff and endobronchial cuff during intubation. To prevent cuff damage against the teeth during insertion into the oral cavity, the teeth can be covered with a moist swab. The FFB is inserted through the tracheal lumen of the DLT after confirming the proper placement by auscultation and capnography and initiation of ventilation (Fig. 10.2a). The FFB is then advanced further until the carina can be identified. Visualization of the bronchial lumen of the tube entering the appropriate main stem bronchus (Fig. 10.2b) (i.e., for a left-sided DLT, the bronchial lumen should be in the left main stem bronchus) and inflation of the bronchial lumen balloon as it lies just distal to the carina confirm correct placement of the DLT. Some DLTs have an indicator line just above the bronchial cuff that should sit at the level of the carina. Direct visualization ensures that neither the bronchial balloon is herniating over the carina nor that the tracheal cuff of the DLT is encroaching on the carina.

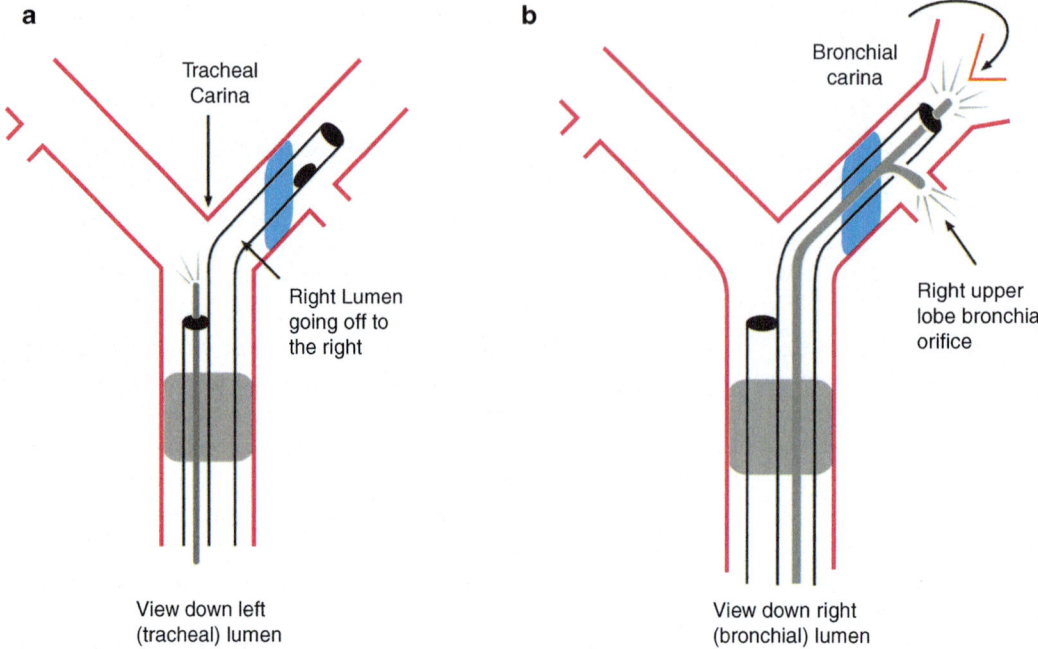

Fig. 10.2 Schematic diagram portrays the use of flexible fibreoptic bronchoscope to determine the precise position of right sided double lumen tube

The determination of right versus left main stem bronchus is done by visualizing the anterior and posterior aspects of the trachea. The tracheal rings, extending throughout the anterior two-thirds of the trachea identify the anterior aspect of the trachea while the membranous component with longitudinal striations identifies the posterior aspect of the trachea. For better placement of an FFB, appropriate use of antisialagogues, suctioning of the DLT, application of lubricating and antifogging agents is done to facilitate manipulation and visualization.

10.5.2 Direct Vision Technique

Here, the FFB is employed as an intubating stylet and is used to guide the bronchial tip of the DLT directly into the appropriate main stem bronchus. The FFB is inserted into the bronchial lumen of the DLT after the bronchial tube tip has passed through the vocal cords, and is slowly advanced down the trachea while maintaining optimal orientation. After identification of the carina and the right and left main stem bronchi, the FFB is advanced into the appropriate main bronchus. The DLT is then threaded over the FFB. The FFB is removed from the bronchial lumen after confirming that the bronchial tip is unobstructed and the tip is proximal to the secondary bronchial branches. The FFB is then inserted in the tracheal lumen to confirm the correct placement of the bronchial cuff position and also to confirm that the lumen of the tracheal tube of the DLT is not resting on the carina. These manoeuvres take time and expertise to perform which may be of concern because this extra time can cause temporary desaturation in some patients having poor pulmonary reserve.

10.6 Confirmation of Proper Placement

Once the tube is in the correct position, a sequence of steps should be performed to confirm its placement:

1. First the tracheal cuff is inflated, and equal ventilation of both the lungs is checked. The breath sounds may not be equal, when the opening of the tracheal lumen is in a main

stem bronchus or at the carina or when the tube is too far down. Withdrawing the tube by 2–3 cm usually restores equal breath sounds.
2. In the second step, the right side is clamped (in the case of the left-sided tube) and the right cap is removed from the connector. This is followed by the slow inflation of the bronchial cuff to prevent any air leak from the bronchial lumen into the tracheal lumen around the bronchial cuff. Inflation of the bronchial cuff should be done to make a seal and may require 2–4 ml of air.
3. In the third step, the clamp is removed and the ventilation of both the lungs is checked with both cuffs inflated. This is to ensure that the bronchial cuff is not too far in, with the bronchial tip in one of the lobe openings.
4. In the final step, each side is clamped selectively and observed for the absence of movement and breath sounds on the clamped side. The ventilated side should have clear breath sounds, and compliant chest movements. If peak airway pressure during two-lung ventilation is 20 cm H_2O, it should not exceed by more than 10 cm H_2O for the same V_T during OLV. If it is more, then one should check tube placement.

FOB is the most important advance in checking and confirming the proper placement of a DLT (Fig. 10.3). Malpositions which are not clinically significant are most commonly missed by the clinician. Smith and colleagues [24] demonstrated that 48% of disposable DLTs whose position was assessed to be in the correct position by conventional auscultation and physical examination by the clinician, on FOB were found to be malpositioned. The bronchoscope is initially introduced through the tracheal lumen to visualize the carina and to ensure that the bronchial cuff is not herniated. The bronchoscope is then passed through the bronchial lumen to identify the left upper lobe bronchial orifices in the left DLT. When using a right-sided DLT, passing the bronchoscope through the right upper lobe ventilating slot of the DLT, the orifice of the right upper lobe bronchus is identified.

It is necessary to recheck the DLT placement when the patient is repositioned, because movement of the tube is common. Airway simulation, and mannequins are found to be useful for training in the use of FFBs [25].

10.7 Malpositioning and Complications

10.7.1 Problems of Malposition of the Double-Lumen Tube

1. At times the DLT may be accidentally misdirected to the opposite side of the desired main stem bronchus. In such a case, there will be collapse of the lung that is opposite to the side of the connector clamp. Inadequate separation, increased airway pressures, and DLT instability usually occur. Tracheal or bronchial lacerations may take place because of the morphology of the DLT curvatures. Ventilation to the right upper lobe is obstructed when a left-sided DLT is inserted into the right main stem bronchus. Therefore, it is essential to recognize and correct such a malposition at the earliest.
2. The DLT may have passed too deep into either main stem bronchus (Fig. 10.4). In such case, breath sounds are not audible over the contralateral side. This is corrected by withdrawing the tube so that the tracheal lumen is just above the carina.

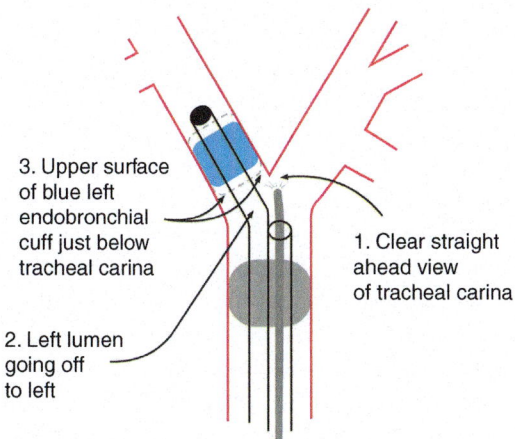

Fig. 10.3 Flexible fibreoptic bronchoscope down the right lumen to determine the precise position of left sided double lumen tube

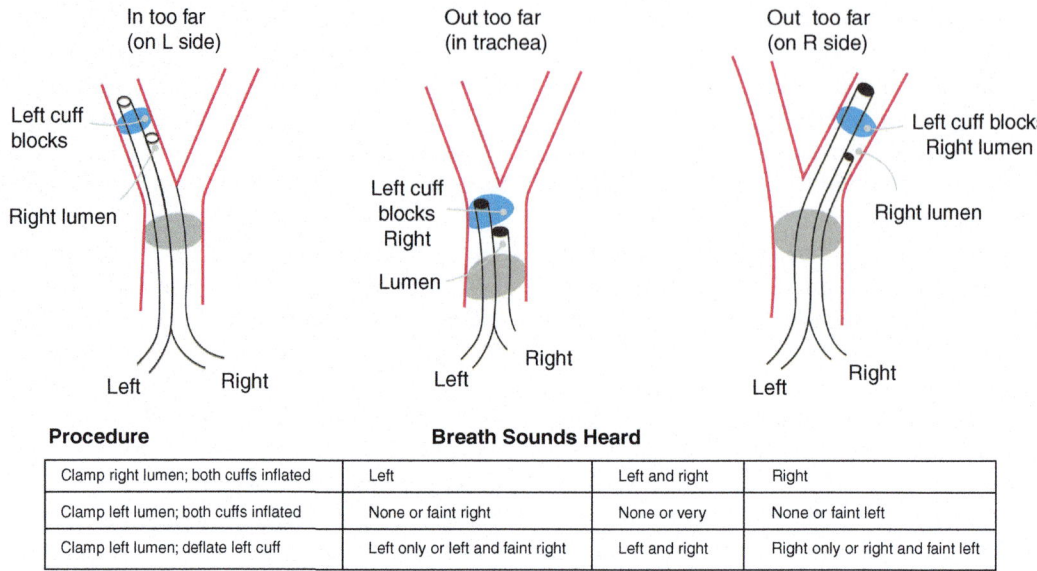

Procedure	Breath Sounds Heard		
Clamp right lumen; both cuffs inflated	Left	Left and right	Right
Clamp left lumen; both cuffs inflated	None or faint right	None or very	None or faint left
Clamp left lumen; deflate left cuff	Left only or left and faint right	Left and right	Right only or right and faint left

Three major malpositions involving a whole lung are possible for a left-sided, double-lumen tube. The tube can be in too far on the left (i.e., both lumens are in the left main stem bronchus), out too far (i.e., both lumens are in the trachea), or down the right main stem bronchus (i.e., at least the left lumen is in the right main stem bronchus). In each of these malpositions, the left cuff, when fully inflated, can completely block the right lumen. Inflation and deflation of the left cuff while the left lumen is clamped creates a breath sound differential diagnosis of tube malposition. L, left; R, right.

Fig. 10.4 Left sided double lumen tube malpositions

3. The DLT may not be inserted far enough so that the bronchial lumen opening is left above the carina. In this position, good breath sounds are heard bilaterally when ventilating through the bronchial lumen. No breath sounds are heard when ventilating through the tracheal lumen because the inflated bronchial cuff obstructs the gas flow from the tracheal lumen. This is corrected by deflating the cuff followed by rotating and advancing the DLT into the desired main stem bronchus.
4. Occlusion of the right upper lobe orifice by a right-sided DLT may occur. The mean distance from the carina to the right upper lobe orifice is 2.1 ± 0.7 cm in women and 2.3 ± 0.7 cm in men. For right-sided DLTs, the ventilating slot in the side of the bronchial catheter must overlie the right upper lobe orifice to facilitate ventilation of this lobe. However, the margin of safety which ranges from 1 to 8 mm is extremely small [26]. Hence, dislocation of the DLT during surgical manipulation should be avoided as it is difficult to ensure proper ventilation to the right upper lobe.
5. On the left side, due to a longer bronchus, tube placement is easier and care should be taken to visualize the openings of both upper and lower lobes.

10.7.2 Complications

Bronchial cuff herniation followed by bronchial lumen obstruction may occur when excessive volumes are used to inflate the cuff. It can herniate over the tracheal carina, and can obstruct ventilation to the right main stem bronchus by obstructing the inlet in the case of a left-sided DLT.

Tracheal laceration or rupture is another complication with DLTs. Bronchial rupture due to overinflation of the bronchial cuff, inappropriate positioning, and intraoperative dislocation were observed with the Robertshaw tube and the disposable DLT [27]. Hence it is important to assess the bronchial cuff pressure and it should be decreased if the cuff is found to be overinflated. In cases where absolute separation of the lungs is not required, the bronchial cuff should be deflated and then reinflated slowly to prevent excessive pressure on the bronchial walls. Unless the lung separation is absolutely required, it is necessary to deflate the bronchial cuff during any repositioning of the patient. Another potential complication with the use of DLTs is airway trauma and rupture of the membranous part of the trachea or the bronchus [28]. An oversized DLT or an undersized DLT that migrates distally into the lobar bronchus and when the main (i.e., tracheal) body of the DLT comes into the bronchus, it can produce lacerations or rupture of the airway. Airway damage during the use of DLTs can present as an unexpected air leak.

When the lung deflation is not completely achieved even if a DLT is in the optimal position, a suction catheter should be passed to the side where lung collapse is supposed to occur to expedite the lung deflation. Then the suction catheter must be removed to avoid including it in a suture line. Tension pneumothorax can develop in the dependent, ventilated lung during OLV. Bilateral bullae or volutrauma can occur due to ventilation with high tidal volume [29].

Sore throat and temporary hoarseness are the most common minor complications. Laryngeal and bronchial injury, tracheo-bronchial tree disruption [30, 31], suturing of DLT to the thoracic structures, and injury to the vocal cord are the other complications that have been reported [32, 33].

10.8 Exchanging the Double-Lumen Tube for a Single-Lumen Tube

10.8.1 Procedure

If the patient has to remain intubated postoperatively, the DLT needs to be replaced with an SLT at the end of the surgical procedure.

Replacement of a DLT with an SLT must be performed with great caution as it can be life-threatening. Before replacing a DLT with an SLT, it must be ensured that the patient is well pre-oxygenated and paralyzed and thorough suctioning has been done. The difficult airway cart should be at hand. An SLT with a stylet is kept ready.

Direct laryngoscopy is performed, preferably using a Miller blade to control the epiglottis. Under direct vision the DLT tracheal cuff should be deflated and the DLT is retracted once the laryngoscope is positioned. The sight of the larynx should not be lost and the laryngoscope blade should not be repositioned while removing the DLT. Once the SLT is beyond the cords, its cuff is inflated, and the tube position is confirmed.

10.8.2 Airway Exchange Catheters

Tube exchange can be done using the airway exchange catheters (AECs). An AEC is placed through the existing DLT followed by the removal of the DLT. The tracheal or bronchial port may be used. Once the DLT is removed, the SLT is guided into the trachea over the AEC. After keeping the SLT in place the AEC is removed. The SLT cuff is then inflated, and the ventilation commenced. Optimal SLT placement is confirmed by capnography [33].

10.8.2.1 Advantages of DLT
- A DLT allows for independent ventilation of each lung. Prevention and management of desaturation are easier with DLTs. This is because CPAP is easy to implement on the nondependent lung while the opposite lung is normally ventilated.
- A larger lumen allows easy access into each mainstem bronchus making suctioning and FOB insertion easier.
- Egress of gases through a DLT and lung deflation for surgical exposure are easier. Improved cuff seals and the solid structure of the DLTs prevent easy dislodgment after it is properly positioned.

10.8.2.2 Disadvantages of DLT
- As compared to an SLT, intubation and proper placement of a DLT may be more difficult, but can be easily performed after adequate training.
- For patients with difficult airway anatomy [34], intubation is even more complex and a bougie meant for a DLT can be used.

- Placement of a DLT can be difficult in cases of a distorted or compressed trachea-bronchial tree, because of the size and rigidity of DLT. In such cases intubation, with the help of an FOB is desirable.
- The larger size of DLT can cause significant airway damage during placement or when it is left in place for a long period; therefore, selection of a proper size is paramount.
- DLTs are often exchanged for SLTs in the ICU because of some management difficulties associated with weaning and pulmonary toileting. However, this process of exchanging can be tedious, especially in the presence of airway edema.
- Familiairty with the DLT anatomy is required to prevent errors in ventilation and management.
- Training in the use of FOB is required for DLT placement.

10.8.2.3 Contraindications for DLT placement

1. Unstable patient
2. Where lung isolation is not mandatory
3. Tracheal or bronchial tumors
4. Anticipated technical difficulty in placing the DLT
5. Small patients in whom the DLT will be oversized

10.9 Single-Lumen Tubes

The use of a DLT may be difficult or not possible in some cases that require lung isolation. In such challenging instances, it will be more appropriate to use either a modified SLT with integrated blockers (i.e., the Univent tube) or to use blockers with a standard SLT (e.g., young patient, unstable patient, anatomical distortion).

10.9.1 Circumstances Where Use of SLT Is Advantageous and Can Give Lung Isolation

1. Lung isolation can be challenging in patients having difficult airway anatomy as it is nearly impossible to place a conventional DLT [35].
2. The safest technique to isolate the involved lung in circumstances where the SLT is in place and the patient has developed significant airway edema or when the patient is placed in the prone position or lateral position and the surgeon is requiring lung isolation mid procedure, would be to use bronchial blockers.
3. DLT insertion may be very difficult in patients with an SLT in situ and have developed traumatized or bloody airways, due to the poor visibility of airway anatomy through an FOB.
4. In young patients, it is often not possible to place a DLT. Bronchial blockers can be accommodated in pediatric size ETTs as small as 5.0 mm. "Main stemming" of the ETT, where we intentionally perform bronchial intubation of the ETT, can be used to achieve lung isolation in pediatric cases requiring ETT less than 5.0 mm.
5. At times selective blockade of specific lung segments may be required. In such cases, the bronchial blocker can be easily positioned into the desired lung segment to be isolated [36, 37].

10.9.2 Disadvantages of Using Single Lumen Tubes

1. Lung deflation
   - Deflating the selectively blocked lung is very slow when bronchial blockers are used. This is because the gas gets trapped in the isolated lung and the only way of removal of this gas is through reabsorption.
   - With the use of the Uninvent tube, deflation of lung is slightly faster through the small lumen of the blocker. Suction can also be applied to the lumen of the Uninvent tube blocker to facilitate lung deflation.
   - Ventilating the lungs with 100% O_2 for a few minutes before inflating the bronchial cuff is done to accelerate lung deflation. By doing this, lung deflation is accelerated as the O_2 is more rapidly reabsorbed compared to air.
   - If the patient's lung functions are conducive, the ventilator circuit can be temporarily disconnected and both the lungs are left

for spontaneous deflation. The cuff of the bronchial blocker is then inflated, and the ventilation is resumed for initiation of SLV.

2. Removal of secretion
   - With bronchial blockers, suctioning the blocked lung beyond the length of the bronchial blocker cannot be done while performing lung isolation.
   - Suctioning the non-blocked lung can be easily done, but due care must be taken to avoid the displacement of bronchial blocker from its final position.
3. Damage to bronchial mucosa
   - The cuffs of bronchial blockers and Univent tube blockers are high pressure and low volume.
   - Prolonged bronchial cuff inflation can cause mucosal ischemia with potentially irreversible ischemic damage. Bronchial cuff should be deflated at the earliest, as soon as the requirement for lung isolation ceases. The technique of "just-seal" bronchial cuff inflation volumes has been encouraged, to reduce mucosal ischemia and damage [38, 39].
   - The bronchial blocker cuff pressure can constantly change with the changes in compliance of the ventilated lung during surgery.
4. Management of desaturation
   - If desaturation occurs during SLV, it is necessary to ensure 100% O_2 to the patient. Adequate ventilation as well as perfusion should be maintained, and tube and blocker placement should be verified using FOB.
   - The nondependent lung cannot receive CPAP as given in SLV with DLT. There is significant occlusion of the luminal space of SLT with the presence of bronchial blocker.
   - As a last option the bronchial cuff can be deflated but this would result in shifting of the bronchial blocker from its location due to lack of stability and will require FOB confirmation each time. Because of this technical issue, full or intermittent-partial inflation of the isolated lung may be cumbersome while using bronchial blockers.

10.10 Univent Tubes

10.10.1 Anatomy

- The Univent tube is a silastic SLT having a built-in chamber for the positioning and advancement of the integrated blocker.
- The integrated Univent blocker has a small lumen along its entire length; this serves two functions. Firstly, it facilitates lung deflation, and secondly, some amount of limited suctioning is possible through it.
- The distal tip of the blocker has a small balloon, and the proximal end of the blocker contains a lumen cap. This cap has to be engaged when the blocker balloon is deflated, for lung ventilation; failing to do this will result in circuit leak. Univent tubes are available in many sizes, all designated by internal lumen size.
- The outer size of the Univent tube is much larger compared to a similarly designated SLT due to thicker tube wall and the presence of an integrated chamber.

10.10.2 Positioning

- It is necessary to check and deflate the cuffs of the bronchial blocker and the main tube.
- The cuffs of both the bronchial blocker and the Univent tube should be checked and fully deflated.
- The Univent tube has to be prepared prior to placement. This includes removal of the proximal and distal tension wires which maintain the shape of the Univent tube during storage.
- The distal tip of the bronchial blocker is shaped like a hockey stick. The distal tip of the bronchial blocker is then retracted into the blocker chamber of the Univent tube to flush the distal tip with the main tube.
- The Univent tube is then passed into the trachea. With the tracheal cuff placed just distal to the cords, the tube must be secured so that a distance between the distal tip of the main tube and the carina is at least 2–3 cm. This will provide enough room for

- manipulation of the bronchial blocker once it is advanced beyond the main tube.
- This is followed by inflation and securing of the main tube cuff to maintain and manipulate the curved shape of the blocker as it advances beyond the tip of the main tube.
- With the use of FOB, the blocker portion of the tube is advanced while maintaining the main tube position under vision.
- The blocker is then placed into the appropriate main stem bronchus by advancing the blocker with a clockwise or a counterclockwise rotation. The entire Univent tube can be rotated in the desired direction if this maneuver is not sufficient to place the blocker in the appropriate bronchus. After correct placement the distance on the blocker should be noted and marked. The cuff present at the proximal end of the blocker should be engaged; else it will result in circuit leak.
- When lung isolation is desired, inflation of the blocker cuff under FOB guidance and the disengagement of proximal cap of the blocker is done to aid in lung deflation.
- Blind placement of the blocker usually results in trauma to the tracheobronchial tree and is often unsuccessful and can lead to complications like bleeding and possibly tension pneumothorax.

10.11 Endobronchial Blockers

- Lung separation can also be achieved with the use of bronchial blockers. They can be placed through a conventional SLT.
- Blockers have a lumen alongside its entire length to permit airway suctioning distal to the blocker tip and for insufflation of oxygen through the lumen.
- The blocker balloon requires a high distension pressure, because of which it can easily slip into the trachea from the bronchus during the change in patient position or surgical manipulation. Slipping of the bronchial blocker will result in ventilation obstruction and loss of the seal between the two lungs. This would lead to a life-threatening situation if the lung isolation was performed to prevent spillage of pus, blood, or fluid from bronchopulmonary lavage.

10.11.1 Indications for the Use of Endobronchial Blockers

1. Patients with difficult airways:
   (a) Patients with history of having undergone any laryngeal or any pharyngeal surgery
   (b) Patients who are tracheotomized
   (c) Patients having a distorted bronchial anatomy (e.g., aneurysmal compression, intrabronchial tumor)
2. Used along with SLT in unstable patients who require postoperative ventilation
3. Patients requiring naso-tracheal intubation
4. Patients having cervical immobility or kyphoscoliosis
5. Special management circumstances:
   (a) Segmental lobe blockade in patients who cannot tolerate one-lung ventilation
   (b) Small adults, pediatric patients
   (c) Patients who are requiring intraoperative lung isolation
   (d) Patients arriving intubated from the intensive care unit to the operating room and change of tube to DLT is not preferred due to possible desaturation or due to significant airway edema

10.12 Types

10.12.1 Coaxial Stand-Alone Endotracheal Blockers

10.12.1.1 Arndt Endobronchial Blocker

- The Cohen Flexitip endobronchial blocker and Arndt blocker were designed for usage through an SLT with the help of a small-sized (4.0-mm) FOB [40–43].
- The Arndt Endobronchial Blocker (Cook Critical Care) was introduced to address the common problem of misdirected FOB for insertion of blocker. It is a wire guided

catheter having a loop snare to hold the FOB during insertion (Fig. 10.5).
- A fiberscope is inserted through the loop snare of the Arndt endobronchial blocker and is guided into the desired bronchus. After the FFB is placed in the desired tip position, the loop snare is released to free the FFB and the blocker is advanced to the tip of the FFB, placing the bronchial blocker in the appropriate position.
- It has a hollow lumen which allows suctioning to aid in the collapse of the lung and can be used to insufflate oxygen into the nondependent lung.
- The set has a multiport adapter through which uninterrupted ventilation can be provided during placement of the blocker under FOB guidance (Fig. 10.6).
- It is available in two sizes: a 7F—adults and a 5F—pediatric size (Table 10.2).
- Drawback of the Arndt blocker is that it is blindly advanced over the FFB into the desired main bronchus. Distal tip of the blocker may get entangled at the carina or at the Murphy eye of the SLT.

10.12.1.2 Cohen Flexitip Endobronchial Blocker

- The blocker has an inbuilt rotating wheel that deflects the distal soft tip by more than 90° and can easily be directed into the desired bronchus (Fig. 10.7). The directional tip makes placement of this device a lot easier when compared to the placement of the Arndt bronchial blocker.
- The blocker cuff is a high-volume, low-pressure balloon. Its pear shape provides an adequate seal of the bronchus. Like with all blockers cuff should be inflated under vision by FOB

10.12.1.3 Uniblocker

- The Uniblocker is essentially the same in design as the blocker that is used in the Univent tube inside the integrated chamber, but a Uniblocker can be used as an independent blocker through a standard ETT.
- Uniblocker has a preformed bend to help in insertion of the blocker into the desired bronchus.

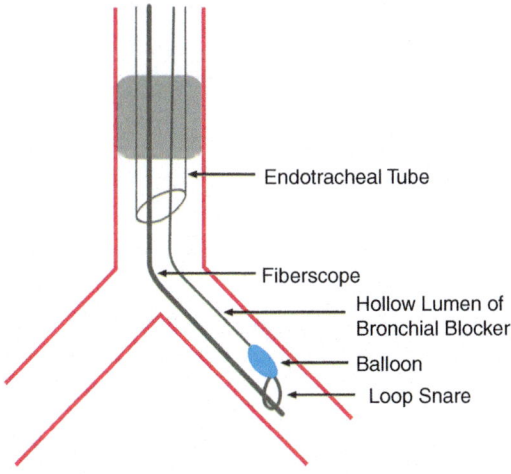

Fig. 10.5 ARNDT endobronchial blocker

Fig. 10.6 Multi port adapter for ARNDT blocker

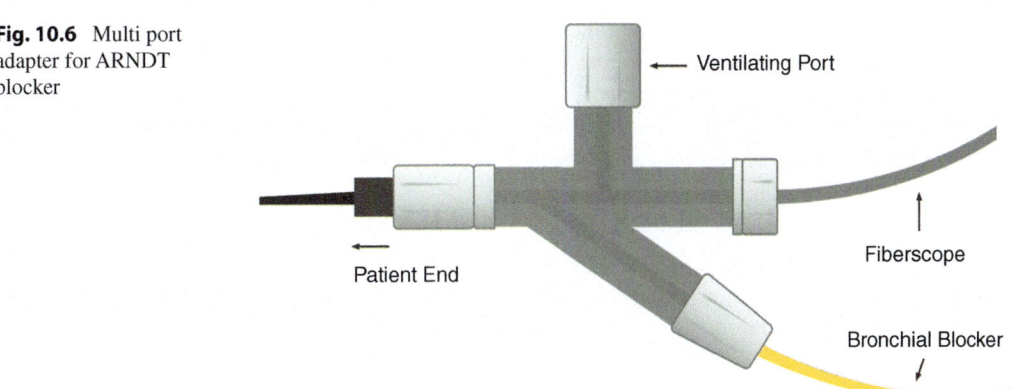

Table 10.2 Characteristics of endobronchial blockers

Characteristics	Arndt blocker	Cohen blocker	Uniblocker	EZ-Blocker
Size	9F, 7F, 5F	9F	9F, 5F	7F
Feature aiding in guidance	Wire loop to snare the FFB	Has a deflecting tip	Has a prefixed bend	Double-lumen bifurcated
Recommended size of ETT (mm)	9F-8 mm ETT 7F-7 mm ETT 5F-4.5 mm ETT	8mm ETT	8mm ETT	8mm ETT
Central lumen	1.8 mm	1.8 mm	2.0 mm	1.4 mm
Murphy eye	Present in 9F device only	Yes	No	No
Disadvantages	Bronchial blocker not visualized during insertion	Expensive	No steering mechanism; it has a prefixed bend	Lumen is very small; impossible to suction

BB, bronchial blocker; *ETT*, endotracheal tube; *FFB*, flexible fiberoptic bronchoscope

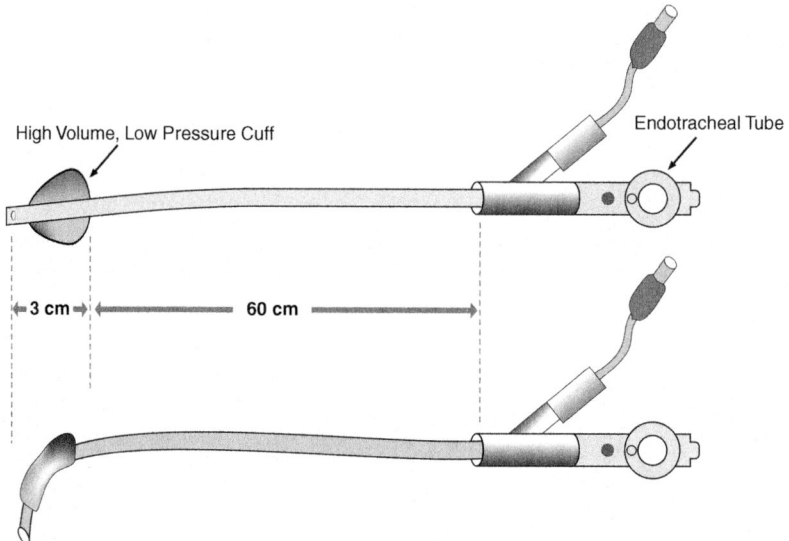

Fig. 10.7 Cohen flexitip endobronchial blocker

10.12.1.4 EZ-Blocker

- It is a 7F, disposable endobronchial blocker used in selective lung ventilation.
- It has a Y-shaped bifurcation at its distal end, and both the limbs of the bifurcation have an individual inflatable cuff and a central lumen.
- It can be inserted through any standard ETT; both the distal cuffed ends are placed into each of the main stem bronchus.
- The desired lung can be isolated by inflating the EZ blocker's balloon on the corresponding side of the main stem bronchus under direct bronchoscopic visualization.
- The clinical experience and evidence with this device is still limited considering it is a new addition to the bronchial blocker family.

10.12.2 Fogarty Embolectomy Catheters

Any device having a balloon-tipped catheter can be efficiently used as a bronchial blocker [44]. Fogarty embolectomy catheters are the most commonly used devices [45].

10.12.2.1 Fogarty Catheter

- The Fogarty catheter has a rigid wire stylet. The wire facilitates the creation of a hockey-stick bend at the distal end, this facilitates directional control of the distal blocker tip.
- When the catheter is positioned under FFB guidance, the stylet is removed. The balloon is inflated until the desired bronchi lumen is occluded under FOB guidance, then the catheter is firmly secured to the ETT.
- The disadvantage of the Fogarty catheter is its inability to suck out the trapped air or secretions or insufflate oxygen distal to the cuff.

10.12.3 Paraxial Endotracheal Blockers

- Placing the bronchial blocker paraxially outside the SLT has the major advantage in allowing the blockers to be placed even with smaller ETTs as the blocker will not share the ETT lumen (Fig. 10.8). There is no opportunity for blocker and the FFB to get entangled within the ETT lumen as the FOB will be inside the lumen and the blocker will be outside the ETT.
- Some of the disadvantages of the para-tube technique include the need to perform laryngoscopy for placing the bronchial blocker into the trachea after ETT placement, the need to deflate the tracheal cuff of ETT while positioning the bronchial blocker on the ETT side, and the potential fear of rupturing the ETT cuff during the bronchial blocker manipulation. Due to these disadvantages, a coaxial placement is more commonly recommended when the ETT lumen size is not an issue.

10.13 Conclusion

The anesthesiologist performing a lung isolation technique should have a good understanding of the underlying primary pathology, knowledge of respiratory physiology, and be well versed in

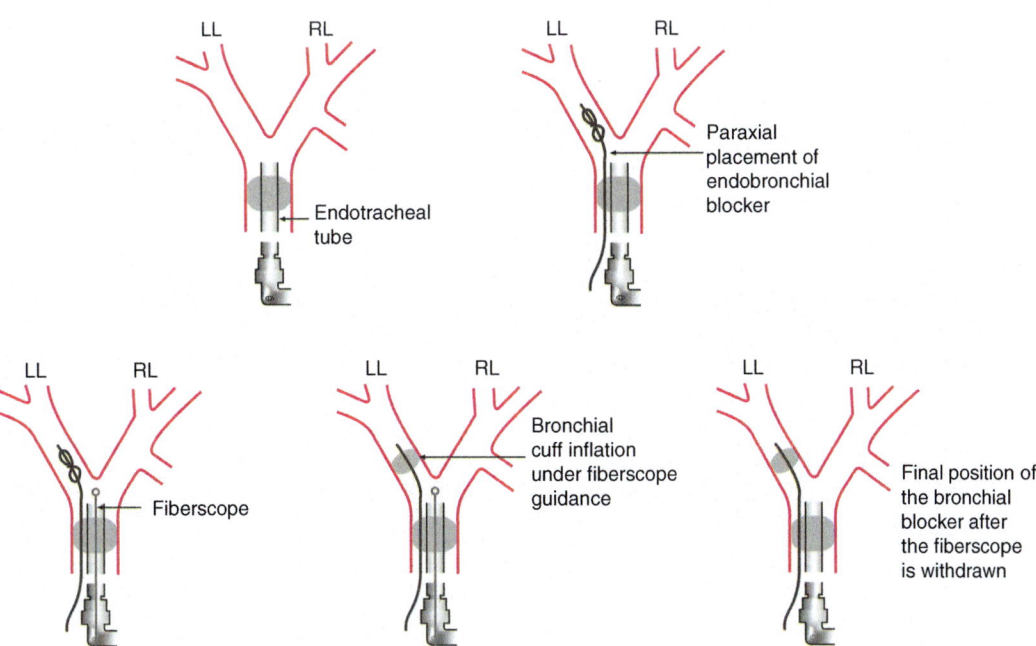

Fig. 10.8 Paraxial placement of endobronchial blocker

planning and executing the most appropriate type of lung isolation technique for the patient needs and surgical exposure.

10.14 Clinical Pearls

1. DLTs are advantageous as they provide bilateral independent lung ventilation, bronchial suctioning, lung deflation, and can switch from one-lung ventilation to both lung ventilation expeditiously.
2. Placement of a DLT can be challenging with distorted or compressed tracheobronchial tree, due to its size and lack of flexibility and intubation over an FOB is desirable in these cases.
3. Selection of a proper size is of paramount importance as a larger size of DLT can contribute to airway damage during placement and when the DLT has to be left in situ for a long period.
4. Bronchial blocker or DLT, the choice of the type of lung separation device selected to provide SLV depends on the clinical circumstances, the anesthesiologist's comfort with a particular device, risk–benefit ratio, and the patient safety.
5. DLTs are often exchanged for SLTs prior to shifting patient to the ICU because of some management difficulties associated with weaning and pulmonary toileting.
6. Postoperative airway edema is inevitable in some cases, and many a times need postoperative ventilation. In such patients replacing a DLT with an SLT postoperatively should be over an airway exchange catheter.
7. Self-sealing diaphragm in elbow connection is essential for continued ventilation during FOB guided DLT or bronchial blocker placement.
8. It is always better to inflate the bronchial cuff under vision by FOB to confirm correct placement and adequate seal.
9. Bronchial blocker may be used par-axially or co-axially for lung isolation.
10. Bronchial blocker group has higher number of cuff dislocations.

References

1. Campos JH. Progress in lung separation. Thorac Surg Clin. 2005;15:71.
2. American Society of Anesthesiologists. Practice guidelines for management of the difficult airway: an updated report. Anesthesiology. 2003;98: 1269–77.
3. Brodsky JB, Adkins MO, Gaba DM. Bronchial cuff pressures of double-lumen tubes. Anesth Analg. 1989;69:608–10.
4. Cohen JA, Denisco RA, Richards TS, et al. Hazardous placement of a Robertshaw-type endobronchial tube. Anesth Analg. 1986;65:100–1.
5. Marasigan BL, Sheinbaum R, Hammer GB, et al. Separation of the two lungs. Benumof and Hagberg airway management; 2013. p. 549–68.
6. Neto PP. Bronchial cuff pressure of endobronchial double-lumen tubes. Anesth Analg. 1990;71:209.
7. Saracoglu A, Saracoglu KT. VivaSight: a new era in the evolution of tracheal tubes. J Clin Anesth. 2016;33:442–9.
8. Slinger PD, Campos JH. Anesthesia for thoracic surgery. Miller's anesthesia, 7th edn. Churchill Livingstone, Philadelphia; 2009.
9. Yasumoto M, Higa K, Nitahara K, et al. Optimal depth of insertion of left-sided double lumen endobronchial tubes cannot be predicted from body height in below average-sized adult patients. Eur J Anaesthesiol. 2006;23:42–4.
10. Brodsky JB, Lemmens HJ. Left double lumen tubes: clinical experience with 1,170 patients. J Cardiothorac Vasc Anesth. 2003;17:289–98.
11. Redford D, Kim A, Barber B. Transesophageal echocardiography for the intraoperative evaluation of a large anterior mediastinal mass. Anesth Analg. 2006;103:578–9.
12. Brooker RF, Zvara DA. Mediastinal mass diagnosed with intraoperative transesophageal echocardiography. J Cardiothorac Vasc Anesth. 2007;21:257–8.
13. Slinger PD, Susssa S, Triolet W. Predicting arterial oxygenation during one-lung anaesthesia. Can J Anaesth. 1992;39:1030–5.
14. Slinger P, Johnston M. Preoperative evaluation of the thoracic surgery patient. Semin Anesth. 2002;21:168.
15. Ehrenfeld JM, Mulvoy W, Sandberg WS. Performance comparison of right- and left-sided double-lumen tubes among infrequent users. J Cardiothorac Vasc Anesth. 2010;24:598–601.
16. Ehrenfeld JM, Walsh JL, Sandberg WS. Right- and left-sided Mallinckrodt double-lumen tubes have identical clinical performance. Anesth Analg. 2008;106:1847–52.
17. Cohen JA, Denisco RA, Richards TS, et al. Hazardous placement of a Robertshaw-type endobronchial tube. Anesth Analg. 1986;65:100–1.
18. Brodsky JB, Benumof JL, Ehrenwerth J, et al. Depth of placement of left double-lumen endobronchial tubes. Anesth Analg 1991;73:570–2.

19. Iwamoto T, Takasugi Y, Hiramatsu K, et al. Three-dimensional CT image analysis of a tracheal bronchus in a patient undergoing cardiac surgery with one-lung ventilation. J Anesth. 2009;23:260–5.
20. Hagihira S, Takashina M, Mashimo T. Application of a newly designed right-sided, double-lumen endobronchial tube in patients with a very short right mainstem bronchus. Anesthesiology 2008; 109:565–8.
21. Hansen TB, Watson CB. Tracheobronchial trauma secondary to a Carlens tube. Presented at the Society of Cardiovascular Anesthesiologists 5th annual meeting, San Diego, CA; 1983.
22. Benumof JL, Partridge BL, Salvatierra C, et al. Margin of safety in positioning modern double-lumen endotracheal tubes. Anesthesiology. 1987;67:729–38.
23. Brodsky JB, Lemmens HJM. Tracheal width and left double-lumen tube size: a formula to estimate left-bronchial width. J Clin Anesth. 2005;17:267.
24. Smith GB, Hirsch NP, Ehrenwerth J. Placement of double-lumen endobronchial tubes: correlation between clinical impressions and bronchoscopic findings. Br J Anaesth. 1986;58:1317–20.
25. McKenna MJ, Wilson RS, Botelho RJ. Right upper lobe obstruction with right-sided double-lumen endobronchial tubes: a comparison of two tube types. J Cardiothorac Anesth. 1988;2:734–40.
26. Benumof JL, Partridge BL, Salvatierra C, et al. Margin of safety in positioning modern double-lumen endotracheal tubes. Anesthesiology. 1987;67:729.
27. Thomas V, Neustein SM. Tracheal laceration after the use of an airway exchange catheter for double-lumen tube placement. J Cardiothorac Vasc Anesth. 2007;21:718.
28. Wagner DL, Gammage GW, Wong ML. Tracheal rupture following the insertion of a disposable double-lumen endotracheal tube. Anesthesiology. 1985;63:698.
29. Yüceyar L, Kaynak K, Canturk E, et al. Bronchial rupture with a left-sided polyvinylchloride double-lumen tube. Acta Anaesthesiol Scand 2003; 47:622.
30. Weng W, DeCrosta DJ, Zhang H. Tension pneumothorax during one-lung ventilation: a case report. J Clin Anesth. 2002;14:529.
31. Zinga E, Dangoisse M, Lechat JP. Tracheal perforation following double-lumen intubation: a case report. Acta Anaesthesiol Belg. 2010;61:71–4.
32. Read RC, Friday CD, Eason CN. Prospective study of the Robertshaw endobronchial catheter in thoracic surgery. Ann Thorac Surg. 1977;24:156–61.
33. Dryden GE. Circulatory collapse after pneumonectomy (an unusual complication from the use of a Carlens catheter): case report. Anesth Analg. 1977;56:451–2.
34. Heike Knoll H, Stephan Ziegeler S, Jan-Uwe Schreiber JU, et al. Airway injuries after one-lung ventilation: a comparison between double-lumen tube and endobronchial blocker: a randomized, prospective, controlled trial. Anesthesiology. 2006;105:471.
35. Saito S, Dohi S, Tajima K. Failure of double-lumen endobronchial tube placement: congenital tracheal stenosis in an adult. Anesthesiology. 1987;66:83–5.
36. Inoue H, Shohtsu A, Ogawa J, et al. New device for one-lung anesthesia: endotracheal tube with movable blocker. J Thorac Cardiovasc Surg. 1982;83:940–1.
37. Murakawa T, Ito N, Fukami T, et al. Application of lobe-selective bronchial blockade against airway bleeding. Asian Cardiovasc Thorac Ann. 2010;18:483–5.
38. Brodsky JB, Adkins MO, Gaba DM. Bronchial cuff pressures of double-lumen tubes. Anesth Analg. 1989;69:608–10.
39. Neto PP. Bronchial cuff pressure of endobronchial double-lumen tubes. Anesth Analg 1990; 71:209.
40. Cohen E. The Cohen Flextip Endobronchial Blocker: an alternative to a double lumen tube. Anesth Analg. 2005;101:1877–9.
41. Campos JH, Kernstine KH. A comparison of a left-sided Broncho-Cath with the torque control blocker Univent and the wire-guided blocker. Anesth Analg. 2003;96:283–9.
42. Campos JH. Progress in lung separation. Thorac Surg Clin. 2005;15:71–83.
43. Narayanaswamy M, McRae K, Slinger P, et al. Choosing a lung isolation device for thoracic surgery: a randomized trial of three bronchial blockers versus double-lumen tubes. Anesth Analg. 2009;108:1097–101.
44. Ginsberg RJ. New technique for one-lung anesthesia using an endobronchial blocker. J Thorac Cardiovasc Surg. 1981;82:542–6.
45. Vale R. Selective bronchial blocking in a small child: case report. Br J Anaesth. 1969;41:453–4.

Ventilation Strategies for Thoracic Surgery

11

Nitin Sethi

11.1 Introduction

One-lung ventilation (OLV) is essential during thoracic surgery to allow a good surgical access and lung isolation [1]. An ideal ventilation strategy during OLV should firstly maintain optimal oxygenation ($SpO_2 > 90\%$) and secondarily, avoid acute lung injury (ALI) [2].

11.1.1 OLV and Hypoxemia

Hypoxemia, defined as an arterial oxygen saturation < 90% or a PaO_2 < 60 mmHg, has an incidence of approximately 10% during OLV [3]. There are multiple factors which contribute to the occurrence of hypoxemia during OLV: (i) creation of intrapulmonary shunts (Qs/Qt) due to blood flow to the non-ventilated, nondependent lung; (ii) hypoventilation of the dependent lung due to mediastinal compression and cranial displacement of the diaphragm, added to it is reduction in functional residual capacity (FRC) due to general anesthesia, overall resulting in lung decruitment; and (iii) high airway pressures during OLV which may accentuate the intrapulmonary shunt [2, 4].

11.1.2 OLV and Acute Lung Injury

The incidence of ALI following thoracic surgery varies from 2% to 4.3% with a mortality rate ranging from 26.5% to 52.5% [2, 4]. Intraoperative ventilator induced lung injury (VILI) is a major contributing factor toward development of ALI following thoracic surgery. Multifactorial causes of VILI during OLV are: (i) use of high tidal volume (V_T) during OLV results in over distention of the alveoli at end inspiration resulting in volutrauma; (ii) high alveolar pressure generated during OLV, i.e., peak airway pressure (Ppeak) > 35–40 cmH_2O or plateau airway pressure (Pplat) > 25 cmH_2O results in barotrauma; and (iii) use of low V_T during OLV results in repeated opening and closing of the alveoli leading to atelectrauma [5, 6]. All the above mentioned factors result in elevation of inflammatory cytokines, interleukin (IL)-6 IL-8 IL-1β, chemokines, and tumor necrosis factor (TNF)-α. Elevated levels of cytokines result in leucocyte migration into the alveoli which causes biotrauma, ultimately resulting in damage to the glycocalyx layer which is the capillary endothelium leading to vascular congestion and alveolar wall thickening. The histological changes mimic those of acute respiratory distress syndrome (ARDS) [7, 8].

N. Sethi (✉)
Institute of Anaesthesiology, Pain and Perioperative Medicine, Sir Ganga Ram Hospital, New Delhi, India

11.2 Management of Ventilation During OLV

The main OLV strategy during thoracic surgery is to provide "protective" lung ventilation based on the "open" lung ventilation concept for ARDS patients. It comprises three key components: use of low V_T, recruitment maneuvers, and application of positive end-expiratory pressure (PEEP) [9]. Use of this strategy prevents repeated opening and closing of the alveoli and keeps them recruited, thereby maintaining gas exchange across the alveolo–capillary membrane which helps in maintaining optimal oxygenation and avoiding ALI. The various ventilation parameters that need to be adjusted for providing optimal OLV are discussed in Table 11.1.

11.2.1 Tidal Volume (V_T)

Use of large V_T was advocated earlier as it was shown to result in end-inspiratory inflation of alveoli, aiding in alveolar recruitment and thereby improving oxygenation. However, excessive V_T can result in elevation of pulmonary vascular resistance (PVR) which leads to increase in intrapulmonary shunt to the non-ventilated lung and thereby worsening oxygenation [10]. Large V_T also results in generation of high Ppeak and both of them are now independent risk factors for developing ALI [11]. In patients receiving OLV with 10 ml/kg V_T, the cytokine levels have been shown to be significantly increased as compared to those receiving 5 ml/kg V_T. Elevated cytokine levels are precursors for developing ALI [5].

Use of 6 ml/kg ideal body weight V_T is recommended during OLV to provide adequate oxygenation while avoiding development of ALI [4]. Furthermore the Ppeak should not exceed 35–40 cmH$_2$O and Pplat limited ≤25 cmH$_2$O. Low V_T ventilation has its own drawbacks, as it can result in FRC falling below the closing capacity thus resulting in increased respiratory dead space and hypercapnia. Compensating for hypercapnia by increasing the respiration rate results in shortening of both inspiratory and expiratory time thereby generating high airway pressures and auto or intrinsic PEEP. Moderate hypercapnia up to PaCO$_2$ ≅ 70 mmHg is well tolerated in majority of the patients and targeting normocapnia by increasing the respiratory rate is not recommended [2]. However, persistent hypercapnia (>70 mmHg) can result in certain adverse effects such as sympathetic stimulation, raised intracranial pressure, cardiac arrhythmias, impaired myocardial contractility, and pulmonary hypertension. Patients who become hemodynamically compromised at elevated carbon dioxide levels will require the use of inotropes [12].

11.2.2 Positive End-Expiratory Pressure (PEEP)

The use of PEEP prevents alveolar collapse as it increases the FRC, thereby maintaining the lung volume above the closing capacity [13]. PEEP has been shown to offset the occurrence of lung injury both during high and low V_T ventilation

Table 11.1 One-lung ventilation strategy

Tidal volume (V_T)	6 ml/kg ideal body weight
Inspired oxygen concentration (FiO$_2$)	Adjusted to maintain SpO$_2$ > 90% FiO$_2$ not to exceed 0.8.
Mode of ventilation	Pressure control ventilation (preferred mode) Volume control ventilation
Respiratory rate	Normal 12–14 breaths per minute; Obstructive lung disease: 8–10 breaths per minute
Inspiratory:expiratory ratio (I:E)	Normal 1:2 Obstructive lung disease 1:2.5 to 1:4 Restrictive lung disease 1:1
Positive end-expiratory pressure (PEEP)	Normal or restrictive lung disease: 5–10 cmH$_2$O Obstructive lung disease: 2–5 cmH$_2$O
Minute ventilation	Adjusted to target PaCO$_2$ 40–70 cmH$_2$O
Target airway pressure	Peak airway pressure < 35–40 cmH$_2$O
Artificial recruitment maneuver	During TLV prior to initiating OLV, during OLV and just prior to reinstating TLV

TLV Two-lung ventilation, *OLV* One-lung ventilation

[14]. Beneficial effects of applied or external PEEP are seen in those patients wherein the intrinsic or auto-PEEP is below the lower inflection point (LIP) [LIP: it is the critical PEEP at which the collapsed alveoli begin to open] commonly seen in patients with normal lung function. In these patients when external PEEP is applied the total end-expiratory pressure (EEP = Intrinsic PEEP + External PEEP) moves towards the LIP thus resulting in effective alveolar recruitment and improved oxygenation. In contrast if the application of PEEP results in EEP being increased appreciably above the LIP then it will result in decrease in oxygenation (Fig. 11.1) [15, 16]. Usually, there is a linear increase in alveolar diameter and its volume till EEP of 10 cmH$_2$O. On achieving an EEP of 15 cmH$_2$O there is a gradual reduction in alveolar diameter and beyond an EEP of 15 cmH$_2$O only alveolar pressures rise without any appreciable increase in diameter resulting in overdistended or hyperinflated alveoli. Overdistention of the alveoli causes compression of the pulmonary capillaries and an increased pulmonary vascular resistance (PVR), diverting the blood from the ventilated towards the non-ventilated lung, causing an increase in intrapulmonary shunt and worsening of oxygenation (Fig. 11.1) [15, 17].

If the intrinsic PEEP can be measured intraoperatively then the appropriate external PEEP required for alveolar recruitment can be determined. However, anesthesia ventilators cannot determine the intrinsic PEEP as it is not possible to apply the end-expiratory hold. Intrinsic PEEP can be interpreted by analyzing the flow volume loops, where in the inspiratory flow starts before the end

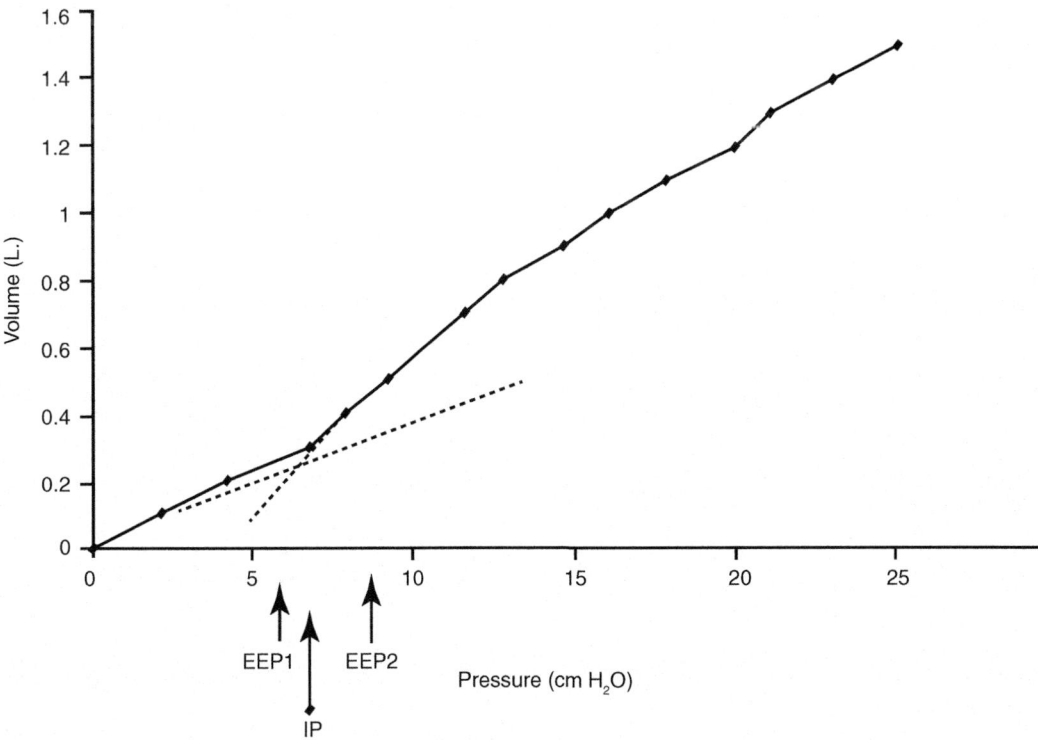

Fig. 11.1 Static compliance curve of the dependent lung during one-lung ventilation (OLV). The inflection point (IP) in this curve 6.6 cmH$_2$O. The initial end-expiratory pressure for this patient during OLV was 6.1 cmH$_2$O. After application of 5 cmH$_2$O of external PEEP the circuit end-expiratory pressure (EEP2) was 8.7 cmH$_2$O. Since the EEP is above the IP, application of PEEP did not improve the arterial oxygen partial pressure. Reproduced with permission from Wolters Kluwer Health, Inc. License Number: 4461230887694. License date: Nov 03, 2018. From: Slinger PD, Kruger M, McRae K, Winton T [2001]. Relation of the static compliance curve and positive end-expiratory pressure to oxygenation during one-lung ventilation. Anesthesiology 95:1096–102

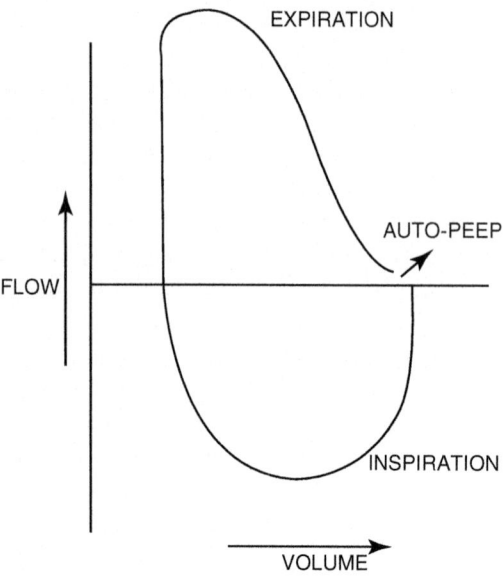

Fig. 11.2 Detection of auto-PEEP by flow volume loop. The expiratory flow curve is not touching the baseline suggesting the presence of auto-PEEP

of the expiratory flow and the expiratory flow curve does not touch the baseline (Fig. 11.2) [18].

An indirect method to determine the effects of auto-PEEP is to calculate the static lung compliance.

(Static compliance = V_T/Pplat − PEEP). A decrease in the measured compliance is an indicator of alveolar hyperinflation or air trapping.

A PEEP of 5–10 cmH$_2$O is beneficial in patients with normal pulmonary function or restrictive lung disease, whereas in patients with severe obstructive airway disease an external PEEP of 2–5 cmH$_2$O can be applied without further aggravating lung hyperinflation [19].

11.2.3 Alveolar Recruitment

Alveolar recruitment involves transient application of controlled high airway pressure of 40 cmH$_2$O to open the collapsed alveoli. Alveolar recruitment maneuvers (ARM) have proven their efficacy in patients with ARDS, wherein ARM not only results in opening of the atelectatic alveoli but also improves oxygenation and decreases dead space ventilation [20].

During OLV the nonoperative lung is highly prone for developing atelectatic lung units due to high FiO$_2$, non-application of PEEP, and external compression of the dependent nonoperated lung by the abdominal contents and mediastinum [19].

ARM should be performed by cyclic stepwise increase in the airway pressures as sudden application of high airway pressures and lung volume typically performed by manual bagging can result in release of proinflammatory cytokines and increased shear stress on the alveoli [20].

During cyclic ARM an alveolar opening pressure of 40 cmH$_2$O is achieved by maintaining the driving pressure of 20 cmH$_2$O (driving pressure = Pplat-PEEP) using pressure control ventilation with gradual increase in PEEP to 20 cmH$_2$O [21]. Current evidence suggests that applying ARM to both the lungs prior to initiating OLV improves oxygenation and gas exchange [22].

A protocol for applying ARM during OLV, a modified combination of protocol described by Tusman et al. [21] and Unzueta et al. [22], is described below (Fig. 11.3a, b):

1. After initiating two-lung ventilation (TLV) the patient is put on volume control ventilation (VCV) with a V_T: 8 ml/kg or on pressure control ventilation (PCV) with pressure adjusted to achieve the target V_T; PEEP: 5 cmH$_2$O; respiratory rate: 12 breaths per minute (bpm) and inspiratory expiration (I: E) 1:2. During OLV, the V_T is reduced to 6 ml/kg or if on PVC, then pressure adjusted to achieve target V_T.
2. ARM is done during TLV 10 mins after lateral positioning of the patient, during OLV, and at the time of reinstating TLV, post OLV.
3. Prior to ARM, PCV is initiated and the pressure is adjusted to obtain the same V_T as during VCV. Ventilation is done for 3 min.
4. Keeping the RR: 12 bpm, the I:E ratio is increased to 1:1 and PEEP is increased to 10 cmH$_2$O for next 5 breaths. The target pressure for PCV is adjusted to 20 cmH$_2$O to maintain

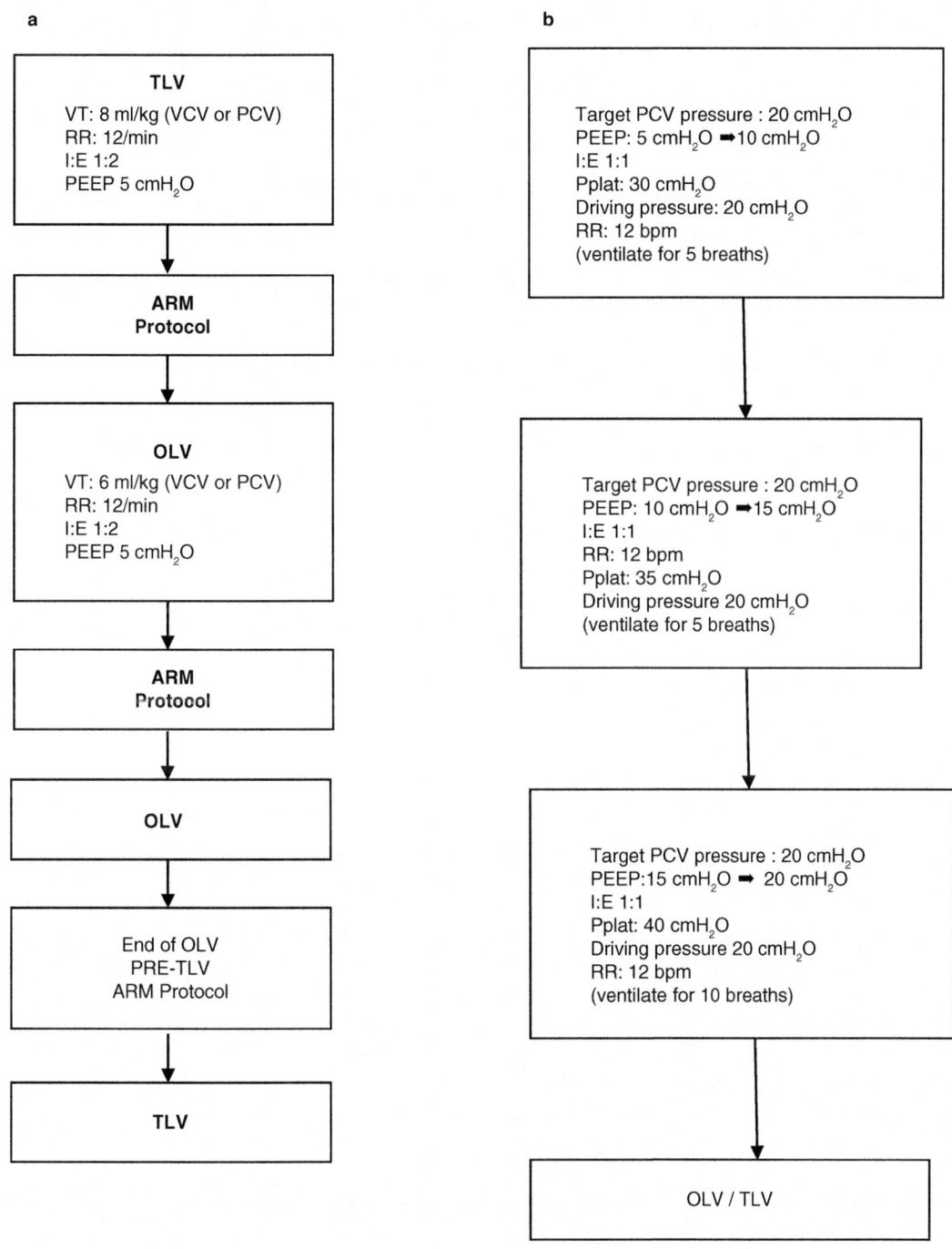

Fig. 11.3 (a) One-Lung Ventilation Management Plan. (b) Artificial Recruitment Maneuver protocol. *TLV* Two-lung ventilation, *ARM* Artificial recruitment maneuver, *OLV* One-lung ventilation, V_T Tidal volume, *RR* Respiratory rate, *I:E* Inspiration:Expiration, *PEEP* Positive end-expiratory pressure

20 cmH$_2$O driving pressure (Target pressure 20 cmH$_2$O + PEEP 10 cmH$_2$O = Pplat 30 cmH$_2$O; Driving pressure = 30 cmH$_2$O [Plat] − 10 cmH$_2$O [PEEP]).
5. At a constant target pressure of 20 cmH$_2$O, the PEEP is increased to 15 cmH$_2$O (Pplat 35 cmH$_2$O) for another 5 breaths.
6. From 15 cmH$_2$O the PEEP is increased to 20 cmH$_2$O with the same target pressure to achieve an alveolar opening of 40 cmH$_2$O (Pplat 40 cmH$_2$O). Ventilation is continued for 10 breaths.
7. The airway pressure is then reduced to achieve the desired V_T [TLV: 8 ml/kg; OLV: 6 ml/kg] and the PEEP kept at 5 cmH$_2$O.

If anytime during the ARM there is worsening of the hemodynamics (change in mean blood pressure and heart rate ± 20% from baseline) then ARM is terminated and a crystalloid bolus of 3 ml/kg is administered [22].

It may be required to limit the Pplat to 30 cmH$_2$O during lung re-expansion at end of OLV duration to avoid any disruption of the staple line post lung resection [19].

Use of alveolar opening pressure or Pplat in the range of 40 cmH$_2$O during ARM may not be tolerated by patients with chronic obstructive airway disease (COAD) wherein lung recruitment will require lower Pplat although no specific alveolar opening pressure range has been described.

A rare complication of lung recruitment is the occurrence of re-expansion of pulmonary edema, which is seen commonly with sudden expansion of long-standing collapsed lung like in patients with lung empyema undergoing decortication [23]. It can be avoided with use of a cyclic ARM instead of manual bagging for lung recruitment. Use of high oxygen concentration should be avoided during ARM as lung recruitment itself is associated with free radical injury [24].

11.2.4 Inspired Oxygen Concentration

Use of inspired oxygen concentration (FiO$_2$) of 1.0 was earlier the norm during OLV, but is not recommended now as exposure to high FiO$_2$ can result in formation of oxygen free radicals thereby resulting in oxidative stress and histopathological changes that mimic ALI [25]. Even a short-term exposure to high FiO$_2$ at time of anesthesia induction can result in absorption atelectasis [24].

An FiO$_2$ of 0.8 can be administered at the start of OLV to improve oxygenation for the initial 15–20 min which should then gradually be decreased to maintain saturation of >90% [19].

11.2.5 Inspiratory: Expiratory (I:E) Time and Respiratory Rate (RR)

The I:E time and respiratory rate has to be adjusted according to underlying condition of the lung parenchyma. In patients with obstructive lung disease the expiratory time needs to be prolonged and RR reduced to the allow complete emptying of the alveoli prior to next inspiration and prevent dynamic hyperinflation of the lung. An I:E ratio in the range of 1:2.5 to 1:4 and RR of 8–10 bpm will provide adequate ventilation in patients with obstructive lung disease [19]. On the other hand, patients with restrictive lung disease have a low lung compliance and require I:E ratio that can minimize the risk of developing barotrauma by decreasing the Ppeak and Pplat. An I:E of 1:1 or if needed use of inverse ratio ventilation along with a low V_T and increased RR (10–15 bpm) to deliver the required minute ventilation will help in reducing the airway pressures although it can result in generation of high intrinsic PEEP.

11.2.6 Mode of Ventilation

VCV has been traditionally used for ventilation under anesthesia during surgery. In VCV, the inspiratory flow follows a square wave pattern, with a gradual increase in airway pressure toward the peak inspiratory pressure and reaches the maximum level when the full V_T is delivered. The airway pressure generated is dependent on the underlying lung compliance; if the compliance is poor then it will result in high Ppeak [26, 27].

PCV has the advantage of a flow pattern wherein the flow is maximal at the beginning of inspiration until the desired pressure is reached and thereafter the flow decreases corresponding with a reduction in lung compliance as the lung expands. Overall, PCV results in more homogenous distribution of V_T in comparison to VCV. Improved oxygenation, reduction in Ppeak and Pplat, enhanced static and dynamic lung compliance are the hallmarks of PCV [28, 29].

A recent meta-analysis confirmed that PCV provides improved oxygenation with lower Ppeak in comparison to VCV in patients undergoing OLV. However, it is difficult to say whether PCV has a clinically relevant benefit over VCV [30].

High-frequency jet ventilation (HFJV) has been employed during thoracic surgery mainly to the operative lung to improve oxygenation in comparison to continuous positive airway pressure (CPAP). HFJV delivery to both the lungs via single-lumen endotracheal tube during thoracic surgery has been shown to result in improved oxygenation with low airway pressures in comparison to conventional OLV [31, 32].

Use of HFJV during routine thoracic surgery is not popular due to its own problems, i.e., difficulty in monitoring airway pressure, delivered V_T and end-tidal CO_2 concentration along with risk of developing barotrauma [33].

11.3 Intraoperative Hypoxemia During Thoracic Surgery

The incidence of hypoxemia during thoracic surgery has declined from an initially reported incidence of 40–50% [34] to a level of 1–10% [35, 36]. Main factors contributing to improved oxygenation during OLV are, firstly, confirmation of proper placement of lung isolation devices using fiberoptic bronchoscopy and secondly, the minimal effect of currently used inhalation anesthetics on hypoxic pulmonary vasoconstriction (HPV).

Despite a reduced incidence of intraoperative hypoxemia, its occurrence during surgery is still a concern because of its effect on non-pulmonary vital organs such as heart and brain. Factors predictive of intraoperative hypoxemia are:

1. Diminished oxygenation during TLV in lateral decubitus position
2. Right sided surgeries due to increased blood flow to the right lung resulting in increased shunt fraction during OLV
3. History of previous surgery to the contralateral or dependent lung
4. Supine position during OLV
5. Obese (BMI > 30 kg/m^2) patients undergoing thoracic surgery
6. An elevated alveolar–arterial CO_2 gradient, which is indicative of V/Q mismatch
7. Normal preoperative spirometry, as normal lung parenchyma will not develop intrinsic or auto-PEEP resulting in significant de-recruitment

11.3.1 Management

The immediate treatment (Fig. 11.4) of a severe hypoxemic (SpO$_2$ < 90%) event is to increase the FiO$_2$ to 1.0 and to resume TLV if permissible. Immediate institution of TLV may not be required if SpO$_2$ 90–95%. The position of the DLT or lung isolation device should be confirmed using fiberoptic bronchoscopy (FOB) as malposition is one of the most common causes of intraoperative hypoxemia. After confirming the position of the lung isolation device, ARM should be applied to the ventilated nonoperative lung. If the hypoxemia is severe then recruitment of both the lungs will be required. Post lung recruitment consider application of continuous positive airway pressure (CPAP) or HFJV to the operative lung. CPAP should start from a level of 5 cmH$_2$O and should not exceed 10 cmH$_2$O [19, 37]. Alternatively, intermittent oxygen insufflation (2–5 lts/min) can be provided to the operative lung via a catheter inserted into the DLT lumen or via the suction port of the fiberoptic bronchoscope. A

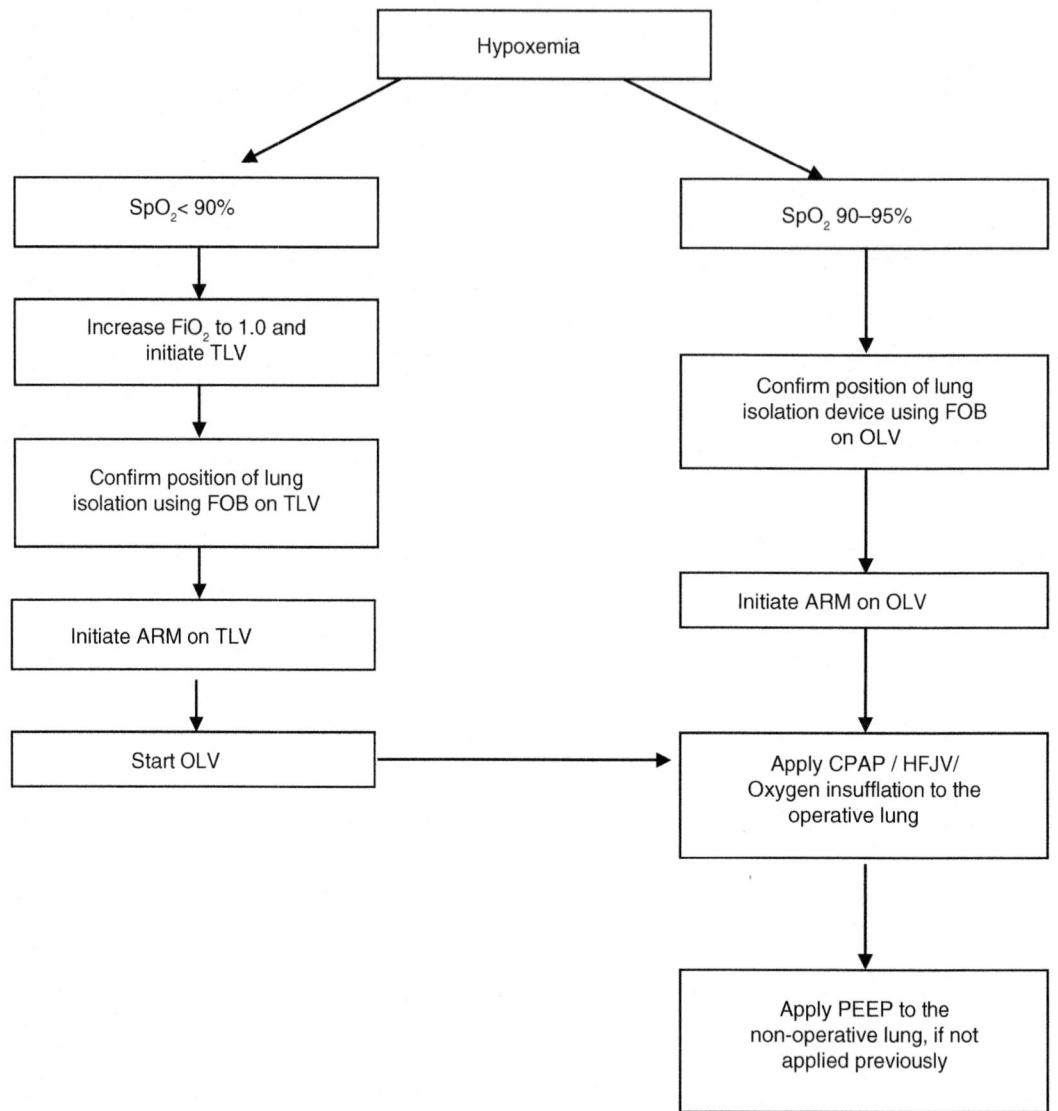

Fig. 11.4 Management of intraoperative hypoxemia. Correct any hemodynamic instability and replace blood loss at all the times. *TLV* Two-lung ventilation, *OLV* one-lung ventilation, *CPAP* Continuous positive airway pressure

limitation of using CPAP, HFJV, and oxygen insufflation is that it can result in partial inflation of the operative lung which can compromise the surgical field especially in patients undergoing thoracoscopic surgery [38, 39].

Post lung recruitment PEEP should be applied to the nonoperative/dependent lung if it was not applied previously. Any hemodynamic instability should be corrected and blood loss should be adequately replaced to ensure proper oxygen delivery to the tissues.

In patients undergoing pneumonectomy who develop severe hypoxemia not responding to above measures, clamping of the pulmonary artery on the operative site can be considered. In addition, use of vasoconstrictors like almitrine, phenylephrine to accentuate the HPV response on the operative side and vasodilatation such as inhaled NO to enhance pulmonary vascular capacitance in the dependent-ventilated lung can be considered if none of the measures to improve oxygenation are helpful [37].

11.4 Conclusion

Protective lung ventilation strategies comprising low tidal volume, use of PEEP, and recruitment maneuvers have evolved the practice of OLV resulting in improved oxygenation and a reduction in incidence of ALI.

References

1. Fischer GW, Cohen E. An update on anesthesia for thoracoscopic surgery. Curr Opin Anaesthesiol. 2010;23:7–11.
2. Bernasconi F, Piccioni F. One-lung ventilation for thoracic surgery: current perspectives. Tumori. 2017;103:495–503.
3. Ishikawa S, Lohser J. One-lung ventilation and arterial oxygenation. Curr Opin Anaesthesiol. 2011;24:24–31.
4. Şentürk M, Slinger P, Cohen E. Intraoperative mechanical ventilation strategies for one-lung ventilation. Best Pract Res Clin Anaesthesiol. 2015;29:357–69.
5. Schilling T, Kozian A, Huth C, et al. The pulmonary immune effects of mechanical ventilation in patients undergoing thoracic surgery. Anesth Analg. 2005;101: 957–65.
6. Kozian A, Schilling T, Röcken C, et al. Increased alveolar damage after mechanical ventilation in a porcine model of thoracic surgery. J Cardiothorac Vasc Anesth. 2010;24:617–23.
7. Alphonsus CS, Rodseth RN. The endothelial glycocalyx: a review of the vascular barrier. Anaesthesia. 2014;69:777–84.
8. Slutsky AS, Ranieri VM. Ventilator-induced lung injury. N Engl J Med. 2013;369:2126–36.
9. Haitsma JJ, Lachmann B. Lung protective ventilation in ARDS: the open lung maneuver. Minerva Anestesiol. 2006;72:117–32.
10. Flacke JW, Thompson DS, Read RC. Influence of tidal volume and pulmonary artery occlusion on arterial oxygenation during endobronchial anesthesia. South Med J. 1976;69:619–26.
11. Jeon K, Yoon JW, Suh GY, et al. Risk factors for postpneumonectomy acute lung injury/acute respiratory distress syndrome in primary lung cancer patients. Anaesth Intensive Care. 2009;37:14–9.
12. Morisaki H, Serita R, Innami Y, et al. Permissive hypercapnia during thoracic anaesthesia. Acta Anaesthesiol Scand. 1999;43:845–9.
13. Schultz MJ, Haitsma JJ, Slutsky AS, et al. What tidal volumes should be used in patients without acute lung injury? Anesthesiology. 2007;106: 1226–31.
14. Tremblay LN, Slutsky AS. Ventilator-induced lung injury: from the bench to the bedside. Intensive Care Med. 2006;32:24–33.
15. Slinger PD, Kruger M, McRae K, et al. Relation of the static compliance curve and positive end-expiratory pressure to oxygenation during one-lung ventilation. Anesthesiology. 2001;95:1096–102.
16. Valenza F, Ronzoni G, Perrone L, et al. Positive end-expiratory pressure applied to the dependent lung during one-lung ventilation improves oxygenation and respiratory mechanics in patients with high FEV1. Eur J Anaesthesiol. 2004;21:938–43.
17. Daly BDT, Edmonds CH, Norman JC. In vivo alveolar morphometrics with positive and expiratory pressure. Surg Forum. 1973;24:217–9.
18. Bardoczky GI, d'Hollander AA, Cappello M, et al. Interrupted expiratory flow on automatically constructed flow-volume curves may determine the presence of intrinsic positive end-expiratory pressure during one-lung ventilation. Anesth Analg. 1998;86:880–4.
19. Lohser J. Evidence-based management of one-lung ventilation. Anesthesiol Clin. 2008;26:241–72.
20. Tusman G, Bohm SH, Suarez-Sipmann F. Alveolar recruitment maneuvers for one-lung ventilation during thoracic anesthesia. Curr Anesthesiol Report. 2014;4:160–9.
21. Tusman G, Böhm SH, Sipmann FS, et al. Lung recruitment improves the efficiency of ventilation and gas exchange during one-lung ventilation anesthesia. Anesth Analg. 2004;98:1604–9.
22. Unzueta C, Tusman G, Suarez-Sipmann F, et al. Alveolar recruitment improves ventilation during thoracic surgery: a randomized controlled trial. Br J Anaesth. 2012;108:517–24.
23. Mahfood S, Hix WR, Aaron BL, et al. Reexpansion pulmonary edema. Ann Thorac Surg. 1988;45:340–5.
24. Misthos P, Katsaragakis S, Theodorou D, et al. The degree of oxidative stress is associated with major adverse effects after lung resection: a prospective study. Eur J Cardiothorac Surg. 2006;29:591–5.
25. Jordan S, Mitchell JA, Quinlan GJ, et al. The pathogenesis of lung injury following pulmonary resection. Eur Respir J. 2000;15:790–9.
26. Campbell RS, Davis BR. Pressure-controlled versus volume-controlled ventilation: does it matter? Respir Care. 2002;47:416–24.
27. Unzueta MC, Casas JI, Moral MV. Pressure-controlled versus volume-controlled ventilation during one-lung ventilation for thoracic surgery. Anesth Analg. 2007;104:1029–33.
28. Schultz MJ, Haitsma JJ, Slutsky AS, et al. What tidal volumes should be used in patients without acute lung injury? Anesthesiology. 2007;106: 1226–31.
29. Nichols D, Haranath S. Pressure control ventilation. Crit Care Clin. 2007;23:183–99.
30. Kim KN, Kim DW, Jeong MA, et al. Comparison of pressure-controlled ventilation with volume-controlled ventilation during one-lung ventilation: a systematic review and meta-analysis. BMC Anesthesiol. 2016;16:72.

31. Dikmen Y, Aykac B, Erolçay H. Unilateral high frequency jet ventilation during one-lung ventilation. Eur J Anaesthesiol. 1997;14:239–43.
32. Ng JM. Hypoxemia during one-lung ventilation: jet ventilation of the middle and lower lobes during right upper lobe sleeve resection. Anesth Analg. 2005;101:1554–5.
33. Ihra G, Gockner G, Kashanipour A, et al. High-frequency jet ventilation in European and North American institutions: developments and clinical practice. Eur J Anaesthesiol. 2000;17:418–30.
34. Hurford WE, Kolker AC, Strauss HW. The use of ventilation/perfusion lung scans to predict oxygenation during one-lung anesthesia. Anesthesiology. 1987;67:841–4.
35. Hurford WE, Alfille PH. A quality improvement study of the placement and complications of double-lumen endobronchial tubes. J Cardiothorac Vasc Anesth. 1993;7:517–20.
36. Brodsky JB, Lemmens HJ. Left double-lumen tubes: clinical experience with 1,170 patients. J Cardiothorac Vasc Anesth. 2003;17:289–98.
37. Lasher J, Ishikawa S. Clinical Management of one lung ventilation. In: Slinger P, editor. Principles and practices of anesthesia for thoracic surgery. New York: Springer; 2011. p. 83–101.
38. Russell WJ. Intermittent positive airway pressure to manage hypoxia during one-lung anaesthesia. Anaesth Intensive Care. 2009;37:432–4.
39. Ku CM, Slinger P, Waddell TK. A novel method of treating hypoxemia during one-lung ventilation for thoracoscopic surgery. J Cardiothorac Vasc Anesth. 2009;23:850–2.

Anesthesia for Lung Resection and Pleural Surgery

12

Himani Chabra and Shikha Sharma

12.1 Introduction

Pulmonary resection and pleural surgeries are the most common thoracic surgical procedures performed in any thoracic surgical unit. Lung resection procedures include wedge resection, segmentectomy, lobectomy, sleeve lobectomy, and pneumonectomy [1], whereas pleural surgeries encompass debridement, decortication, and pleurodesis [2]. Other miscellaneous thoracic surgical procedures include thoracic duct ligation, closure of bronchopleural fistula sympathectomy and several others. These procedures can be performed either by open thoracotomy or video-assisted thoracoscopic surgery (VATS). Advancement in surgical techniques and instrumentation has led to increased interest in thoracoscopic, especially VATS, procedures. VATS was initially used only for minor procedures, but recently it has gained popularity in lung resection and pleural surgeries as well [3]. In fact they are considered to be of choice in most cases due to enhanced recovery, decreased length of stay, and sparing of mechanical chest wall function [4, 5].

Most of the lung resections are related to lung malignancy, tuberculosis (TB) and its clinical sequelae, fungal infections and trauma. However, pleural pathologies like presence of pneumothorax, pleural effusion, hemothorax, chylothorax, empyema, or pleural-based tumors (malignant mesothelioma) warrant surgical intervention to treat the pathology.

The factors to be considered while managing these patients include:

1. Age
2. Pack year smoking
3. Preexisting lung disease
4. Preoperative chemotherapy
5. Baseline lung function
6. Additional comorbidities
7. Nature of surgical procedure
8. Amount of pulmonary resection
9. Open vs VATS (surgical approach)

However, the risk of postoperative respiratory complications (atelectasis, pneumonia, and ARDS) increases to a greater extent in lobectomy and pneumonectomy, where more extensive lung resection is done.

Surgical procedures on and around the lungs require proper knowledge of techniques for lung isolation, ventilation and oxygenation. Knowing tracheobronchial anatomy and airway equipment for one-lung ventilation is of paramount importance [6].

During pulmonary resection surgery, the pulmonary artery, vein, and bronchus are identified and divided at various levels according to the type of resection performed. It is done at the segmental level in segmentectomy,

H. Chabra (✉) · S. Sharma
Institute of Anaesthesiology, Pain and Perioperative Medicine, Sir Ganga Ram Hospital, New Delhi, India

bronchial level in lobectomy, and at main stem bronchus level in pneumonectomy.

12.2 Lobectomy

Currently, it is the standard form of therapy for most patients with lung cancer (Fig. 12.1) [3]. It is also performed for an infective pathology (post tubercular sequelae, lung abscess and fungal infections). It can be performed via open thoracotomy or VATS. Once the surgeon has dissected the lobe and blood vessels, the anesthesiologist is asked to perform a maneuver to confirm whether the surgeon has clamped the correct bronchus or not. The anesthesiologist unclamps the DLT or deflates the bronchial blocker and inflates the operative lung to see that the correct lobe has been clamped while the remaining lung gets ventilated. In addition, prior to division of any structure by surgeon, the anesthesiologist has to make sure that no object (endotracheal tube, suction catheter) is present at the site of surgical resection.

12.3 Sleeve Lobectomy

It is a parenchymal sparing surgery in patients with limited pulmonary reserve where otherwise a pneumonectomy is indicated. The diseased lobe is removed with sleeve of main stem bronchus and the remaining lobe with its bronchus is re-anastomosed with the proximal mainstem bronchus [7]. This is commonly performed in bronchogenic carcinomas, carcinoid tumors of bronchus, endobronchial metastasis, and bronchial adenomas. The surgery demands lung isolation to be done by using contralateral DLT so that it does not interfere with the surgical field.

12.4 Pneumonectomy

It is a high risk thoracic surgical procedure performed for large central tumors, distal main stem bronchus involvement, tumors with transfissural extension, advanced bronchiectasis and invasive infections with parenchymal destruction not responding to antibiotic therapy (Fig. 12.2) and a massive hemoptysis [8]. It is associated with higher incidence of complications (cardiac, acute lung injury (ALI), and ARDS) and mortality (8–10% vs 2% for lobectomy) [9].

It is traditionally performed via a posterolateral thoracotomy incision, but minimally invasive approaches are also gaining popularity. Here pulmonary artery, superior and inferior pulmonary veins, and main stem bronchus are evaluated for resectability, looped and divided. After dividing the bronchus, the test for air leak

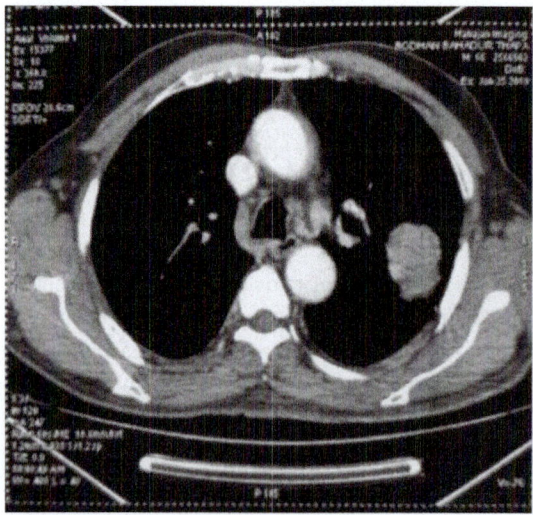
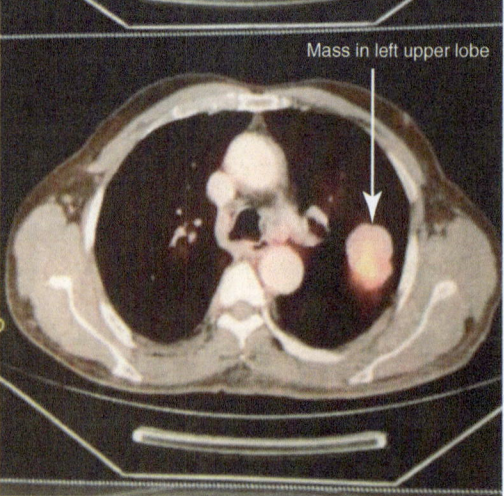

Fig. 12.1 Adenocarcinoma left upper lobe posted for left upper lobectomy

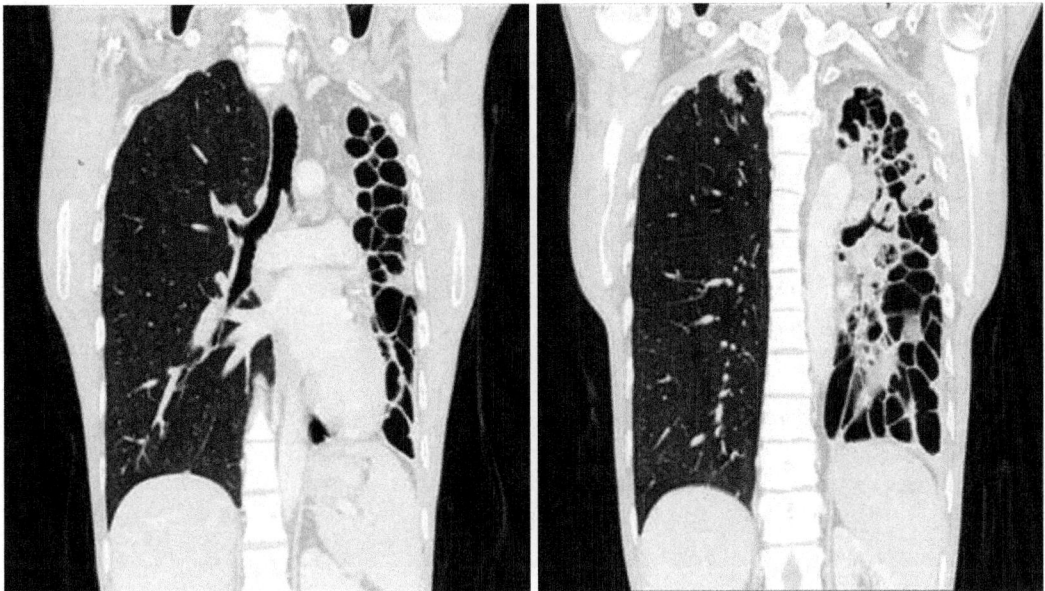

Fig. 12.2 CT image showing left-sided post tubercular destroyed lung requiring pneumonectomy

is performed and bronchial stump reconstruction done to prevent the formation of bronchopleural fistula. In these cases also the lung has to be isolated using contralateral DLT or if the same sided DLT is used, it is to be withdrawn before dividing the bronchus.

ALI (post-pneumonectomy pulmonary edema) is the most dreaded complication after pneumonectomy ultimately leading to respiratory failure. Incidence of ALI is up to 4–8% and is associated with upto 40%mortality [3]. Risk factors include right-sided pneumonectomy, increased perioperative fluid administration, decrease in ventilatory function, increase in pulmonary artery pressure and pulmonary vascular resistance and therefore an increase in RV afterload [10–12].

Focus should be on restrictive use of perioperative fluid therapy and protective lung ventilation strategies to decrease morbidity and mortality associated with pneumonectomy.

There is no standard consensus among surgeons for the best management of post pneumonectomy residual space. Immediately post surgery, some prefer to place an intercostal tube with continuous drainage while others prefer to clamp the same for 1–2 postoperative days.

12.5 Limited Pulmonary Resection (Segmentectomy and Wedge Resection)

Segmentectomy involves anatomical resection of a bronchopulmonary segment. This procedure is usually done in patients with smaller peripheral tumors with limited pulmonary reserves. Wedge resection is nonanatomical resection of a portion of lung parenchyma [13]. This is usually performed for diagnosis of lung nodules for frozen section or as a palliative procedure in patients with metastatic lesions.

12.6 Pleurodesis

This procedure involves fusion of parietal and visceral pleura causing obliteration of pleural space. Indications include recurrent pneumothorax, persistent pleural effusion, and pneumothorax with prolonged air leak. This could be done either by chemical pleurodesis using sclerosing agents such as talc, doxycycline or by mechanical pleurodesis by abrading the parietal pleura with a dry gauze or prolene mesh [2].

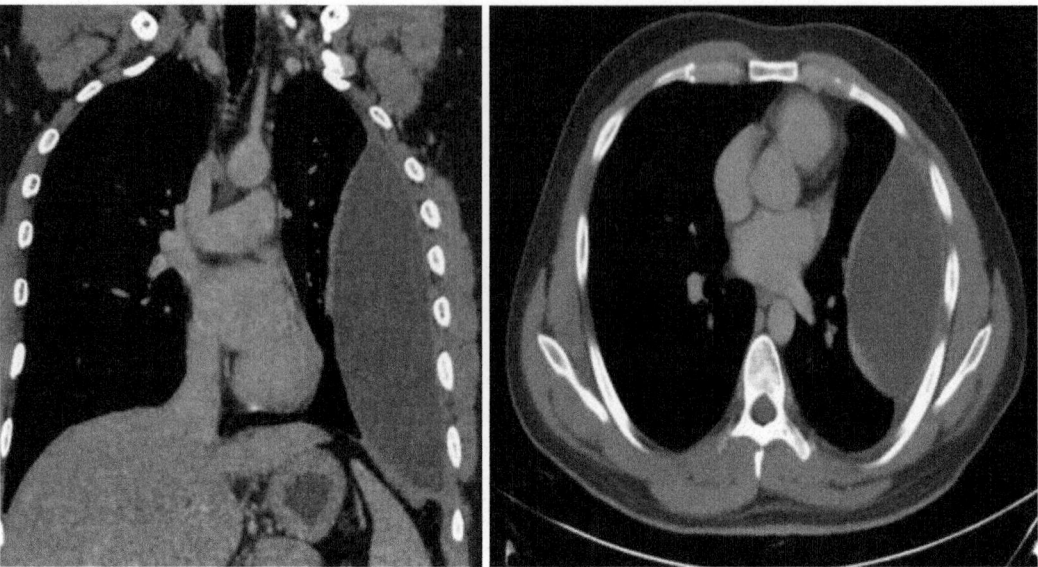

Fig. 12.3 CT image showing left-sided tubercular empyema compressing the left lung, necessitating decortication surgery

12.7 Debridement

This may be required in patients of empyema (Fig. 12.3) with tube thoracostomy not improving with antibiotics, multiloculated empyema and retained clots [2].

12.8 Decortication

It involves removal of fibrotic pleura (due to malignant, infectious or traumatic process) from the lung to allow expansion of lung. At the end of procedure, full re-expansion of the lung should happen to fill the pleural cavity to prevent any future recurrences. Common problems associated with this are lung injury and significant bleeding [2].

12.9 Urgency of Lung Resection Surgeries

In general, these surgeries are largely elective except for few situations where the risk of morbidity and mortality increases to a great extent.

Emergent procedures: Patients with massive hemoptysis where conservative and other modalities have failed.

Urgent procedures: In patients with lung abscess and bronchiectasis to provide source control when the patient is in severe sepsis.

Elective procedure: Lung carcinomas after proper preoperative evaluation and optimization done.

12.10 Preoperative Evaluation

The two main concerns to be addressed in preoperative evaluation include whether or not the patient will tolerate OLV intraoperatively and how will be the postoperative recovery profile [6]. Evaluation of the cardiopulmonary status is of paramount importance. Pulmonary function test and gas exchange are not indicated in every patient except in lung resections. The base line clinical status/functional capacity of the patient and the extent of the planned surgery guide the physicians for preoperative evaluation. All patients should be assessed according to the three-legged tool including: (1) respiratory mechanics, (2) pulmonary gas exchange, and (3) cardiopulmonary reserve (See Chap. 6).

All patients should be evaluated as per the AHA/ACC guidelines for patients with cardiac disease for noncardiac surgery, as thoracotomy/lung resection surgeries are considered high risk procedures for cardiac complications, > 5% [14].

Patients having active cardiac conditions should be evaluated and treated before undergoing any thoracic surgery. Patients who are with baseline decreased pulmonary function scheduled for extensive lung resection should undergo cardiopulmonary exercise stress testing to predict their ability to tolerate the surgery [15].

Following conditions require the patient to be evaluated and optimized before taking up for surgery [1]:

1. Decompensated heart failure
2. Severe valvular disease
3. Significant arrhythmias
4. Recent MI (< 30 days)
5. Unstable angina, COPD exacerbation
6. Active tracheobronchial/lung infection
7. Active infection/sepsis of any source
8. DVT and/or pulmonary embolism
9. AKI on CKD

12.11 Implications of Coexisting Diseases on Perioperative Care

A. Cardiovascular system

Incidence of perioperative MI during lung surgery is nearly 4%, which increases up to 20% in patients with previous MI [16]. If history and/or ECG suggests previous MI, the patient should be evaluated by exercise stress testing. If stress testing shows myocardial ischemia, this situation requires further evaluation by coronary angiography. Invasive procedures like PCI and CABG should be considered only if indicated, regardless of the planned lung resection surgery [17–21].

Lung resection surgeries should be deferred for at least 4–6 weeks post CABG and if percutaneous coronary intervention is required (PCI), bare metal stents should be implanted instead of drug eluting as then the patient can undergo surgery after 3 months [22]. In patients with increased risk of perioperative myocardial ischemia, maintain oxygen demand/supply by heart rate control, maintaining coronary perfusion pressure, preventing hypoxemia, and optimizing oxygen carrying capacity.

Beta blockers should be either continued in patients already taking them or should be started well before rather than immediate preoperative [23].

Pneumonectomy can significantly cause right ventricular dysfunction with immediate increase in right ventricular afterload after clamping the ipsilateral pulmonary artery. It is most pronounced on first postoperative day but may present later as well.

These changes can also be seen in lobectomy, but are generally well tolerated unless patient has baseline pulmonary hypertension [24].

B. Pulmonary system

Pulmonary complications are the major cause of morbidity and mortality in patients undergoing thoracic surgery:

Severity of pulmonary complications depends on various factors such as,

1. Baseline pulmonary function
2. Degree of lung tissue resected
3. Mechanics of chest wall (Thoracotomy/VATS)
4. Adequate postoperative analgesia

(i) COPD

Patients should be assessed for COPD/ILD and severity of its symptoms.

Risk reduction

Patients should be optimized before surgery with medical therapy. This includes treatment with bronchodilators, treatment of active airway infection by specific antibiotics and pre- and postoperative chest physiotherapy to prevent retention of secretions and atelectasis.

(ii) Bronchial Asthma

Optimization to achieve minimal airway reactivity and peak expiratory flow more than 80% of the patient's baseline. Short acting bronchodilators and corticosteroids should be continued until the day of surgery. In symptomatic patients a short course of oral prednisolone is effective.

(iii) Smoking

Risk of pulmonary complications associated with smoking is directly proportional to pack years and inversely proportional to time since last use. Ideally it should be stopped at least 8 weeks prior to surgery to reduce the complications, but even short-term cessation is beneficial than smoking up to the time of surgery, as it decreases the level of carboxy hemoglobin and thus there is less hypoxemia [25, 26].

C. Renal System

Patients undergoing thoracic surgery, especially pneumonectomy are at high risk of acute kidney injury [27]. Multiple risk factors include perioperative hemodynamic instability with hypotension and decreased renal perfusion pressure (Fig. 12.4), hypovolemia due to fluid restriction, peripheral vascular disease, diabetes mellitus, hypertension, large volume of colloids, lower hematocrit values, SIRS triggered by ALI and neuroendocrine/metabolic response to surgery [1].

Presence of preoperative CKD or pre- and peroperative risk factors for AKI can make these patients highly susceptible for developing perioperative AKI.

Risk reduction measures:

1. Maintain preoperative normovolemia in patients with high risk
2. Avoid acute on chronic anemia
3. Correct hypotension and vasodilatation by using vasopressors to maintain renal perfusion pressure
4. Avoid nephrotoxic drugs

D. Gastrointestinal system

Patients with GERD/hiatus hernia are assessed for severity of symptoms. LFTs and albumin are part of preoperative evaluation of cancer patients, who those with infective pathologies and are on ATT [1].

Risk reduction measures:

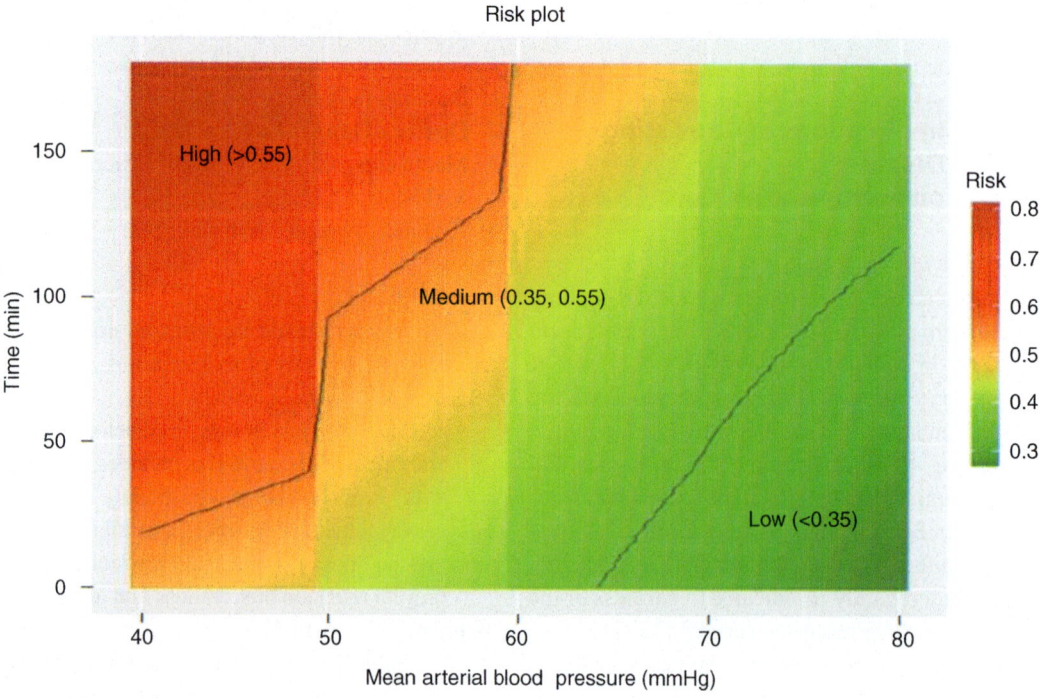

Fig. 12.4 Correlation between intraoperative blood pressure and risk of AKI

1. Consider giving H2 blockers and prokinetics in those with poorly controlled reflux symptoms
2. Titrate dosage of anesthetic medications in patients with hypoalbuminemia and malnutrition and expect longer duration action of medications in these patients

12.12 Preoperative Concerns Specific to Pleural Surgeries

1. Septicemia may be present in patients with empyema/BPF, so optimal antibiotic therapy should be started preoperatively.
2. Patients with infective pathologies or chylothorax may be malnourished and hypovolemic. So, preoperative TLC, serum electrolytes, total protein and albumin levels should be evaluated.
3. Decortication surgeries where significant blood loss is anticipated, blood and blood products should be arranged [2].

12.13 Intraoperative Management

The goal of any anesthetic technique for lung resection and pleural surgery is to provide earliest extubation with fast return of spontaneous ventilation and best possible respiratory mechanics with minimal alteration of sensorium.

12.14 Equipment Required

Equipment for lung isolation e.g. double lumen tube, bronchial blockers or univent tubes should be arranged. Fibreoptic bronchoscope to check tube placement and intraoperative use should be ready. Bougie and airway exchange catheter are desirable. A circuit for delivering CPAP bean bags, warming devices including warn air blankets and IV fluid warmers should all be available.

12.15 Monitoring

Once patient's identity is confirmed, consent obtained, and site marked, an IV line preferably 18G should be secured on the nondependent side

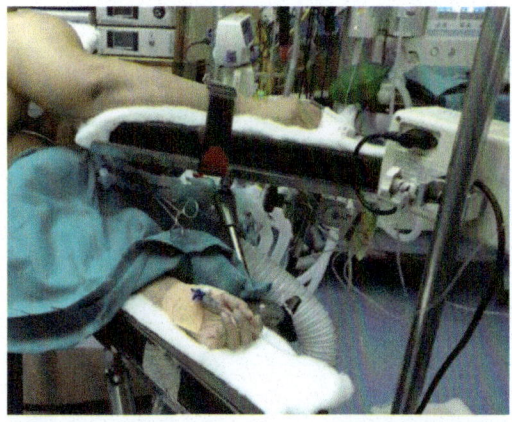

Fig. 12.5 Final lateral positioning of the patient showing IV access on nondependent limb and arterial line on dependent limb and cotton padding done

(Fig. 12.5). After induction of anesthesia, another 18 gauge IV line is secured. Blood loss is usually minimal except for surgery in patients, post radiotherapy, extra pleural pneumonectomy and decortication. If surgical dissection around great veins (vena cava/subclavian vein) is expected, then contralateral venous access, central line, or lower limb access should be taken.

An invasive arterial line should be put in the dependent limb usually after induction of anesthesia for beat-to-beat blood pressure and arterial blood gas monitoring (Fig. 12.5).

Central line insertion is routinely not required but may be indicated in patients with cardiac comorbidities, CKD, anticipated large volume blood loss, extensive pulmonary resections and patients requiring hyper alimentation in postoperative period.

Use of pulmonary artery catheter is not routinely recommended due to its unreliable measurements, but if used, care to should be taken to withdraw the catheter to the pulmonary valve before clamping and ligating the PA.

TEE is more sensitive than pulmonary artery catheter for monitoring intraoperative cardiac function and fluid administration. Urinary catheterization is done for urine output monitoring.

In lateral positioning, an axillary roll (Fig. 12.6) is placed under upper chest and not in the axilla to prevent brachial plexus injury and head is supported to avoid any traction on neck (Fig. 12.7). A cotton roll is placed between neck and shoulder joint to

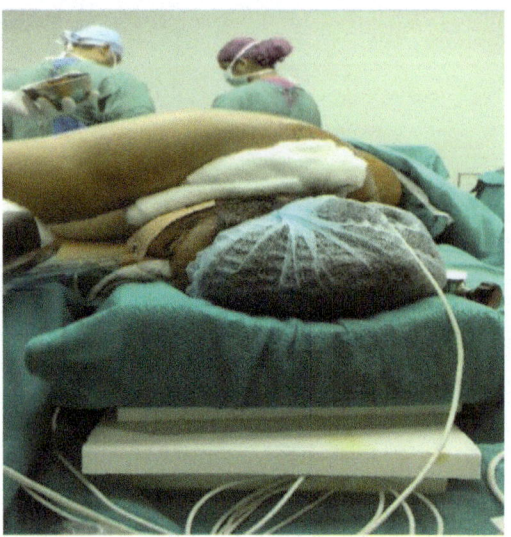

Fig. 12.6 Lateral positioning showing axillary roll kept under the upper chest

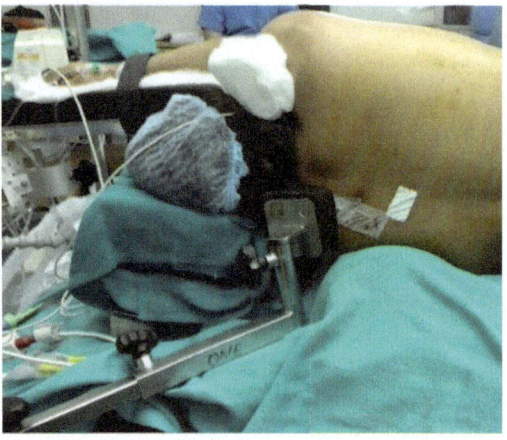

Fig. 12.7 Final positioning of patient showing head supported and cotton roll kept between neck and shoulder

prevent postoperative shoulder pain (Fig. 12.7). Cotton is placed under all bony prominences to prevent peripheral nerve injuries.

12.16 Anesthesia Technique

General anesthesia with preoperative insertion of thoracic epidural catheter for perioperative analgesia is technique of choice. However, at author's institute, the epidural is inserted post induction after counselling the patient.

Avoid preoperative use of sedatives, especially in patients with lung disease and limited respiratory reserve. Titrate the dose of induction agents, opioids, and neuromuscular blockers to ensure minimal respiratory dysfunction at end of procedure. Opioids to be used by epidural route preferably. Avoid use of epidural opioids less than 1 hour before end of procedure. Use short acting inhalational/intravenous agents for prompt extubation.

There is no proven benefit for use of intravenous versus inhalational agents for maintenance of anesthesia when either one is used with thoracic epidural. Short acting volatile agents decrease air way irritability, obtund air way reflexes and can be eliminated rapidly allowing early extubation, but should not be used in more than one MAC concentration as they prevent HPV.

12.17 Lung Isolation Techniques

Proper separation of lung ventilation requires placing a DLT or bronchial blockers. DLT allows rapid lung collapse and ventilation, allows suctioning and applying CPAP to operating lung which is not possible with a bronchial blockers. It is a practice at the author's institute to put DLT on contralateral side in surgeries involving main stem bronchus (for example pneumonectomy or main bronchus sleeve resections).

12.18 Ventilatory Settings

At author's institute, it is usual practice to ventilate the patient using pressure control mode as it is more physiological.

After confirmation of DLT placement, airway pressures on two-lung ventilation in lateral position are noted and then are seen again after clamping the operative side. The airway pressures should normally increase by up to 10 cm of water after clamping. If the increase is more than that, then suspect tube misplacement and reconfirm the position of the tube.

Pressure control ventilation for OLV is preferred as every patient has a different lung compliance. This mode gives breaths, which are almost similar to physiological breaths, the tidal volume varying with each breath and according to lung compliance, thus reducing lung damage due to pressure.

Hypoxemia and acute lung injury are the major concerns with OLV. Hypoxemia is usually due to alveolar hypoventilation and increased shunt fraction, whereas ALI is caused by ventilatory stress (volutrauma, barotrauma, atelectrauma), re-expansion pulmonary injury, massive transfusion and lung surgery itself. High intraoperative tidal volume (more than 6 ml/kg) is an independent risk factor for developing ALI following lung resection surgery especially pneumonectomy [28, 29]. Following pneumonectomy, FRC of the residual lung increases, so using larger tidal volumes combined with increased FRC could result in volume-induced lung injury.

Lung protective strategy includes tidal volume of 4–6 ml/kg ideal body weight with peak pressures of <35 cm water and plateau pressure of <25 cm water with respiratory rate adjusted to maintain normocapnia to mild permissive hypercapnia and PEEP as needed to improve oxygenation [30–32].

12.19 Ventilation in Special Situations

12.19.1 Obstructive Lung Disease

Besides the concerns discussed above, avoiding dynamic hyperinflation has to be taken care of in these patients. Dynamic hyperinflation occurs when there is inadequate expiratory time. This can be prevented using I:E ratio in the range of 1:3 to 1:5 and lower respiratory rates and avoiding extrinsic PEEP.

In patients with bullous emphysematous lung disease, where there is loss of structural integrity, using larger tidal volume or high airway pressures during OLV, will lead to complications like rupture, pneumothorax, and injury to non-bullous emphysematous lung as well. So, after completion of OLV, lung should be re-expanded with very low tidal volumes and airway pressures and gradually increasing them to achieve desired lung expansion.

12.19.2 Interstitial Lung Disease

ILD results in diffuse scarring and fibrosis of smaller airways and alveolar walls. It leads to increased elastic recoil of lungs with less distensible alveoli and contracted lung volume. High I:E ratio (1:1 or 1:2) with low tidal volume (around 4 ml/kg of predicted body weight) with high respiratory rates should be used to prevent increased airway pressures and its consequences.

12.20 Fluid Therapy

Perioperative fluid therapy in lung resection surgeries remains controversial. Reducing perioperative fluid administration and minimizing the hydrostatic pressure in pulmonary capillaries is of utmost importance in thoracic surgery in preventing ALI. A conservative fluid approach, i.e., zero balance is strongly suggested.

Restrictive fluid regime often warrants concomitant use of vasopressors to counteract the vasodilator effects of anesthesia and thoracic epidural blockade and to maintain renal perfusion pressure while maintaining intravascular normovolemia and stable hemodynamics [3].

Patients should be encouraged to take carbohydrate drinks up to 2 h before surgery. Intraoperative balanced crystalloids should be limited to 1–4 ml/kg/h to replace losses by perspiration, evaporation, and urine output. Replacement of third space losses is no more justified. Consider blood transfusion, to replace lost blood. Administer vasopressors to maintain hemodynamics rather than giving fluid boluses. Keeping the lung dry and circulatory compartments close to normovolemia remains a dictum in lung resection surgeries [33, 34].

Patients undergoing pneumonectomy have the highest possibility of developing right ventricular dysfunction. So, restricted fluid therapy has the utmost importance in preventing this complication. Pulmonary edema following pneumonectomy has a mortality rate of 20–40%.

12.21 Analgesia

Pain control is a significant goal to be achieved especially in patients with poor baseline lung function and with more extensive lung resections. Adequate postoperative analgesia helps decreasing respiratory complications.

Thoracic epidural (Fig. 12.8) is the mainstay technique used for providing intraoperative as well as postoperative analgesia. It is a common practice at author's institute to tunnel the epidural through the subcutaneous tissue before fixation to prevent its accidental removal while movement of the patient (Fig. 12.9). It can be used either as bolus technique, or patient controlled epidural analgesia (PCEA). Advantages include:

1. Decreased incidence of cardiac arrhythmias
2. Early tracheal extubation
3. Decreased duration of ICU stay
4. Decreased intraoperative requirement of anesthetic drugs
5. Improved postoperative respiratory mechanics with better ability to cough
6. Early mobilization and chest physiotherapy
7. Suppression of neuroendocrine stress response [35–38]

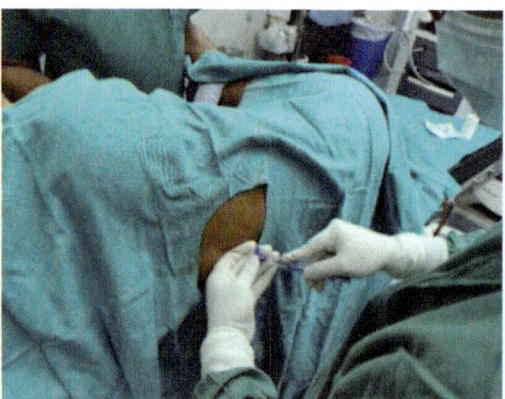

Fig. 12.8 Thoracic epidural placement

12.22 Drawbacks

1. Technique related: dura puncture, spinal cord injury, hematoma
2. Hypotension
3. Bradycardia
4. Potential to decrease inspiratory effort with high level of motor blockade
5. Opioid-related nausea, vomiting, sedation, respiratory depression, pruritis and ileus

A combination of low concentration of local anesthetics and opioids is most commonly used. It is a common practice at author's institute to give epidural morphine in the intraoperative period followed by 0.0625% bupivacaine plus 2.5 mcg/ml fentanyl in postoperative period by PCEA pump. As nowadays, there is increased trend for minimally invasive surgical approaches, postoperative requirement for analgesia also decreases. Other techniques which can be used include thoracic paravertebral block, intercostal nerve blocks, and intrapleural analgesia [1].

12.23 Intraoperative Events

The following events are commonly encountered during lung resection and pleural surgeries:

1. During VATS procedure, surgeon generally uses CO_2 insufflation for collapsing the lung at a pressure approximately 6 mmHg which

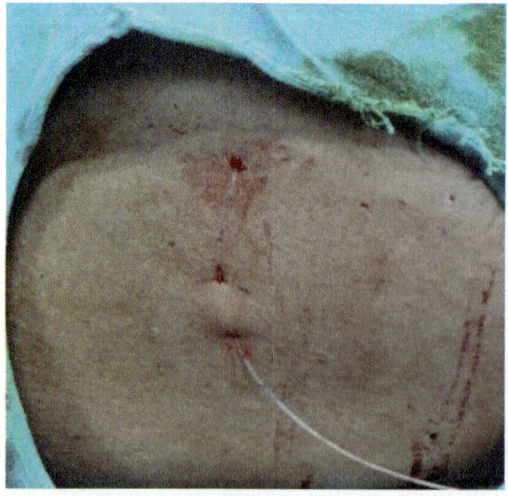

Fig. 12.9 Epidural tunneling done before fixation

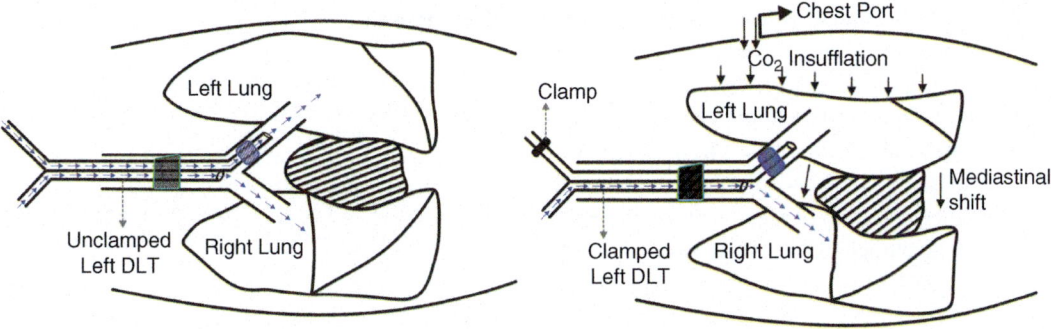

Fig. 12.10 Effect of CO_2 insufflation compressing the mediastinum and opposite lung

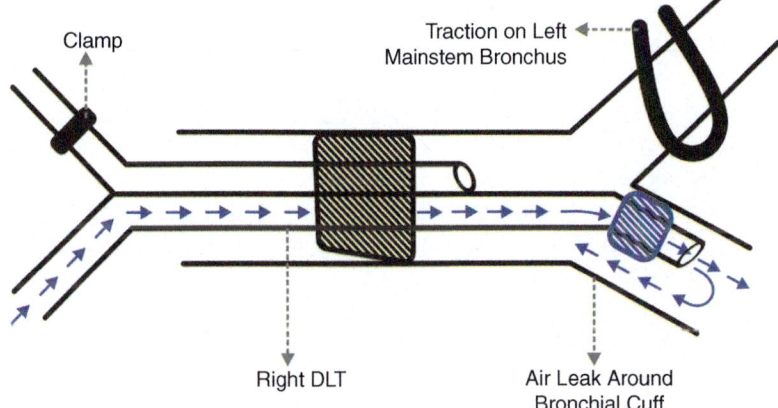

Fig. 12.11 Leak in ventilation when traction is put on the operative main stem bronchus

rarely may go up to 8 mmHg for 5–10 min. CO_2 insufflation causes the mediastinum to shift to contralateral side thus compressing the ventilated lung (Fig. 12.10) and decreasing the tidal volume delivery in PCV mode or increasing airway pressure if VCV is being used. So it is advisable to keep a watch on delivered tidal volume and titrate the settings accordingly.

2. During surgical dissection, when the surgeon loops the main stem bronchus in pneumonectomy, it pulls the endobronchial part of DLT in the contralateral bronchus thus causing leak in ventilation (Fig. 12.11). So a counter traction on the DLT should be maintained that time.
3. Before the surgeon divides the main stem bronchus and pulmonary artery, ensure that the DLT, suction catheter tip and PA catheter have been pulled back to make sure they are not included in the stapler line.
4. The anesthesiologist should be cautious, while the surgeon is performing hilar dissection or pericardial dissection as major vessel injury, arrhythmias, and hypotension can occur.
5. Once the lobe or lung has been removed, the surgeon tests for bronchial stump leak by asking the anesthesiologist to give sustained 25–30 cm of H_2O positive pressure in the circuit. The anesthesiologist should slowly expand the lung over 1–2 min starting with lower airway pressures and gradually increasing to prevent lung injury and chances of re-expansion pulmonary edema.
6. Hypotension is commonly encountered intraoperatively as there is decreased venous return due to surgical manipulation, super-added by hypovolemia and vasodilatation. It should not be treated with excessive fluid administration, rather use vasopressors and blood products if required.
7. During decortication more blood loss can occur as compared to lung resection surgery due to blunt dissection of pleura away from

chest wall. Patients with empyema or infective pathology may present with sepsis or sequelae.
8. In extrapleural pneumonectomy for malignant pleural mesothelioma, there is dissection of parietal pleura away from chest wall, diaphragm, and mediastinum followed by en-bloc resection of lung, pleura, pericardium and diaphragm [39]. This surgery involves more blood loss, major vessel injury, and cardiac complications. Manipulation during surgery can cause restriction to ventilation of the opposite lung leading to atelectasis.
9. Cardiac herniation can occur, when patient returns to supine position in patients who have undergone pneumonectomy and in patients where pericardium is partially removed and not reconstructed. It leads to kinking of great vessels and hemodynamic collapse which does not respond to chest compressions or pharmacological treatment. Immediate returning to lateral position or sternotomy should be done in such situations.
10. In patients undergoing surgery where the diseased lung was collapsed for quite some time, sudden re-expansion of that lung may lead to re-expansion pulmonary edema on the operating table. The anesthesiologist should be aware of this complication and expand the chronically collapsed lung very gradually.

12.24 Extubation

At the end of surgery, the patient should be completely awake with no residual neuromuscular blockade and optimal analgesia before extubation. Careful assessment of vocal cords should be done immediately after extubation in selected cases where there is suspicion of recurrent laryngeal nerve injury.

12.25 Conclusion

Patients undergoing lung resection and pleural surgeries are at high risk. Adequate precautions regarding intravenous fluids and ventilator strategies should be practiced.

References

1. Rio JMD. Pulmonary resection – pneumonectomy, lobectomy and segmentectomy/standard and thoracoscopic. Available from https://www.clinicalpainadvisor.com/home/decision-support-in-medicine/anesthesiology. Accessed 29 June 2019.
2. Pawlowski J, Ott Q. Overview of anesthesia for patients with pleural disease. Available from https://www.uptodate.com/contents.Accessed on 29 June 2019.
3. Ochroch EA, Lambright E, Kertai M, et al. Anesthesia for open pulmonary resection: a systems approach. In: Slinger P, editor. Principles and practice of anesthesia for thoracic surgery. 1st ed. New York: Springer; 2011. p. 309–31.
4. Whitson BA, Groth SS, Duval SJ, et al. Surgery for early-stage non-small cell lung cancer: a systematic review of the video-assisted thoracoscopic surgery versus thoracotomy approaches to lobectomy. Ann Thorac Surg. 2008;86:2008–18.
5. Mahtabifard A, DeArmond DT, Fuller CB, et al. Video-assisted thoracoscopic surgery lobectomy for stage I lung cancer. Thorac Surg Clin. 2007;17:223–31.
6. Weigel WA, Hoaglan CD. The practical management of one lung ventilation. Adv Anesth. 2013;31:61–85.
7. Hoffman H. Bronchial sleeve resection. In: Dienemann HC, Hoffmann H, Detterbeck FC, editors. Chest surgery. 1st ed. Springer: Berlin; 2015. p. 185–209.
8. Demmy TL, Dexter EU. Thoracotomy pneumonectomy. In: Dienemann HC, Hoffmann H, Detterbeck FC, editors. Chest surgery. 1st ed. Springer: Berlin; 2015. p. 137–47.
9. Allen MS, Darling GE, Pechet TT, et al. Morbidity and mortality of major pulmonary resections in patients with early stage lung cancer: initial results of the randomized, prospective ACOSOG Z0030 trial. Ann Thorac Surg. 2006;81:1013–20.
10. Zeldin RA, Normandin D, Landtwing D, et al. Postpneumonectomy pulmonary edema. J Thorac Cardiovasc Surg. 1984;87:359–65.
11. Licker M, de Perrot M, Spiliopoulos A, et al. Risk factors for acute lung injury after thoracic surgery for lung cancer. Anesth Analg. 2003;97:1558–65.
12. Foroulis CN, Kotoulas CS, Kakouros S, et al. Study on the late effect of pneumonectomy on right heart pressures using Doppler echocardiography. Eur J Cardiothorac Surg. 2004;26:508–14.
13. Oizumi H, Kato H, Endoh M, et al. Techniques to define segmental anatomy during segmentectomy. Ann Cardiothorac Surg. 2014;3(2):170–5.
14. Fleisher LA, Beckman JA, Brown KA, et al. ACC/AHA 2007 guidelines on perioperative cardiovascular evaluation and care for noncardiac surgery. J Am Coll Cardiol. 2007;50:1707–32.
15. British Thoracic Society; Society of Cardiothoracic Surgeons of Great Britain and Ireland Working Party. BTS guidelines: guidelines on the selection

16. of patients with lung cancer for surgery. Thorax. 2001;56: 89–108.
16. von Knorring J, Lepäntalo M, Lindgren L, et al. Cardiac arrhythmias and myocardial ischemia after thoracotomy for lung cancer. Ann Thorac Surg. 1992;53:642–7.
17. Garcia S, Moritz TE, Ward HB, et al. Usefulness of revascularization of patients with multi-vessel coronary artery disease before elective vascular surgery for abdominal aortic and peripheral occlusive disease. Am J Cardiol. 2008;102:809–13.
18. Garcia S, McFalls EO. CON: preoperative coronary revascularization in high-risk patients undergoing vascular surgery. Anesth Analg. 2008;106:764–6.
19. McFalls EO, Ward HB, Moritz TE, et al. Predictors and outcomes of a perioperative myocardial infarction following elective vascular surgery in patients with documented coronary artery disease: results of the CARP trial. Eur Heart J. 2008;29:394–401.
20. McFalls EO, Ward HB, Moritz TE, et al. Clinical factors associated with long-term mortality following vascular surgery: outcomes from the Coronary Artery Revascularization Prophylaxis (CARP) trial. J Vasc Surg. 2007;46:694–700.
21. McFalls EO, Ward HB, Moritz TE, et al. Coronary-artery revascularization before elective major vascular surgery. N Engl J Med. 2004;351:2795–804.
22. ASA Committee on Standards and Practice Parameters. Practice alert for the perioperative management of patients with coronary artery stents. Anesthesiology. 2009;110:22–3.
23. Devereaux PJ, Yang H, Yusuf S, et al. Effects of extended-release metoprolol succinate in patients undergoing non-cardiac surgery (POISE trial): a randomised controlled trial. Lancet. 2008;371:1839–47.
24. Pedoto A, Amar D. Right heart function in thoracic surgery: role of echocardiography. Curr Opin Anaesthesiol. 2009;22:44–9.
25. Vaporciyan AA, Merriman KW, Ece F, et al. Incidence of major pulmonary complications after pneumonectomy; association with timing of smoking cessation. Ann Thorac Surg. 2002;73:420–5.
26. Akrawi W, Benumof JL. A pathophysiological basis for informed preoperative smoking cessation counseling. J Cardiothorac Vasc Anesth. 1997;11:629–40.
27. Slinger PD. Postpneumonectomy pulmonary edema: good news, bad news. Anesthesiology. 2006;105:2–5.
28. Fernandez-Perez ER, Keegan MT, Brown DR, et al. Intraoperative tidal volume as a risk factor for respiratory failure after pneumonectomy. Anesthesiology. 2006;105:14–8.
29. Grichnik KP, D'Amico TA. Acute lung injury and acute respiratory distress syndrome after pulmonary resection. Semin Cardiothorac Vasc Anesth. 2004;8:317–34.
30. Malhotra A. Low-tidal-volume ventilation in the acute respiratory distress syndrome. N Engl J Med. 2007;357:1113–20.
31. Petrucci N, Iacovelli W. Lung protective ventilation strategy for the acute respiratory distress syndrome. Cochrane Database Syst Rev. 2007;28:CD003844.
32. The Acute Respiratory Distress Syndrome Network. Ventilation with lower tidal volumes as compared with traditional tidal volumes for acute lung injury and the acute respiratory distress syndrome. N Engl J Med. 2000;342:1301–8.
33. Slinger P. Update on anesthetic management for pneumonectomy. Curr Opin Anaesthesiol. 2009;22:31–7.
34. Jackson TA, Mehran RJ, Thakar D, et al. Case 5–2007 postoperative complications after pneumonectomy: clinical conference. J Cardiothorac Vasc Anesth. 2007;21: 743–51.
35. Yeager MP, Glass DD, Neff RK, et al. Epidural anesthesia and analgesia in high-risk surgical patients. Anesthesiology. 1987;66:729–36.
36. Clemente A, Carli F. The physiological effects of thoracic epidural anesthesia and analgesia on the cardiovascular, respiratory and gastrointestinal systems. Minerva Anestesiol. 2008;74:549–63.
37. Spray SB, Zuidema GD, Cameron JL. Aspiration pneumonia; incidence of aspiration with endotracheal tubes. Am J Surg. 1976;131:701–3.
38. Sackner MA, Hirsch J, Epstein S. Effect of cuffed endotracheal tubes on tracheal mucous velocity. Chest. 1975;68:774–7.
39. Tsai FC, Liu CWY, Shitalkumar S. Extrapleural pneumonectomy perioperative anaesthetic conduct. Sri Lankan J Anaesthesiol. 2018;26:156–8.

Mediastinal Masses

Mahinder Singh Baansal

13.1 Introduction

Tumors arising in or around the vicinity of the mediastinum are rare, but, if present they pose significant challenges to the anesthesiologist, as they may involve/compress vital structures in and around mediastinum [1–5].

Mediastinal tumors vary considerably in their nature (benign/malignant) and site of occurrence. They may be found in the anterior, middle, or posterior mediastinum. Mediastinal masses can occur in any age group and usually 50% are asymptomatic, diagnosed first on routine X-rays [6].

13.2 Anatomy

The term mediastinum is derived from Latin meaning "midway." Hence it is the middle space in the thoracic cavity, between the two lungs. Within the thoracic cavity—the mediastinum is divided into four compartments as defined by Classic model and Shields' model [7–10].

In Classic model the mediastinum is divided into four compartments namely superior, anterior, middle, and posterior.

Shields described an alternative model dividing mediastinum in three compartments namely anterior, middle (visceral) and posterior [8].

The division of mediastinum into various compartments helps in determining the incidence, location and planning the approach of medical/surgical management of the masses (Fig. 13.1, Tables 13.1 and 13.2) [11].

Mediastinal masses can be benign or malignant, developing from the structures (Table 13.3):

(1) Normally present in mediastinum
(2) That pass through mediastinum during development phase
(3) Or may be metastasis of the malignancies that arise elsewhere in the body

13.3 Clinical Presentation

As masses increase in size the symptoms and signs result from direct compression or infiltration of the vital structures present in the mediastinum, e.g., heart, lung, superior vena cava, trachea, or bronchi [12, 13].

13.3.1 Systemic Symptoms

Systemic symptoms viz. fever, night sweats, and weight loss can be present in cases of lymphoma or may be due to variety of paraneoplastic

---

M. S. Baansal (✉)
Institute of Anaesthesiology, Pain and Perioperative Medicine, Sir Ganga Ram Hospital, New Delhi, India

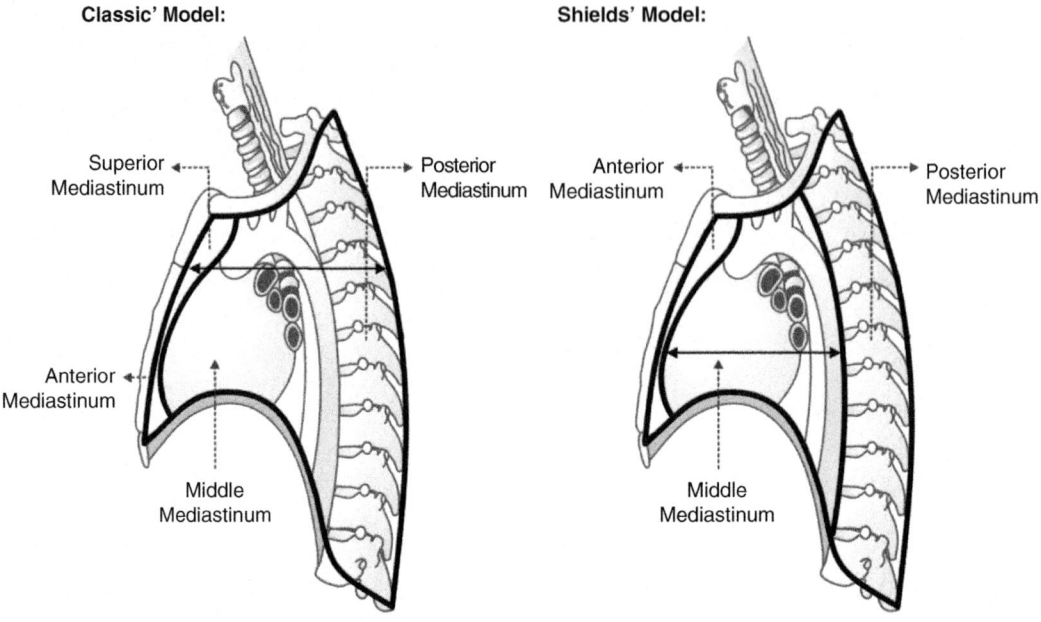

Fig. 13.1 Classic and Shields' model for compartmentalization of mediastinum

Table 13.1 Division of mediastinum

Compartment	Anterior	Posterior
Anterior	Sternum	Anterior aspect of trachea and anterior margin of heart
Middle	Anterior aspect of trachea and posterior margins of heart	A vertical line drawn along the thoracic vertebra 1 cm behind the anterior margin
Posterior	Vertical line drawn along the thoracic vertebra 1 cm behind their anterior margin	Costo vertebral junctions

Table 13.2 Contents in each mediastinal compartment

Compartment	Contents
Anterior	Fat, thymus, lymph nodes, heart, descending aorta, esophagus
Middle	Lymph nodes, esophagus, descending aorta, trachea, bronchi
Posterior	Paravertebral soft tissue/neurogenic tissues

syndromes, such as myasthenia gravis with thymoma [14].

13.3.2 Symptoms and Signs of Anterior Mediastinal Mass

Usually the cardiovascular system is less affected than the respiratory system by an anterior mediastinal mass (Fig. 13.2).

Respiratory symptoms and signs occur due to compression of trachea, carina, bronchi, or involvement of pleura and are as follows (Table 13.4).

Cardiovascular symptoms and signs due to compression or infiltration of heart or blood vessels (Table 13.5).

13.3.3 Respiratory System

Most common finding in cases of large mediastinal mass is extrinsic compression of tracheobronchial tree which depending on degree and

13 Mediastinal Masses

Table 13.3 Types of masses which may be seen in each compartment

Anterior	Middle	Posterior
Thymus • Thymoma • Thymic cyst • Thymic hyperplasia • Thymic carcinoma	Bronchogenic cyst	Neurogenic tumors • Neurofibroma • Neurilemmoma • Neurosarcoma • Ganglioneuroma • Ganglioneuroblastoma • Neuroblastoma • Chemodectoma • Pheochromocytoma
Lymphoma	Pericardial cyst	Meningoceles
Germ cell tumor • Teratoma/dermoid cyst • Seminoma • Non-seminoma – Yolk sac tumor – Embryonal carcinoma – Choriocarcinoma	Lymphadenopathy • Lymphoma • Sarcoid • Metastatic lung cancer	Thoracic spine lesions (e.g., Pott's disease)
Intrathoracic thyroid • Substernal goiter • Ectopic thyroid tissue	Enteric cyst	
Parathyroid adenoma	Esophageal tumors	
Hemangioma	Vascular masses and enlargement	
Lipoma		
Liposarcoma		
Fibroma		
Fibrosarcoma		
Foramen of Morgagni hernia		

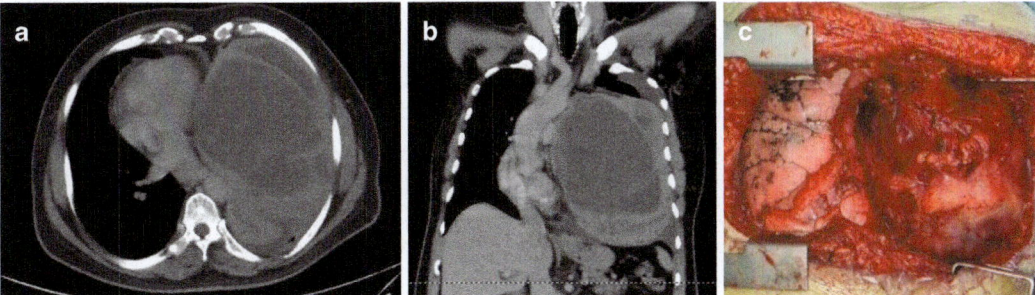

Fig. 13.2 CT scan image of large anterior mediastinal mass compressing heart and mediastinal structures (**a**) and (**b**) and intra-operative picture of same mass (**c**)

Table 13.4 Respiratory symptoms and signs

History	Physical examination
Cough	Decreased breath sounds
Dyspnea on lying supine or excretion	Stridor
Orthopnea	Cyanosis
Cyanosis	Rhonchi

Table 13.5 Cardiovascular symptoms and signs

History	Physical examination
Fatigue	Neck or facial edema
Syncope	Jugular venous distension
Shortness of breath	Blood pressure instability
Orthopnea, cough	Postural changes in blood pressure or pulsus paradoxus
Headache	Papilloedema

chronicity of compression, may lead to narrowing of tracheal lumen, deformity or tracheomalacia.

The weight, size, location of the mass and duration of compression determine the severity of tracheobronchial tree changes, signs and symptoms.

While a small size tumor has minimal effects on tracheobronchial tree, but it can compress the trachea or carina as it grows resulting in weakness in wall of trachea (tracheomalacia), narrowing (tracheal compression) or bending (scabbard trachea). The degree of the compression also depends on the position of the patient. In sitting position tracheal compression will be minimal. However, in supine position tracheal compression can be severe due to effect of gravity on the mass and the end expiratory increase in intra pleural pressure which approaches nearly zero. Hence this type of positional compression is called as "dynamic compression." Static tests (e.g., X-ray, CT) may not give the true picture of physiological effects of compression.

A fixed narrowing of tracheal, which limits the air flow during both inspiration and expiration, produces inspiratory and expiratory stridor. These patients may have breathing difficulty even at rest.

Symptoms at different phases of respiration depend on location and degree of tracheal narrowing or obstruction produced by the mediastinal mass. If variable compression is intrathoracic, then symptoms are produced only during expiratory phase of respiration due to compression of trachea by positive intrathoracic pressure generated during expiration. While extrathoracic variable obstruction produces symptoms only during inspiratory phase of respiration due to generation of negative intrathoracic pressure that accentuate tracheal narrowing and may lead to tracheal collapse. These patients have exertional dyspnea or orthopnea due to compression of trachea/bronchus which can be all mitigated by elevating the head end of the bed with one or more pillows or lying down in propped up position [15–17].

Patients with tracheomalacia usually present with dry cough, dyspnoea, dysphagia (due to esophageal compression), chest pain or recurrent pulmonary infections.

Pleural involvement presents either as pleural effusion or pleural and chest wall pain which may be due to direct pleural involvement or due to obstruction of lymphatic drainage by the tumor.

13.3.4 Cardiovascular

The heart and great vessels may be involved by the mass resulting in cardiovascular dysfunction. The mass may infiltrate or compress pericardium/myocardium, superior vena cava or pulmonary artery. Due to its thick muscular wall, location and large intraluminal pressure the aorta is usually spared.

Pericardial effusion may be due to pericardial involvement which may progress to cardiac tamponade or lead to constrictive pericarditis. Right heart function and pulmonary artery is compromised due to mass effect or direct infiltration, which results in an increase in jugular venous pressure, hepatomegaly and orthostatic changes.

Compression of a major intrathoracic vessel and fixed or limited cardiac output is suggested by a history of syncope or syncope during a Valsalva maneuver.

(A) Compression of pulmonary artery or a major intrathoracic vessel

Due to shielding effect of the aorta, in an awake patient the pulmonary artery is rarely compressed by an anterior mediastinal mass. However, supine position and loss of negative intrapleural pressure during anesthesia may cause compression of pulmonary arteries which may manifest as sudden onset of hypoxemia, hypotension, which may lead to cardiac arrest. In such cases, patient should be repositioned to lateral decubitus or prone position, which helps in restoring the cardiac output by offsetting the gravitational effects of the tumor on pulmonary artery. However, when repositioning is not possible or in pediatric patients, tumor can be lifted by inserting one finger behind the sternal notch and other behind the xiphoid process, to lift the sternum.

In cases where the above measures fail, extracorporeal membrane oxygen (ECMO) or femoro-femoral bypass can be started.

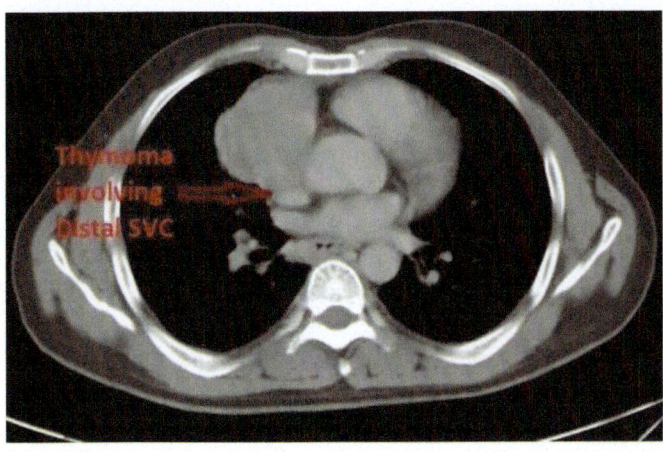
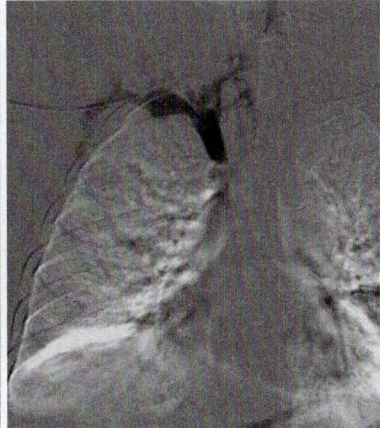

Fig. 13.3 CT scan of superior vena cava syndrome and venography

However, ECMO is ineffective unless a major vein and artery has been cannulated before induction of anesthesia [18–21].

(B) Superior vena cava compression (Fig. 13.3)

Superior vena cava syndrome (SVCS) refers to the signs and symptoms which develop due to an impaired venous drainage from forehead and neck due to obstruction by the mass [22].

The signs and symptoms of SVCS increase in the supine position and when patient is sitting, leaning forward.

In slow developing SVCS, compensatory mechanisms may attenuate the symptoms; however, when there is sudden obstruction in venous drainage, resulting in rapid development of SVS, it is often poorly tolerated and requires emergency intervention.

Radiation is the treatment of choice in cases of tumor-associated mediastinal syndrome. However, in lymphoma associated with SVCS, chemotherapy and steroids with or without radiation is treatment of choice. Usage of steroids may result in necrosis of tumor which may lead to delay in diagnosis and treatment.

13.4 Diagnosis and Evaluation of Mediastinal Mass

Mediastinal mass is usually diagnosed on a plain chest X-ray which may have been taken for another reason as majority of patients are asymptomatic. In a minority of cases, patients may present with symptoms referable to the anterior mediastinal mass that requires further investigations.

13.4.1 X-ray

Chest X-ray is an initial investigation of choice. A good quality postero-anterior and lateral chest X-ray can localize the mass, delineate the borders of the mass as well as provide evidence of compression of airways. Intrinsic or extrinsic compression of the esophagus may be differentiated by Barium swallow by studies.

13.4.2 Computerized Axis Tomography (CAT)

CT scan is the next imaging modality of choice. Modern CAT scan is extremely rapid and provides detailed information. CT scan with or without contrast localizes the mass within the compartments of the mediastinum and helps to plan the best approach for biopsy/surgery. It also provides information regarding nature of mass whether solid/cystic and presence of calcification/fluid or fat, staging of tumor, location or extent of compression or involvement of vital or mediastinal structures.

A contrast enhanced CAT scan facilitates detailed identification of organs, e.g., major blood vessels, airways, heart/lungs, soft tissue perfusion of organs and intracardiac anatomy. High-resolution CT with 3-D reconstruction helps in determining the collateral circulation and to plan for optimal surgical strategy.

However, CT scans do not provide information about dynamic or position related compression of airways or blood vessels. In a retrospective study by Azizkhan et al., the severity of pulmonary symptoms do not corelate with the extent of tracheal narrowing on CAT scan. However, reduction in tracheal diameter nearly equal to 50% on CT scan has been associated with higher rate of complications under general anesthesia. Hence CT scan corelates more with complications under general anesthesia rather than severity of pulmonary symptoms.

The findings by Azizkhan et al. is reconfirmed by retrospective analysis by Shamberger et al [27].

13.4.3 Magnetic Resonance Imaging (MRI)

It is usually used as a secondary investigational tool after CT scan. MRI is often used for specific indications such as neurogenic tumors or when involvement of spinal or mediastinal nerves is suspected, for classification of equivocal CAT findings and to differentiate between mass and cardiovascular structures. To decrease the motion artifacts produced by movement of heart, an **ECG gated CT or MRI** has been used which produces superior images than conventional CT or MRI for evaluating structures close to the heart. This examination can also be performed in recumbent and lateral position, to determine any changes produced by the mass due to change in position of the patient.

13.4.4 Angiography or Myelography

To determine the source of blood supply of the tumor which may cause major intraoperative bleeding, angiography or myelography may be used. It has also been used when spinal or paraspinal involvement, obstruction, or invasion of vascular structures is suspected, e.g., superior vena cava, pulmonary artery.

13.4.5 Transthoracic and Transesophageal Echocardiography

Role of transthoracic and transesophageal echocardiograph for the evaluation of mediastinal masses (TEE) is not firmly established. Echocardiography offers complimentary information regarding invasion of great vessels and heart and to distinguish between pericardial and intracardiac tumors with depressed cardiac function and pericardial effusion.

One should however remember that even in presence of normal preoperative ECHO, great vessel compression and myocardial dysfunction can occur upon assuming supine position and during anesthesia induction.

13.4.6 Positron Emission Tomography (PET) Scan

Fluorodeoxyglucose positron emission tomography (FDG-PET) has a definitive role in diagnosis, staging, and prognosis, though it provides little additional information regarding the anatomical assessment of the mass. FDG-PET can help to determine metabolic activity of the tumor which will help in predicting the response of tumor to chemotherapy.

13.4.7 Bronchoscopy

Fiberoptic flexible bronchoscopy can provide valuable information during preoperative assessment regarding location and amount of extrinsic airway compression and also its severity in different positions. Thus it can provide information regarding dynamic compression of airway.

13.4.8 Pulmonary Function Tests and Flow Volume Loops [23, 24]

Pulmonary function tests and flow volume loops were used extensively during workup of an anterior mediastinal mass.

However, subsequent studies failed to demonstrate any correlation between changes in spirometry and flow volume loops with perioperative airway complication rates. Neither do they give any additional information about intraoperative morbidity and mortality beyond the information obtained from imaging studies, hence nowadays they are not routinely performed during evaluation.

13.5 Risk Assessment and Risk Stratification (Fig. 13.4)

Risk of intraoperative complications during anesthesia is determined by risk assessment and risk stratification [25].

Risk Assessment is done by:

a. Clinical signs and symptoms
b. Radiological studies

13.5.1 Clinical Signs and Symptoms

Assessment of severity and rate of progression with emphasis on presence any symptoms in supine position is done.

13.5.1.1 Grading Scale for Symptoms in Patients with Mediastinal Mass Syndrome

- Asymptomatic—can lie supine without symptoms.
- Mild—Can lie supine with some cough/pressure sensation.
- Moderate—can lie supine for short periods but not indefinitely.
- Severe—cannot tolerate supine position.

Positional dyspnea or orthopnea and stridor are ominous signs and may predict degree of tracheal compression and likelihood of complications.

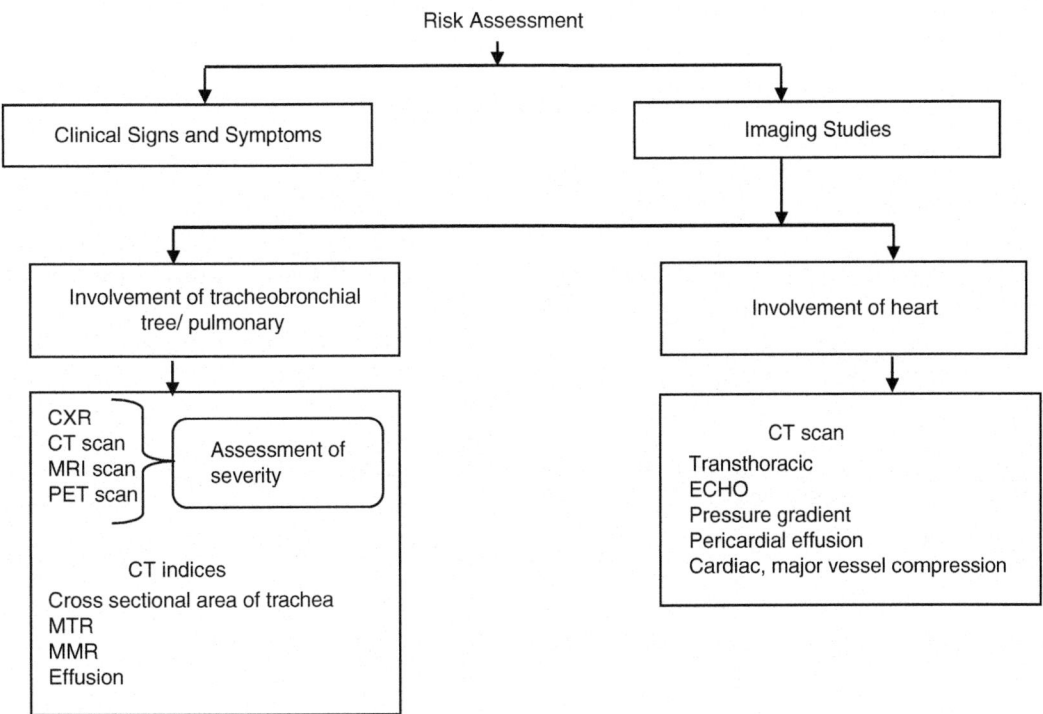

Fig. 13.4 Risk assessment of mediastinal mass

In cases of postural symptoms, efforts should be made to determine the position in which symptoms are minimal. Significant obstruction to right ventricular filling or ejection is indicated by a paradoxical decrease in blood pressure with a change in position from upright to supine. SVC syndrome is suggested by plethora of head and neck and prominent cutaneous veins.

13.5.2 Radiological Studies [26]

CXR/CT chest, MRI, PET scan helps to quantify the degree and extent of mediastinal vital structures involvement also echocardiography is used when cardiac or vascular compression is suspected.

13.5.2.1 CT Scan Indices [26–28]
1. Tracheal diameter
    Tracheal compression is measured by dividing the smallest anteroposterior diameter by that of thoracic inlet.
    A decrease in the diameter of trachea by 35% is associated with symptoms, while more than 50% decrease may lead to complete airway obstruction during induction of anesthesia.
2. Tracheal cross-sectional area
    The widest diameter is usually taken at thoracic inlet with lung apices appearing in the picture while the narrowest point is determined by CT sections above the carina.

Mediastinal thoracic ratio (MTR) and mediastinal mass ratio (MMR)

$$\frac{\text{Maximum width of mediastinal mass}}{\text{Maximum thoracic width}}$$

Mediastinal mass ration may either be <0.3, between 0.31 and 0.43 or greater than or equal to 0.44. Greater the MMR, more are the chances of complications.

MTR is calculated by comparing the size of the mediastinal mass with thoracic diameter, MTR > 50% has higher risk of intraoperative complications.

13.6 Risk Stratification

The patient can be divided into three risk groups on the basis of clinical and imaging findings.

1. Safe (no/low risk)
    a. Clinical signs and symptoms—asymptomatic
    b. Imaging—minimal/no tracheal compression
2. Uncertain (intermediate risk)
    a. Mild/moderate symptomatic child
        Imaging tracheal diameter > 50% of normal
    b. Mild/moderate symptomatic adult
        Imaging tracheal diameter < 50% of normal
    c. Adult unable to give history
        Imaging with abnormal dynamic evaluation
3. Unsafe (high risk)—severely symptomatic adult child
    Imaging tracheal compression >50% with symptoms of SVC obstruction

13.7 Perioperative Management to Reduce Pre, Intra and Postoperative Surgical and Anesthetic Complications

13.7.1 Reducing Size of Tumor

Depending on the histological diagnosis, preoperative neoadjuvant chemotherapy, steroids or radiation therapy can be given to reduce the tumor mass and surrounding infiltration and facilitating the surgical resection. However, this approach is considered controversial as it may cause rapid tumor lysis, adversely affecting the accuracy of tissue diagnosis.

However, for making a histopathological diagnosis taking a fine needle aspiration (FNA) or core needle biopsy is essential in addition to radiological imaging [29–31].

Depending on location of the mass various methods are employed for obtaining tissue diagnosis which include ultrasound or CT guided lymph node or mass biopsy, transthoracic biopsy, tracheobronchial USG guided, transesophageal or surgical methods, such as mediastinoscopy, thoracoscopy, and mediastinotomy.

In evaluation of mediastinal masses role of tissue diagnosis remains controversial as it can lead to seeding of tumor tissue in the biopsy tract especially in cases of thymic neoplasms.

According to National Comprehensive Cancer Network Guidelines on thymic malignancies, if a resectable thymoma is suspected on the basis of clinical and radiological features, surgical biopsy should be avoided.

Decision regarding approach to the tumor should include a multidisciplinary team approach involving surgeon, respiratory physician, oncologist, pathologist, and radiation experts.

13.7.2 Preoperative Embolization of the Tumor Feeding Blood Vessels

Role of preoperative embolization of the tumor feeding blood vessels in cases of mediastinal mass is still work in progress as some studies show it can lead to decrease in size of the tumor as well as reduced intraoperative bleeding. Blood supply of these tumors is usually derived by internal mammary artery, bronchial arteries, thyrocervical trunk, intercostal vessels pulmonary artery, and even from coronary arteries.

13.7.3 Preoperative Maintenance of Airway [6]

In severe dynamic airway obstruction, stenting of the trachea or bronchi can be used to maintain an adequate airway. After during chemotherapy/radiation therapy for allowing normal spontaneous ventilation as tumor responds to therapy the stents can be later removed.

13.7.4 Perioperative Optimization of Systemic Effects of Tumor

Patients having intrathoracic goiter (Fig. 13.5) may require optimization of thyroid function, similarly in patients having thymoma nearly 30% of the patients may have myasthenia gravis as well which may require further optimization.

13.8 Anesthetic Management

Anesthesia in patients with mediastinal mass is usually required for conducting diagnostic and therapeutic procedures.

The decision for the choice of anesthetic technique depends on the risk stratification (safe, unsafe intermediate); urgency and type of procedure, i.e., whether the procedure is diagnostic or therapeutic in nature.

Usually *adult* patients who are in *safe* group, and scheduled to undergo a diagnostic or therapeutic procedure, can safely undergo general anesthesia with muscle relaxant aided tracheal intubation.

However, in all other groups of patients "NPIC" anesthesia technique *"Noli" Pontes Igni Consumere,* i.e., "do not burn your bridges" technique is followed. i.e *maintain spontaneous ventilation as for as possible during anesthesia.*

Extra care must be taken in cases of asymptomatic or mildly symptomatic children as they have higher rate of complications due to the smaller size of thoracic cavity, more compressible and smaller tracheobronchial tree. As children are unable to give their history of positional symptoms, reduced FRC and cardiopulmonary reserve, hence the anesthesia and surgical team should be ready to rapidly change the patient's position during initiation of anesthesia or during surgery if signs of cardiorespiratry compromise develops.

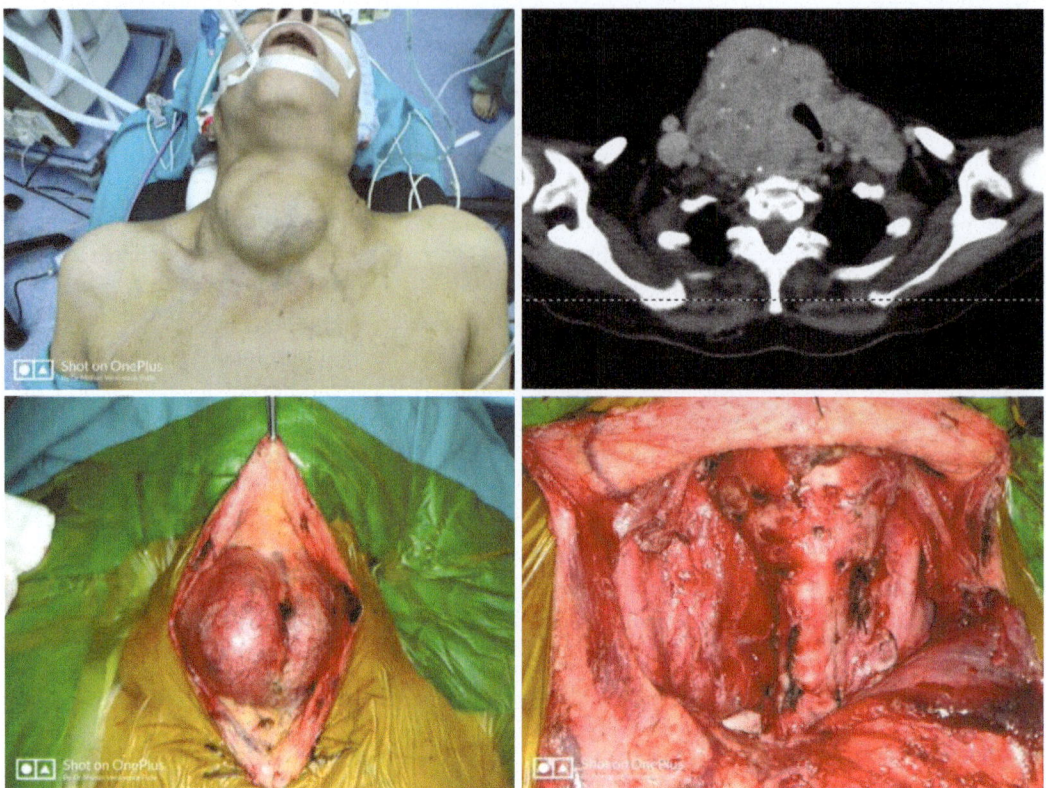

Fig. 13.5 Large retrosternal thyroid compressing trachea and its surgical resection

In *uncertain* or *unsafe* patients coming for *diagnostic* procedures local or regional anesthesia is preferred.

13.8.1 Effect of GA in Mediastinal Mass

13.8.1.1 Respiratory Effects

Patency of airways depends on balance between gravity and negative intrathoracic pressure.

During general anesthesia there is reduction in thoracic volume up to 1000 ml and FRC decreases by 20% which may be due to decreased transverse diameter of thorax as well as cephalad displacement of abdominal contents due to absence of craniocaudal movement of diaphragm. Relaxation of bronchial musculature which reduces the transpleural pressure gradient which result in greater compressibility of the airways from the overlying mass. This leads to reduced airway diameter resulting in turbulent flow and thus greater resistance to airflow.

However patients with spontaneous ventilation, even in supine position, maintain sufficient negative intrathoracic pressure even in supine position to mitigate the effects of gravity. Neuromuscular blockade and IPPV augment the effects of gravity and may lead to enhanced compressive effects due to the mass.

13.8.1.2 Cardiovascular Effects

Direct compression of major blood vessels may lead to severe hemodynamic compromise while direct cardiac compression may lead to arrhythmias and low output syndrome.

During general anesthesia an increase in intrathoracic pressure due to IPPV may further hamper venous return.

13.8.1.3 Effect of Position

In supine position of the tumor is maintained by two opposing forces, i.e., the negative intrathoracic pressure (negative recoil of lungs and rib cage) pulling it upward and gravity pulling it downward.

The negative intrathoracic pressure is the sum of both anatomical (including intercostal and other muscular tone) and physiological (respiration) forces which pull the tumor in an upward direction, whereas opposing the negative intrathoracic pressure is gravity which pulls the tumor in downward direction.

Any intervention, which makes the intrathoracic pressure less negative shifts the balance of pressure in favor of gravity thus pulling the vital structures, such as right side of heart (RA and pulmonary artery) and tracheobronchial tree downward. Examples of such maneuvers include induction of anesthesia, cessation of spontaneous ventilation and institution of positive pressure ventilation. Supine position leads to further increase in tumor mass due to increase in central blood volume, preferential ventilation of the poorly perfused anterior lung sections, and dorsal atelectasis which leads to an increase in V/Q mismatch, thus increasing the shunt fraction. Combination of one-sided main stem bronchial compression and other side pulmonary artery compression can cause catastrophic complete V/Q mismatch.

13.8.2 Sedation

Judicious use of sedation in high or intermediate risk population is recommended. Usually short acting drugs with minimal cardiorespiratory depression are used, e.g., ketamine.

Nowadays dexmedetomidine has also been used due to its minimal effects on hemodynamics and respiration [32].

13.8.3 Induction and Intubation

The anesthesiologist should know the exact location of the mass and its effect on surrounding anatomy. Unsafe patients should be shifted in sitting or semi-sitting (Fowler's) position with minimal or no sedation. Induction should be performed in stepwise manner and is usually a team approach with effort to maintain adequate ventilation and circulation.

Spontaneous ventilation should be kept as far as possible [33].

Presence of adequate and trained staff for rescue positioning should be ensured [34].

Awake fiberoptic intubation in sitting or lateral position under local anesthesia of the airway with or without minimal sedation is the preferred technique as it is the most reversible technique which can be aborted at any point. The endotracheal tube should be placed beyond the site of tracheal compression, have largest possible inside diameter and ability to resist extrinsic compression (e.g., reinforced tube). If lung isolation is desired, the use of bronchial blocker or a double-lumen tube using airway exchange catheter is performed.

If fiberoptic intubation fails, then airway can be maintained with rigid bronchoscope via venturi injector and maintenance of anesthesia through intravenous route. Once sternotomy is performed and tumor is lifted and the degree of airway obstruction decreases, the rigid bronchoscope can be replaced by endotracheal tube (Table 13.6).

Table 13.6 Airway management during anesthesia for mediastinal masses

Patient position
• Induction in sitting position
• Change supine position to lateral or prone position which is best tolerated by the patient
Preserve spontaneous breathing
• Inhalational induction
• Awake fiber bronchoscopic intubation
• Intravenous induction (ketamine, dexmedetomidine)
Airway intubation use of
• Long endotracheal tube
• Double-lumen endobronchial tube
• Rigid bronchoscope
• Tracheobronchial stents
Cardiopulmonary bypass
• Under local anesthesia before induction of anesthesia

13.8.4 Anesthetic Preparation

Apart from standard ASA monitoring, preinduction invasive arterial and CVP lines are secured in intermediate or high-risk patients.

If the mass is involving superior vena cava with signs and symptoms of SVC obstruction, there is increased central venous pressure resulting in decreased blood flow in the superior vena cava which may delay the onset of anesthetic and emergency drugs and make their efficacy uncertain. Hence IV in upper extremity is not an effective form of drug administration in SVCS; in such patients central and peripheral lines should be placed in lower half of the body (femoral artery and veins) prior to induction of anesthesia. It is important to use same side femoral vessels, reserving the other side for cardiopulmonary bypass. In patients with SVC syndrome or with severe compressive symptoms or when heart and major blood vessels are involved, preoperative cardiopulmonary bypass should be established as there is no role of standby bypass nowadays as even with a primed ECC circuit and perfusionist present in the operating room, it still takes at least 5–20 mins to cannulate the femoral vessels and initiate ECC resulting in significant neurological injury. Hence it is now recommended to do femoral cannulation and initiation of ECC before induction of anesthesia in uncertain or high-risk group of patients.

Pulse oximeter should be placed on the right hand to monitor brachiocephalic trunk injury intraoperatively.

Short acting medications should be used for induction of anesthesia, i.e., sevoflurane and etomidate, while remifentanil is the preferred choice of opioid.

Use of BIS monitoring is helpful to adjust depth of anesthesia.

13.8.5 Management of Acute Airway Obstruction (Fig. 13.6) [35, 36]

Loss of airway due to subglottic obstruction is most common and most feared complication in patients with anterior mediastinal mass syndrome.

It can occur at any stage during induction of anesthesia or even intraoperatively. As the lower airway may be involved, a possibility exists that emergency tracheostomy will not relieve the airway obstruction in these patients.

The first step should be to minimize or reverse the deleterious effects of GA and IPPV any by changing the patient position.

Cardiopulmonary bypass can be initiated if already kept ready and emergency thoracotomy/ median sternotomy and tumor debulking done.

13.8.6 Helium–Oxygen Mixture

It can reduce the resistance to the airflow through the compressed airway; however, it limits the amount of inspired fraction of oxygen in cases of severe hypoxemia [6].

13.8.7 Intraoperative Management

Intraoperatively spontaneous ventilation should be maintained as long as possible.

If muscle relaxation is required then short acting muscle relaxants, e.g., succinylcholine may be used. After giving succinylcholine, if significant rise in airway pressure is not there, i.e., maximum ventilation pressure < 40 cmH_2O, then longer acting muscle relaxant may be given.

In case of severe respiratory or hemodynamic compromise the operating table should be tilted to the rescue position after ruling out the possibility of surgical bleeding.

While the basic principles of administering appropriate fluids (colloid or crystalloids) are followed, vasopressor and inotropic medications should be administered simultaneously.

The surgeon should be asked to elevate the mass physically to relieve the compression.

If not relieved, the definitive rescue modality extracorporeal circulation (ECC) should be started which provides both oxygenation and circulatory support.

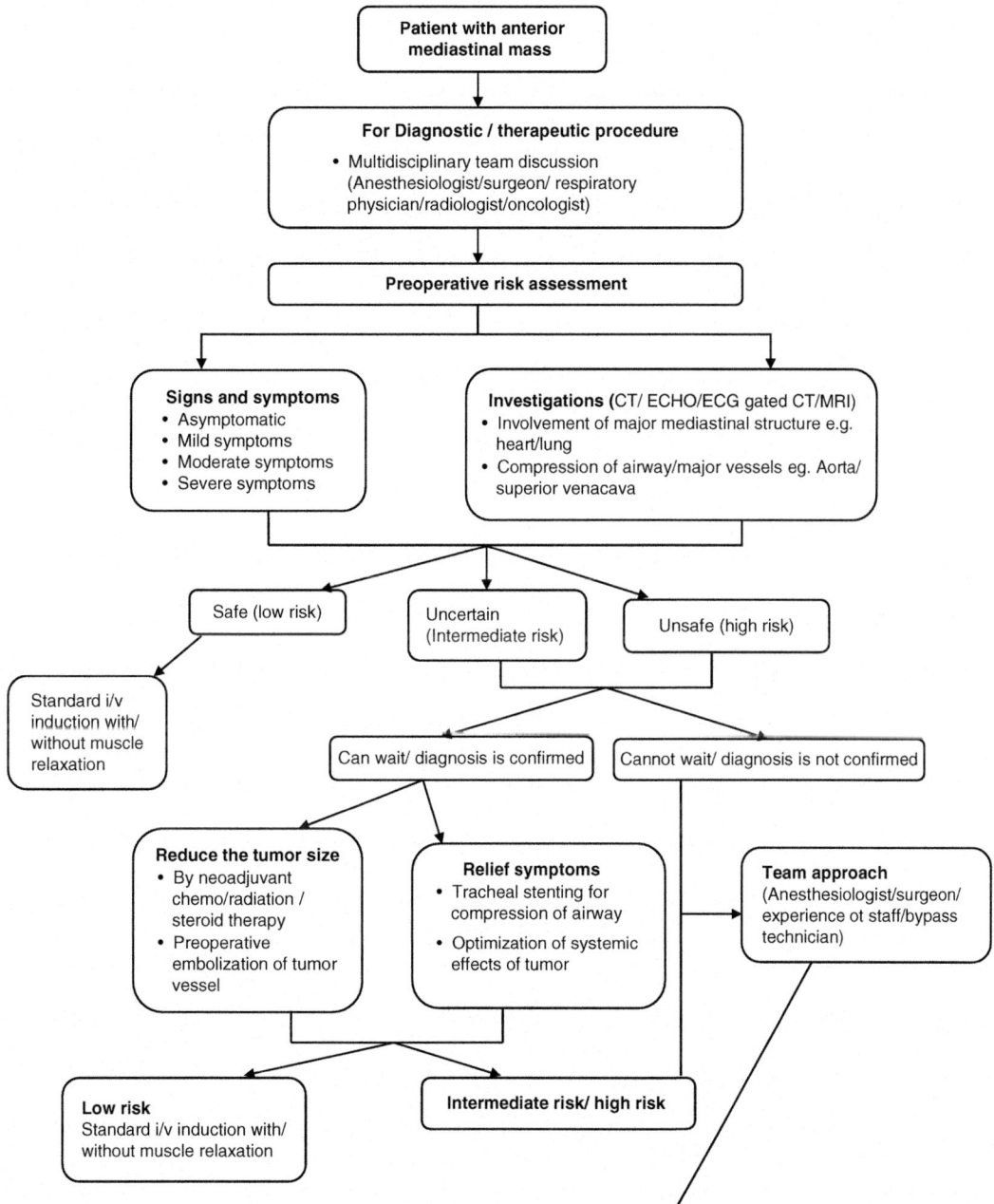

Fig. 13.6 Anesthetic management strategies of patient with anterior mediastinal mass

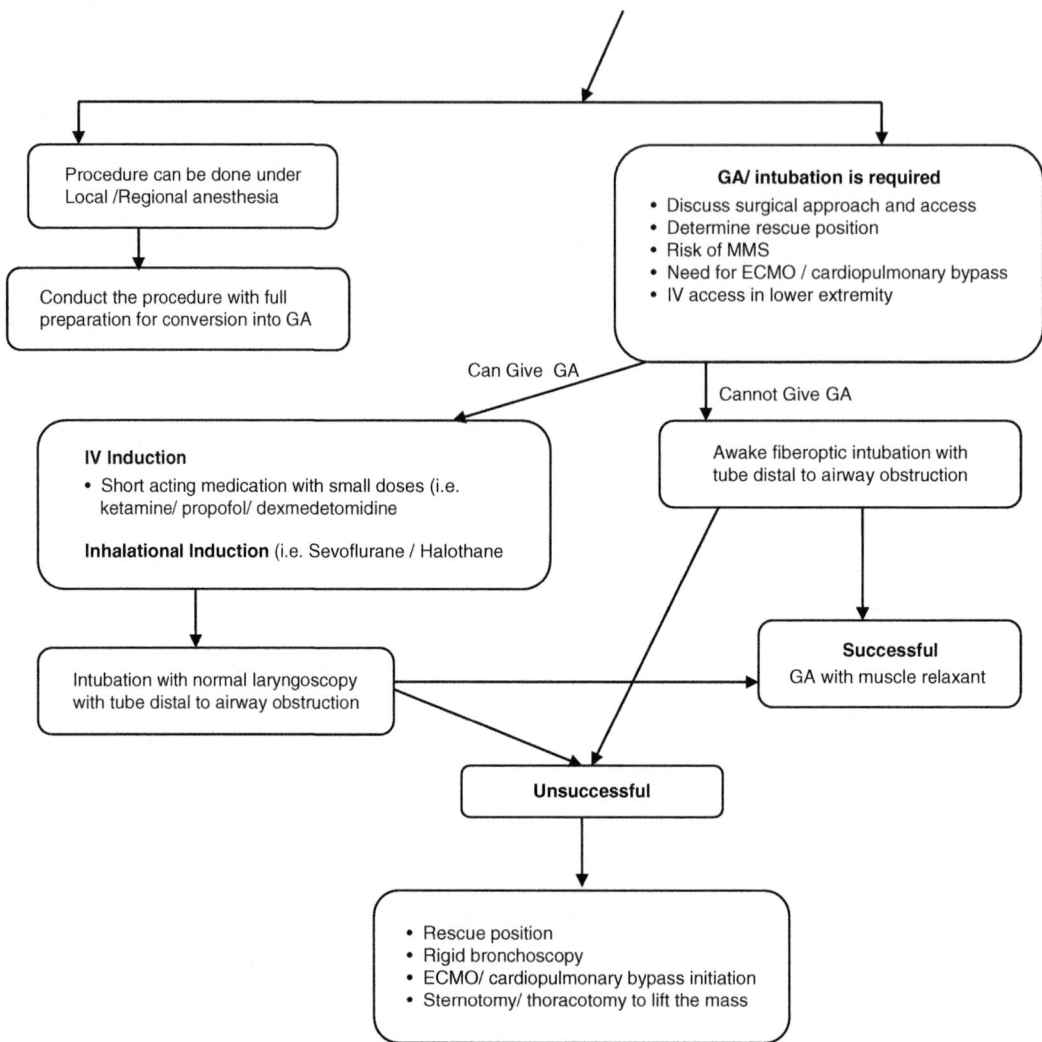

Fig. 13.6 (continued)

Intraoperative regular ABG sampling should be done to check for blood gases, adequacy of ventilation, Hb, and electrolytes.

Blood loss should be monitored carefully and availability of blood products and rapid infusion devices should be ensured in OT [37].

13.8.8 Pain Management

Preinduction thoracic epidural block to cover T2–T12 dermatomes is given in all cases. Administration of only epidural opioids avoiding use of local anesthetics to reduce possibility of hemodynamic instability is practised [38].

13.8.9 Emergence and Recovery

In patients who have undergone diagnostic studies and in surgeries where the mass is not removed completely emergence and recovery may be complicated by airway obstruction. Glottic edema and postoperative stridor may occur in patients with SVC obstruction and prolonged surgeries.

Airway complications are more common during emergence and recovery period. Extubation should only be attempted when patient is fully awake and there is complete recovery of muscle strength. Even with apparently successful extubation the patient should be monitored carefully in post-anesthesia care unit with entire team fully prepared to perform emergency reintubation if there is rapid deterioration after extubation. Postoperative surgical bleeding should also be ruled out in cases of rapid deterioration, as it is quite common [39].

13.9 Nerve Section [2]

Anterior mediastinal tumors may invade phrenic and/or recurrent laryngeal nerve. Surgical division of these nerves may lead to vocal cord palsy and diaphragmatic paresis/paralysis leading to partial or complete airway obstruction with decreased respiratory efforts.

Tracheomalacia may occur after resection of tumor [39].

13.10 Effect of Chemotherapy [2]

Bleomycin used in the treatment of variety of mediastinal masses may cause pulmonary toxicity, hence one should have baseline pulmonary function tests in such patients, and intraoperative low inspired FiO_2 should be used to prevent further pulmonary damage.

13.11 Role of Intraoperative TEE [40–44]

Intraoperative transesophageal echocardiography should be considered in patients with unexplained persistent hypotension or hypoxemia, as it provides real-time imaging of the heart and nearby structures. TEE also provides information regarding degree of rigid ventricular outflow tract (RVOT) obstruction, contractility or compression, pericardial effusion and volume status of the patient.

13.12 Conclusion

A clear and detailed understanding of the pathophysiology of anterior mediastinal mass is key to the management of such cases.

Prior knowledge of potential problems is essential in order to anticipate cardiorespiratory complications which may be exacerbated by general anesthesia.

Three principles should be kept in mind: (1) a thorough preoperative assessment, i.e., history, physical examination, radiological and laboratory examination which helps in classification of the patient into low, middle, or high risk; (2) maintenance of spontaneous ventilation; and (3) determination of rescue positioning.

A collective team approach (surgeon, radiologist, cardiopulmonary bypass technician, oncologist and other OT staff) is required which should understand the risk involved in anesthetizing a patient with an anterior mediastinal mass and type of interventions required to mitigate the effects of tumor (rigid bronchoscopy/positioning) that may be required during emergency.

There is no role of standby bypass nowadays.

References

1. Piro AJ, Weiss DR, Hellman S. Mediastinal Hodgkin's disease: a possible danger for intubation anesthesia. Int J Radiat Oncol Biol Phys. 1976;1:415–9.
2. Keon TP. Death on induction of anesthesia for cervical node biopsy. Anesthesiology. 1981;55:471–2.
3. Bray RJ, Fernandes FJ. Mediastinal tumour causing airway obstruction in anaesthetised children. Anaesthesia. 1982;37:571–5.
4. Mackie AM, Watson CB. Anaesthesia and mediastinal mass. Anaesthesia. 1984;39:899–903.
5. Goh MH, Liu XY, Goh YS. Anterior mediastinal masses: an anaesthetic challenge. Anaesthesia. 1999;54:670–4.
6. Gothard JWW. Anesthetic considerations for patients with anterior mediastinal masses. Anesthesiol Clin. 2008;26:305–14.
7. Johnson D, Shah P. Mediastinum. In: Standring S, editor. Gray's anatomy: thorax. 29th ed. Edinburgh: Elsevier Churchill Livingstone; 2005. p. 976.
8. Shields TW. General thoracic surgery: the mediastinum, its compartments and the mediastinal lymph nodes. 5th ed. Philadelphia: Lippincott Williams & Wilkins; 2000.

9. Daniel P, Raymond T, Daniel M. Mediastinal anatomy and mediastinoscopy. In: Sellke MD, Nido PJD, Swanson SJ, editors. Sabiston & Spencer Surgery of the chest: mediastinum. 7th ed. Philadelphia: Elsevier Saunders; 2005.
10. Neuman GG, Weingarten AE, Abramowitz RM. et al. The anesthetic management of the patient with an anterior mediastinal mass. Anesthesiology. 1984;60:144–7.
11. Warren WH. Chapter 122: Anatomy of the mediastinum with special reference to surgical access. In: Pearson's thoracic and esophageal surgery. 3rd ed. Milton, ON: Elsevier; 2009. p. 1472.
12. Prakash UB, Abel MD, Hubmayer RD. Mediastinal mass and tracheal obstruction during general anesthesia. Mayo Clin Proc. 1988;63:1004–11.
13. Miller RD, Hyatt RE. Obstructing lesions of the larynx and trachea: clinical and physiologic characteristics. Mayo Clin Proc. 1969;44:145–61.
14. Sungur Z, Sentürk M. Anaesthesia for thymectomy in adult and juvenile myasthenic patients. Curr Opin Anaesthesiol. 2016;29:14–9.
15. Erdos G, Tzanova I. Perioperative anaesthetic management of mediastinal mass in adults. Eur J Anaesthesiol. 2009;26:627–32.
16. Li WWL, Boven WJP, Annema JT, et al. Management of large mediastinal masses: surgical and anesthesiological considerations. J Thorac Dis. 2016;8(3):E175–84.
17. Slinger PD, Campos JH. Anesthesia for thoracic surgery. In: Miller RD, Eriksson LI, Fleisher LA, et al. editors. Miller's anesthesia. 7th ed. Amsterdam: Elsevier; 2009. p. 1856.
18. Said SM, Telesz BJ, Makdisi G, et al. Awake cardiopulmonary bypass to prevent hemodynamic collapse and loss of airway in a severely symptomatic patient with a mediastinal mass. Ann Thorac Surg. 2014;98(4):e87–90.
19. Wang G, Lin S, Yang L, et al. Surgical management of tracheal compression caused by mediastinal goiter: is extracorporeal circulation requisite? J Thorac Dis. 2009;1(1):48–50.
20. Hong T, Jo KW, Lyu J, et al. Use of venovenous extracorporeal membrane oxygenation in central airway obstruction to facilitate interventions leading to definitive airway security. J Crit Care. 2013;28: 669–74.
21. Herring K, Sreelatha P, Roy S, et al. Perioperative airway management of a mediastinal mass through early intervention with extracorporeal membrane oxygenation (ECMO). Int J Clin Anesthesiol. 2014;2(1):1022–4.
22. Chaudhary K, Gupta A, Wadhawan S, et al. Anesthetic management of superior vena cava syndrome due to anterior mediastinal mass. J Anaesthesiol Clin Pharmacol. 2012;28(2):242–6.
23. Van der Els NJ, Sorhage F, Bach AM, et al. Abnormal flow volume loops in patients with intrathoracic Hodgkin's disease. Chest. 2000;117:1256–61.
24. Hnatiuk OW, Corcoran PC, Sierra A. Spirometry in surgery for anterior mediastinal masses. Chest. 2001;120:1152–6.
25. Li WW, van Boven WJ, Annema JT, et al. Management of large mediastinal masses: surgical and anesthesiological considerations. J Thorac Dis. 2016;8(3):E175–84.
26. Brooker RF, Zvara DA, Roitstein A. Mediastinal mass diagnosed with intraoperative transesophageal echocardiography. J Cardiothorac Vasc Anesth. 2007;21:257–8.
27. Shamberger RS, Holzman RS, Griscom NT, et al. CT quantitation of tracheal cross-sectional area as a guide to the surgical and anesthetic management of children with anterior mediastinal masses. J Pediatr Surg. 1991;26:138–42.
28. Anghelescu DL, Burgoyne LL, Liu T, et al. Clinical and diagnostic imaging findings predict anesthetic complications in children presenting with malignant mediastinal masses. Pediatr Anesth. 2007;17:1090–8.
29. Borenstein SH, Gerstle T, Malkin D, et al. The effects of prebiopsy corticosteroid treatment on the diagnosis of mediastinal lymphoma. J Pediatr Surg. 2000;35:973–6.
30. Greenstein S, Ghias K, Krett NL, et al. Mechanisms of glucocorticoidinduced apoptosis in hematological malignancies. Clin Cancer Res. 2002;8:1681–94.
31. Frankfurt O, Rosen ST. Mechanisms of glucocorticoid induced apoptosis in hematological malignancies: updates. Curr Opin Oncol. 2004;16:553–63.
32. Abdelmalak B, Marcanthony N, Abdelmalak J, et al. Dexmedetomidine for anesthetic management of anterior mediastinal mass. J Anesth. 2010;24:607–10.
33. Thakur P, Bhatia PS, Sitalakshmi N, et al. Anesthesia for mediastinal mass. Indian J Anaesth. 2014;58(2):215–7.
34. Gardner JC, Royster RL. Airway collapse with an anterior mediastinal mass despite spontaneous ventilation in an adult. Anesth Analg. 2011;113(2): 239–42.
35. DeSoto H. Direct laryngoscopy as an aid to relieve airway obstruction in a patient with mediastinal mass. Anesthesiology. 1987;67:116–7.
36. Azizkhan RG, Dudgeon DL, Buck JR. Life-threatening airway obstruction as a complication to the management of mediastinal masses in children. J Pediatr Surg. 1985;20(6):816–22.
37. Park BJ, Flores R, Downey RJ, et al. Management of major hemorrhage during mediastinoscopy. J Thorac Cardiovasc Surg. 2003;126:726–31.
38. Kiss G, Castillo M. Nonintubated anesthesia in thoracic surgery : general issues. Ann Transl Med. 2015;3:110.
39. Bechard P, Letrouneau L, Lacasse Y, et al. Perioperative cardiorespiratory complications in adults with mediastinal mass. Anesthesiology. 2004;100:826–34.
40. Yang YL, Lu HI, Huang HW, et al. Mediastinal tumor resection under the guidance of transesopha-

geal echocardiography. Anaesth Intensive Care. 2007;35(2):312.
41. Lin CM, Hsu JC. Anterior mediastinal tumour identified by intraoperative transesophageal echocardiography. Can J Anaesth. 2001;48:78–80.
42. Oneglia C, Di Fabio D, Bonora-Ottoni D. Is transesophageal echocardiography useful in planning surgery of mediastinal thymomas? Int J Cardiol. 2007;121:312–4.
43. Redford DR, Kim AS, Barber BJ, et al. Transesophageal echocardiography for the intraoperative evaluation of a large anterior mediastinal mass. Anesth Analg. 2006;103(3):578–9.
44. Thys DM, Abel MD, Brooker RF, et al. Practice guidelines for perioperative transesophageal echocardiography. Anesthesiology. 2010;112:1.

Anesthesia Considerations for Tracheal Reconstruction

14

Ashwin Marwaha

Keywords

Tracheal stenosis · Tracheal resection · Reconstruction · Cross-field ventilation · Total Intravenous anesthesia · Ventilation strategies

14.1 Introduction

The trachea was the last unpaired organ of human body to be considered by surgeons for surgical intervention. The belief that cartilage heals poorly prevented the surgeons from exploring trachea [1]. It was only in the 1950s that tracheal surgery was attempted. Earliest reports of tracheal resection have been described by Belsey [2] and carinal resection by Barclay [3]. Initially it was believed that 2 cm was the maximum length that could be resected safely [4]. This belief led to complex tracheal reconstruction methods using tissue flaps. Over the years there has been advancement in technology and equipment, better understanding of airway physiology, and improvement in surgical and anesthesia techniques. This has enabled complex tracheal surgeries in patients previously deemed unfit. Currently, more than 50% of tracheal length may be safely resected and anastomosed [5].

A. Marwaha (✉)
Institute of Anaesthesiology, Pain and Perioperative Medicine, Sir Ganga Ram Hospital, New Delhi, India

Tracheal resection and reconstruction is a complex procedure, which requires precise planning and coordination between the surgical and anesthetic teams. These patients have compromised airway, with/without suboptimal respiratory function along with coexisting medical comorbidities. The proposition becomes more challenging by virtue of airway sharing and the dynamic nature of airway compromise. These procedures require multidisciplinary care. There are few centers with the requisite infrastructure for conducting such complex procedures. Therefore, there is relative lack of literature on anesthetic management and airway control/ventilation strategies for these surgeries.

14.2 Anatomy (Fig. 14.1)

The upper airway is composed of the nose, pharynx, and larynx, while the trachea, bronchi, and distal bronchial segments form the lower airway. The adult trachea measuring 10–11 cm extends from the larynx to carina, corresponding to the sixth cervical vertebra to fifth thoracic vertebra. Eighteen to twenty C-shaped cartilaginous rings form the anterolateral wall of trachea, while the posterior wall is membranous. The upper one-third is extrathoracic and lower two-third is intrathoracic. Since the trachea is mobile, these individual lengths can vary with respiration and neck movement. The adult tracheal diameter is about 2 cm in males and 1.5 cm

Fig. 14.1 Tracheal anatomy (Reproduced from Celine P (5). With permission from Springer nature. Copyright 1999)

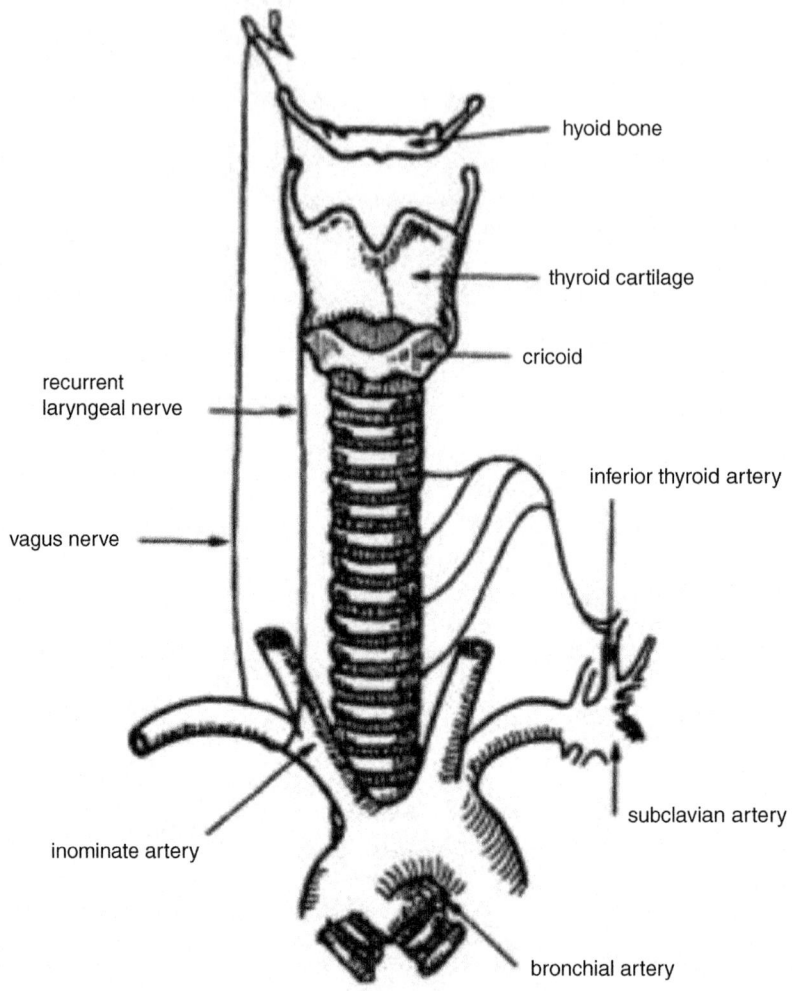

in females, while in children it is smaller, more mobile, and deeply situated. Carina marks the division of right and left main bronchi. The right main bronchus is shorter, wider, and more vertical. It divides into right upper lobe bronchi before continuing as bronchus intermedius, terminating in the right middle and lower lobe bronchi. The left main bronchus is narrower and more in line with trachea and branches into left upper and lower bronchi.

Blood supply to the trachea is extensive and segmental, via a network of vessels from inferior thyroid artery and bronchial artery (Fig. 14.2). Pressure against the tracheal mucosa (endotracheal tube cuff) can compromise the blood

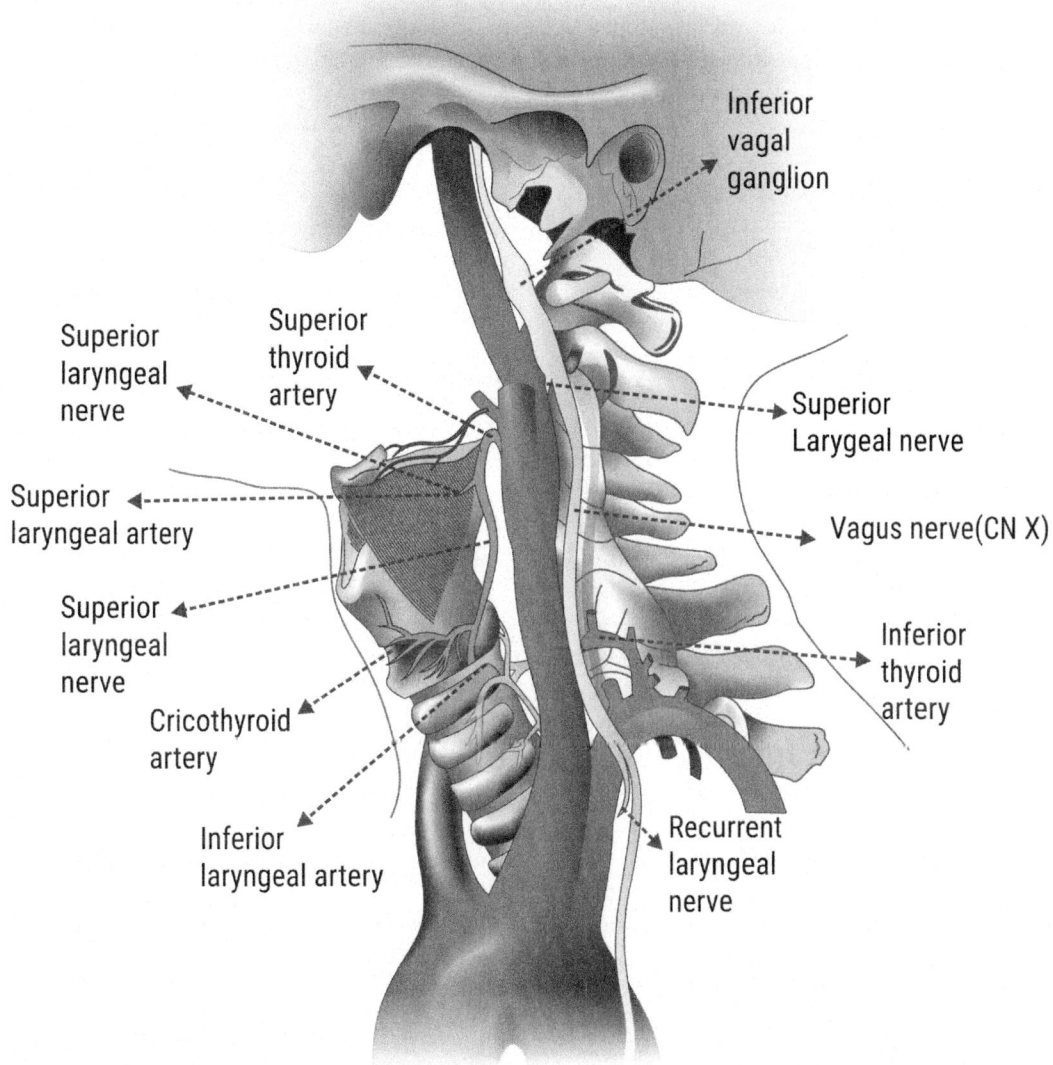

Fig. 14.2 Tracheal blood supply

supply. This can cause pressure necrosis, which on healing leads to fibrosis resulting in stenosis. Microangiopathies associated with conditions like diabetes mellitus and radiation may aggravate this process. Nerve supply of trachea is through the superior and recurrent laryngeal nerves, which are branches of the vagus nerve. Recurrent laryngeal nerve is prone to injury during laryngotracheal surgeries because of its anatomical location in the trachea-esophageal groove. This also makes it vulnerable to involvement in tracheal pathology, i.e., malignancy.

14.3 Physiology of Airway Obstruction

The airflow in a normal trachea is laminar. The major determinants of this normalcy are tracheal diameter and pressure gradient across the trachea. A normal airflow despite a tracheal narrowing is possible, but this requires a higher pressure proximal to the narrowing. This translates to increased work of breathing and reduced exercise capacity. With intrathoracic lesions, spontaneous ventilation is better tolerated as the pressure in the thorax drops below the tracheal pressure during inspiration. A 50% reduction in the tracheal lumen (8 mm or less) will cause symptoms such as stridor and dyspnoea to appear on exertion [6]. Any further reduction of this (5–6 mm or less) will cause these symptoms to appear even at rest [7, 8]. The other determinants of the symptoms and their severity are:

(a) The *exact etiology of obstruction*.
(b) The *rate of progression of the obstruction*.
(c) *Location of the obstruction*—a fixed airway narrowing at larynx and upper trachea manifests as inspiratory obstruction whereas lower airway obstructions manifest as expiratory symptoms, e.g., dynamic collapse.

Flow volume loops help us to better understand the minutiae of airway obstruction. Fixed obstructions reveal reduction of both inspiratory and expiratory peak flows. The effect of dynamic collapse varies with different phases depending upon the location of the collapse, i.e., inspiratory attenuation in extrathoracic and expiratory attenuation in intrathoracic lesions. Emphysematous collapse, however, manifests with collapse of small airways and appears first in expiration and later in inhalation [9–11]. Flow volume loops no longer have the same importance now, as imaging techniques have improved and the pathophysiology of tracheal stenosis is better understood.

Improved imaging techniques and better clinical observations are now favored to study the desired dynamic respiratory components.

14.4 Etiology

Table 14.1 enumerates various causes of tracheal obstruction [12, 13]. Patients who require tracheal resection and reconstruction commonly

Table 14.1 Etiology of tracheal stenosis

Tumors
Primary tumors
Malignant
Adenoid cystic carcinoma (cylindroma), squamous cell carcinoma, others
Benign
Neurofibroma, chondroma, chondroblastoma, hemangioma, pleomorphic adenoma
Secondary tumors
Direct extension
Thyroid, larynx, lung, esophagus
Metastasis
Lung, breast, lymphoma
Inflammatory lesions
Post-intubation lesion
Stricture, granuloma, malacia, tracheoesophageal fistula
Post-traumatic stenosis
Blunt trauma, penetrating injury, emergency tracheostomy
Postinfectious strictures
Tuberculosis, diphtheria, histoplasmosis, rhinoscleroma
Burns
Connective tissue disease
Systemic lupus erythematosus, Wegener's granulomatosis, amyloidosis
Compressive lesions
Goitre
Vascular compression
Thoracic aneurysm, congenital vascular rings, innominate artery aneurysm, anomalous right innominate artery, double aortic arch, complete tracheal rings and associated aberrant origin of left pulmonary origin
Miscellaneous
Sarcoidosis, relapsing polychondritis, osteoplastica tracheopathy, idiopathic

Reproduced from Celine P (5). With permission from Springer nature. Copyright 1999

have post-intubation stenosis or tumors. The incidence of post-intubation tracheal stenosis has decreased with the current use of high-volume, low-pressure cuffed ET tubes [14]. Over inflated cuff, large bore tracheal tube, tube movement, prolonged intubation, steroids, hypotension, infection, diabetes, and nasogastric tube are the risk factors associated with post-intubation strictures. The site of stenosis varies with respect to whether patient was intubated (oral/nasal) or tracheotomized (Fig. 14.3). Primary tracheal tumors although rare in adults, are malignant with squamous cell carcinoma and adenoid cystic histopathological subtypes being the commonest.

14.5 Clinical Presentation

The symptoms are nonspecific and vague. Onset is usually insidious with progressive dyspnoea on exertion being the predominant symptom. There may be associated wheezing and stridor. The nonspecific nature of symptoms often delays the diagnosis [12, 13, 15]. An acute respiratory infection can be the precipitating event. Dyspnoea on exertion appears typically when 50% of tracheal diameter is narrowed while 75% narrowing leads to dyspnoea at rest corresponding to 8 mm [6] and 5–6 mm [7, 8] respectively. Other symptoms may include hemoptysis, persistent cough (productive/nonproductive),

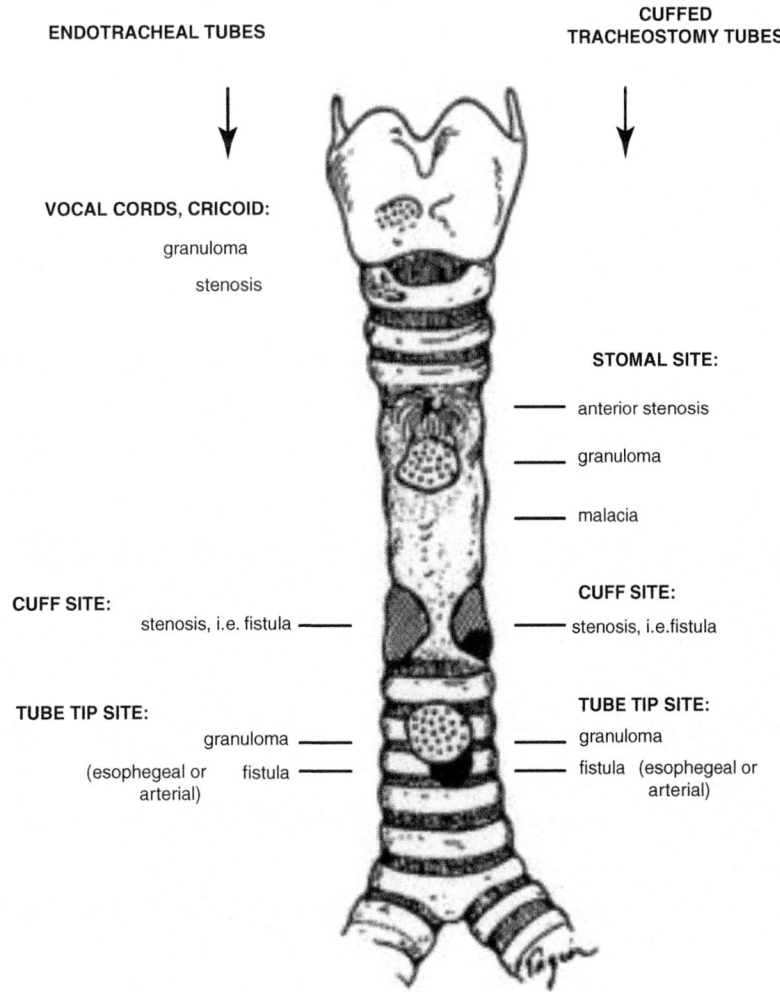

Fig. 14.3 Type and location of tracheal lesions (Reproduced from Celine P (5). With permission from Springer nature. Copyright 1999)

dysphagia, and hoarseness (involvement of recurrent laryngeal nerve) according to underlying pathology. Wheezing and stridor are often treated for asthma till symptoms become nonresponsive to bronchodilators and/or associated symptoms manifest or tracheal lumen reduces to critical diameter. Patients of tracheal stenosis may range from those with no associated comorbidities to those having multiple associated comorbidities. Cyanosis is a dangerous sign implying complete airway occlusion, and these patients require tracheostomy before any corrective procedure can be contemplated.

Pediatric patients require a separate mention. Children with congenital tracheal stenosis may present with biphasic stridor, tachypnea, retractions, nasal flaring, apnea, cyanosis, wheezing, noisy breathing, recurrent upper respiratory symptoms, persistent croup, and pneumonia. Dysphagia with apnea and cyanotic spells may occur with attempts to swallow solid food. Failure to thrive is common. Patients with respiratory symptoms following intubation (irrespective of the duration of intubation) require high suspicion index for diagnosing tracheal stenosis.

14.6 Anesthesia Considerations

Patients with tracheal obstruction are managed according to the severity and etiology of obstruction. The goal of treatment is cure or palliation. Anesthesiologists may be involved at the time of diagnostic workup or therapeutic interventions.

Bronchoscopy is vital for diagnostic workup of tracheal stenosis (Fig. 14.4). It helps assess the nature, length, location, extent of lesion, and degree of obstruction. Macroscopic appearance of stenotic segment helps identify the possible etiology, e.g., stenosis secondary to tuberculosis has granulation tissue while cobblestone appearance of mucosa points to sarcoidosis. Bronchoscopy also allows tissue biopsy for definitive diagnosis and helps evaluate vocal cord function along with evaluation of dynamic airway collapse with respiration. Patients presenting with moderate to severe obstruction are treated with emergency tracheal dilatation (with or without stenting) or tracheostomy. Bronchoscopy in these patients is deferred and is generally a part of definitive treatment [16]. Depending on the etiology, presentation, and patient various treatment options are available.

14.6.1 Irradiation

The common adult carcinoma histological subtypes that cause tracheal stenosis (squamous cell and adenoid cystic) respond well to irradiation [13]. However, due to recurrence after a few years, this modality is not the definitive treatment, but is good as a postoperative adjunct

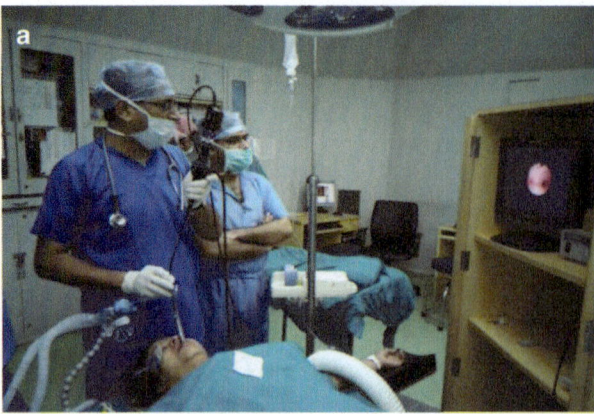
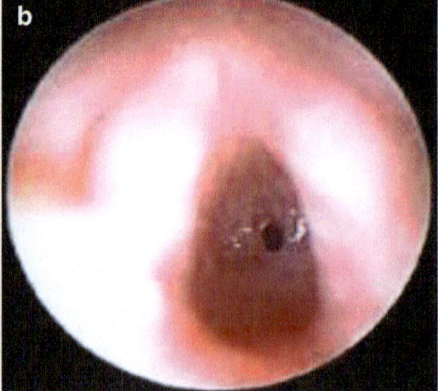

Fig. 14.4 Diagnostic bronchoscopy. (**a**) bronchoscopy procedure; (**b**) bronchoscopy view of tracheal stenosis

[12, 13]. A high incidence of tracheal dehiscence discourages its use preoperatively [17].

14.6.2 Laser

Malignant lesions not amenable to surgical resection are treated by laser therapy with CO_2 or YAG [18] in adults and KTP laser in the pediatric age group [17].Endoscopic laser treatment provides the ability to cut and vaporize the tumor and is used to achieve radial incision, dilatation, and excision [19]. Nd:YAG laser is the laser of choice because of its better reach in the tracheobronchial tree. However, as its depth cannot be controlled with precision, there is a risk of perforation [20]. Lasers are unable to destroy the root of tumors, hence there is recurrence after tumor ablation. Also, lasers are not recommended prior to definitive surgery, as they destroy the adjacent healthy tissue, which compromises the anastomosis [21].

From the anesthesia point of view, before any use of laser/cautery, the standard precautions of airway fire protocol need to be taken. General anesthesia is mandatory in patients where the laser is being used, as undue movement of patients can be disastrous. Anesthesia is induced with propofol in titrated doses and the airway is secured with a supraglottic device (i-gel). A flexible bronchoscope is passed through the catheter mount to enable laser ablation. At the time of laser use, FiO_2 is lowered and air is used along with protective laser gear.

14.6.3 Dilatation

Tracheal dilatation is being used as a planned procedure to evaluate the need for surgical resection or just prior to a tracheal resection and anastomosis, to facilitate airway control in the operation theater. It can also be an emergency procedure for management of the obstructed airway. Mature, firm tracheal stenoses and those with cartilaginous components are unsuitable for dilatation [16]. Tracheal dilatation is a temporary procedure to buy time for workup, achieve control of infection/inflammation/associated medical comorbidity [5]. Tracheal dilatation is performed under general anesthesia, induced with dexmedetomidine/propofol in carefully titrated does, with the airway secured with a supraglottic device like i-gel/PLMA which provides the access to bronchoscope. Dilatation is done by round dilators with progressively increasing diameter passed through the working channel of bronchoscope [21]. Multiple dilatations increase the risk of edema and iatrogenic trauma.

14.6.4 Tracheal Stents

Tracheal stenting may be used as a palliative measure in patients with extensive tumors unsuitable for surgical resection. It is definitive treatment for patients with extensive benign strictures unsuitable for surgery, patients with trachea destroyed by multiple reconstruction attempts, or those patients in whom associated comorbidities make surgery unfeasible. Tracheal stents maybe used as temporary measures (in patients under preparation for surgery) or as adjuncts (to protect fresh tracheal anastomosis) [22]. Tracheal stents can be metallic or made of silicon. Silicon stents may migrate while metallic stents can collapse with external pressure or have granulation tissue ingrowth leading to luminal occlusion. Generally silicon stents are used for benign strictures while metallic stents are preferred for malignant lesions [23, 24].

Tracheal stent placement is performed by the surgeon or an intervention pulmonologist. An experienced anesthesiology team is essential as we deal with unprotected compromised airway and run the danger of partially/near complete obstructed airway turning into a completely obstructed airway. Sedative premedication is avoided, except for extremely anxious patients, as there is a high probability of hypoventilation in a partially obstructed airway. Dexmedetomidine is a good sedative, if required. An anticholinergic may be given to decrease the airway secretions [25]. Preoxygenation (longer than in normal patients) is mandatory. Local anesthetics are used to anesthetize the airway, keeping in mind the possibility of exacerbation of inspiratory airflow limitation, secondary to inhibition of dilator responses and absorption of local anesthetics. For patients presenting with respiratory compromise, an initial tracheal dilatation under local anesthesia provides the vital margin of safety for further procedure. Induction of anesthesia is titrated as per patient's condition, lesion and associated comorbidities. TIVA with propofol and titrated doses of opioids is the technique of choice. The golden rule is to avoid neuromuscular blockade and maintain spontaneous ventilation [26, 27]. Various techniques are used for airway control, depending on the lesion, location, patient's condition and user comfort. Nasal airway and oxygen supplementation, supraglottic device and an ETT are the options available. At the author's institution induction of anesthesia is done with propofol and titrated doses of opioids, while the airway is maintained with a nasal airway with oxygen supplementation and a rigid bronchoscope is used to deploy stents and confirm position. Ventilation maybe assisted through the ventilating port with slower rate and longer inspiratory and expiratory times. In cases where a silicon stent is to be deployed, an i-gel may be used. Anesthesia is maintained with propofol infusion to maintain anesthetic depth during periods where ventilation maybe interrupted. At the end of the procedure, infusion is stopped and the patient is allowed to wake up fully with intact airway reflexes. Patients are monitored in the PACU.

14.6.5 Tracheostomy

Some patients require tracheostomy to secure the airway. In these patients, tracheostomy is performed preferably at the damaged part, in an attempt to preserve the healthy tracheal wall to achieve anastomosis [12, 14, 28]. This may not be always possible, as the person performing tracheostomy and the person performing subsequent tracheal resection anastomosis are usually different.

14.6.6 Surgery

Tracheal resection and primary anastomosis is the definitive treatment for tracheal stenosis. For malignant lesions extensive tracheal involvement, deep mediastinal invasion, and metastasis needs to be ruled out. Adenoid cystic carcinomas are an exception as long survival is seen even in patients with metastasis [12].

14.7 Preoperative Evaluation

Pre-anesthetic evaluation is similar to that for any other patient scheduled for surgery under general anesthesia and comprises of thorough history, physical examination, and appropriate laboratory investigations. Associated comorbidities, if any, should be optimized. Preoperative ECG provides a baseline as surgery of airway and mediastinal structures can initiate the sympathoadrenal response. Patients over 40 years or with significant risk factors predisposing to coronary artery disease should undergo detailed cardiac assessment (echo, stress test, and angiography, if required). Special emphasis is given to airway and pulmonary system assessment. Bag and mask ventilation and intraoperative airway management should be assessed and planned. Physical examination should stress on tracheal palpation and assessment of neck mobility (flexion and extension).

History of dyspnea, especially dyspnea at rest, should be elicited as the pattern of dyspnea helps gauge the location as well as diameter of stenosis. Inspiratory symptoms indicate fixed obstruction of larynx and upper trachea, while expiratory symptoms are associated with lower airway pathology (dynamic collapse/tracheomalacia/tumors). The position in which the patient is comfortable should be documented and preferably anesthesia should be induced in the same position. Airway obstruction with forced respiratory efforts should be assessed. Extrathoracic lesions worsen with forced inspiration, while forced expiration worsen intrathoracic lesions. Pulmonary function tests and spirometry can be done in elective procedures. Flow volume loops are not reliable indicators of the degree of obstruction as they are effort dependent [8].

Bronchoscopy is the most helpful modality for the anesthesiologist as it helps identify the site, length, and diameter of tracheal narrowing. As tracheal stenosis is progressive, the possibility of

14 Anesthesia Considerations for Tracheal Reconstruction

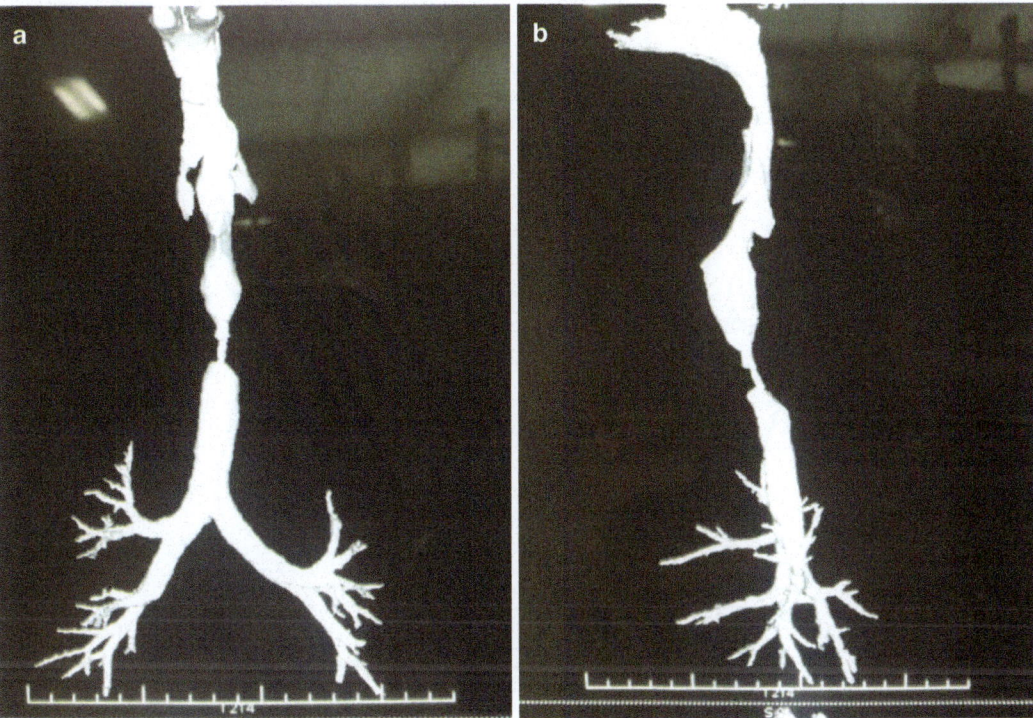

Fig. 14.5 High-resolution CT of neck and thorax with three-dimensional reconstruction (**a**) AP view, (**b**) lateral view

stenosis having worsened between bronchoscopy and surgery needs to be kept in mind. Therefore, bronchoscopy should be done as close to the date of surgery as possible. Chest X-ray, standard CT scan, and MRI are not very helpful. High resolution CT of neck and thorax with three-dimensional reconstruction (Fig. 14.5) aid in both, initial assessment and postoperative follow-up.

For lung parenchymal resection cases, ventilation and perfusion scans should be considered [29]. All possible reversible pulmonary conditions contributing to morbidity should be identified and addressed. Cessation of smoking is important with respect to the detrimental effects of smoking on ciliary activity leading to difficulty in mobilizing secretions with respect to postoperative period.

14.7.1 Patient Selection

Patients with a resectable lesion, and functional glottis have favorable outcome with surgery. Surgery is best avoided in patients with neuromuscular disorders, severe pulmonary dysfunction likely to require postoperative ventilation, ventilator-dependent patients with severe pulmonary dysfunction, steroid dependent, patients with invasive tumors, and those who have undergone neck and chest radiation therapy.

14.8 Surgical Considerations

The location and extent of stenotic lesion determines the site and extent of surgical incision, the length of trachea which will be resected and the position of patient. Grillo [5] investigated cadaveric studies and determined that 4.5 cm, i.e., seven tracheal rings could be removed and end-to-end anastomosis achieved without compromising the blood supply or causing excessive traction. The blood vessels enter the lateral tracheal wall in segmental fashion; therefore, anteroposterior dissection prevents devascularization. Figure 14.6 shows the various surgical incisions.

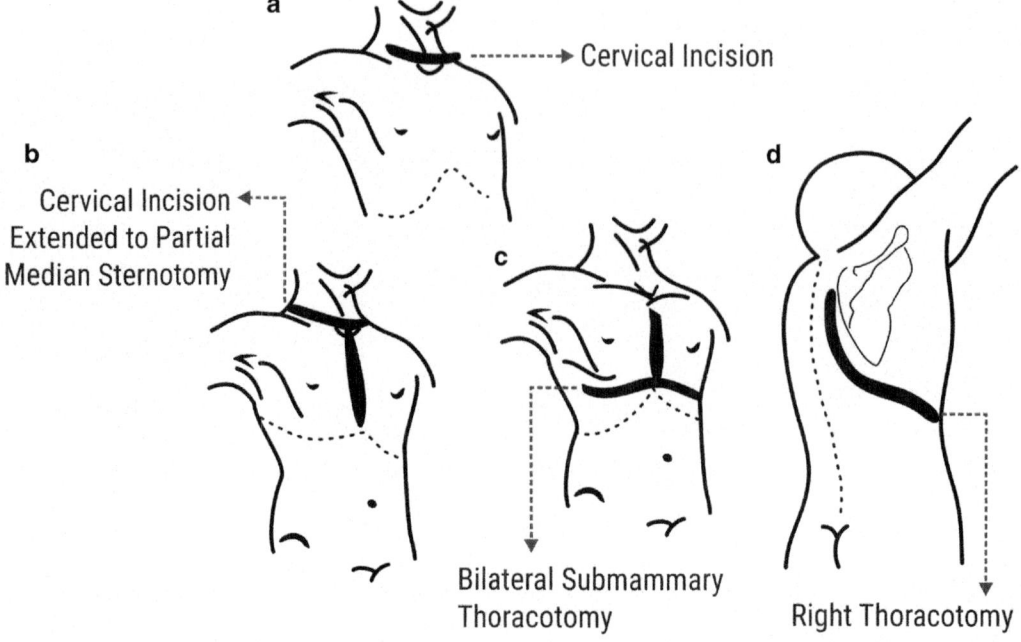

Fig. 14.6 Surgical approaches for tracheal resection anastomosis. (**a**) Cervical incision; (**b**) Cervical incision extended to partial median sternotomy; (**c**) Bilateral submammary thoracotomy; (**d**) Right thoracotomy

14.8.1 Subglottic and Upper Tracheal Lesions

These lesions are best approached via cervical/collar incision with or without upper sternotomy in supine position and neck extended. Posterior shell of the cricoid cartilage is preserved, if possible, to protect the recurrent laryngeal nerves. Most subglottic stenosis (1–4 cm length) are managed with segmental resection and primary anastomosis. Malignancies require more extensive surgeries (laryngectomy). Lesions very close to the glottis risk vocal cord edema; therefore, a Montgomery T-tube is placed. After primary anastomosis the head is maintained in flexion, to minimize traction on the anastomosis. This is achieved by a *Guardian* suture (Fig. 14.7) between the chin and the anterior chest wall.

14.8.2 Mid Trachea

These lesions are operated on via a cervicomediastinal incision. The upper trachea can be explored through the cervical incision and if required a laryngeal drop may be performed to get an additional 1 cm for reducing traction on the anastomosis. The mediastinal incision includes a mini-sternotomy extending up to the angle of sternum and allows exploration of the anterior carina and both tracheobronchial angles.

14.8.3 Carina

The type of carinal resection planned determines the incision. Isolated carinal resection is approached via sternotomy. Carinal resection of

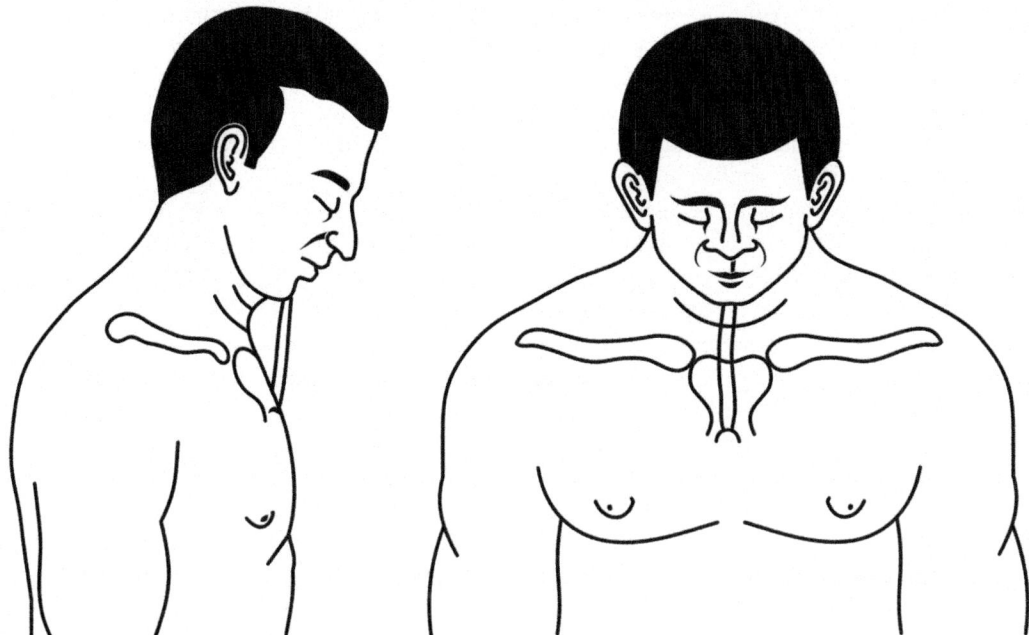

Fig. 14.7 Guardian suture

up to 4 cm can be done without laryngeal release. Carinal resection along with parenchymal resection is operated via a posterolateral thoracotomy or a "Clamshell incision".

14.9 Anesthetic Management

14.9.1 Operating Room Setup

In addition to the equipment usually present in the operating room, special ones are endotracheal tubes of various sizes particularly smaller sizes (2.5–6.5), reinforced ETT for ventilation through surgical field and flexible fiberoptic bronchoscope (adult and pediatric).

14.9.2 Intravenous Access and Monitors

Generally the blood loss is minimal. Since the arms are tucked by the side of the patient and under drapes, two wide bore (18 g) IV cannula should be secured. In most cases the standard ASA monitoring (ECG, SpO_2, NIBP, and $EtCO_2$) is sufficient. Intra-arterial catheter is indicated in selected scenarios, i.e., use of jet ventilation, apnea during tracheal anastomosis, and monitoring in hilar release (hemodynamic changes resulting from retraction of the heart). Central venous line (CVL) is rarely indicated except in patients with severe cardiomyopathy. Central venous line when established is preferably via femoral or subclavian approach to keep the neck free for tracheal resection.

Anesthesia depth monitor (BIS) is mandatory, as these procedures are performed (either fully or in part, i.e., open tracheal anastomosis) under total IV anesthesia. Neuromuscular monitoring (TOF) should be used to ensure motionless surgical field for precise suturing, and complete recovery at the end, which is imperative to mitigate stress on the anastomosed trachea. Urine output monitoring helps assess adequate organ perfusion.

14.9.3 Induction and Maintenance

A clear and well discussed plan for induction and airway control should be formulated preoperatively in consultation with surgeon and pulmonologist involved. Close communication is of paramount importance. All the equipment for airway management should be arranged and checked for functionality.

Preoxygenation for longer than the usual 3 minutes is mandatory. Anesthetic induction maybe performed in the sitting, semi-sitting, or supine positions, the determining factor being the position in which airway obstruction is the least and the patient is most comfortable. Previous bronchoscopy findings help guide the induction and airway control strategy. Anesthesia technique needs to be modified according to severity of stenosis. In cases with minimal obstruction, anesthesia is induced with intravenous agent, neuromuscular blockade achieved and trachea is intubated as per standard practice [30, 31]. Propofol with or without ketamine is the agent of choice.

In patients who have significant stenosis, rigid bronchoscopy and tracheal dilatation is performed after anesthesia induction to facilitate placement of endotracheal tube. Inhalation induction is achieved by gradually increasing the concentration of sevoflurane with oxygen. Spontaneous breathing is preferred during bronchoscopy although ventilation may be assisted. Propofol infusion maybe used along with sevoflurane to increase the depth. Opioids are used to blunt the noxious stimuli. Airway should be topicalized prior to instrumentation. For patients who are already tracheostomized, routine intravenous induction is followed by ventilation through the tracheostomy tube.

Intravenous induction with propofol and with short acting muscle relaxant and an awake fiberoptic is the other option available to facilitate bronchoscopy and secure the airway. However, airway instrumentation without muscle relaxant can be a tricky proposition as it can put the patient at risk of negative pressure pulmonary edema (patient breathing against a nearly obstructed airway). Once the trachea is intubated muscle relaxant is given (if not given earlier) and positive pressure ventilation is instituted. Anesthesia is maintained with inhalational agent in oxygen. Provision for cross-field ventilation is made and during the open airway phase (which is explained further) anesthesia is maintained with TIVA, i.e., propofol infusion.

Dexmedetomidine, administered by infusion, is a useful agent as it provides analgesia, anxiolysis, and amnesia with minimal respiratory depression [32]. It has the potential to be the sole anesthetic agent for induction and controlled emergence [33].

14.9.4 Ventilation Strategies

Surgery of the airway is a challenging proposition for the anesthesiologist. The aim is to ensure satisfactory gas exchange without hindering the surgical field, preventing movement and minimizing the spray of blood and secretions. The various options practiced are as follows:

1. *Distal Tracheal Intubation with Cross-Field Ventilation*—For a mid-tracheal lesion an appropriate sized endotracheal tube is negotiated beyond the stenosis. For distal lesions the tube is placed proximally (Fig. 14.8a). As tracheal resection commences the surgeons intubate the distal trachea with a sterile reinforced tube (Fig. 14.8b). A new sterile anesthetic circuit is passed over the drapes and connected to the anesthesia machine (cross-field ventilation Fig. 14.9). The oral endobronchial tube, used at the start of case, is replaced with a new regular size endotracheal tube, which is inserted through the glottis and kept there (Fig. 14.8c). The stenosed part is resected and posterior anastomosis between the two ends is done utilizing apnea–ventilation–apnea technique (Fig. 14.10). The new endotracheal tube is positioned distal to the anastomotic site by the surgeons and the last part of anastomosis (anterior sutures) is done over the tube (Figs. 14.8d and 14.11). Variation of cross-field ventilation has been described by Geffin [7]. Lower tracheal tumors and carinal tumors require improvisation (Figs. 14.12 and 14.13). The cross-field ventilation tube is positioned in the left main bronchus, while the surgeons resect the lower trachea and/or carina, and anastomose the right main bronchus with the resected tracheal margin. The tube is then repositioned distal to the anastomosis to ventilate the right lung while the left main bronchus is anastomosed with the newly anastomosed trachea and right main bronchus creating a new carina. The tube is withdrawn and placed above the suture line till the trachea is extubated. The apnea–ventilation–apnea technique results in some hypercapnia which is acceptable. Propofol

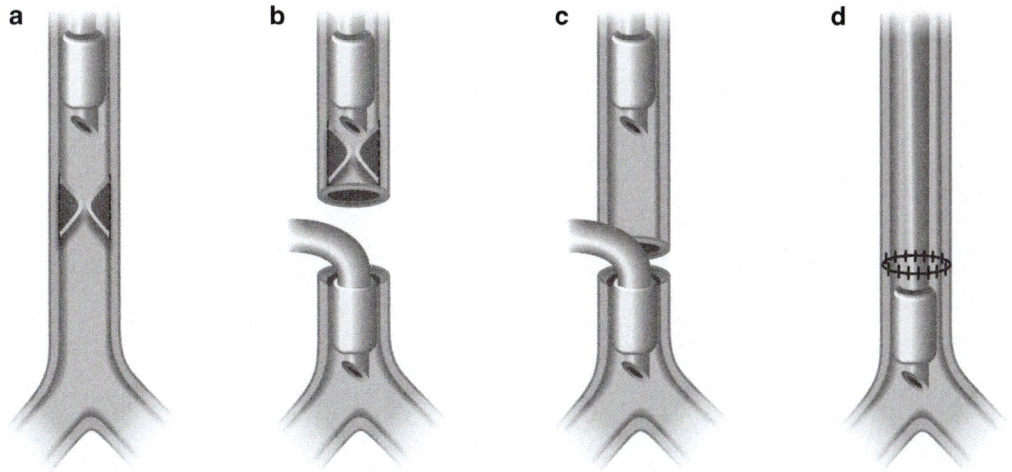

Fig. 14.8 Tracheal resection with distal tracheal with sterile reinforced tube

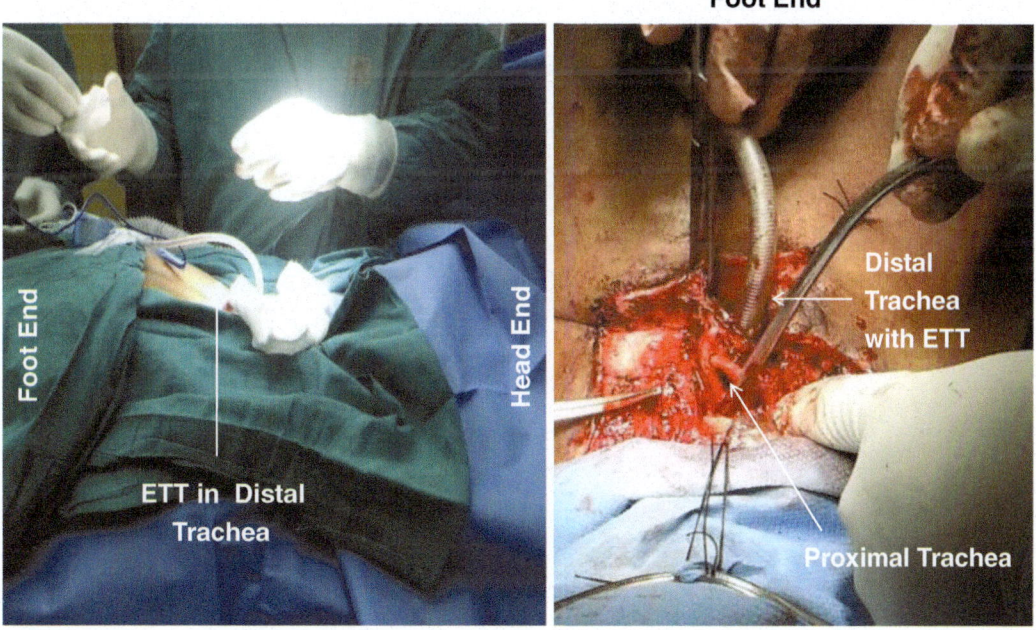

Fig. 14.9 Cross-field ventilation (lateral and head end view)

infusion during the open airway phase provides good anesthesia.

2. *Low Frequency Jet Ventilation*—Jet ventilation for clinical use was demonstrated by Sanders [34]. It allows ventilation with adequate tidal volumes without obstructing the surgical field. This is achieved by release of gas under pressure (50–60 psi) through a narrow aperture (catheter). The jet pulses at rate of 10–20/min, used with lengthy small orifice catheters, can ventilate distal airways, monitored by visible chest rise. This modality of ventilation for tracheal resection was first described in the 1970s [35, 36]. Independent catheters for each bronchus ventilation can be used for carinal lesions [37]. Advantages of this mode of ventilation are the simplicity, minimal interference with surgical field, and

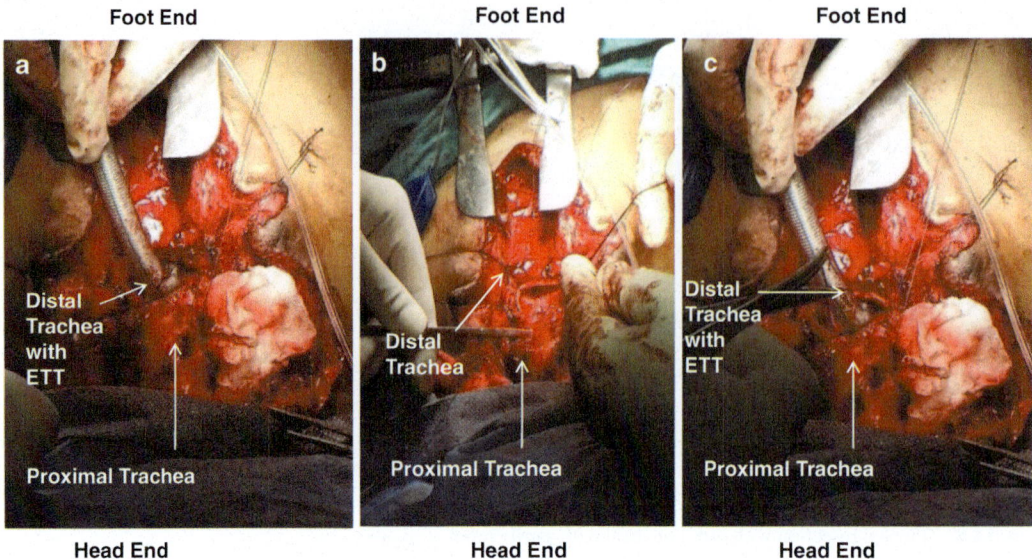

Fig. 14.10 Apnea–ventilation–apnea technique. (**a**) distal tracheal ventilation; (**b**) apnea and tracheal suturing; (**c**) resumed tracheal ventilation

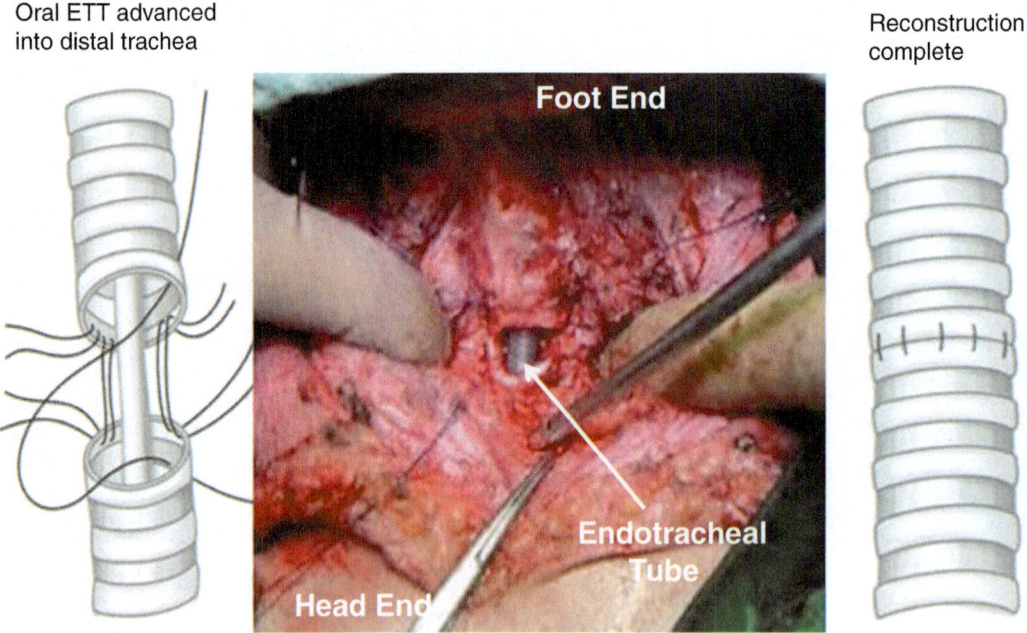

Fig. 14.11 Anterior-lateral tracheal suturing over endotracheal tube

non-requirement of specialized equipment. Disadvantages are entrainment of blood and debris from surgical field in distal airway, and lack of monitoring of $EtCO_2$, inspired oxygen, and anesthetic gas concentration.

3. *High Frequency Jet Ventilation*—Tidal volumes generated are in the range of 2–5 ml/kg, being smaller compared to the conventional tidal volumes [38]. Rate ranges between 100 and 400/min. This is achieved by delivering gas from a high pressure source through a stiff narrow orifice catheter. The position of catheter is determined by nature of lesion and procedure planned. A pneumatic/electronically controlled flow interrupter regulates the air jet. Additional gas is entrained with high

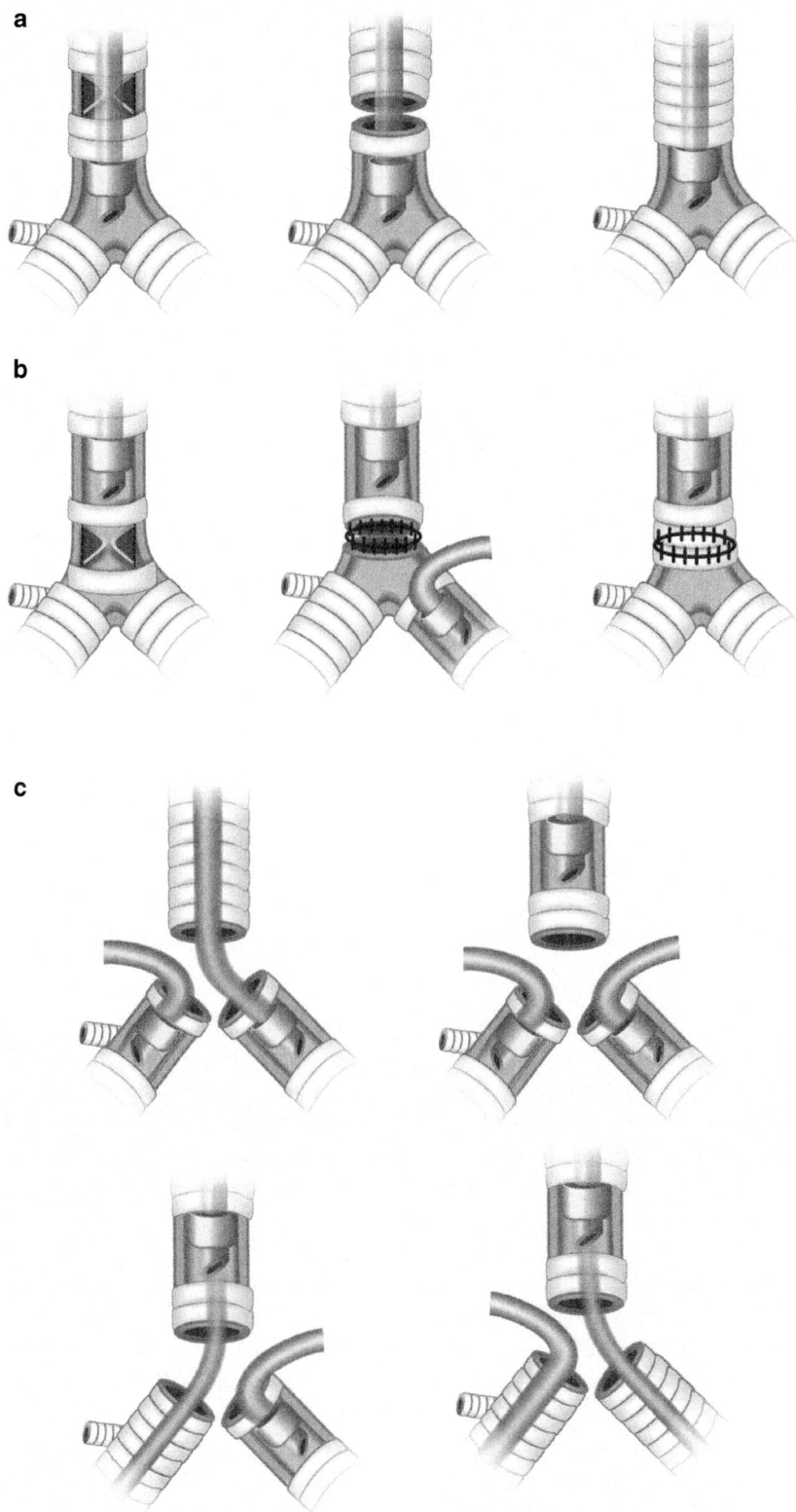

Fig. 14.12 Variations of endotracheal tube for lower tracheal tumor

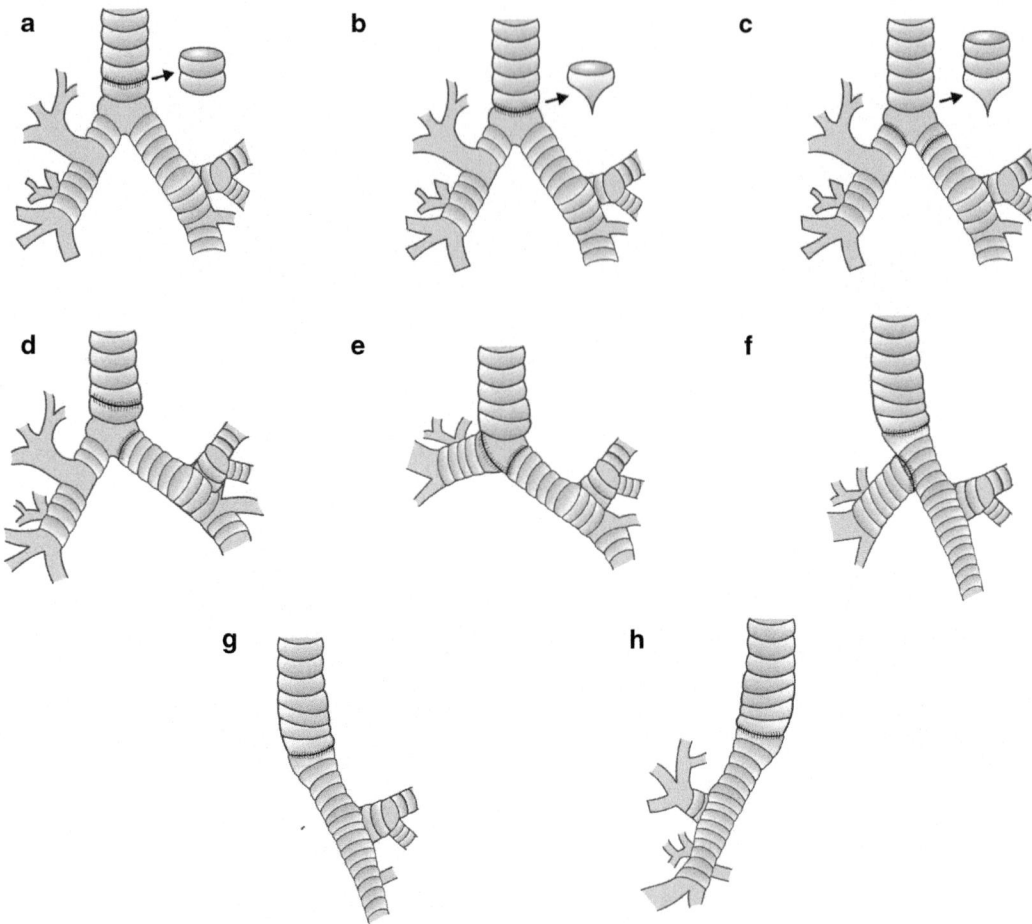

Fig. 14.13 Variations of tracheobronchial anastomosis for carinal tumors

velocity gas jet. Adjustable variables are driving pressure, frequency, and inspiratory time. High respiratory rates hamper lung deflation, thus a distended lung is maintained. This constant state of distention of lung results in peripheral airway pressures being positive while peak and mean airway pressures remain low [38–41]. Advantages of this technique are near motionless operative field and uninterrupted lung ventilation during surgery. Disadvantages are auto-PEEP generation, impaired CO_2 elimination, and tracheal laceration with pneumothorax by catheter tip ("whip motion" injury).

4. *High Frequency Positive Pressure Ventilation*—HFPPV aims to provide motionless surgical field by minimizing the tidal volume of 3–5 ml/kg at a rate of 60 breaths/min. This can be achieved with a multi-orifice insufflation catheter positioned at the tip of endotracheal tube and a conventional ventilator. Whip motion injury chances are minimized with multi-orifice catheter. Biggest advantage is uninterrupted access for anastomosis of the whole circumference of trachea. Main disadvantages are the possibility of barotrauma and the challenge of monitoring ventilation.

5. *Cardiopulmonary Bypass and Extracorporeal Oxygenation*—Cardiopulmonary bypass (CPB) was first used in 1959 for carinal tumors [42]. The need for systemic anticoagulation has resulted in CPB being used

in very specific situations: small children for tracheoplasty of long segments [43], malignant conditions in adults requiring combined cardiac and pulmonary procedure [44], complex tracheobronchial injuries [45], tracheal lesion causing occlusion not amenable to be bypassed by either rigid bronchoscopy or tracheotomy [46]. Recently extracorporeal membrane oxygenation (ECMO) has shown considerable promise for use in adults as well as pediatric patients, particularly with the possibility of peripheral vascular cannulation rather than the central one [47, 48]. This translates into reduced anticoagulation and associated complications.

14.9.5 Extubation and Emergence

Prompt extubation after tracheal reconstruction is desirable, to mitigate the stress of positive pressure ventilation or trauma by endotracheal tube cuff, to the fresh tracheal anastomosis. Prior to extubation a check bronchoscopy for tracheobronchial toileting and inspection of anastomosis is required/desirable (Fig. 14.14). Bucking by the patient should be strictly prevented. Switching over to propofol infusion (if on inhalational agent) is helpful as it allows rapid emergence without agitation. Tapering of the neuromuscular block is the norm. After thorough suctioning of the oropharynx, the neuromuscular blockade is reversed and trachea is extubated with the patient in an awake state where airway patency is assured.

Another option is to extubate the spontaneously breathing anesthetized patient and place a laryngeal mask. The aim is to avoid bucking and coughing. Maintenance of normothermia is mandatory to prevent postoperative shivering and increased oxygen consumption. Humidification of gases prevents drying of airway and postoperative airway irritation.

It is important to counsel the patient in the preoperative period about maintenance of head in flexed position, avoiding abrupt neck extension, and placement of guardian stitch in the postoperative period. The need for reintubation can be challenging. The neck is positioned in flexed position, operated airway may be edematous and

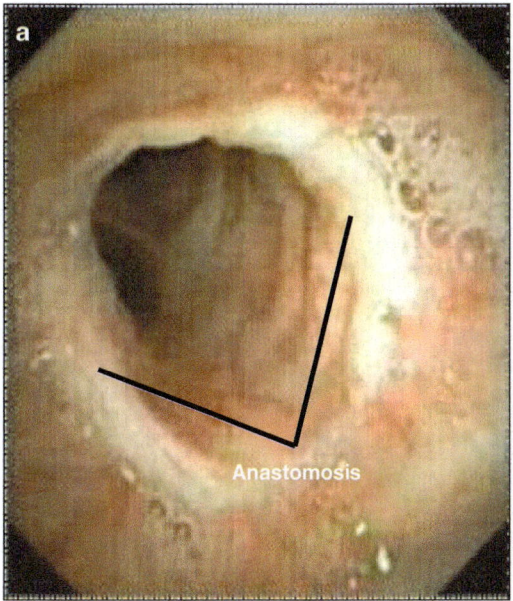
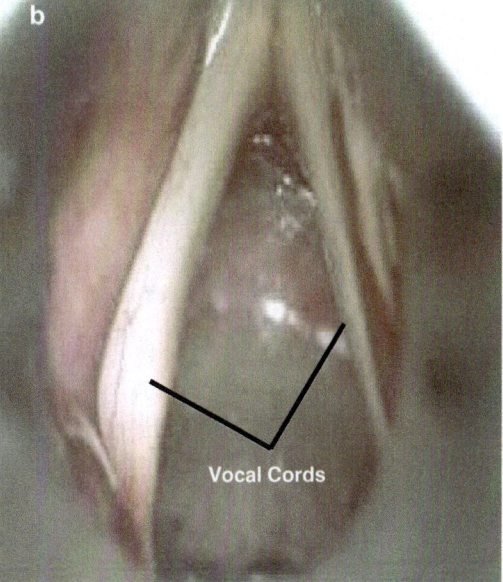

Fig. 14.14 Check bronchoscopy after surgery. (**a**) tracheal anastomosis; (**b**) vocal cord movement

blood smudged, and there is possibility of injury to new anastomosis and/or dislodgment of stent, if placed. Reintubation, if required, should be done with a bronchoscope.

14.9.6 Post-operative Care

Postoperatively these patients must be monitored in the ICU. Constant respiratory monitoring is warranted, to detect any complication of fresh anastomosis. Clinical observation is supplemented by periodic ABG analysis. Patients should be kept in a sitting position (to prevent abdominal contents from hampering movement of the diaphragm) with the head flexed (to minimize traction on fresh tracheal anastomosis). Pain needs to be managed effectively depending on the incision used. Thoracotomy incisions are best managed with epidural and PCEA pumps. Other incisions can be managed with multimodal analgesia to lessen the need for opioids. Opioid sparing pain relief regimes prevent a delirious patient with respiratory depression. Aggressive pulmonary toileting, physiotherapy, antitussives, nebulization, and humidified oxygen are important to ensure a good outcome.

Table 14.2 Complications of tracheal resection

Complications related to the surgical site
Granulation tissue
Stenosis (partial or complete)
Dehiscence
Failure of wound healing
Recurrent laryngeal nerve dysfunction
Wound infection
Persistent stoma
Hemorrhage
Malacia
Simple air leak with subcutaneous emphysema
Laryngeal edema
Aspiration
Deglutition problems
Tracheoesophageal fistula
Tracheoinnominate fistula
Esophagocutaneous fistula
Non-tracheal surgery related
Respiratory failure
Pneumonia
Pulmonary embolism
Pneumothorax
Myocardial infarction
Deep vein thrombosis
Atrial fibrillation
Tetraplegia
Guillain–Barré syndrome

Reproduced from Celine P (5). With permission from Springer nature. Copyright 1999

14.9.7 Complications

Tracheal resection and anastomosis is a complex procedure. Common complications pertaining to all surgeries, i.e., residual effect of analgesics, neuromuscular blockers, and atelectasis due to secretions apply to these procedures as well. The pathology behind the lesion and the surgical extent (degree of dissection and mobilization) further present specific complications. Complications can be related to surgery and non-surgery related as enumerated in Table 14.2. Of the non-surgery related complications, tetraplegia needs special mention. Four cases have been reported till date [49–53]. Hyperflexion of neck in postop period compromising the blood supply of vertebral artery has been implicated. Three of the four cases recuperated on reducing flexion of neck. Relative hypotension due to sitting position could be a contributory factor. The author recommends the use of a *guardian roll* to prevent complications of excessive neck flexion [49].

14.10 Regional Anesthesia

Regional anesthesia for tracheal resection has been explored since 2010 [54]. Literature mentions the use of four different regional anesthesia techniques:

1. *Cervical epidural catheters*—Tracheal resection and anastomosis under cervical epidural placed at C7/T1 level with a local anesthetic like ropivacaine 0.5% has been reported [55]. In addition to epidural block, surgical site infiltration and airway topicalization with local anesthetic is required. These patients

may need supplementation with analgesics and/or sedatives. Patients remain spontaneously breathing throughout the procedure with oxygen supplementation. On tracheal incision there may be desaturation which requires oxygen insufflation through a catheter inserted into the distal trachea. Only patients without cardiac comorbidity with subglottic lesions not requiring median sternotomy can be chosen for cervical epidural. They must also have no contraindications to neuraxial anesthesia.
2. *Cervical plexus block*—Bilateral cervical plexus block with ultrasound guidance has been reported in two patients to safely allow tracheal resection and anastomosis [56, 57]. Approximately 7 ml of ropivacaine 0.5% has been shown to be adequate. Patients require additional intravenous analgesics and/or sedatives. However, one patient required LMA insertion and the other was intubated.
3. *Local infiltration*—A case with subglottic hamartoma occluding the airway was operated by stepwise local infiltration of local anesthetic. Analgesia and sedation was supplemented with drugs like ketamine and midazolam [58].
4. *Thoracic epidural*—Thoracic epidural anesthesia by catheter placed at T7/8 level can provide adequate operating conditions [59]. The epidural block has to be supplemented with analgesics including opioids and/or intercostal nerve blocks. Patients are sedated and LMA is inserted using propofol. Spontaneous ventilation is maintained throughout the procedure.

14.11 Conclusion

Tracheal resection and anastomosis is a complex and challenging surgery. Advances in both surgical techniques and anesthesia management have made this complex procedure safer. This procedure requires immaculate planning, and coordination between the surgical and anesthesia teams. Importance of out of the box thinking and improvisation on the spot cannot be overemphasized. New airway management approaches have been used, although in a lesser number of cases. These can be beneficial in some select group of patients, where they might be an acceptable alternative to conventionally used airway approaches.

References

1. Grillo HC. The development of Tracheal surgery: an historical review. Techniques of tracheal surgery. Ann Thorac Surg. 2003;75:610–9.
2. Belsey R. Resection and reconstruction of the intrathoracic trachea. Br J Surg. 1950;38:200–8.
3. Barcley RS, McSwan N, Welsh TH. Tracheal reconstruction without the use of grafts. Thorax. 1957;12:177–83.
4. Heitmiller RF. Tracheal release maneuvers. Chest Surg Clin N Am. 1996;6:675–82.
5. Pinsonneault C. Tracheal resection and reconstruction. Can J Anesth. 1999;46(5):439–55.
6. Al-Bazzaz F, Grillo H, Kazemi H. Response to exercise in upper airway obstruction. Am Rev Respir Dis. 1975;111(5):631–40.
7. Geffin B, Grillo HC, Cooper JD, et al. Stenosis following tracheostomy for respiratory care. JAMA. 1971;216(12):1984–8.
8. Lavelle TF Jr, Rotmann HH, Weg JG. Isoflow-volume curves in the diagnosis of upper airway obstruction. Am Rev Respir Dis. 1978;117(5):845–52.
9. Jungebluth P, Moll G, Baiguera S, et al. Tissue-engineered airway: a regenerative solution. Clin Pharmacol Ther. 2011;91(1):81–93.
10. Delaere PR. Tracheal transplantation. Curr Opin Pulm Med. 2012;18(4):313–20.
11. Fung D, Devitt J. Anatomy, physiology, and innervation of Larynx. Anesth Clin North Am. 1995;13:259–76.
12. Grillo HC, Mathisen DJ. Diseases of trachea and bronchi. In: Paprella MM, Shumrick DA, Gluckman JL, Meyerhoff WL, editors. Otolaryngology, head and neck, vol. III. 3rd ed. Philadelphia: WB Saunders; 1991. p. 2385–97.
13. Grillo HC. Benign and malignant diseases of the trachea. In: Shields TW, editor. General thoracic surgery. 3rd ed. Philadelphia: Lea & Febiger; 1989. p. 667–79.
14. Grillo HC, Donahue DM. Post intubation tracheal stenosis. Semin Thorac Cardiovasc Surg. 1996;8:370–80.
15. Mathisen DJ. Tracheal tumors. Chest Surg Clin N Am. 1996;6:875–98.
16. Shapshay SM, Valdez TA. Bronchoscopic management of benign stenosis. Chest Surg Clin N Am. 2001;11:749–68.
17. Muehrcke DD, Grillo HC, Mathisen DJ. Reconstructive airway operation after irradiation. Ann Thorac Surg. 1995;59:14–8.

18. Grillo HC. Management of idiopathic tracheal stenosis. Chest Surg Clin N Am. 1996;6:811–8.
19. Bolliger CT, Sutedja TG, Strausz J, et al. Therapeutic bronchoscopy with immediate effect: laser, electrocautery, argon plasma coagulation and stents. Eur Respir J. 2006;27:1258–71.
20. Lando T, April MM, Ward RF, et al. Minimally invasive techniques in larnygotracheal reconsruction. Otolaryngol Clin N Am. 2008;41:935–46.
21. Pinsonneault C, Fortier J, Donati F, et al. Tracheal resection and reconstruction. Can J Anaesth. 1999;46:439–55.
22. Geraldine D, Stacey S, Ochroch EA. Anesthesia for patients with tracheal stenosis. Anesthesiol Clin. 2010;28:157–74.
23. Chin CS, Litle V, Yun J, et al. Airway stents. Ann Thorac Surg. 2008;85:S792–6.
24. Shin JH, Song HY, Shim TS, et al. Management of tracheobronchial strictures. Cardiovasc Intervent Radiol. 2004;27:314–24.
25. Brodsky JB. Anesthesia for pulmonary stent insertion. Curr Opin Anaesthesiol. 2003;16:3.
26. Conacher ID. Anesthesia and tracheobronchial stenting forcentral airway obstructionin adults. Br J Anaesth. 2003; 90: 367-74.
27. Finlayson GN, Brodsky JB. Anesthetic considerations for airway stenting in adult patients. Anesthesiol Clin. 2008;26:281–91.
28. Couraud L, Jougon J, Velly JF, et al. Iatrogenic stenosis of the airways. Surgical indications in a series of 217 cases. (French) Ann de Chir. 1994;48:277–83.
29. DePerrot M, Fadel E, Mercier O, et al. Long term results after carinal resection for carcinoma. J Thorac Cardiovasc Surg. 2006;131:81–9.
30. Anesthesia and Airway Management for Tracheal Resection and Reconstruction, Sandberg & Warren, Lippincott Williams and Wilkins. Vol 38 (1), 2000.
31. Anesthesia for tracheal resection: a new techniques of airway management in a patient of severe stenosis of the mid-trachea; S D Mentzelopoulos; July 6, 1999.
32. Abdelmalak B, Makary L, Hoban J, et al. Dexmedetomidine as sole sedative for awake intubation in management of critical airway. J Clin Anesth. 2007;19:370–9.
33. Hammer GB, Philip BM, Schroeder AR, et al. Prolonged infusion of dexmedetomidine for sedation following tracheal resection. Pediatr Anaesth. 2005;15:616–20.
34. Sanders RD. Two ventilating attachments for bronchoscopes. Del Med J. 1967;39:170–3.
35. Lee P, English ICW. Management of anesthesia during tracheal resection. Anesthesia. 1974;29:305–10.
36. Ellis RH, Hinds CJ, Gadd LT. Management of anesthesia during tracheal resection. Anesthesia. 1976;31:1076–9.
37. Clarkson WB, Davies JR. Anesthesia for carinal resection. Anesthesia. 1978;33:815–7.
38. Howland WS, Carlon GC, Goldiner PL, et al. High frequency jet ventilation during thoracic surgical procedures. Anesthesiology. 1987;67:1009–12.
39. Carlon GC, Kahn RC, Howland WS, et al. Clinical experience with high frequency ventilation. Crit Care Med. 1981;9:1.
40. Sjostrand U. High frequency positive-pressure ventilation: a review. Crit Care Med. 1980;8:345–51.
41. Glenski JA, Crawford M, Rehder K. High-frequency, small volume ventilation during thoracic surgery. Anesthesiology. 1980;59:577–80.
42. Louhimo I, Leijala M. Cardiopulmonary bypass in tracheal surgery in infants and small children. Prog Pediatr Surg. 1987;21:58–63.
43. Benca JF, Hickey PR, Dornbusch JN, et al. Ventilatory management assisted by cardiopulmonary bypass for distal tracheal reconstruction in a neonate. Anesthesiology. 1988;68:270.
44. Ernst M, Koller M, Grobholtz R, et al. Both atrial resection and superior vena cava replacement in sleeve pneumonectomy for advanced lung cancer. Eur J Cardiothorac Surg. 1999;15:530.
45. Symbas PN, Justicz AG, Ricketts RR. Rupture of the airways from blunt trauma: treatment of complex injuries. Ann Thorac Surg. 1992;54:177–80.
46. Wilson RF, Stieger Z, Jacobs J, et al. Temporary partial cardiopulmonary bypass during emergency operative management of near total tracheal occlusion. Anesthesiology. 1984;61:103.
47. Hasegawa T, Oshima Y, Matsuihisa H, et al. Clinical equivalency of cardiopulmonary bypass and extracorporeal membrane oxygenation support for pediatric tracheal reconstruction. Pediatr Surg Int. 2016;32:1029–36.
48. Kim CW, Km DH, Son BS, et al. The feasibility of extracorporeal membrane oxygenation in the variant airway problems. Ann Thorac Cardiovasc Surg. 2015;21:517–22.
49. Kumar A, Marwaha A, Pappu A, et al. Regressive quadriparesis following tracheal resection anastomosis. J Clin Anesth. 2018;44:42–3.
50. Borrelly J, Simon CI, Bertrand P. Cases of regressive paraplegia after repeated resection of the trachea. One case. (French) Ann de Chir. 1981;35:618–9.
51. Pitz CCM, Duurkens VAM, Goossens DJA, et al. Tetraplegia after a tracheal resection procedure. Chest. 1994;106:1264–5.
52. Dominguez J, Rivas JJ, Lobato RD, et al. Irreversible tetraplegia after tracheal resection. Ann Thorac Surg. 1996;62:278–80.
53. Grillo HC, Mathisen DJ. Primary tracheal tumors: treatment and results. Ann Thorac Surg. 1990;49:69–77.
54. Macchiarini P, Rovira I, Ferrarello S. Awake upper airway surgery. Ann Thorac Surg. 2010;89:387–90. discussion 390–381.
55. Vachhani ST, Tsai JY, Moon T. Tracheal resection with regional anesthesia. J Clin Anesth. 2014;26:697–8.

56. Cho AR, Kim HK, Lee EA, et al. Airway management in a patient with severe tracheal stenosis: bilateral superficial cervical plexus block with Dexmedetomidine sedation. J Anesth. 2015;29:292–4.
57. Liu J, Li S, Shen J, et al. Non-intubated resection and reconstruction of trachea for the treatment of a mass in upper trachea. J Thorac Dis. 2016;8:594–9.
58. Loizzi D, Sollitto F, De Palma A, et al. Tracheal resection with patient under local anesthesia and conscious sedation. Ann Thorac Surg. 2013;95:e63–5.
59. Li S, He J, et al. Video-assisted transthoracic surgery resection of a tracheal mass and reconstruction of trachea under non-intubated anesthesia with spontaneous breathing. J Thorac Dis. 2016;8:575–85.

Awake/Non-intubated Thoracic Surgery

Mahinder Singh Baansal

Awake thoracic surgery encompasses usage of various local or regional anesthesia techniques, with or without sedation, in patients undergoing surgical or diagnostic procedures with open or video-assisted thoracoscopic technique, who are breathing on their own and are also cooperative during the procedure [1]. Technically awake thoracic surgery is more challenging for the anesthesiologist and surgeon, than when general anesthesia is used for the surgery. However, this method can be of great benefit to the patients, as the normal physiology of a patient in terms of cardiopulmonary, neurologic and muscular systems is maintained while complications of general anesthesia, tracheal intubation, one-lung ventilation and prolonged mechanical ventilation are avoided, thus reducing the postoperative complications, providing better pain relief and enhanced recovery, particularly in high-risk patients [2].

Non-intubated anesthesia for thoracic surgery is commonly used for thoracoscopic procedures, such as thymectomy, wedge resections and lung volume reduction surgery.

However, awake thoracic surgery is not completely risk free. These procedures require the making of an open pneumothorax, which hinders both oxygenation and ventilation. Surgical maneuvering is also technically demanding under spontaneous ventilation. Clinical evidence continues to grow with time and the results of the awake technique are encouraging; however, more studies are required to clearly demarcate indication, limitations and benefits [3–8].

15.1 History of Awake Thoracic Surgery (ATS)

The start of the twentieth century saw thoracic surgery being carried out under local or regional anesthesia. Creation of surgical pneumothorax was associated with increased morbidity and mortality [9]. World War I (1914–1918) led to many casualties, but it also led to the finding that even bilateral large open chest wounds did not necessarily lead to the demise of a soldier. This fact and the concurrent advances in anesthesia techniques in the early 1920s introduced local or regional anesthesia techniques in thoracic surgery [10–15].

Jacobaeus used regional anesthesia for thoracoscopic procedures and sedated anxious patients with the help of bromide or phenobarbital [16]. In 1946, paravertebral blocks were combined with local novocaine infiltration for more effective pain control and dampening reflexes. In 1950, Buckingham et al. proposed and used thoracic epidural anesthesia for awake thoracic surgery in 607 patients [17]. A few years later,

M. S. Baansal (✉)
Institute of Anaesthesiology, Pain and Perioperative Medicine, Sir Ganga Ram Hospital, New Delhi, India

Vischnevski created a multistep protocol for using local analgesia which he used in over 600 surgeries including major procedures such as esophagectomies and lung resections [18].

However, advances in anesthesia techniques (double-lumen tube, one-lung ventilation) led to rapid decline in non-intubated/awake thoracic surgery.

Subsequent refinements in surgical techniques like multi- and uniportal VATS procedures led to the reintroduction of awake (non-intubated) anesthetic techniques in thoracic surgery.

15.2 Surgical Pneumothorax: Pathophysiology

Open pneumothorax created for awake thoracic surgery results in drop of the lung volume on the operating side, since the lung is no longer held open by negative intrapleural pressure; also the unopposed elastic recoil of lung tissue tends to collapse the lung, creating adequate space for ergonomic surgical maneuvering [19]. The lung collapse during inspiration is enhanced due to: (a) the descent of diaphragm on the side of surgery (open pneumothorax) resulting in air from the environment rushing in to enter the pleural cavity of same side, and filling the space around the exposed lung; (b) gas entering in the dependent closed chest (lung with more negative pressure) from nondependent open chest (lung at atmospheric pressure) which results in further reduction in the size of the open lung. The opposite occurs during expiration. This reversal of nondependent (open) lung movements during different phases of respiration is called as paradoxical respiration (Fig. 15.1) [19]. Paradoxical respiration is increased if surgical incision is large and when there is increased airway resistance in the intact lung.

In the awake, lateral position, surgical opening of the nondependent (operative) hemithorax, leads to imbalance of the pleural pressures (more in the open lung where pleural pressure is at atmospheric pressure, than the dependent lung where pleural pressure is more negative) causing a downward displacement of the mediastinum into the dependent hemithorax. Inspiration accentuates this mediastinal shift, due to caudad movement of diaphragm making intrapleural pressure in the dependent lung relatively more negative. Thus the decrease in tidal volume of the dependent lung is directly proportional to the

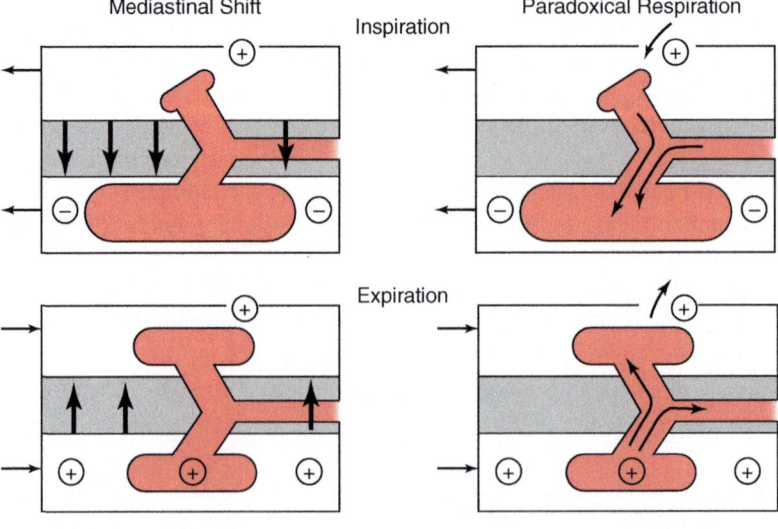

Fig. 15.1 Schematic representation of paradoxical respiration and mediastinal shift (Source: Modified from Benuof Elsevier 1995 (Sketch (Lungs))

mediastinal displacement during inspiration. During expiration, diaphragm moves cephalad, resulting in relatively positive pressure in the dependent hemithorax, thus pushing up the mediastinum. This shifting of mediastinum during different phases of respiration is called as mediastinal shift (Fig. 15.1) which results in hypoxia and hypercapnia and may also result in circulatory changes, i.e., decreased venous return, and increased sympathetic responses, resembling shock [19]. Infiltration of the pulmonary plexus at hilum by local anesthetics and vagal nerve block can diminish these reflexes [20].

Since the diaphragmatic mobility is unaffected by the open thorax, the compression by abdominal contents on the dependent lung is contained and adequate ventilatory exchange is maintained despite the physiological changes associated with an open thoracic cavity.

Patients having normal lungs, i.e., in cases where the normal lung elastic recoil is functional, surgical pneumothorax may result in near total lung collapse; however, in patients having pleural adhesions and hyperinflated lungs, e.g., emphysema, the degree of lung collapse may be limited.

Spirometry performed in awake and lateral position in the open versus closed chest found that there was a decrease in the forced expiratory volume in 1 second (FEV1) and forced vital capacity in all phases of respiration but this drop was less profound in patients with emphysema as compared to those with relatively normal lungs (Fig. 15.2) These contradictory readings are a result of positive end-expiratory pressure in the peripheral alveolar regions and prolonged exhalation times which could counteract the deleterious physiological effects of pendular ventilation in patients having emphysematous disease of lung [2].

15.3 Indications for Awake Thoracic Surgery

For better patient outcome, it is imperative for anesthesiologists, chest physicians, surgeons and intensivists to work in close coordination and discuss the important issues regarding patient management

- Pleural space surgery [1, 8, 21–26]:
  - Pleural effusion drainage [23]
  - Pleurodesis under TEA/thoracic paravertebral/local anesthesia
  - Pleurostomy [1]
  - Decortication
  - Pneumothorax, including pleurectomy
  - Empyema drainage
  - Bleb resection

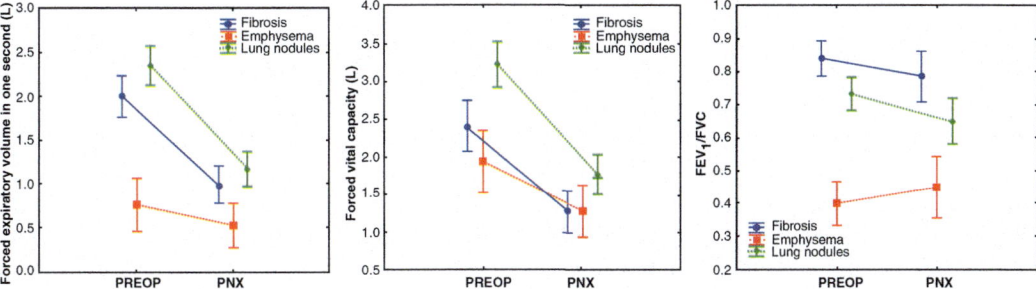

Fig. 15.2 Behavior of arterial oxygen tension to fraction of inspired oxygen ratio (PO_2/FiO_2) and arterial carbon dioxide tension ($PaCO_2$) measured preoperatively (PREOP), and after creation of a surgical pneumothorax (PNX) in patients with interstitial lung disease (fibrosis), emphysema, and normal lung function (lung nodules) (Reprinted with permission from Pompeo.) (Permission awaited)

- Biopsies of different thoracic structures [1, 21–23, 25]:
  - Anterior mediastinal mass biopsy
  - Pleural/lung biopsy
- Surgery on the lung [3, 27–32]:
  - Pneumonectomy
  - Lobectomy via thoracotomy and thoracoscopy
  - Bilobectomy
  - Wedge resection
  - Thoracoscopic lobectomy and segmentectomy
  - Lung metastasis resection
  - Lung volume reduction surgery and bullectomy
- Surgery on the mediastinum [22]:
  - Pericardial window
  - Tracheal resection under cervical epidural [30]
  - Thymectomy under TEA [3]
- Other indications:
  - Thoracic sympathectomy for palmer hyperhidrosis
  - Tracheal resection under cervical epidural anesthesia

15.4 Advantages of Awake Thoracic Surgery

Awake thoracic surgery avoids general anesthesia-related injuries to teeth or vocal cords, barotrauma, volutrauma, atelectasis and prolonged ventilation [33, 34].

Awake thoracic surgeries also show not only decrease in postoperative complications but also decrease in operating room time and hospital stay. A large RCT by Liu et al. in 2015 which included 354 patients, showed reduction in respiratory complications from 10% to 4.2% ($P = 0.039$), and also lower postoperative complications 6.7% were reported in non-intubated group than in the intubated group (16.7%) ($P = 0.004$) [35].

Other benefits have included no PONV, superior postoperative analgesia, more effective coughing, reduced thrombotic complications, better hemodynamic stability, faster resumption of oral intake along with reduction in stress and immunologic responses and hence faster recovery.

Higher patient satisfaction, especially in patients suffering from severe chronic pulmonary disease is reported as they have already experienced prolonged ICU stays and weaning problems. Higher patient satisfaction may also be due to feeling of better sense of self control.

Thus awake thoracic surgery apart from offering many advantages to the patient also results in improved operation theater utilization and hospital efficacy resulting in overall cost effectiveness [35–38].

15.5 Contraindications to Awake Thoracic Surgery

15.5.1 Patient Related

Patient refusal, coagulopathy (INR greater than 1.5, antiplatelet therapy), increased chances of aspiration, septicemia, hemodynamic instability, neurological disorders, cerebral edema, history of severe anxiety or panic attacks, obesity (BMI > 35) and spinal deformity.

15.5.2 Anesthesia Related

Anticipated difficult airway, local anesthesia allergy and inexperience.

15.5.3 Surgery Related

Anticipated prolonged duration of surgery, difficult anatomy, extensive adhesions, previous same side surgery, and phrenic nerve paralysis of non-operated side.

15.6 Complications and Pitfalls

These can be divided into those caused by local or regional techniques and those due to untoward hemodynamic, respiratory and neurological events.

In patients undergoing awake thoracic surgery not only airway and respiratory management is crucial, but also certain intraoperative complications which may develop namely hypoxia, hypercapnia, coughing and patient movement, all of which the anesthesia and surgical team should be aware of. The creation of the surgical pneumothorax leads to a decrease in arterial oxygenation which is easily controlled by an oxygen supplementation and is compensated by increase of oxygenation and ventilation by the dependent lungs efficiency [39, 40]. In addition there are suprapontine compensatory mechanisms which preserve ventilation in awake patients who have been subjected to increased inspiratory load.

Arterial hypoxemia combined with hypercapnic acidosis can cause marked sympathetic stimulation resulting in decreased glomerular filtration and increased fluid retention which could lead to CCF. The deleterious effects of hypercapnia are seen in patients with CCF, arrhythmias, elevated pulmonary or intracranial pressures. Restricted surgical access to the diaphragm, patient movement, coughing, diaphragmatic or lung movement could pose problems to surgeons. To counteract these concerns a local anesthetic spray on the surface of the lung, vagal, and phrenic nerve blocks or a remifentanil infusion could also be used [39, 40].

15.7 Patients Selection for Awake Thoracic Anesthesia

A thorough informed consent should be taken informing the anesthetic risks and benefits and availability of various techniques of awake thoracic surgery as not all patients are willing to being awake or sedated during surgery.

As there are no absolute contraindications for GA, it always remains the last resort in regional anesthesia failure. For ATS, patients must be carefully selected as it requires more experience and preparation. Previously ATS was performed mostly in ASA I-II patients without anticipated difficult airway (Mallampati grade I-II) having body mass index <30, a tumor size of less than 6 cm, and with good cardiopulmonary function and fewer comorbidities [41]. However, indications are nowadays extended to very high-risk patients having severe cardiac and respiratory issues which are usually a contraindication for awake thoracic surgery [42, 43].

ATS is reported in high-risk cases such as patients with advanced diffuse interstitial lung fibrosis on home oxygen treatment, patients having restrictive chronic respiratory failure on nasal NIV and in patients with severe obstructive pulmonary disease having FEV1 27% [43].

Non-intubated thoracic surgery is also reported in cases of history of difficult weaning from the ventilator, inflammatory alveolitis, multiple bilateral lung metastases, pneumomediastinum, pyothorax, recurrent unilateral or bilateral pneumothorax, severe emphysema having atrial fibrillation with severe pulmonary hypertension, and in cases of advanced limb girdle myopathy which is a contraindication for use of volatile anesthetics and muscle relaxant.

In patients with advanced terminal chronic respiratory disease, carrying high risk of ventilator dependency under GA with increased morbidity and mortality, GA can present an ethical dilemma. In such cases when contraindications to regional anesthetic techniques are not there, ATS could help if risk–benefit ratio favors surgery for reversing an acute pathology, thus avoiding early death and could contribute to patient well-being, enhancing the quality of life.

Surgical issues can also be a contraindication for ATS which include major bleeding, major lung surgery, when stripping of interlobular vessels and handling of incomplete fissures despite inflation of affected lung may be difficult. Conversion to GA should be performed without hesitation [44].

Feasibility of ATS generally depends both on comfort level/experience of the anesthesiologist and surgeon. This can explain the relatively less number of patients, varying from 8.6% to 19.7% per year at various institutions undergoing ATS as compared those undergoing thoracic surgery under GA [45].

15.8 Techniques for ATS; Local/Regional

Anesthetic techniques used for ATS are:

- Local infiltration of wound
- Serratus anterior plane (SAP) block
- Intercostal nerve block supplying the surgical site
- Thoracic paravertebral block (PVB) with or without catheter placement
- Thoracic epidural analgesia (TEA) with or without local anesthesia
- Lidocaine administration in the pleural space

Benefits of all the above anesthetic techniques can be extended during intraoperative or even in postoperative period by use of catheter placement, e.g., local wound catheter placement, in either the local wound, thoracic or paravertebral space.

15.9 Local Anesthesia Technique of Diego Gonzalez-Rivas [46, 47]

A technique was described by Gonzalez-Rivas in patients undergoing thoracoscopic lobectomy in which entire surgery was done using only single-port which resulted in reduced surgical trauma as compared to a standard VATS approach thus reducing the need for more invasive anesthesia techniques. The single-port VATS can be done under LA without intubating the patient also obliviating requirement of epidural anesthesia or vagal blockade.

For surgery, a single intercostal space is utilized after infiltration with long-acting local anesthetic (5 ml, 5 mg/ml of L bupivacaine) resulting in single intercostal nerve block providing sufficient analgesia for the entire duration of surgery.

15.10 Local Anesthetic Technique by Hung [29]

This technique is similar to Gonzalez-Rivas technique but they infiltrated multiple intercostal spaces (from T3 to T8) thus mitigating the need of thoracic epidural during VATS surgery.

15.11 Thoracic Paravertebral Block for Awake Thoracic Surgery (PVB) [25]

Piccioni et al. first described the usage of thoracic PVB as a sole anesthetic technique for patients undergoing video-assisted thoracoscopic surgery providing pain relief comparable to thoracic epidural during and after thoracic surgery with lesser complications and side effects. PVB offers the advantage of providing unilateral block without producing bilateral sympathetic blockade. PVB not only reduces the incidence of hypotension, urinary retention and pulmonary complications but also reduces the chances of neurological damage associated with thoracic epidural [25]. Hence PVB can be used where thoracic epidural is contraindicated such as in septicemia, coagulopathy, neurological disorders, or deformity of spine.

Thoracic paravertebral block when compared to thoracic epidural is relatively easier to learn and can be performed by various methods such as using the landmark technique and loss of resistance technique, with or without use of nerve simulation. In addition, ultrasound guidance has improved the chances of successful blockade with lower complication rate.

15.12 Epidural Anesthesia

If the awake thoracic surgery is expected to be of long duration, then a thoracic epidural should be placed. Like the PVB, a thoracic epidural has the advantage of providing postoperative pain relief using boluses or an infusion of a local anesthetic agent, unlike a technique where only a single injection has been employed. An article on ATS mentions that TEA provided adequate pain relief for a surgery that lasted 219 min [21]. Dural puncture, neurological injury, and rarely paraplegia are some of the complications associated with TEA, therefore PVB which has fewer contraindiaction is an alternative that can be used. The usual site for placing the TEA is between T3 and T7, and the final placement would depend upon the surgical site and discussion with the operating surgeon. The volume of a local anesthetic to be used would take into account the length of the incision and the patient's size and weight and should achieve somatosensory anesthesia between the second and twelfth thoracic vertebrae. The choice of local anesthetic depends on surgical requirements: if rapid onset is needed then lidocaine 20 mg/ml is used, otherwise ropivacaine 7.5 mg/ml, which has a slower onset, but a much longer half-life is an alternative. Both low and high concentrations of local anesthetics have drawbacks. The first could result in an inadequate sensory block, causing the patient to react to the intrathoracic surgical manipulations leading to pain, anxiety, and panic. On the other hand, higher concentrations of the local anesthetic would result in a motor block of the intercostal nerves and muscles and a consequent decrease in the tidal volume. Gruber and coworkers found that 0.25% bupivacaine used for TEA had no deleterious effects on ventilatory mechanics and gas exchange even in patients with severe COPD and was well tolerated [48].

Surgery should be commenced only when the surgical site has been completely anesthetized. This is done by testing the area using ice cubes or maximal painful tactic stimuli produced via a neurotransmitter.

It is important to remember that epidural anesthesia causes hypotension because of vasodilatory action. Whenever the mean arterial pressure drops below 65 mm Hg and/or systolic arterial pressure is less than 90 mm Hg, fluid bolus can be given and vasoactive drugs, if required, can be added. In an article on nine patients who underwent ATS, ephedrine or phenylephrine was used in 50% to treat hypotension (MAP below 65 mm Hg or systolic less than 90 mmHg). If phenylephrine requirements become too high, it may be replaced by norepinephrine [21].

15.13 Serratus Anterior Plane (SAP) Block [49]

In 2013, Blanco and coworkers first described the ultrasound-guided serratus anterior plane block. In their study the block was performed in healthy volunteers by blocking the lateral branches of intercostal nerves and prolonged effective surgical anesthesia from T2 to T9, which lasted 750–840 min. Employing the same technique for SAP block, Kunhabdulla and coworkers used it for patients who had multiple rib fractures. After placing the block, catheter insertion was done to provide continuous infusion of local anesthetic. The technical details of SAP were as follows. Block is performed by using a high-frequency ultrasound probe placed over the fifth rib in the posterior axillary line in the vertical axis and then rotated the aligned along the long axis of the rib; this helps in identification of the serratus anterior muscle. Next, the skin is anesthetized using 1% lignocaine, followed by 18 G Touhy needle introduction, between the posterior and mid-axillary line, under the serratus anterior muscle and over the surface of the rib. For confirmation of the position of the tip of the Touhy needle, 3 ml saline was used for hydrodissection, then 20 ml, 0.125% bupivacaine was injected via the needle. A 20 G epidural catheter was introduced via the Touhy needle and advanced to 4 cm beyond the tip of the needle and tunneled subcutaneously to guard against displacement. A continuous infusion of bupivacaine 0.0625% with 1 mg/ml of fentanyl at 7 ml/h is started in the postoperative period, 4 hours after completion of the surgery. Some clinicians avoid the addition of opioids to the continuous infusion of local anesthetics in those with obstructive sleep apnea to avoid respiratory depression [50].

15.14 Sedation During ATS

Short acting drugs, e.g., remifentanil and propofol are preferred. Remifentanil, having ultra-short context-sensitive half-time of nearly 3 min not only provides excellent analgesia, but also its effects can be reversed by naloxone in case of overdosage.

Propofol TIVA has advantages such as its dosage can be rapidly titrated thus maintaining spontaneous respiration and airway reflexes. Propofol can be used either alone or as combination with remifentanil. In several studies, target controlled infusions (TCI) of either propofol, or remifentanil, alone or in combinations are used to provide light sedation, resulting in responsive, but less anxious patients during surgery [21].

There are no definitive recommendations to measure propofol plasma concentration to obtain anxiolysis as its plasma concentration has to be titrated according to the needs of patients and can vary from one patient to another and also depends on the anesthesiologist's expertise. However, one can monitor the depth of anesthesia using BIS monitoring to titrate the sedation levels. Nasopharyngeal airway along with oxygen supplementation via cannula or Venturi mask should be used in cases of airway obstruction and desaturation arising due to oversedation.

In patients having severe COPD when sedation is required use of ketamine is preferred as it preserves the inspiratory muscle tone thus maintaining the functional residual capacity and thus reducing the chances of hypercapnia [51]. Nowadays dexmedetomidine, an α2-adrenoceptor agonist, is also used as a sedative during ATS which not only decreases anesthetic and opioid requirements during perioperative period but also attenuates sympathetic, neuroendocrine, hemodynamic responses preserving respiratory and psychomotor functions. However, it can produce mild to moderate cardiovascular depression resulting in fall in blood pressure and heart rate [51].

15.15 Perioperative Monitoring for ATS

Standard ASA monitoring including ECG, pulse oximetry, noninvasive blood pressure monitoring, respiratory rate, and capnography is recommended. BIS monitoring is done when sedation is given to monitor depth of anesthesia. Measurement of end-tidal CO_2 can be done by attaching expiratory CO_2 ($EtCO_2$) detector to the oxygen mask or nasal cannula. At least two IV lines should be secured in patients undergoing ATS for IV fluids and medications separately. Constant communication with the patient intraoperatively (if not sedated) is a perfect physiological monitor.

15.16 Lung Recruitment During ATS

The open pneumothorax created during ATS results in shifting of mediastinum, while dependent lung compression leads to atelectasis, making spontaneous breathing difficult, thus worsening hypoxemia and hypercarbia. Noninvasive ventilation can be applied to mitigate the effects of open pneumothorax such as atelectasis and mediastinal shift. NIV also leads to reduction in left ventricular afterload resulting in increased cardiac output.

Lung re-expansion, if desired by the surgeon, can be done using progressive application of PEEP using NIV. If no air leaks are present in the surgical lung, NIV should be continued in the immediate postoperative period and in the recovery room and postoperative ICU to prevent atelectasis and pneumonia. Postoperatively, lung re-expansion can be monitored with physical examination, X-rays of chest or ultrasound of the lung [52].

NIV application not only reduces atelectasis, but also reduces chances of postoperative nosocomial infections, decreased ICU and hospital stay, and reduction in overall morbidity and mortality [53].

15.17 Conversion to GA and Emergency Intubation

Given the limitations of ATS, caution must be exercised while conducting ATS. The risk of conversion to GA is determined not only by the patient's health status and comorbidities, but also by the anticipated complications during the surgery. When complications begin to emerge, patients must be intubated early to reduce the risks of emergency intubation.

Factors responsible for conversion to GA can be anesthesia or surgery related. Anesthesia factors are severe hypoxemia, hypercarbia, panic attack, tachypnoea, and failure of regional anesthesia technique and poor pain control, while major bleeding, difficult anatomy, dense adhesions, requirement of immobile surgical field, complex hilar dissection, including silicosis or tuberculous patients are the surgical factors responsible for conversion.

When emergency arises, conversion to GA should be done quickly and has to be performed by an experienced and well prepared team of anesthesiologists, surgeons, and operation theater staff in a coordinated manner. Understanding and coordination between the team members are keys for success. Preoperatively, to allow rapid change of patient position needed during emergency, an additional bedsheet must be put under the patient while positioning the patient for surgery. The dilemma faced by the operating team to induce general anesthesia in such a scenario requires quick covering of the surgical incision with a surgical suture or sterile dressing only.

There should be coordination and discipline among operating room team members while turning the patient supine to facilitate conversion to GA and tracheal intubation. Induction of anesthesia can be performed quickly by using a fast acting drugs propofol and muscle relaxants such as succinylcholine or rocuronium [54].

15.18 Cough During ATS

Manipulation of the lung during surgery can lead to stimulation of cough reflex, which can be a hindrance during surgery due to movements of surgical field. Techniques to suppress cough reflex are the inhalation of aerosolized lidocaine or application of local anesthetic spray on surface of the lung, stellate ganglion block or a vagus nerve block and administration of remifentanil to blunt the cough reflex. However, one should be aware of pulmonary aspiration and resultant respiratory tract infection that may result with suppression of the cough response (Table 15.1) [54].

Table 15.1 Anesthesia protocol

Type	Spontaneous ventilation	Consciousness	Regional anesthesia	IV anesthesia	BIS monitoring	Need for stellate ganglion or vagal block (thoracic)
Non-intubated anesthesia with sedation	Yes	No	Yes TEA/local	Yes	Yes/no	Yes/no
Non-intubated awake anesthesia	Yes	Yes	TEA/local	No	No	No
Non-intubated anesthesia with LMA	Yes	No	TEA/local	Yes	No	Yes/no

15.19 Conclusion

In carefully selected patients, awake thoracic surgery can be successfully performed by an experienced anesthetic and surgical team and can be offered as an option to the patient. Apart from reducing morbidity and facilitating early recovery, awake thoracic surgery can be performed in patients deemed high risk or unfit for undergoing surgery under general anesthesia. It is postulated that awake thoracic procedures decrease the chances of recurrence in cancer patients due to its positive effects on immune system and decreased surgical stress response than general anesthesia. Further these procedures can help in development of fast track and ambulatory thoracic surgery programs. Thus certain thoracic procedures can be safely performed with awake or non-intubated anesthetic techniques, improving patient outcome and reducing cost.

References

1. Pompeo E, Mineo D, Rogliani P, et al. Feasibility and results of awake thoracoscopic resection of solitary pulmonary nodules. Ann Thorac Surg. 2004;78:1761–8.
2. Pompeo E. Pathophysiology of surgical pneumothorax in the awake patient. In: Pompeo E, editor. Awake thoracic surgery (ebook). Sharja: Bentham Science Publishers; 2012. p. 9–18.
3. Al-Abdullatief M, Wahood A, Al-Shirawi N, et al. Awake anaesthesia for major thoracic surgical procedures: An observational study. Eur J Cardiothorac Surg. 2007;32:346–50.
4. Macchiarini P, Rovira I, Ferrarello S. Awake upper airway surgery. Ann Thorac Surg. 2010;89:387–90.
5. Mineo TC, Pompeo E, Mineo D, et al. Awake nonresectional lung volume reduction surgery. Ann Surg. 2006;243:131–6.
6. Pompeo E, Mineo TC. Two-year improvement in multidimensional body mass index, airflow obstruction, dyspnea, and exercise capacity index after nonresectional lung volume reduction surgery in awake patients. Ann Thorac Surg. 2007;84:1862–9.
7. Rusch VW, Mountain C. Thoracoscopy under regional anesthesia for the diagnosis and management of pleural disease. Am J Surg. 1987;154:274–8.
8. Tacconi F, Pompeo E, Fabbi E, et al. Awake video-assisted pleural decortication for empyema thoracis. Eur J Cardiothorac Surg. 2010;37:594–601.
9. Sauerbruch F, O'Shaughnessy L. Thoracic surgery. London: Edward Arnold; 1937. p. 324–86.
10. Birbeck LH, Lorimer GM, Gray HM. Removal of a bullet from the right ventricle of the heart. Br Med J. 1915;2:561–2.
11. Eloesser L. Recent advances in regional (local) anesthesia. Cal State Med J. 1912;10:90–7.
12. Eloesser L. Local anesthesia in major surgery: its uses and limitations. Cal State Med J. 1923;21:412–5.
13. Kergin FG. The treatment of chronic pleural empyema. Ann R Coll Surg Engl. 1955;17:271–90.
14. Lambert A. Axillary approach to Schede thoracoplasty. Surg Gynecol Obstet. 1947;84:56–61.
15. Sauerbruch F. The nature and history of the treatment of tuberculosis. Zentralbl Chir. 1951;76:421–30.
16. Moisiuc FV, Colt HG. Thoracoscopy: origins revisited. Respiration. 2007;74:344–55.
17. Buckingham WW, Beatty AJ, Brasher CA, et al. An analysis of 607 surgical procedures done under epidural anesthesia. Mo Med. 1950;47:485–7.
18. Petrovsky BV. Role of local anesthesia according to Vischnevsky in thoracic surgery. Anesth Analg. 1952;9:75–9.
19. Benumof JL. Distribution of ventilation and perfusion. In: Benumof JL, editor. Anesthesia for thoracic surgery. 2nd ed. Philadelphia, PA: WB Saunders; 1995. p. 35–52.
20. Grichnik KP, Clark JA. Pathophysiology and management of one-lung ventilation. Thorac Surg Clin. 2005;15:85–103.
21. Kiss G, Claret A, Desbordes J, et al. Thoracic epidural anaesthesia for awake thoracic surgery in severely dyspnoeic patients excluded from general anaesthesia. Interact Cardiovasc Thorac Surg. 2014;19:816–23.
22. Klijian AS, Gibbs M, Andonian NT. AVATS: awake video assisted thoracic surgery-extended series report. J Cardiothorac Surg. 2014;9:149.
23. Migliore M, Giuliano R, Aziz T, et al. Four-step local anaesthesia and sedation for thoracoscopic diagnosis and management of pleural diseases. Chest. 2002;121:2032–5.
24. Nezu K, Kushibe K, Tojo T, et al. Thoracoscopic wedge resection of blebs under local anaesthesia with sedation for treatment of a spontaneous pneumothorax. Chest. 1997;111:230–5.
25. Piccioni F, Langer M, Fumagalli L, et al. Thoracic paravertebral anaesthesia for awake video-assisted thoracoscopic surgery daily. Anaesthesia. 2010;65:1221–4.
26. Pompeo E, Tacconi F, Mineo D, et al. The role of awake video-assisted thoracoscopic surgery in spontaneous pneumothorax. J Thorac Cardiovasc Surg. 2007;133:786–90.
27. Chen JS, Cheng YJ, Hung MH, et al. Nonintubated thoracoscopic lobectomy for lung cancer. Ann Surg. 2011;254:1038–43.
28. Guo Z, Shao W, Yin W, et al. Analysis of feasibility and safety of complete video-assisted thoracoscopic resection of anatomic pulmonary segments under non-intubated anesthesia. J Thorac Dis. 2014;6:37–44.
29. Hung MH, Hsu HH, Chan KC, et al. Non-intubated thoracoscopic surgery using internal intercostal

nerve block, vagal block and targeted sedation. Eur J Cardiothorac Surg. 2014;46:620–5.
30. Pompeo E, Mineo TC. Awake pulmonary metastasectomy. J Thorac Cardiovasc Surg. 2007;133:960–6.
31. Pompeo E, Tacconi F, Mineo TC. Comparative results of non-resectional lung volume reduction performed by awake or non-awake anesthesia. Eur J Cardiothorac Surg. 2011;39:e51–8.
32. Wu CY, Chen JS, Lin YS, et al. Feasibility and safety of nonintubated thoracoscopic lobectomy for geriatric lung cancer patients. Ann Thorac Surg. 2013;95:405–11.
33. Deng HY, Zhu ZJ, Wang YC, et al. Non-intubated video-assisted thoracoscopic surgery under loco-regional anaesthesia for thoracic surgery: a meta-analysis. Interact Cardiovasc Thorac Surg. 2016;23:31–40.
34. Tacconi F, Pompeo E. Non-intubated video-assisted thoracic surgery: where does evidence stand? J Thorac Dis. 2016;8:S364–75.
35. Liu J, Cui F, Li S, et al. Nonintubated video-assisted thoracoscopic surgery under epidural anesthesia compared with conventional anesthetic option: a randomized control study. Surg Innov. 2015;22:123–30.
36. Irons JF, Miles LF, Joshi KR, et al. Intubated versus nonintubated general anesthesia for video-assisted thoracoscopic surgery-a case-control study. J Cardiothorac Vasc Anesth. 2017;31:411–7.
37. Kanni G, Tacconi F, Sellitri F, et al. Impact of awake videothoracoscopic surgery on postoperative lymphocyte responses. Ann Thorac Surg. 2010;90:973–8.
38. Tacconi F, Pompeo E, Sellitri F, et al. Surgical stress hormones response is reduced after awake videothoracoscopy. Interact Cardiovasc Thorac Surg. 2010;10:666–71.
39. Irons JF, Martinez G. Anaesthetic considerations for non-intubated thoracic surgery. J Vis Surg. 2016;2:61.
40. Sunaga H, Blasberg J, Heerdt P. Anesthesia for non-intubted video-assisted thoracic surgery. Curr Opin Anaesthesiol. 2017;30:1–6.
41. Dong Q, Liang L, Li Y, et al. Anesthesia with non-tracheal intubation in thoracic surgery. J Thorac Dis. 2012;4:126–30.
42. Guarracino F, Gemignani R, Pratesi G, et al. Awake palliative thoracic surgery in a high-risk patient: one-lung, non-invasive ventilation combined with epidural blockade. Anaesthesia. 2008;63:761–3.
43. Mukaida T, Andou A, Date H, et al. Thoracoscopic operation for secondary pneumothorax under local and epidural anesthesia in high-risk patients. Ann Thorac Surg. 1998;65:924–6.
44. Nakanishi R, Yasuda M. Awake thoracoscopic surgery under epidural anesthesia: is it really safe? Chin J Cancer Res. 2014;26:368–70.
45. Pompeo E, Rogliani P, Tacconi F, et al. Randomized comparison of awake nonresectional versus nonawake resectional lung volume reduction surgery. Awake thoracic Surgery Research Group. J Thorac Cardiovasc Surg. 2012;143:47–54.
46. Gonzalez-Rivas D, Fernandez R, de la Torre M, et al. Thoracoscopic lobectomy through a single incision. Multimed Man Cardiothorac Surg. 2012; 2012
47. Gonzalez-Rivas D, Fernandez R, de la Torre M, et al. Single-port thoracoscopic lobectomy in a nonintubated patient: the least invasive procedure for major lung resection? Interact Cardiovasc Thorac Surg. 2014;19:552–5.
48. Gruber EM, Tschernko EM, Kritzinger M, et al. The effects of thoracic epidural analgesia with bupivacaine 0.25% on ventilatory mechanics in patients with severe chronic obstructive pulmonary disease. Anesth Analg. 2001;92:1015–9.
49. Blanco R, Parras T, McDonnell JG, et al. Serratus plane block: a novel ultrasound-guided thoracic wall nerve block. Anaesthesia. 2013;68:1107–13.
50. Etches RC. Respiratory depression associated with patient-controlled analgesia: a review of eight cases. Can J Anaesth. 1994;41:125–32.
51. Tokics L, Strandberg A, Brismar B, et al. Computerized tomography of the chest and gas exchange measurements during ketamine anaesthesia. Acta Anaesthesiol Scand. 1987;31:684–92.
52. Lichtenstein D, Mezière G, Seitz J. The dynamic air bronchogram. A lung ultrasound sign of alveolar consolidation ruling out atelectasis. Chest. 2009;135:1421–5.
53. Jaber S, Michelet P, Chanques G. Role of non-invasive ventilation (NIV) in the perioperative period. Best Pract Res Clin Anaesthesiol. 2010;24:253–65.
54. Kiss G, Castillo M. Nonintubated anesthesia in thoracic surgery: general issues. Ann Transl Med. 2015;3(8):110.

Anesthetic Considerations for Procedures in Bronchoscopy Suite

16

Naresh Dua

The infrastructure of the bronchoscopy room suite, where a variety of interventional procedures are done by interventional pulmonologists has been fine-tuned to accommodate the advances and innovations of medical science irrespective of diagnostic, curative, or palliative trends. Consequently, there has been increasing demand for the specialized anesthesia services required for bronchoscopic procedures.

The anesthesia team handling the suite requires a high level of expertise to handle emergencies that arise as a result of sharing the airway with the pulmonologist; blood, secretions, and noxious stimuli originating from various instruments. Underlying patient comorbidities add to the challenge. Better equipment available today has ensured that these complex procedures can be done more safely.

In the bronchoscopy suite the procedures done may be classified into:

1. Diagnostic thoracoscopic/bronchoscopic biopsy for detecting precancerous lesions or the early staging neoplasms.
2. Medical thoracoscopy.
   a. Pleurodesis.
   b. Spontaneous pneumothorax.
   c. TOF closure (plug).
3. Palliative procedures.
   a. Airway stents.
   b. Tumor ablation (cryo-resection).
4. Miscellaneous procedures—argon plasma cautery, laser application, endobronchial electrosurgery, balloon bronchoplasty, and bronchial thermoplasty.
5. Future procedures may include interventional pulmonologists in minimally invasive lung volume reduction surgery for severe asthma with placement of endobronchial valves.

16.1 Diagnostic Intervention Procedures

Bronchoscopy and thoracoscopy play major roles in identifying different disease entities such as tuberculosis, sarcoidosis, previously inhaled foreign bodies, and infiltrative lung disease. The main challenge faced by the anesthesiologist is to ensure that there are no complications intraoperatively and to make a patient comfortable during the procedure. Before undertaking bronchoscopy the underlying comorbid conditions have to be optimized first before induction of general anesthesia.

Diagnostic bronchoscopy is the investigative modality where a biopsy is taken to determine the second line of treatment options [1].

The patient is fasted for 6–8 h prior to bronchoscopy. The choice of anesthesia depends on

N. Dua (✉)
Institute of Anaesthesiology, Pain and Perioperative Medicine, Sir Ganga Ram Hospital, New Delhi, India

© Springer Nature Singapore Pte Ltd. 2020
J. Sood, S. Sharma (eds.), *Clinical Thoracic Anesthesia*,
https://doi.org/10.1007/978-981-15-0746-5_16

the general condition of the patient. GA/TIVA and MAC are the modalities available for anesthetic management.

16.2 Thoracoscopy and Therapeutic Indications

Pleural effusion is prevalent in clinical practice, the causes being malignancy or tuberculosis in 10–30% of these patients (Fig. 16.1). To make definitive diagnosis a closed pleural biopsy (CPB) is required which can be done under local anesthesia, total intravenous anesthesia (TIVA), or general anesthesia.

16.2.1 Spontaneous Pneumothorax

Patients with COPD or emphysema may, after a vigorous bout of cough, develop life threatening spontaneous pneumothorax and present in the casualty with severe hypotension and respiratory discomfort.

Treatment:

1. Optimize the basal condition.
2. Chest tube insertion.
3. Treat the underlying cause: medical and surgical management.

16.3 Diagnostic Bronchoscopy (Fig. 16.1)

Bronchoscopy is an endoscopic technique to visualize the interior of the airways for diagnostic and therapeutic procedures. It may be rigid or flexible (Fig. 16.2).

Rigid bronchoscopy is usually done for diagnosis and foreign body removal in adults and children, as it allows the passage of large instruments for removal of inhaled bulky objects and at the same time provides means for positive pressure ventilation.

Advantages and disadvantages for rigid and flexible bronchoscopy are listed in Table 16.1 [2].

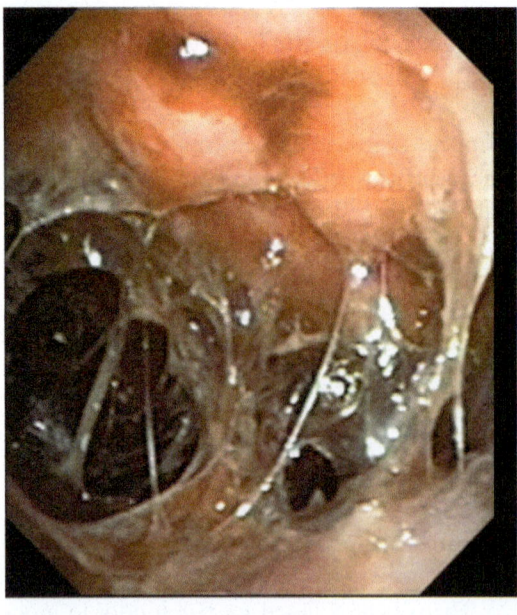
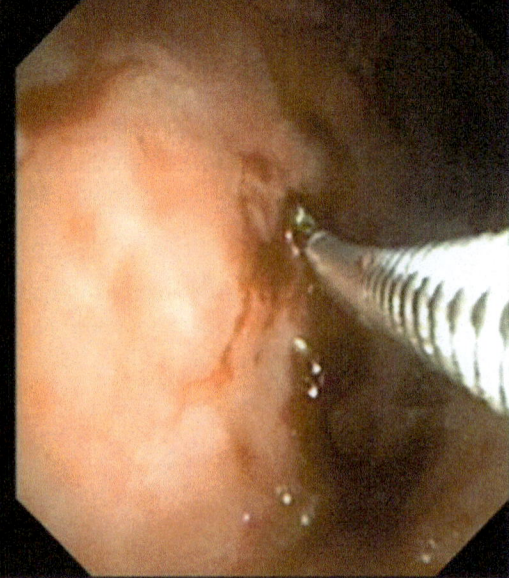

Fig. 16.1 Thoracoscopy

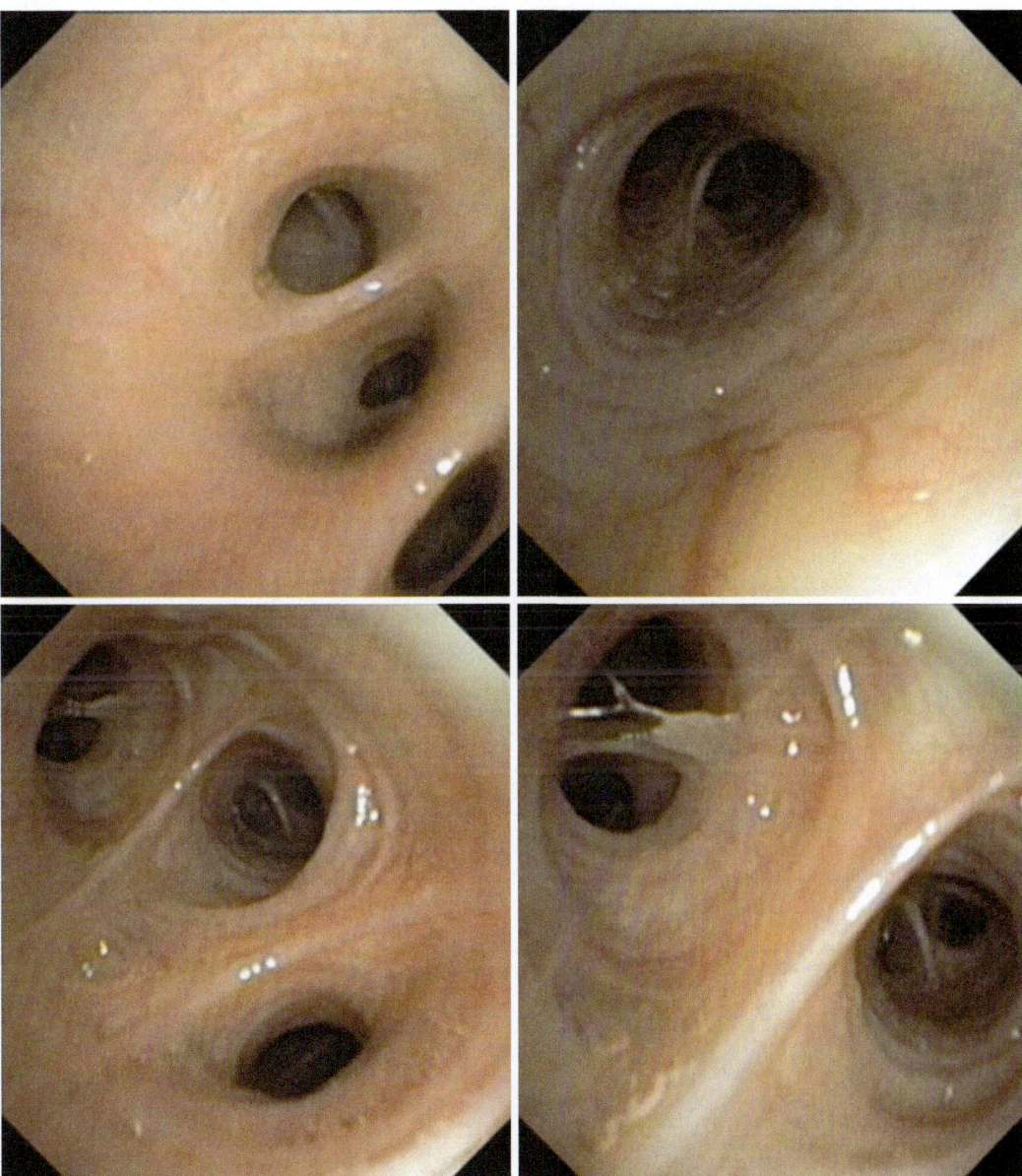

Fig. 16.2 Diagnostic bronchoscopy

Rigid bronchoscopy is done under general anesthesia. An exhaustive preoperative evaluation is mandatory and includes medical history, routine laboratory investigations, diagnostic imaging studies, PFT (if required) should be done and a coagulation profile. Past medical records, if available must be scrutinized and pertinent information about anesthesia management, airway access size of endotracheal tube, the bronchoscope to be used, and intraoperative difficulties anticipated must be noted. A thorough assessment of the upper airway is a prerequisite to prevent injury during instrumentation.

Table 16.1 Pros and cons of flexible and rigid bronchoscope

Bronchoscope	Pros	Cons
Flexible	• It can be done at bedside. • It does not require general anesthesia and can be done under conscious sedation. • It requires spontaneous ventilation. • Done in upright position. • It can be maneuvered to the peripheral zones of the lung for better visualization.	• Risk of laryngeal edema, bleeding, and pneumothorax. • Needs fragmentation of foreign body before removal. • Small size of aspiration channel.
Rigid	• When patency of the airway is compromised by granulation tissue of tumor, rigid bronchoscope is the only instrument that can be inserted past the obstruction. • Done in supine position.	• Done in operating room. • Requires ventilation. • Teeth may be damaged. • Limited visualization.

All elective patients for rigid bronchoscopy can be premedicated with antisialagogues, benzodiazepines, and bronchodilators. Anesthetic considerations include the operative indication, patient comorbidities, and complications associated with a particular procedure.

Airway obstruction remains the most frequent indication for bronchoscopic intervention and these procedures are typically performed on an emergency basis in patients in respiratory distress. Patients encountered on an emergent basis have the additional risk associated with full stomach and unsecure airway.

The patient is customarily kept in a supine position at the edge of the operating table and head extension is done by using a sand bag or a shoulder roll. The head is placed on a ring with the chin pointing upward. This is the shaving chin position (Fig. 16.3).

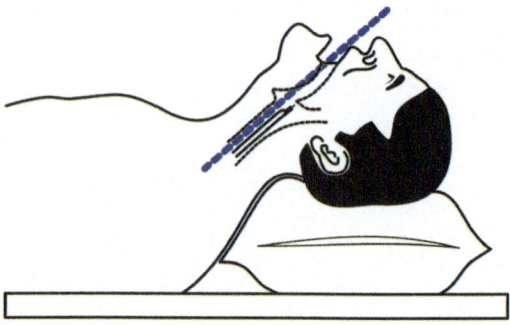

Fig. 16.3 Shaving chin position

Standard intraoperative monitoring should be done with specific requirements for sick patients, e.g., ABG analysis via an arterial line in place. The type of anesthesia varies from procedure to procedure: for rigid bronchoscopy, general anesthesia with muscle relaxation, hypnosis and analgesia is the ideal choice. It is advisable to insert a cuffed ETT or an LMA. ETT is the preferred choice of airway control, to prevent aspiration of regurgitated material [3].

N_2O is contraindicated in these patients to prevent air trapping causing over inflation of lungs. Use of short acting muscle relaxants is preferred.

In flexible bronchoscopy total intravenous anesthesia (TIVA) is the choice, where one can titrate and regulate the level of sedation, from conscious sedation to deep sedation, while maintaining protective airway reflexes. Benzodiazepines along with fentanyl and target controlled infusion of propofol and dexmedetomidine are the available choices for TIVA. Bradycardia, hypotension, and respiratory depression are a possibility, thus extensive monitoring is mandatory.

16.4 Postoperative Care

It is advisable to check that all extubation criteria are met before extubating trachea, particularly the complete reversal of muscle relaxant, allowing the patient to control his own airway and avoiding hypoxia.

In the recovery room, monitoring of vitals includes the respiratory rate, SpO_2, and lookout for episodes of bronchospasm or laryngospasm.

16.5 Anesthesia for Thoracoscopy

Overnight fasting, preoperative anxiolytics, and nebulization must be prescribed for the patient posted for thoracoscopy.

16.5.1 Anesthetic Considerations

In the critical patient, where room air saturation is below 90% ($SpO_2 < 90\%$), interventional procedures should be done under local anesthesia with mild sedation. Constant intraoperative monitoring and readiness for appropriate action (tracheal intubation and ventilation) must be kept ready.

In morbid patients who are maintaining their room air saturation above 90% may be administered total intravenous anesthesia (TIVA) with proper care of vitals.

The use of muscle relaxants has to be done judiciously. For some of the interventional procedures where the bronchoscopist/pulmonologist request for complete control of respiration, short acting muscle relaxants are used.

16.6 Palliative Procedures

1. Tracheal stenting: Tracheal dilatation (Fig. 16.4) and stenting (Fig. 16.5) is a relatively new procedure for the treatment of tracheal stenosis and used as palliative measure for the shortened life expectancy in cancer patients while tracheal dilatation is common in noncancerous patients who have tracheal stenosis due to miscellaneous causes like ventilator-dependent trauma, prolonged tracheal intubation, Wegener's granulomatosis, amyloidosis, and relapsing polychondritis.
2. Benign lesions are the commonest form of the obstructive type of tracheal lesions, mainly due to prolonged intubation, inhalational injury, or may be idiopathic (Table 16.2).

16.6.1 Symptoms

Symptoms differ from patient to patient depending upon the variability of the tracheal lumen available for ventilation, whether the growth is intra-luminal, or if there is extra-luminal pressure (by secondaries, growth etc.). In benign cases, patients may complain of intractable cough leading to difficulty in breathing and weight loss. In severe cases, SVC obstruction and chances of syncope may be present.

Patient may present with cachexia and malnutrition endocrine abnormality as hyperparathyroidism, inappropriate secretion of antidiuretic hormone (SIADH) and Cushing's syndrome and increased chances of venous thrombosis.

16.7 Airway Stents

Montgomery pioneered the application of airway stents for the management of subglottic stenosis in the 1960s [4]. In 1990, Dumon introduced a silicone stent positioned completely within the tracheal lumen [5]. Nowadays, pulmonologists and interventional bronchoscopists use airway stents to restore the patency of the central airway in cases where obstruction is arising from prolonged intubation or post-traumatic tracheal reconstruction as tracheal stricture or malignancy-related causes. Contemporary airway stents are made up of silicone, metal, or a combination of the two [6].

Although no ideal stent is manufactured till now but of available options, silicone stents are useful for benign conditions of central airway obstruction as they are easy to remove and reposition but require rigid bronchoscopy for placement and have the limitations of migration, flammability, and reduced inner diameter.

Although the metal stents can be placed under local anesthesia, they have much better mucociliary transport, large inner diameter, easier placement technique, and do not migrate but their use is still restricted to malignant conditions for palliation due to concerns relating to difficulty in extraction, granuloma formation, and stent obstruction.

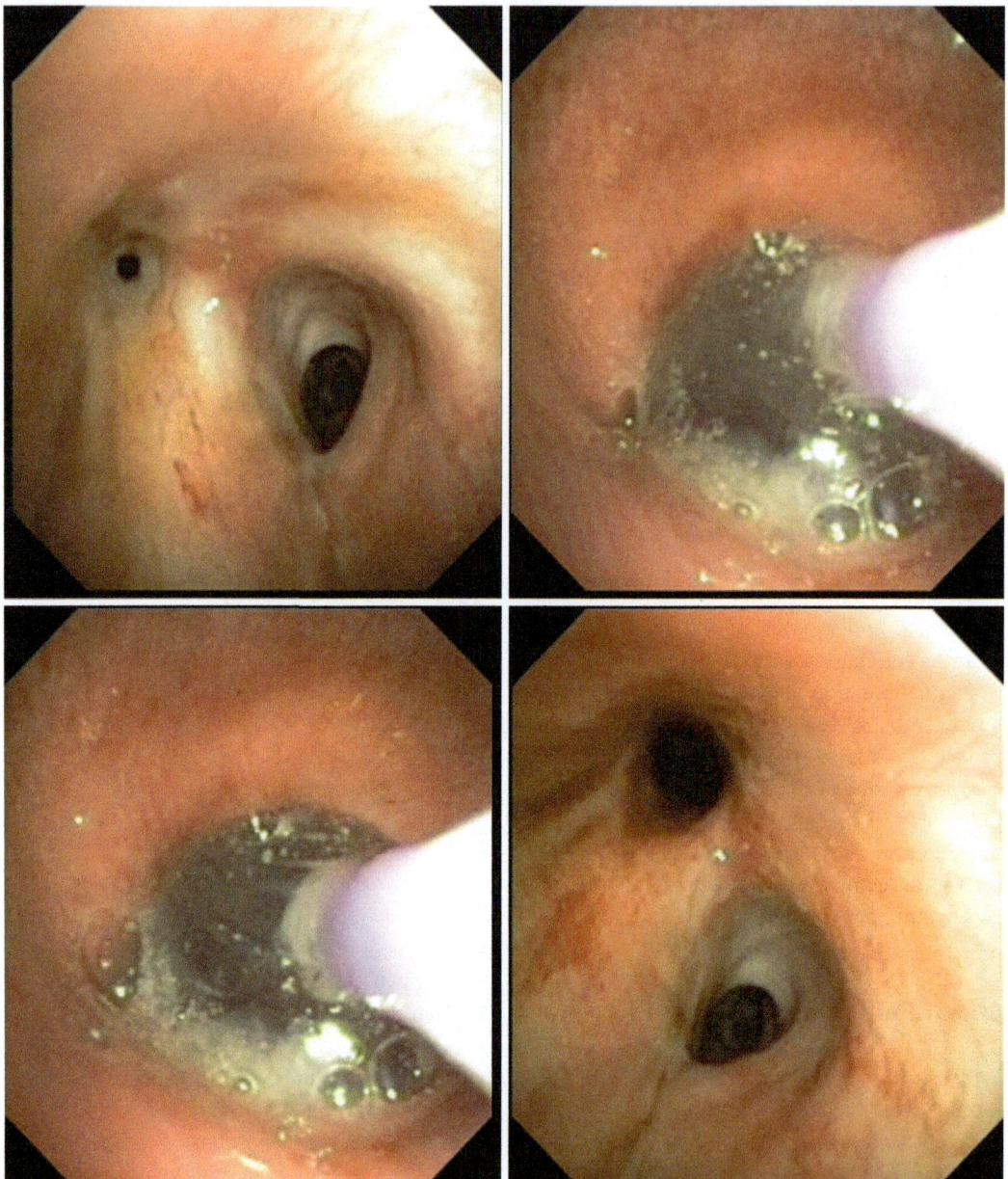

Fig. 16.4 Tracheal dilatation

The primary aim for safe and balanced anesthetic technique for airway stenting lies in optimization of patent airway availability during induction of anesthesia, at the same time making sure that coughing is kept to a minimum to provide a stable surgical field. All precautions should be taken for any unexpected total airway obstruction.

Team work between anesthesiologist, surgeon, bronchoscopist, and theater staff has to be coordinated for Plan A and Plan B for rescuing from any kind of emergency.

Various techniques of anesthesia can be utilized to achieve the guide wire placement and tracheal stenting, as long as airway is secure and oxygenation and ventilation are adequate.

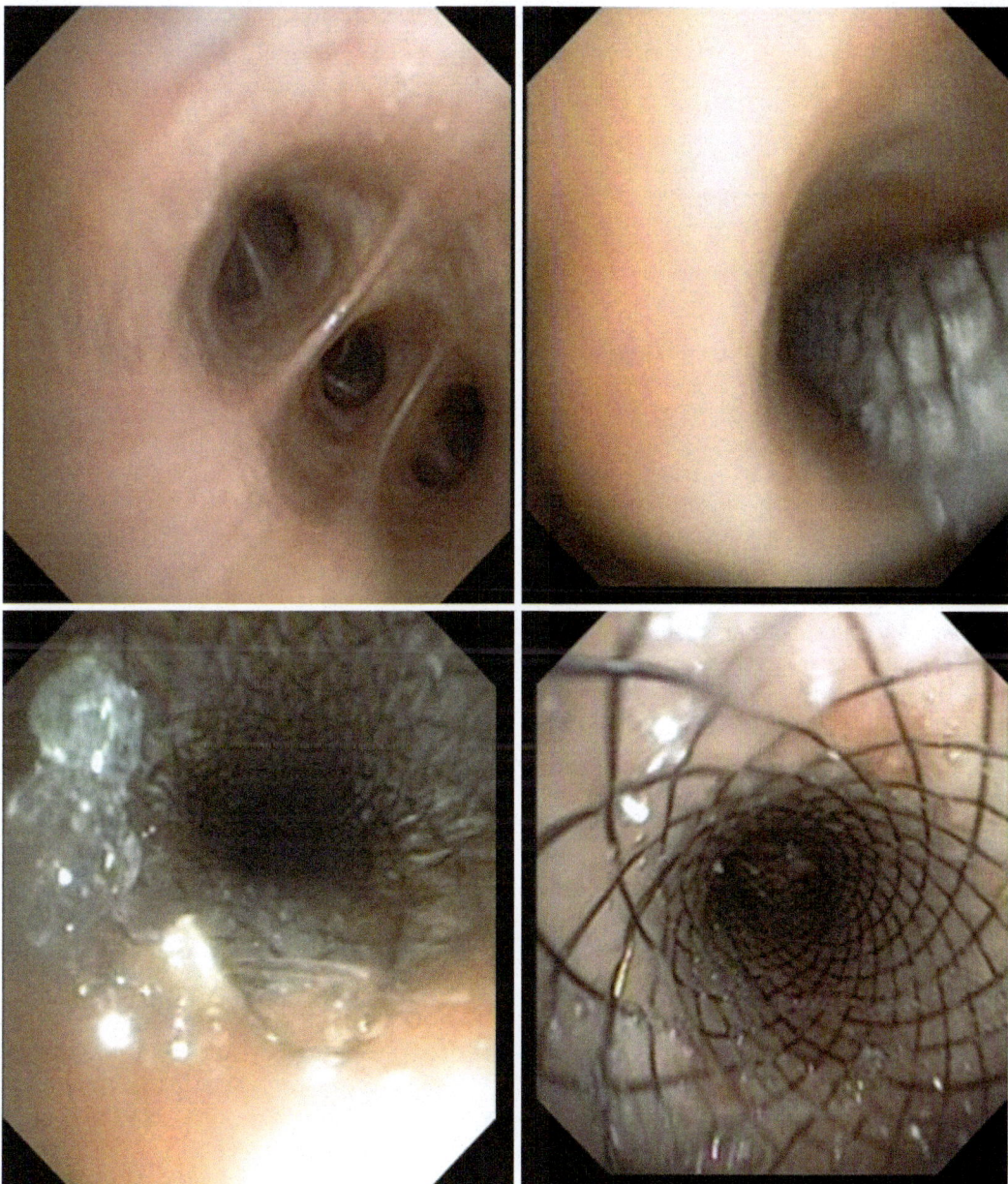

Fig. 16.5 Tracheal Stenting

Preanesthetic decisions between rigid and flexible determine the anesthetic technique to be used.

Rigid bronchoscopy requires neuromuscular block with agents such as atracurium with maintenance of paralysis throughout the procedure. In case of tracheal stenosis, high frequency jet ventilation via a catheter can be employed but only if expiration can be ensured. For flexible bronchoscopy, neuromuscular relaxation may be avoided and anesthesia can be maintained with inhalational or TIVA. The LMA is the preferable airway device over ETT. Maintenance of anesthesia is with TIVA using propofol, dexmedetomidine, fentanyl, or sufentanil [4]. Cough response should be obtunded by using topical

Table 16.2 Causes of tracheal stenosis

Nonmalignant conditions	Malignant conditions
Tracheo/bronchomalacia	Primary endoluminal carcinoma
Goiter	Metastatic carcinoma
Webs	Esophageal carcinoma
Granulation tissue (tracheal tube, foreign body, anastomosis, Wegener's granulomatosis, post-transplant)	Mediastinal tumors (thymus, thyroid, teratoma)
Lymphadenopathy (infectious, sarcoid)	Lymphadenopathy (malignancy)
	Lymphoma

local anesthesia. Other IV drugs, e.g., lidocaine, steroid, and deriphyllin also play a significant role in reducing the cough stimulus. Bronchoscopy has its own drawbacks: hemorrhage, obstruction, perforation leading to pneumothorax or pneumomediastinum, but these can be minimized by excellent team work.

16.8 Recovery

As airway handling leads to irritability and edema of the airway, postoperative safety measures are essential. A patient who is conscious with normal neurological function, supplemental oxygen, nebulization, and steroid cover suffice. Heliox should be available as it can improve gas flow in situations of critical airflow limitation.

16.8.1 Laser

Lasers are light sources which emit light coherently so that it can center on a particular spot which leads to photocoagulation and vaporization of the tissue in focus. From the variety of lasers available, the two usually employed in medical practice are the Nd:YAG (neodymium/yttrium aluminum garnet, wave length 1064 nm) and CO_2 (wave length 10 μm) types. The Nd:YAG is used by bronchoscopists because it is compatible with the flexible and rigid bronchoscopes and has an excellent coagulation profile. The incisions made with this laser are however less precise [7].

For the anesthesiologists, the chance of an airway fire is an ever present danger and extreme vigilance is required at the time of laser ablation. Oxygen delivery can be switched off for short period [8]. Laser protective gears must be used by the entire team. Smoke evacuation systems have been advocated in papilloma excision [9]. The choice of anesthesia depends on extensive of procedure from sedation to TIVA and complete general anesthesia.

16.9 Endobronchial Electrosurgery (EBES)

In this surgery which is used for therapeutic interventions, alternating high frequency current generates heat that can be used for coagulation, vaporizing, or cutting tissue, according to the power applied to the device used [10]. This leads to tissue destruction which is dependent on the power applied to the device, contact time with the tissue, electrical properties of the tissue, and the surface area of the contact. EBES can be used for both, pedunculated or sessile, lesions employing wire loops or debulking probes, respectively. It is cheaper than laser and easier to use than other interventional pulmonology equipment. The indications and contraindications of EBES are similar to the Nd:YAG laser (pacemakers and internal defibrillators), the potential for airway fires is also present with it. It can be done in conscious sedation to deep sedation as per the procedure time requirement [11].

16.10 Argon Plasma Cautery (APC)

In this technique argon gas is forced out of a probe tip where it meets a high voltage current. This ionizes the gas into a plasma which acts as a conductor for monopolar electric current which grounds itself into the nearest lesion [12]. This non-touch technique delivers thermal energy to a depth of approximately 2–3 mm. The outcome is that the heat produced evaporates intra- and extracellular water and coagulates the protein resulting in tissue destruction [13]. The hazards associated with APC are air embolism and electromagnetic interference. The APC is an efficacious modality especially for areas within the airway that are highly vascular and can even be used near endobronchial stents. However, the shallow penetration means it is not as efficient as the laser in debulking tissue [14].

16.11 Balloon Bronchoplasty

Treatment of symptomatic airway stenosis can be done via balloon bronchoplasty. In this a silicone balloon is maneuvered into the stenotic area by means of rigid or flexible bronchoscopy alone or combined with fluoroscopic guidance and then applying increasing pressure by inflating the balloon. Balloon bronchoscopy is generally used in conjunction with other modalities like stent deployment or electrocautery [15].

16.12 Delayed Resection Techniques

The delayed mode techniques used in interventional pulmonology are cryotherapy, brachytherapy, and photodynamic therapy. These are commonly used in patients with non-obstructing lesions who will not be operated, those with advanced malignancy as part of palliative treatment and for early stage carcinomas. The delayed mode therapies are done via fiber-optic bronchoscopy and associated complications are less than with the more invasive modalities (Figs. 16.6 and 16.7).

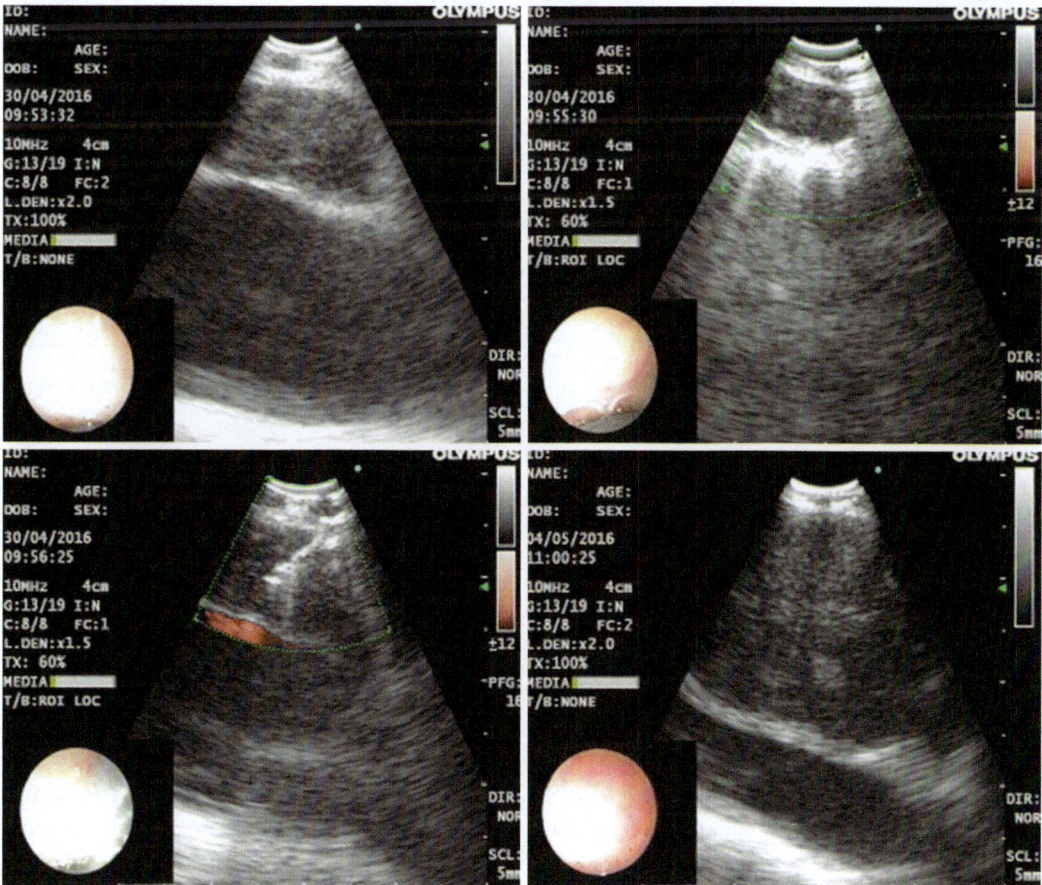

Fig. 16.6 Endobronchial ultrasonography

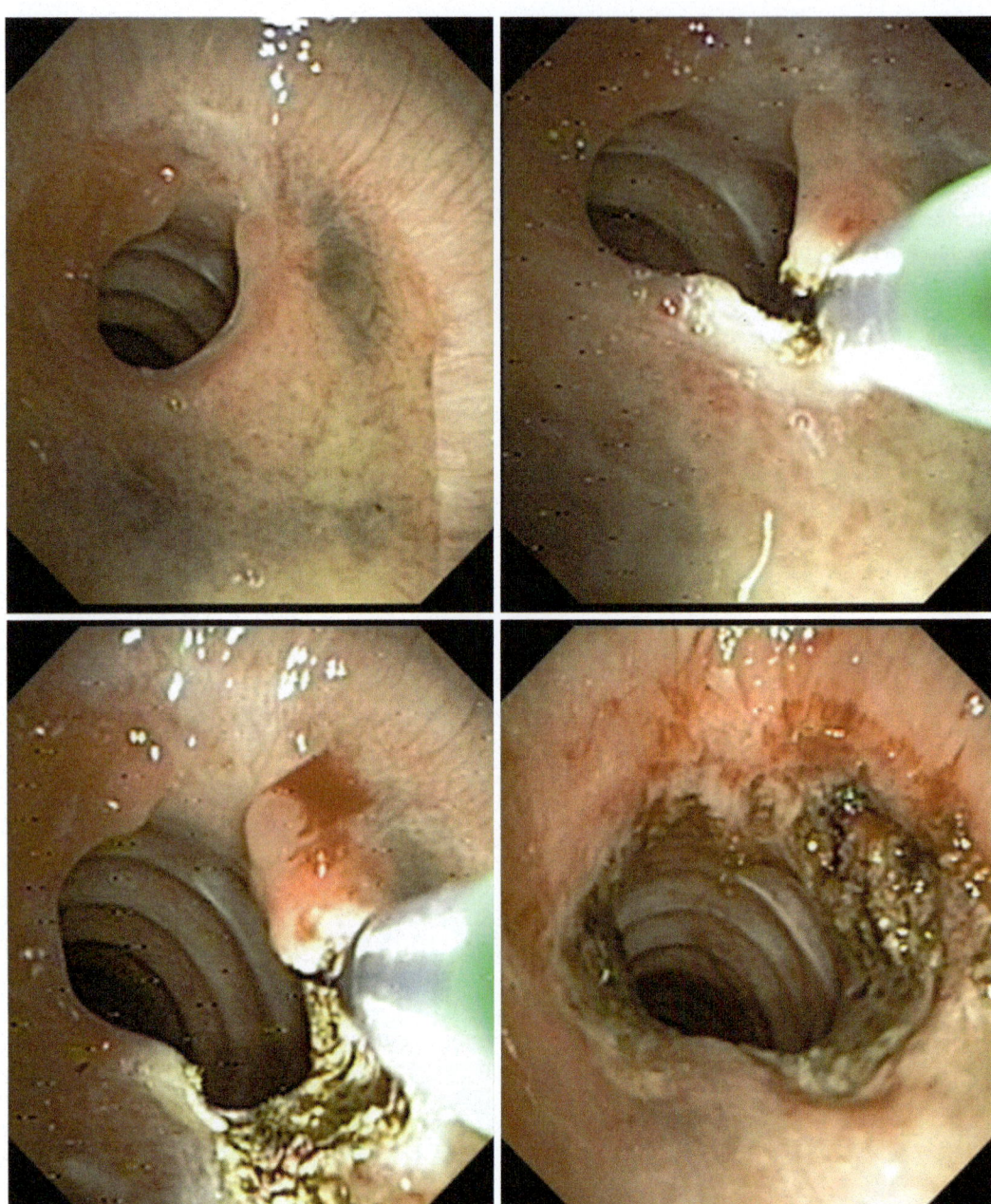

Fig. 16.7 Endobronchial electrosurgery

Cryotherapy is the most commonly used among the delayed mode modalities (Fig. 16.8). It is based on the cytotoxic effects of freezing. It can destroy (cryoablation), adhere to (cryoadhesion), and take a biopsy (cryobiopsy) from the tissue to which the modality is applied. This therapeutic and diagnostic tool works via rapid freezing and thawing cycles which lead to damage at several levels like molecular, cellular, and structural. It works on the Joule–Thomson effect where a gas or a liquid when forced through a valve under high pressure to a low pressure area cools down (Fig. 16.9). Some tissues with higher water content such as tumors, skin, granulation,

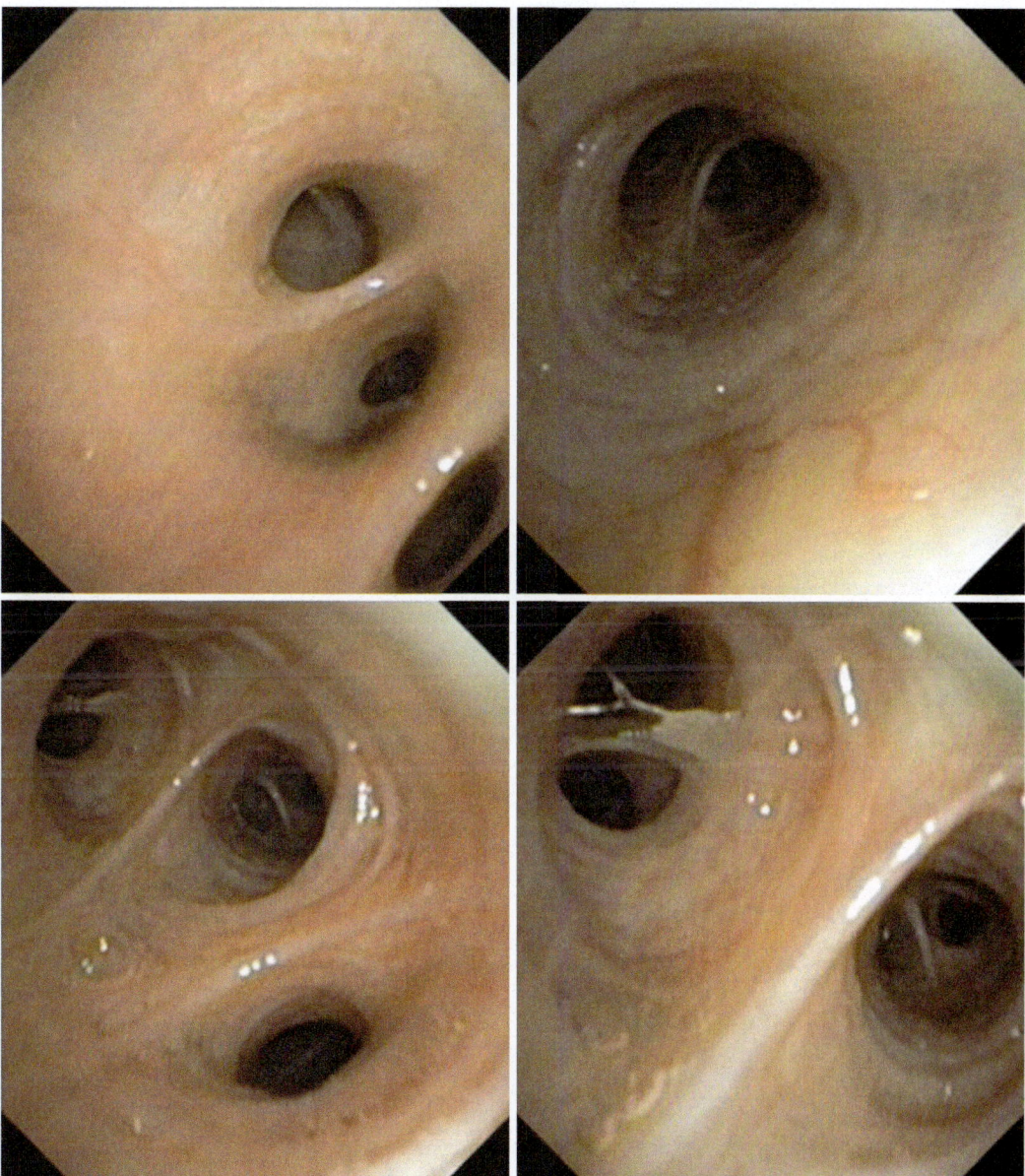

Fig. 16.8 Diagnostic bronchoscopy

or mucous membranes are more cryosensitive in contrast to others namely fat, cartilage, connective, and fibrous tissue which are cryoresistant. It is used mainly as palliative and adjunctive therapy in the treatment of benign and malignant central airway obstruction with 90% relief as per some studies. It can also be used for foreign body removal, endobronchial and transbronchial biopsy (Fig. 16.10) [16, 17].

Recently the metered cryospray has been introduced where the cryogen is liquid nitrogen instead of nitrous oxide. A cold resistant catheter is placed into the airway for passage of the liquid nitrogen which rapidly expands and vaporizes and causes intense cooling of the target tissue. This means that the anesthesiologist has to respond to a unique situation resulting from barotrauma because of gas

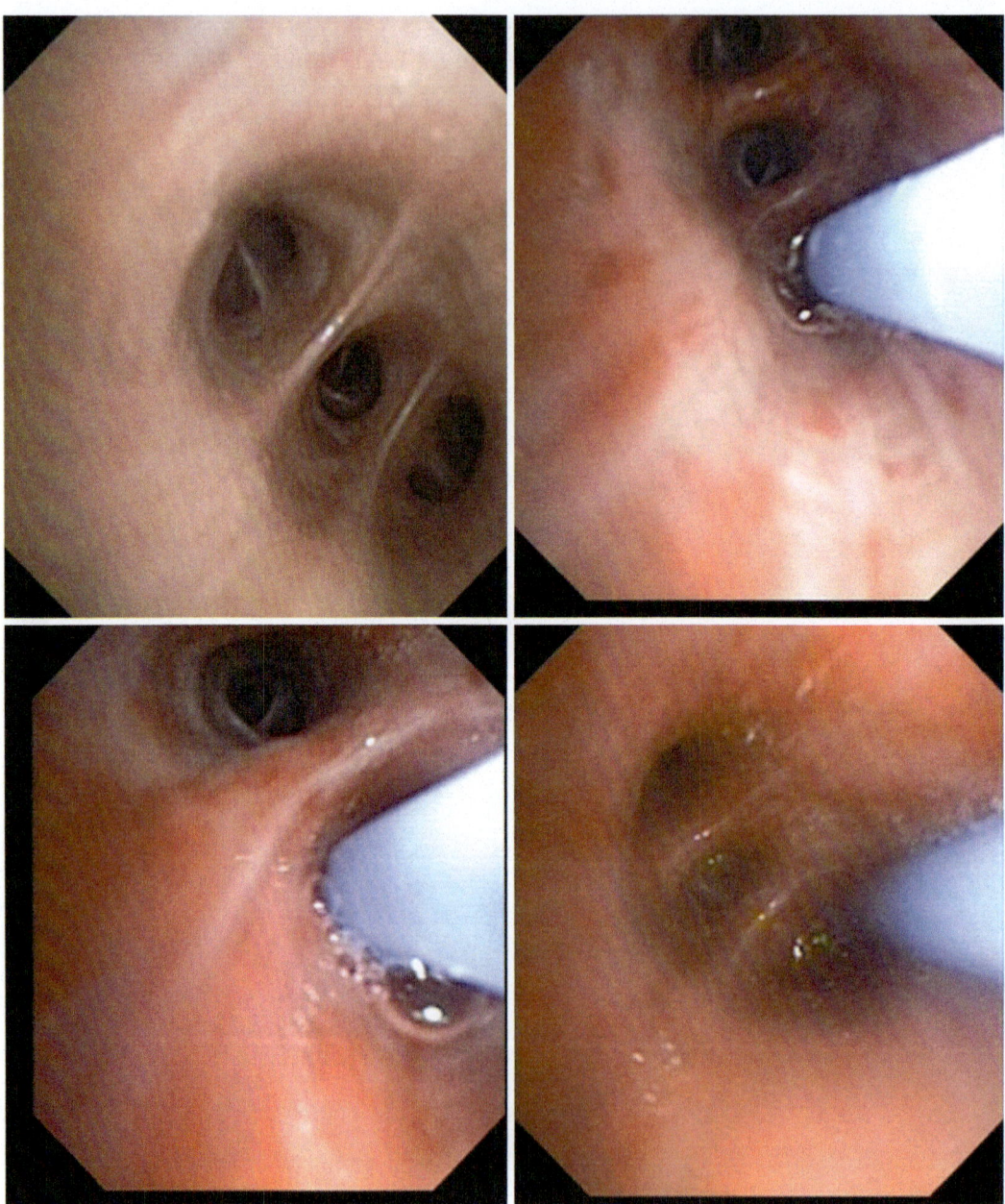

Fig. 16.9 Cryotherapy

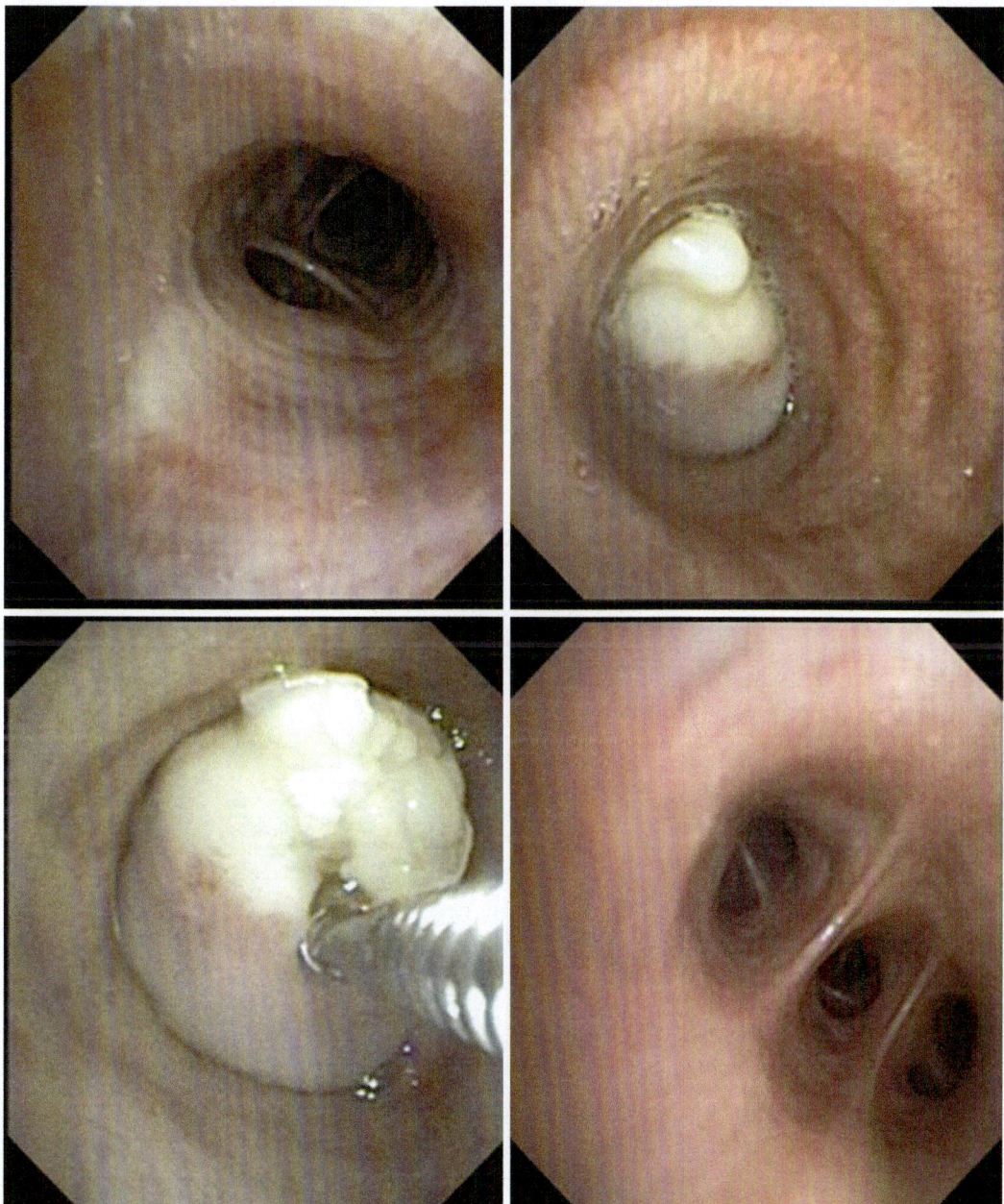

Fig. 16.10 Tumor resection

expansion and hypoxia due to displacement of oxygen by the nitrogen gas [18].

16.13 Bronchial Thermoplasty

This is a recent interventional bronchoscopic technique employed in the treatment of severe asthma. The procedure entails the application radiofrequency to airway wall to generate a temperature of ~65 °C, the result being a reduced muscle mass without scarring or destruction of the tissue. There has been improvement in the airflow of asthmatics after the application of this technique; however, further studies are needed to assess its safety profile and efficacy (Fig. 16.11) [19, 20].

These miscellaneous procedures as APC, balloon bronchoplasty, cryotherapy, and bronchial thermoplasty may be done under conscious to deep sedation and as per the procedure specific requirement. General anesthesia with or without muscle relaxation with LMA and ILMA or ETT are always an option with complete backup of postoperative ventilation and care.

16.14 Total Lung Lavage

In diagnostic bronchoscopy, pulmonologist usually take bronchoalveolar fluid and lavage for diagnostic purpose but total lung lavage is indicated in indicator for the patients who are suffering from pulmonary alveolar proteinosis (PAP). It is a rare pulmonary disease where alveolar accusation of surfactant occurs. It is made up of protein and lipids.

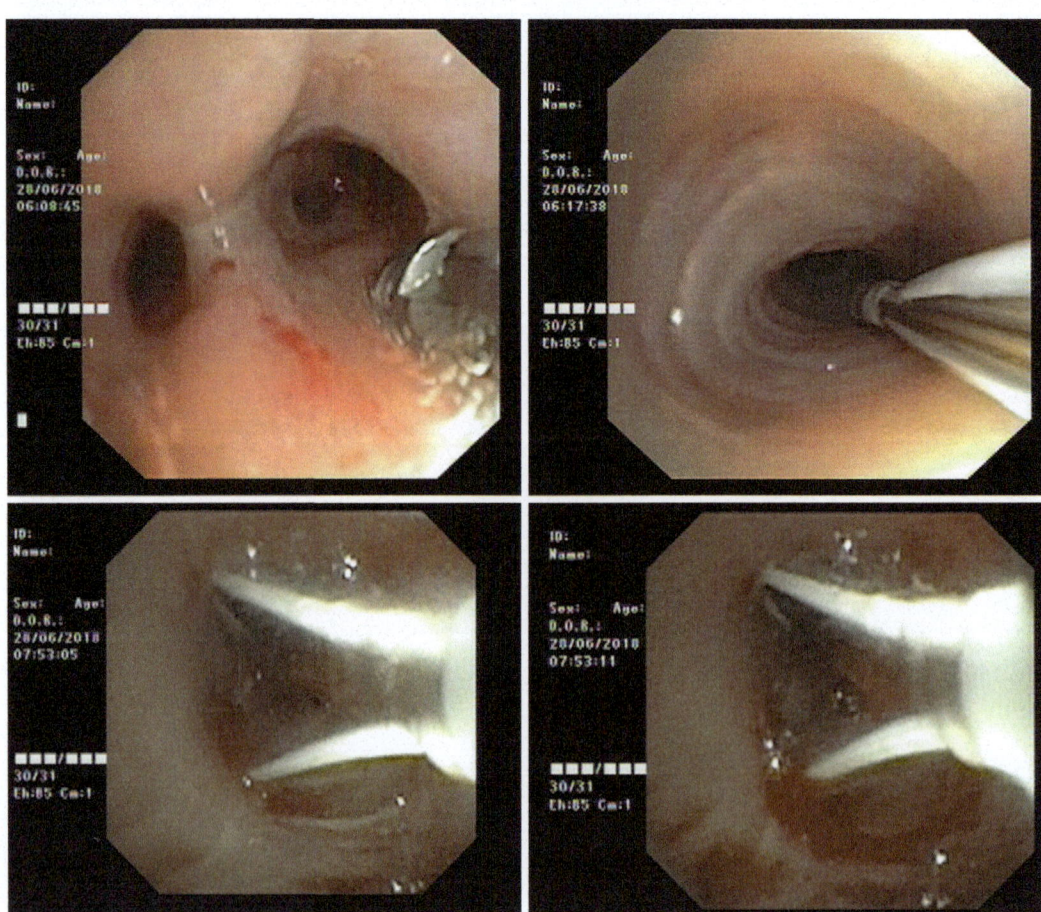

Fig. 16.11 Bronchial thermoplasty

The main etiology PAP is primarily neonatal, congenital, idiopathic, neonatal, and secondarily because of exogenous or environmental exposure.

Diffuse ground glass opacities with intralobular and interlobular septum thickening may be seen radiologically. The diagnosis of PAP can be made if bronchoalveolar lavage (BAL) fluid has a milky appearance and Periodic Acid Schiff (PAS) positive globular in biopsy.

For total lung lavage, anesthesiologist has to be well equipped for postoperative ventilation.

16.15 Foreign Body Impingement and Extraction

It is one of the commonest reasons for bronchoscopy. The children and old aged patients are at greatest risk owing to immature or blunted airway and swallowing reflexes [21].

The complications of foreign body aspiration depend on components and biogradients of inhaled foreign body. The anesthetic consideration involves general condition of patient with keeping in mind the irritability of airway, episodes of desaturation, hacking cough etc. Any complication has to be dealt with accordingly.

Diagnostic imaging, e.g., chest X-ray and computed tomography scan has promising role but limitations are always there.

Foreign body extraction in adult patients may be done under topical intravenous anesthesia or deep sedation while in pediatric population, it is done under GA. Appropriate fasting guidelines have to be followed before foreign body extraction.

16.16 Conclusion

With the advances and innovation of medical sciences there are a lot of procedures done in bronchoscopy suite. Diagnostic and therapeutic procedures varying from diagnostic bronchoscopy to bronchial thermoplasty have to be done under sedation varying for mild to deep and general anesthesia.

Utmost care has to be taken regarding from desaturation spells to postoperative complication which have to be dealt with complete backup plan. Skilled anesthesiologist with prompt decision-making power will counterfoil any life threatening emergencies. Maintaining protective airway reflexes is the key point for successful completion of procedure.

References

1. Sakuraba M, Masuda K, Hebisawa A, et al. Diagnostic value of thoracoscopic pleural biopsy for pleurisy under local anaesthesia. ANZ J Surg. 2006;76(8):722–4.
2. Chadha M, Kulshrestha M, Biyani A. Anaesthesia for bronchoscopy. Indian J Anaesth. 2015;59(9):565–73.
3. Murphy GS, Brull SJ. Residual neuromuscular block: lessons unlearned. Part I: definitions, incidence, and adverse physiologic effects of residual neuromuscular block. Anesth Analg. 2010;111(1):120–8.
4. Guha A, Mostafa SM, Kendall JB. The Montgomery t-tube: anesthetic problems and solutions. Br J Anesth. 2001;87(5);787–90.
5. Dumon JF. A dedicated tracheobronchial stent. Chest. 1990;97(2):328–32.
6. Saito Y. Endobronchial stents: past, present, and future. Semin Respir Crit Care Med. 2004;25(4):375–80.
7. Van Der Spek AF, Spargo PM, Norton ML. The physics of lasers and implications for their use during airway surgery. Br J Anaesth. 1988;60(6):709–29.
8. Geffin B, Shapshay SM, Bellack GS, et al. Flammability of endotracheal tubes during Nd-YAG laser application in the airway. Anesthesiology. 1986;65(5):511–5.
9. Moghissi K, Dixon K, Hudson E, et al. Endoscopic laser therapy in malignant tracheobronchial obstruction using sequential and YAG laser Nd photodynamic therapy. Thorax. 1997;52(3):281–3.
10. Barlow DE. Endoscopic applications of electrosurgery: a review of basic principles. Gastrointest Endosc. 1982;28(2):73–6.
11. Ernst A, Silvestri GA, Johnstone D. Interventional pulmonary procedures: guidelines from the American college of chest physicians. Chest J. 2003;123(5):1693–717.
12. Grund KE, Storek D, Farin G. Endoscopic argon plasma coagulation (APC) first clinical experiences in flexible endoscopy. Endosc Surg Allied Technol. 1994;2(1):42–6.
13. Sheski FD, Mathur PN. Endobronchial electrosurgery: argon plasma coagulation and electrocautery. Semin Respir Crit Care Med. 2004;25(4):367–74.
14. Morice RC, Ece T, Ece F, et al. Endobronchial argon plasma coagulation for treatment of

hemoptysis and neoplastic airway obstruction. Chest. 2001;119(3):781–7.
15. McArdle JR, Gildea TR, Mehta AC. Balloon bronchoplasty: its indications, benefits, and complications. J Bronchol Interv Pulmonol. 2005;12(2):123–7.
16. Schumann C, Hetzel M, Babiak AJ, et al. Endobronchial tumor debulking with a flexible cryoprobe for immediate treatment of malignant stenosis. J Thorac Cardiovasc Surg. 2010;139(4):997–1000.
17. Mohamed AS, El-Din MAA. Fiberoptic bronchoscopic cryo-ablation of central bronchial lung cancer. Egypt J Chest Dis Tuberc. 2016;65(2):527–30.
18. Browning R, Turner JF, Parrish S. Spray cryotherapy (SCT): institutional evolution of techniques and clinical practice from early experience in the treatment of malignant airway disease. J Thorac Dis. 2015;7(Suppl 4):S405–14.
19. Bel EH. "Hot Stuff" bronchial thermoplasty for asthma. Am J Respir Crit Care Med. 2006;173:941–2.
20. Cox G. New interventions in asthma including bronchial thermoplasty. Curr Opin Pulm Med. 2008;14(1):77–81.
21. Rafanan AL, Mehta AC. Adult airway foreign body removal. What's new? Clin Chest Med. 2001;22(2):319–30.

Overview of Lung Transplant

Akhil Kumar

17.1 Introduction

Over the last three decades, lung transplantation has evolved from an experimental procedure to definitive treatment option for patient with end-stage pulmonary disease, especially when all other therapeutic measures have been unsuccessful. Lung transplant (LT) has provided to a large number of patients an increased survival benefit [1] along with improved health-related quality of life [2], as observed after other solid organ transplantations [3]. Lung transplantation encompasses lobar, single lung, sequential bilateral lung and combined heart lung transplantation. Double lung transplant is a more frequently performed procedure worldwide, [4] with better long-term survival observed in comparison to single lung transplantation when done for certain specific diseases [5].

The first human LT was performed by Hardy and co-workers after years of research in 1963 [6]. The recipient had carcinoma of lung and had received a single left lung transplant. The patient survived only 18 days and succumbed to malnutrition and renal failure. In the next two decades approximately 44 lung transplants were performed worldwide without long-term clinical survival. The first successful unilateral lung transplant with long-term survival was performed by Joel Cooper and team on 7 November 1983. The patient was discharged after 6 weeks of hospitalisation and maintained an active life for 5 years [7]. Due to a complication following a transbronchial lung biopsy he died in the sixth postoperative year. In the last three decades major advancements like newer immunosuppressants, better organ preservation, technical refinements in surgical skills, advanced anesthesia care, improved postoperative care, earlier diagnosis of rejection and enhanced surveillance of infection has led to an improved survival of LT recipients.

17.2 Indications of Lung Transplant

The number of lung transplants performed has steadily increased over the decades and a total of 4122 procedures were performed worldwide in 2015 as reported to International Society of Heart and Lung Transplant Registry [4]. LT is now offered for a myriad of diseases including:

1. Chronic obstructive pulmonary disease with or without α_1 antitrypsin deficiency
2. Interstitial lung disease
3. Bronchiectasis with or without cystic fibrosis
4. Idiopathic interstitial pneumonia
5. Idiopathic pulmonary arterial hypertension
6. Connective tissue disease

A. Kumar (✉)
Institute of Anaesthesiology, Pain and Perioperative Medicine, Sir Ganga Ram Hospital, New Delhi, India

7. Obliterative bronchiolitis
8. Lymphangioleiomyomatosis
9. Retransplant

Till date COPD, interstitial lung disease, bronchiectasis with or without cystic fibrosis, and idiopathic pulmonary arterial hypertension have accounted for 89.1% of lung transplants performed worldwide [4]. The remaining 10.9% of the lung transplants were performed for disease which included connective tissue disease, cancer, sarcoidosis, lymphangioleiomyomatosis and retransplant.

17.3 Patient Selection for Lung Transplant [8]

Lung transplant should be considered for patients who meet the following criteria:

1. High: >50% risk of death from lung disease within 2 years, if LT is not performed
2. High: >80% likelihood of surviving at least 90 days after LT
3. High: >80% likelihood of 5 years post-transplant survival from a general medical perspective, provided that there is adequate graft function

17.4 Disease-Specific Timing of Listing for Transplant [8]

A consensus document released in 2014 gave broad guidelines for listing of patients for LT, although wide inter-institutional variations are often encountered.

17.4.1 Interstitial Lung Disease

- Decline in FVC ≥10% during 6 months of follow-up
- Decline in DLCO ≥15% during 6 months of follow-up
- Desaturation to <88% or distance <250 m on 6 min walk test or >50 m decline in 6 min walk distance over a 6-month period
- Pulmonary hypertension on right heart catheterisation or 2-dimensional echocardiography
- Hospitalisation because of respiratory function decline, pneumothorax or acute exacerbation

17.4.2 Cystic Fibrosis

- Chronic respiratory failure
  - With hypoxia alone [partial pressure of oxygen (PaO_2) <8 kPa or <60 mm Hg]
  - With hypercapnia [partial pressure of carbon dioxide ($PaCO_2$) >6.6 kPa or >50 mm Hg]
- Long-term noninvasive ventilation therapy
- Pulmonary hypertension
- Frequent hospitalisation
- Rapid lung function decline
- World Health Organisation functional class IV

17.4.3 Chronic Obstructive Pulmonary Disease (COPD)

- BODE (Body-mass index, airflow obstruction, dyspnea and exercise) index ≥7
- FEV_1 (Forced expiratory volume-1 s) <15–20% predicted
- Three or more severe exacerbations during the preceding year
- One severe exacerbation with acute hypercapnic respiratory failure
- Moderate to severe pulmonary hypertension

17.4.4 Pulmonary Vascular Disease

- NYHA functional class III or IV despite a trial of at least 3 months of combination therapy including prostanoids
- Cardiac index of <2 l/min/m^2
- Mean right atrial pressure of >15 mm Hg
- 6 min walk test <350 m

- Development of significant hemoptysis, pericardial effusion, or signs of progressive right heart failure (renal insufficiency, increasing bilirubin, brain natriuretic peptide or recurrent ascites)
- Infection with *Burkholderia cenocepacia, Burkholderia gladioli* and MDR (Multidrug resistant) *Mycobacterium abscessus.*
- Atherosclerotic disease sufficient to put candidate at risk post transplant.

17.5 Contraindications to Lung Transplant

It is an ever evolving list and varies from centre to centre. With advances in medical science an ever increasing number of patients are receiving LT.

17.5.1 Absolute

- Recent history of malignancy
- Untreatable significant dysfunction of other major organ systems
- Acute medical instability like sepsis, myocardial infarction and liver failure
- Bleeding diathesis
- Chronic infection which is poorly controlled
- Significant chest wall or spinal deformity
- Class II or III obesity (BMI > 35 kg/m^2)
- Current non-adherence to medical therapy
- Psychiatric or psychological condition with poor rehabilitation potential

17.5.2 Relative

- Increasing age should not be a limiting criterion for transplant, but patients with age >65 years are associated with low physiological reserve.
- Class I obesity (BMI 30.0–34.9 kg/m^2), with particularly truncal obesity.
- Severe malnutrition and osteoporosis.
- Extensive prior chest surgery or lung resection (as it may cause technical difficulty).
- Preoperative mechanically ventilated patients and/or patient on extracorporeal life support.
- Infection with hepatitis B or C and HIV.

17.6 Lung Allocation

Initially donor lungs were allocated on the basis of time accumulated on the waitlist which was assumed to correspond to disease severity. There is a huge demand–supply gap between the available organs and patients awaiting transplant. In 2005, lung allocation score (LAS) was implemented to preferentially allocate organs on the basis of medical urgency and to provide maximum post-transplant survival benefit. LAS is a numerical scale from 0 to 100 and is calculated as the difference between perceived transplant survival benefit and waitlist urgency [9]. From, pre-LAS era to 2007 the number of active waitlisted candidates declined by 54% and simultaneously reduction in median waiting time from 792 days to 141 days was observed [10]. After introduction of LAS the waitlist mortality dropped significantly by 40% and an increased number of patients with restrictive lung disease were allocated organs [11]. The LAS can be calculated online (https://optn.transplant.hrsa.gov/resources/allocation-calculators/las-calculator/).

17.7 Donor Selection and Management

17.7.1 General Management

After certification of brain death and obtaining consent from donor's family, appropriate donor management protocols should be initiated to maintain viability of precious organs. A single patient is a potential multiorgan donor, catering to the tailored requirements of each individual organ, pose challenges in the donor management. While liberal fluid administration protocol is beneficial for renal transplant outcome, it may prove to be hazardous for lung transplantation. Neurohormonal homeostatic balance is disrupted after brain death and can lead to detrimental effects on organ system, particularly causing lung injury.

Some form of shock invariably follows brain death and adequate haemodynamic management forms the foundation of donor management. Euvolemia should be maintained by adequate crystalloid infusion to target a mean arterial pressure (MAP) of 60 mm Hg and central venous pressure (CVP) of 6–8 mmHg [12]. If required vasopressin (0.01–0.04 IU/min) is the agent of choice to maintain haemodynamics [13] and it additionally helps in reversing diabetes insipidus. Hormone replacement therapy should be initiated at the earliest to correct thyroid deficiency, adrenal insufficiency and diabetes insipidus [14]. Normothermia should be maintained and hyperglycaemia (>180 mg/dl) avoided. Ongoing continuous medical care is the norm to maintain donor organ function.

17.7.2 Pulmonary Management

All potential lung donors should have a nasogastric tube in place to prevent a possible aspiration of gastric contents. Baseline chest X-ray and if possible a CT scan of the chest should be obtained to rule out pneumonia, contusion or pulmonary edema. A bronchoscopy is done to look for gross anatomical examination, presence of hyperaemia, foreign bodies, blood and secretions. Presence of bronchial secretions is not a contraindication but reappearing after proper suctioning denotes an ongoing pathological process. A lung protective ventilation strategy comprising of low tidal volume (6–8 ml/kg), positive end expiratory pressure (PEEP) less than 8 cm of H_2O with a peak inspiratory pressure of less than 30 cm of H_2O is advocated [15, 16]. Neurogenic pulmonary edema is common after brain death, so judicious use of crystalloid and blood products is practised to maintain lowest possible CVP and simultaneously maintain adequate organ perfusion with good urine output. Broad spectrum antibiotics are commonly administered prophylactically along with methyl-prednisolone 15 mg/kg bolus to be repeated every 6 h for decreasing inflammation [17].

The ideal criteria for selection of brain dead donors for lung transplantation are as follows [18, 19]:

- Age <55 years
- Less than 20-pack-year smoking
- Absence of significant abnormality on chest radiograph
- Absence of purulent secretions or signs of aspiration during bronchoscopy
- PaO_2 > 300 mm Hg on FiO_2 1 and PEEP 5 cm of H_2O
- Negative Gram staining
- Appropriate size matching
- Intubation period <5 days
- Ischaemia times less than 4 h
- No pulmonary edema or asthma

To overcome organ shortage, centres are now performing lung transplant with donors beyond the ideal criteria (extended or marginal donors) [20]. These donors are older, history of greater duration of smoking, lower PaO_2/FiO_2 ratio and possibly some infiltrates on chest X-ray. On the basis of presently available data there seems to be no contraindication for the use of marginal donors [21, 22].

17.8 Intraoperative Donor Management

The guiding principles of intraoperative management are decided by the organs to be harvested. A repeat bronchoscopy is performed and an arterial blood gas sample obtained. A midline sternotomy is performed to open up the pleural spaces and a visual inspection of the lungs done, to rule out consolidation, emphysema or trauma. The ventilator is disconnected to allow for deflation of lungs and manual palpation to check for masses or nodule is also done. After acceptability of the organ, heparin 300 U/kg is given as an intravenous bolus [23]. A cannula is inserted in pulmonary artery, de-aired and 500 μg of PGE1 (alprostadil) is infused to dilate the pulmonary vascular bed to enhance flushing and also provide protection against graft dysfunction [24]. Perfadex (low K+ dextran), 60 ml/kg, is used as lung preservative solution worldwide with satisfactory results [25]. It is infused at a temperature of 4–8 °C with pressure of 10–15 mm Hg aided by gravity. After mobilisation of the surrounding structures, the lungs are hand ventilated with FiO_2 0.5 and then allowed to deflate to half the total lung capacity [26]. 4–8 mm staples are deployed twice around the trachea, and the trachea is transected between the staple lines. After removal of lungs, gravity-dependent retrograde infusion of perfadex (250 ml) in each pulmonary vein is done, to flush out any small pulmonary emboli [27].

17.9 Donation After Cardiac Death

It is of utmost importance to clear the contents of stomach to mitigate the risk of aspiration. Intravenous heparin is administered prior to declaration of death before cessation of life support or may be administered post-mortem [28]. Cold perfadex (4C) via chest tube is infused in both pleural cavities to bring lung temperature below 21 °C (topical cooling) [29]. Rest of the procedure is same as for donation after brain death.

17.10 Preservative Solution

Extracellular solutions [Perfadex/Celsior/Histidine-tryptophan-ketoglutarate (HTK)] containing low potassium and high sodium are better than intracellular solutions like Euro-collins [30]. Perfadex is the most commonly used solution for lung preservation. It leads to homogenous flushing of the lung, accompanied by less chances of pulmonary edema in the graft tissue [31]. Perfadex yields a better oxygenation [32], superior lung compliance [33] and increased intracellular metabolic activity of alveolar cells when compared to Euro-collins [34]. It has also shown to improve 30 days and 1 year post-transplant survival [25].

17.11 Ischaemia Time

Median allograft ischaemia times have increased over the last 25 years from 4 h in the 1990s to more than 5 h in the recent years [4]. Cold ischaemia time greater than 6 h did not have any adverse outcome on graft function in either intraoperative, early post-operative or long-term follow-up period [35]. In the current scenario prolonged ischaemia time allows for farther transportation and better donor–recipient matching. For non-heart beating donors, maximum permissible warm ischaemia time (absence of circulation until establishment of effective topical cooling) is 90 min. After topical cooling, the graft may remain viable for another 4 h [28, 29].

17.12 Choice of Procedure

Underlying lung pathology is the prime determinant of the type of procedure to be performed, but other factors like age, functional status, institutional preferences, presence of pulmonary hypertension and infection also play a pivotal role. Single lung transplantation provides great societal benefit by allowing more patients to be transplanted, but also offers less lung reserve in scenario of graft dysfunction. Patients undergoing single lung transplant have shorter waiting and operating times with a possible rapid recovery profile. Single lung transplant was commonly performed for non-suppurative diseases such as those with idiopathic pulmonary fibrosis, specifically in the absence of secondary pulmonary hypertension [36, 37]. However, now a large percentage of patients are undergoing bilateral lung transplantation. An analysis of patients undergoing transplant for idiopathic pulmonary fibrosis found that bilateral lung transplant is associated with better graft survival than single lung transplant (62 vs. 50 months) [38]. Older patients (>60 years) with COPD might be suitable candidates for single lung transplant [39], although bilateral lung transplant avoids complications like native lung hyperinflation. Bilateral lung transplant is the procedure of choice for septic lung disease and cystic fibrosis in order to avoid contamination of the transplanted lung from the native infected lung. It is also the preferred option for idiopathic pulmonary arterial hypertension or secondary pulmonary hypertension from other pulmonary conditions. Bilateral lung transplant allows equal distribution of cardiac output to both the lungs. In single lung transplant, high vascular resistance of the native lung directs the entire cardiac output to allograft with a possible threatening risk of impending pulmonary edema. Bilateral lung transplantation might also allow for better utilisation of marginal donors who are otherwise deemed unsuitable for single lung transplant. Irrespective of the primary pathology, bilateral lung transplant has better long-term survival when older donors (>60 years) are used for younger patients [40].

17.13 Expanding the Donor Pool

17.13.1 Deceased Donor

Brain death leads to physiological alterations resulting in neurogenic pulmonary edema [41]. which can potentially be avoided in donation after cardiac death. Although utilisation of lungs after cardiac death is increasing, the numbers are considerably less as compared to other solid organ transplants [42]. Recipients from donation after cardiac death donors have not shown inferior outcome in terms of primary graft dysfunction (PGD) and survival at 72 h in comparison to brain dead donors [43].

17.13.2 Ex Vivo Lung Perfusion

Ex vivo Lung Perfusion (EVLP) is one of the most important advancements in the field of lung transplant in recent times and is a promising technique to increase the number and quality of allograft. The components of EVLP circuit are shown in Fig. 17.1 [44]. This technique is used to assess lung function of a suboptimal or marginal donor (who would have been outrightly rejected) and donation after cardiac death. EVLP allows lungs to be re-evaluated over a considerable time period for physiological, radiological and bronchoscopic parameters which helps in determining whether the lungs can be transplanted. Pre-transplant viability analysis improves the decision-making process, to accept earlier discarded organs, or reject organs that were accepted earlier. Normothermic EVLP allows for preservation of lung homeostasis, metabolic functions and optimise donor organs. Currently three different EVLP protocols are employed worldwide, namely, The Toronto, Lund and Organ Care System (Transmedic, Andover, MA) with variation in methodology as outlined in Table 17.1 [45]. Donor lung initially deemed unfit for transplant can be reconditioned following EVLP use by alveolar recruitment, clearance of bronchial secretions, removal of clots in pulmonary circulation, reduction in pulmonary edema by high oncotic pressure of the perfusate and removal of inflammatory cells, thereby decreasing inflammation [46]. A large number of potential donor lungs are considered injured, and successful repair can possibly revolutionise lung transplantation. Use of high risk donor lungs after EVLP had similar results in comparison to lungs obtained after satisfying conventional donation criteria [47, 48]. EVLP also allows for various therapeutic interventions to be carried out for treatment of donor lung injuries [45]. It has been recently utilised for individualised lung repair by providing ex vivo thrombolysis [49], treatment of infected lung [50] and surfactant administration to restore lung function loss caused by gastric aspiration [51].

17.13.3 Living Donor Lobar Transplantation

To overcome the shortage of lung allograft, the technique of living donor related lobar lung transplantation was developed for patients awaiting lung transplant, especially in regions where deceased donation rates are low. Two healthy and ABO compatible donors are selected. After functional and anatomical size matching with the recipient, donor lobectomies are performed. The right lower and left lower lobes are harvested from

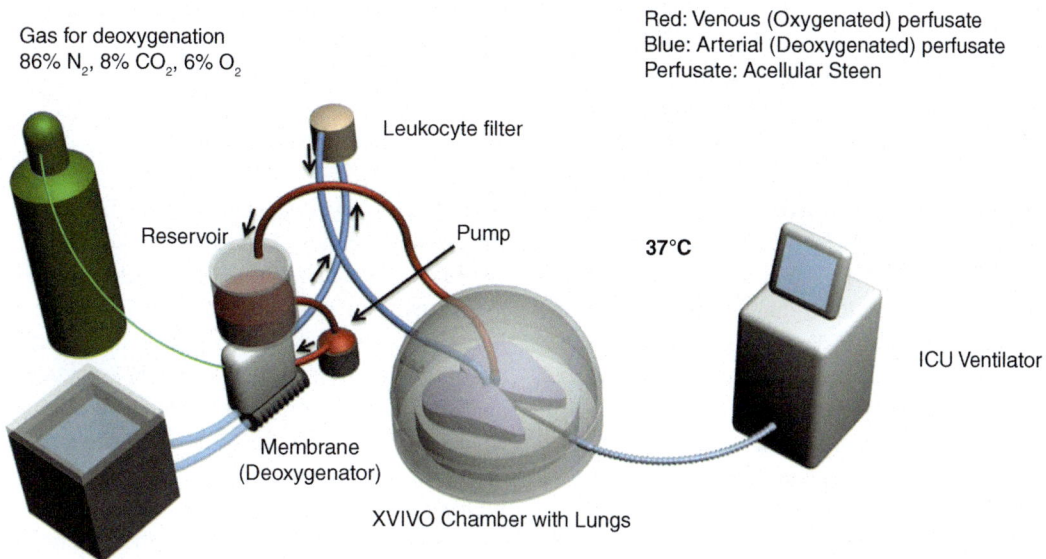

Fig. 17.1 Components of ex vivo lung perfusion circuit. The perfusate is circulated by a centrifugal pump passing through a membrane gas exchanger and a leukocyte-depletion filter before entering the lung block through the pulmonary artery. A filtered gas line for the gas-exchange membrane is connected to an H-size tank with a specialty gas mixture of oxygen (6%), carbon dioxide (8%) and nitrogen (86%). A heat exchanger is connected to the membrane gas exchanger to maintain the perfusate at temperature. Pulmonary artery flow is controlled by the centrifugal pump and measured using an electromagnetic flow metre. The outflow oxygenated perfusate returns through the left atrial cannula to a hard-shell reservoir. Lungs are ventilated with a standard ICU-type ventilator. The lungs are contained in a specifically designed lung enclosure (XVIVO; Vitrolife, Goteborg, Sweden). Reproduced from Cypel M, Yeung JC, Keshavjee S. Novel approaches to expanding the lung donor pool: donation after cardiac death and ex vivo conditioning. Clin Chest Med 2011;32(2):233–44 [44]. With permission from Elsevier. Copyright 2011

Table 17.1 Ex vivo lung perfusion protocols

Parameter	Methodology		
	Toronto	Lund	OCS[a]
Perfusion			
Target flow	40% cardiac output	100% cardiac output	2.0–2.5 l/min
Flow characteristic	Continuous	Continuous	Pulsatile
PAP	Flow dictated	≤20 mmHg	≤20 mmHg
LA	Closed	Open	Open
Perfusate	Steen solution	Steen solution + RBC's hct 14%	OCS solution + RBC's hct 15–25%
Ventilation			
Start temperature	32 °C	32 °C	34 °C
Tidal volume	7 ml/kg donor bw	5–7 ml/kg donor bw	6 ml/kg donor bw
Respiratory ratio (bpm)	7	20	10
PEEP	5 cmH$_2$O	5 cmH$_2$O	5–7 cmH$_2$O
FiO$_2$ (%)	21	50	12
Beginning of EVLP	Static device: recipient site or specialised centres	Static device: recipient site	Mobile device: donor site

Reproduced from Reeb J, Keshavjee S, Cypel M. Expanding the lung donor pool: advancements and emerging pathways. Curr Opin Organ Transplant 2015; 20(5):498–505 [45]. With permission from Wolters Kluwer Health, Inc. Copyright 2014
bpm breaths per minute, *bw* body weight, *FiO$_2$* inspired fraction of oxygen, *LA* left atrium, *PAP* pulmonary artery pressure, *PEEP* positive end-expiratory pressure, *RBCs* red blood cells
[a]*OCS* Organ Care System (Transmedics)

two donors. These lobes are transplanted in the recipient and act as surrogates for the whole right and left lung. The major problem with lobar lung transplant is the size disparity of the graft with recipient, as for an adult patient the graft might be small, on the contrary a paediatric patient might receive an oversized graft. Additionally full cardiac output supplying relatively undersized lobes add to the complexities of the procedure [52]. The survival rate at 30 days, 1 year and 3 years following living donor lobar lung transplantation are similar to those after deceased donations [53].

Downsized deceased donors are utilised primarily to shorten the waiting times for critically ill or small patients. Earlier studies suggested no difference in outcome following deceased donor lobar lung transplantation [54], but recent data indicates inferior survival when compared with other forms of lung transplantation [55].

17.14 Extracorporeal Life Support as Bridge to Transplant

A significant number of patients develop complications like life threatening hypoxia, hypercapnia and pulmonary hypertension, and eventually die while waiting for a transplant. Extracorporeal Life Support (ECLS) has now allowed patients to survive such critical period and undergo lung transplant. ECLS restores homeostasis, prevents initiation of mechanical ventilation thereby preventing complications like ventilator-induced lung injury and ventilator-associated pneumonia and also decreases respiratory distress in an awake patient thus allowing for active physical therapy possible. The best ECLS strategy in majority of patients is single site VV-ECMO (veno-venous extracorporeal membrane oxygenation) but it needs to be tailored as per individual patients and their physiological requirements (Fig. 17.2) [56]. In patients having significant pulmonary artery hypertension, VV-ECMO is best avoided. The best strategy is to use a peripheral veno-arterial (VA)-ECMO followed by pulmonary artery–left atrium (PA-LA) nova lung, if subsequent hypoxia develops [57]. Recent evidence supports the use of ECMO as an alternating bridging therapy to mechanical ventilation. Patients managed with ECMO preoperatively have showed acceptable 1 year post-transplant survival [58].

17.15 Recipient

A successful lung transplant programme requires close co-ordination between various medical specialists like pulmonologist, anesthesiologist, psychiatrist, infective disease specialist, surgeon, intensivist, perfusionist, transfusion specialist and medical social worker. Pertinent aspects like availability of organ, exigent nature of surgery, chances of survival, duration of post-operative hospital stay, possible complications, need for lifelong immunosuppression and financial implications should be discussed with the patient and their relatives well in advance.

17.15.1 Preoperative Evaluation

Standard evaluation and testing for patients undergoing lung transplant are listed in Table 17.2 [59]. A significant time usually elapses between the initial assessment and the day of surgery, so the attending anesthesiologist needs to perform a quick re-evaluation. Apart from the routine concerns like fasting status, aspiration prophylaxis, airway examination (selecting an appropriate size of double-lumen tube) and checking for vascular access sites, special emphasis should be given to the level of deterioration of lung function, available cardiopulmonary reserve and medications of the patient.

Patients presenting with pulmonary artery hypertension may have host of other impairments including renal dysfunction with fluid retention, ascites formation due to hepatic congestion and altered platelet function due to prostaglandin treatment [60]. Patients with mean pulmonary artery pressure greater than 25 mm Hg poorly tolerate hypoxia, hypercarbia and intraoperative pulmonary artery clamping, necessitating emergent ECLS use. Decision for elective use of ECLS depending upon the individual patient characteristics can be made in advance [61].

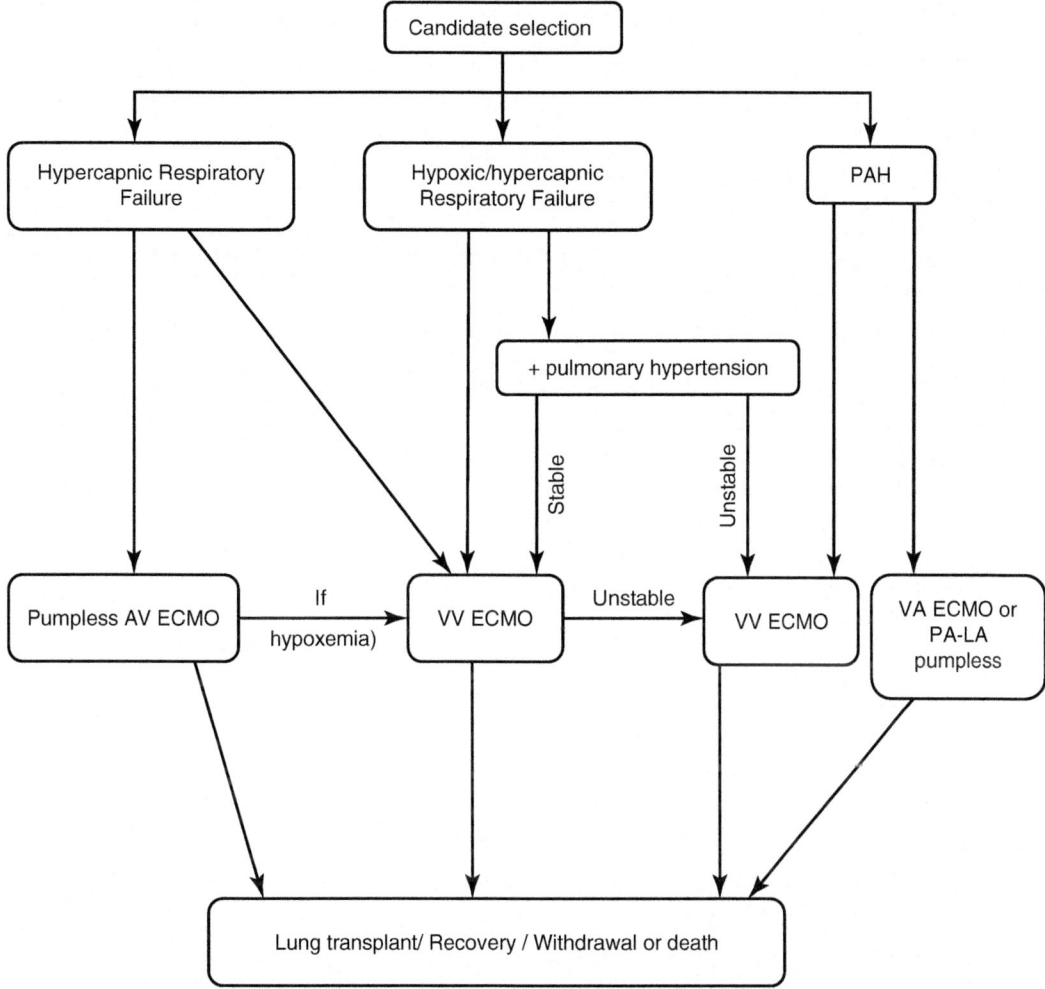

Fig. 17.2 Algorithm for selection of ECMO support configuration. *PAH* pulmonary artery hypertension; *AV* arteriovenous; *VV* venovenous; *ECMO* extra corporeal membrane oxygenation; *PA-LA* pulmonary artery-left atrium. Reproduced from Crotti [56]. With permission from Springer Nature. Copyright 2014.

Patients with cystic fibrosis have usually undergone multiple prior surgical procedures (chest tube insertion, pleurodesis, pleurectomy etc.) leading to extensive adhesions and distortion of anatomy, complicating the procedure of native lung pneumonectomy and predisposing to intraoperative bleeding. There is high incidence of chronic suppurative infections with the most commonly isolated organisms being *Pseudomonas aeruginosa* (often MDR) [62], *Burkholderia cepacia* complex (confers heightened mortality) [63], *Aspergillus fumigatus* and non-tuberculous mycobacterium [64]. Cystic fibrosis related diabetes mellitus is present in 50% of the patients [65]. Vitamin D deficiency, low BMI, osteoporosis and osteopenia are usually present in patients with cystic fibrosis. Gastro-oesophageal reflux and intestinal dysmotility are common preoperative findings [66].

Increasing number of lung transplants are now performed for patients aged greater than 65 years with improved early outcomes [67]. There is increased incidence of coronary artery disease in this subset of patients. Selective patients with significant coronary artery disease may undergo preoperative percutaneous coronary intervention or simultaneous coronary artery by-pass grafting along with lung transplant with acceptable early and medium-term outcomes [68].

Table 17.2 Components of lung transplant evaluation

1. Complete history and physical, including detailed family history
2. Consultations: (a) Transplant surgery   (b) Psychosocial evaluation   (c) Nutrition   (d) Transplant infectious disease   (e) Transplant pharmacy   (f) Financial coordinator   (g) Transplant coordinator: This visit will include a detailed orientation of the pre and post lung transplant process, including post-operative risks, management, outcomes etc.   (h) Contraceptive counselling for women of child-bearing potential   (i) Other consultations as dictated by clinical scenario, e.g. rheumatology for connective tissue disease assessment
3. Pulmonary evaluation: (a) PA and lateral chest X-ray   (b) Spiral CT of chest with contrast   (c) Pulmonary function test with DLCO   (d) Arterial blood gases on room air   (e) 6 minute walk distance with pre and post saturation   (f) V/Q scan with differential quantitation for single lung transplant cases   (g) Diaphragmatic sniff test: ultrasound or fluoroscopy   (h) QuantiFERON test/T-Spot test
4. Cardiovascular evaluation: (a) EKG   (b) Echocardiogram   (c) Right heart catheterisation   (d) Left heart catheterisation with coronary angiography for patient age >50 or >45 and strong family history or clinical suspicion.   (e) Consider stress testing (dobutamine echo) if known CAD   (f) Carotid Doppler for high risk patients >60 years, h/o neurologic event, and patients found to have CAD   (g) Lower extremity ABI for high risk >60 years, history or exam suggestive of PVD, diabetes, and patients found to have CAD

5. GI evaluation:
 (a) Spiral CT of abdomen and pelvis with contrast
 (b) Colonoscopy or CT colonography for age >50 years
 (c) Cine-esophagogram on all patients
    (i) If reflux and/or esophageal dysmotility, consider 24 h pH/impedance probe and esophageal manometry
    (ii) Consider gastric emptying study
    (iii) Consider GI consultation

6. Other testing: (a) 24 h urine for creatinine clearance   (i) If the calculated GFR is <40   (b) Bone mineral density (DXA scan)   (c) Mammogram for women >40   (d) PAP smear annually   (e) Dental clearance
7. Laboratory tests: (a) Full chemistry panel, CBC with differential, uric acid, lipid panel, thyroid function, iron, TIBC, ferritin, vitamin D level, PT/PTT, pre-albumin, Hgb A1C   (b) Urine drug screen   (c) Blood cotinine level   (d) Urinanalyis, with micro   (e) Urine albumin to creatinine ratio if diabetic   (f) Hypercoagulable workup if there is a personal or family history of venous and/or arterial thrombosis   (g) Stool for occult blood if no colonoscopy   (h) PSA in males >40 or younger if family history of prostate cancer   (i) Sputum gram stain and culture (routine, fungal and AFB) if productive cough present and in all CF/bronchiectasis patients   (j) MRSA nasal swab   (k) Anti-HLA antibodies (PRA)   (l) Blood type, tissue typing (prior to listing)   (m) Serology: CMV IgG, HIV, viral hepatitis, EBV, RPR, HSV, VZV, MMR, toxoplasmosis

Reproduced from an open access article by Girgis RE, Khaghani A. A global perspective of lung transplantation: part 1-recipient selection and choice of procedure. Global cardiology science and practice 2016:5 [59]

17.16 Induction Immunosuppression

Induction therapy is now routinely utilised in up to 70% of the cases. The three induction agents currently in use are anti-thymocyte globulin (ATG), anti CD52 monoclonal antibody (alemtuzumab) and IL-2 (interleukin-2) receptor antagonist (basiliximab). Choice of agent is centre specific but more than 80% of recipients getting induction therapy receive IL-2 receptor antagonist [4], which has resulted in improved survival as compared to those transplanted without induction therapy [69]. All recipients with significant panel reactive antibodies receive intravenous immunoglobulins and undergo preoperative or intraoperative plasmapheresis depending upon institutional protocols [70].

17.17 Pre-induction and Monitoring

Prophylactic antibiotics, antifungal and antiviral medications are given as per protocol. Availability of blood products is checked. Fasting status is determined and aspiration prophylaxis is administered accordingly. Patients who are on domiciliary oxygen therapy continue to receive it prior to induction. Premedication with opioids in the holding area is generally avoided for the fear of developing respiratory depression and consequent worsening of hypoxia, hypercarbia and right ventricular dysfunction. Informed consent is checked and viability of donor organs confirmed from the surgical team. Two large bore (16G or 18G) peripheral lines are inserted. Mandatory monitoring includes 5-lead electrocardiography, pulse oximetry, capnography, urinary output via indwelling catheter, spirometry, temperature and anesthetic agent analysis. Invasive arterial line (radial) allows for continuous blood pressure monitoring and repeated arterial blood gas sampling. Patients with severe pulmonary artery hypertension require pre-induction arterial line and pulmonary catheter placement. Multi-lumen central line is secured often from the left subclavian site. Pulmonary artery catheter allows for monitoring of cardiac output, pulmonary artery pressure, right ventricular loading conditions and mixed venous oxygen saturation. If desired, as per institutional preference thoracic epidural catheter may be placed preoperatively. Near-infrared reflectance spectroscopy is a useful tool for monitoring cerebral oxygenation during periods of extracorporeal haemodynamic support. Frequent intraoperative haemodynamic depression warrants titration of volatile anesthetic, making bispectral index monitoring an integral part of awareness surveillance.

17.18 Induction

Induction is one of the most critical periods of anesthesia. Prior to induction, recipient is preoxygenated for at least 5 min. The major goals are rapid control of airway, adequate oxygenation and maintenance of haemodynamic stability. Factors leading to increased pulmonary vascular resistance (hypoxia, hypercapnia, acidosis and light anesthesia) are to be avoided to prevent development of pulmonary hypertension and consequent right ventricular failure. Avoidance of myocardial depression and maintenance of systemic vascular resistance is also of utmost importance. All induction agents can be used safely provided they are utilised in a titrated and judicious manner. Rapid sequence intubation is seldom employed and slow titration of opioids (fentanyl) to reduce the effects of sudden withdrawal of sympathetic tone along with etomidate can be a useful choice. Intubation is achieved after a short period of gentle positive pressure ventilation accompanied with cricoid pressure while titrating inhalational anesthetics. Muscle relaxation may be achieved by a non-histamine releasing agent like vecuronium bromide and in cases with high aspiration risk, use of succinylcholine or high dose rocuronium is recommended. In patients with raised pulmonary artery pressure, a pre-induction inhaled pulmonary vasodilator [inhaled nitric oxide (NO)] and commencing β_1 and α_1 agonist infusion may be imperative for haemodynamic optimisation.

Post-induction hypotension may be due to deleterious effects of positive pressure ventilation on venous return, epidural local anesthetic, and negative inotropic and vasodilatory effects of induction agents. Vasopressor and inotropic agents should be ready for use in situation of worsening hypotension. All patients at risk of cardiovascular collapse should have femoral site prepared and ready for emergency cannulation for extracorporeal support. At induction, for all patients surgeon and perfusionist should be on standby for ready institution of extracorporeal support in case of haemodynamic collapse.

17.19 Airway Management

A left-sided double-lumen tube (DLT) is the preferred lung isolation technique for lung transplantation. A right-sided DLT needs to be withdrawn in the trachea during conduct of right bronchial anastomosis due its relatively short length. A single-lumen tube with a bronchial blocker is an alternative, but is prone to frequent dislodgement and requires repositioning during surgery. Double-lumen tubes allow for greater surgical ease, irrigation of the divided bronchus, differential lung ventilation after graft reperfusion, postoperative independent lung ventilation in patients with single lung transplant for emphysema and direct fibre-optic guided visualisation of bronchial anastomosis site. In cases of difficult intubation, a rapid control of airway with single lumen tube may precede a DLT insertion. A single-lumen tube allows for conduct of bronchoscopy for obtaining cultures and allows clearance of secretions in patients with suppurative diseases.

17.20 Positioning

A single lung transplant is performed either through an anterolateral thoracotomy (supine position), or, via, posterolateral thoracotomy (lateral decubitus) approach. Bilateral sequential lung transplant is performed in supine position with bilateral transverse thoracosternotomy (clamshell) incision or bilateral anterolateral thoracotomies sparing the sternum [71]. Arms are kept abducted and placed over the head with adequate support to facilitate exposure to both axillary area and chest. Care must be taken to avoid excessive stretching of arms to prevent inadvertent brachial plexus injury.

17.21 Ventilation Strategy and Maintenance of Anesthesia

The management of one lung ventilation is particularly difficult due to native lung pathology which is compounded by increased shunts in supine position, due to the absence of observed beneficial effects of gravity in lateral position. Underlying lung conditions pose unique challenges to one lung ventilation and strategies for management are described in Table 17.3 [72]. After initiation of positive pressure ventilation in patients of COPD it is important to avoid hyperinflation. High airway pressure can cause barotrauma with rupture of bullous emphysema leading to tension pneumothorax. Additionally, due to expiratory flow obstruction gas trapping may occur, leading to dynamic hyperinflation causing circulatory collapse as a result of decreased venous return. In such a scenario the circuit is disconnected till the airway pressure decreases to zero and blood pressure starts to increase. The ventilatory strategy to minimise such mishaps are: tidal volume 6–8 ml/kg, reduced respiratory rate to 4–10 breaths per minute, inspiratory to expiratory ratio ≥1:3, titrate FiO_2 to maintain SpO_2 90%, increased inspiratory flow rate to about 60–100 l/min, keeping plateau pressure less than 30 cm of H_2O and use of pressure control ventilation [73].

Patients with interstitial lung disease and pulmonary fibrosis are particularly difficult to ventilate. For delivering adequate tidal volume, higher ventilatory pressures are required. A strategy employing low tidal volume, increased respiratory rate and sufficient PEEP would seem appropriate for such patients [74]. One lung ventilation is required for all patients except

Table 17.3 Challenges and intraoperative management strategies for different underlying lung pathologies

Recipient pathology	Intraoperative complications	Management strategies
Obstructive (COPD, BOS)	• Dynamic hyperinflation • Tension pneumothorax	• Use pressure control ventilation to minimise dynamic hyperinflation • Maximum exhalation time (I:E 5 1:3–1:4) to minimise auto-PEEP • Check for auto-PEEP: interrupted inspiratory flow on the flow–volume curve • No or low extrinsic PEEP (3–4 cm H_2O)
Suppurative (cystic fibrosis, bronchiectasis)	• Thick, profuse secretions • Severe hypercapnia • Difficult dissection due to prior thoracic procedures	• Initial SLT intubation for BAL and suctioning • May require higher airway pressures • May require higher level of PEEP • Frequent suctioning
Restrictive (pulmonary fibrosis, hypersensitivity pneumonia)	• Severe pulmonary hypertension • May not tolerate OLV	• May need high peak inspiratory pressures (40 cm H_2O) • Maximise inspiratory time (I:E = 1:1–1:2) • Higher extrinsic PEEP (8–10 cm H_2O)
Primary pulmonary hypertension	• Severe hemodynamic instability due to right ventricular failure	• Central venous access before induction • Inotropic/vasopressor/inhaled pulmonary vasodilators on induction • Continue perioperative intravenous prostaglandins • Prepare for extracorporeal mechanical circulatory support

BAL bronchoalveolar lavage, *BOS* bronchiolitis obliterans syndrome, *COPD* chronic obstructive pulmonary disease, *I:E* inspiratory time to expiratory time ratio, *OLV* one-lung ventilation, *PEEP* positive end-expiratory pressure, *SLT* single-lumen tube
Reproduced from Nicoara A, Anderson-Dam J. Anesthesia for Lung Transplantation. Anesthesiol Clin 2017; 35(3):473–89 [72]. With permission from Elsevier. Copyright 2017

those on extracorporeal support. Institution of one lung ventilation worsens hypoxia and hypercarbia. To improve oxygenation during one lung ventilation, maneouvers like intermittent lung inflation, non-ventilated lung continuous positive airway pressure, PEEP on ventilated lung and allowing permissive hypercapnia are employed. Patients unable to tolerate one lung ventilation will require initiation of cardiopulmonary bypass (CPB) or ECMO. Maintenance of anesthesia can be achieved by a balanced technique with a combination of opioids (fentanyl or equivalent), muscle relaxants and inhaled anesthetics or propofol infusion. The fear of inhibition of hypoxic pulmonary vasoconstriction and significant worsening of oxygenation with the use of volatile agents has not been seen in clinical settings and should not preclude their use [75, 76]. On the contrary, ischaemic preconditioning and decreased alveolar inflammatory response seen with volatile anesthetics may be useful [77]. The need for frequent airway access (bronchoscopy, suctioning) accompanied with native lung disease and pneumonectomy renders uptake of volatile anesthetic unreliable, making propofol infusion an attractive choice for maintenance of anesthesia. Nitrous oxide is best avoided during lung transplantation due to several reasons; first, it can expand air cavities, like in emphysematous disease and in presence of occult pneumothorax; second, possibility of catastrophic expansion of air emboli; third, it has a propensity to increase pulmonary vascular resistance thereby worsening pulmonary hypertension and, lastly, due to high inspired FiO_2 used during one lung ventilation it is generally not possible to add nitrous oxide to the inspired gas mixture.

17.22 Surgical Procedure

The lung receiving lesser perfusion of the two as observed in ventilation perfusion scan is transplanted first in bilateral sequential lung transplant. Pneumonectomy of the native lung can be cumbersome, especially in case of suppurative lung diseases or in patients who have had prior thoracic surgery with extensive pleural adhesions. Large amount of blood loss can occur. Frequent hilar manipulations and cardiac compression can lead to reduced cardiac output and hypotension which requires vasopressor support and active fluid management. After the hilar structures are exposed, the pulmonary artery catheter is withdrawn in proximal pulmonary artery and test clamping of the pulmonary artery of the operative lung is carried out. It will improve the oxygenation by reducing shunt, but will divert the entire cardiac output to the opposite lung leading to increased pulmonary artery pressure and possible right ventricular dysfunction. If there is significant haemodynamic instability accompanied with increase in pulmonary artery pressure without right ventricular failure, as observed by echocardiography, treatment with inotropes, vasopressors and inhaled pulmonary vasodilators (NO or prostacyclin) to decrease pulmonary vascular resistance can possibly allow off-pump transplantation. In patients with pre-existing right ventricular dysfunction and pulmonary hypertension, pulmonary artery clamping invariably leads to right ventricular failure (ballooning of right ventricle as seen on TEE), necessitating extracorporeal support with either ECMO(V-A) or CPB.

17.23 Anastomosis of Allograft and Reperfusion

During implantation bronchial anastomosis is completed first, following which the anesthesiologist performs bronchoscopy to visualise anastomotic integrity and carries out pulmonary toileting. The pulmonary artery anastomosis is fashioned next, followed by venous anastomosis done by attaching a cuff of donor atrium containing upper and lower pulmonary veins to the recipient atrium. High degree of vigilance is required with use of atrial clamp as it can lead to arrhythmias, impede ventricular filling and occlude the flow in a coronary vessel. Methyl prednisolone 500 mg and mannitol 25 g are administered intravenously once the venous anastomosis is about to complete. Before completing the venous anastomosis, the atrial clamp is partially released to allow de-airing of the graft and TEE is monitored for the presence of left-sided air bubbles. Lung reperfusion is carried out slowly (low pressure perfusion) over a period of 15–20 min avoiding hyperperfusion of the graft [78]. During reperfusion, significant blood loss can occur due to leaks from vascular anastomotic sites. Severe hypotension due to myocardial stunning consequent to venous return of cold pneumoplegia, ischaemic metabolites and air embolism in superiorly placed right coronary artery is observed. Small boluses of adrenaline and calcium are generally required to restore myocardial contractility. Primary graft dysfunction occurring immediately in the transplanted lung is clinically, histopathologically and radiologically similar to acute respiratory distress syndrome, so initial ventilation should involve lung protective strategy. Ventilation is started with lowest possible FiO_2 <30% with an aim to maintain PaO_2 >70 mm Hg. Tidal volume of 6 ml/kg (consider using donor body weight, if graft is undersized) while not exceeding peak inspiratory pressure of 30 cm of H_2O. PEEP of 6–8 cm of H_2O is applied with gentle recruitment manoeuvres to recruit atelectatic segments. Respiratory rate is kept at 8–10 breaths per minute [79]. At this time, the native lung is ventilated with FiO_2 1 with a self-inflating bag. During off support bilateral sequential lung transplant the next step is to maintain oxygenation with one lung ventilation on the transplanted lung, while contralateral lung pneumonectomy is performed. Patients might need extracorporeal support this time due to graft failure, haemodynamic instability or right ventricular dysfunction. For transplant performed on CPB or ECMO, the transplanted lung is ventilated with initial setting and some perfusion via right ventricular ejection is allowed by partially clamping the venous drainage line. After ventilation and perfusion of the second lung is established, the extracorporeal support is gradually weaned off. Patients might require continuation of ECMO postoperatively, the type primarily decided by haemodynamic instability (V-A) or gas exchange abnormality (V-V).

17.24 Transesophageal Echocardiography

As advocated by the American Society of Anesthesiologists [80], TEE has a well-defined role in management of lung transplant and now constitutes an essential component of monitoring. It is placed immediately after intubation to note any deterioration of preoperative echocardiographic parameters. An initial assessment involves, but is not limited to left and right ventricular function, pulmonary artery pressure, identification of intracardiac shunts (patent foramen ovale/atrial septal defect), visualisation of pulmonary veins, tricuspid regurgitation, intracardiac thrombus, ascending aorta atheroma and regional wall motion abnormalities. Transesophageal Echocardiography (TEE) guides in the optimal placement of pulmonary artery catheter prior to transection of pulmonary artery. In comparison to pulmonary artery catheter, TEE is more reliable for estimating fluid status and preload thereby proving invaluable during periods of haemodynamic instability. Surgical clamping of pulmonary artery increases right ventricular afterload which may precipitate right ventricular failure. In such a scenario TEE examination can greatly facilitate the decision of whether to institute extracorporeal support [81]. Post-reperfusion TEE examination often reveals air as microbubbles in the left heart after incomplete de-airing of pulmonary veins. This leads to coronary air embolism [82] with new onset regional wall motion abnormalities consequent to transient myocardial ischaemia. After implantation, TEE is used to evaluate the patency and functioning of the pulmonary vein and pulmonary artery anastomosis. Significant narrowing of pulmonary arterial anastomosis leads to persistent pulmonary hypertension, whereas pulmonary venous anastomotic site stenosis manifests as pulmonary congestion and hypotension.

17.25 Fluid Management

Adequate fluid administration to optimise preload is necessary for stable haemodynamics. In models of acute respiratory distress syndrome [83] and allograft lungs [84], the alveolar fluid clearance is reduced thereby making them susceptible to low pressure edema. So a restrictive fluid therapy seems attractive. After excluding patients with poor myocardial contractility, presence of CVP >7 mm Hg was associated with prolonged mechanical ventilation and increased mortality after lung transplantation [85]. A retrospective analysis found that the probability of developing PGD grade 3 increased by 13% for each additional litre of fluid administered [86]. The goal of blood transfusion should be to optimise tissue oxygen delivery. Mixed venous oxygen saturation <65%, rising lactate levels and acidosis can act as triggers of blood transfusion. It is reasonable to carry out blood transfusion to maintain haemoglobin levels between 8 and 10 g/dl. Blood transfusion has also been observed as an independent predisposing factor for PGD [86, 87], possible mechanisms being fluid overload, increased intrapulmonary hydrostatic pressure and transfusion related acute lung injury. A univariate and multivariate analyses by Weber and colleagues [88] showed increased mortality among recipients given blood transfusions, with greater than 4 units having a hazard ratio of 3.8.

17.26 Extracorporeal Support

Although two-thirds of cases of lung transplant can be performed without ECLS (CPB or ECMO) their use is not uncommon. Planned use of Extracorporeal Support (ECS) during the conduct of lung transplantation involves continuation of ECMO from the preoperative period, when a concomitant cardiac surgery is also planned, presence of severe pre-existing pulmonary artery hypertension and if there is a requirement of intraoperative plasmapheresis. Exigent use of ECS can arise during sudden cardiovascular collapse with induction of anesthesia; inability to maintain oxygenation during one lung ventilation for pneumonectomy; haemodynamic instability along with right ventricular failure following transection of pulmonary artery; poor oxygenation due to graft dysfunction; and development of unstable haemodynamics during conduct of second lung pneumonectomy. Traditionally CPB was the preferred modality of intraoperative ECS but recently ECMO (V-A configuration) has emerged as the first choice at many centres. In comparison to CPB the use of ECMO has shown better patient outcomes as observed in recent studies [89, 90]. ECMO circuits are small requiring lesser priming volumes and low dose heparinisation; moreover there is absence of blood–air interface and cardiotomy suction. All these factors potentially contribute in mitigating the rise of systemic inflammatory response and coagulopathy [89, 90]. Additionally CPB is an independent risk factor for PGD [87], whereas the use of ECMO did not increase the incidence of severe PGD within 72 h postoperatively [91]. In comparison to CPB, ECMO use is associated with fewer re-explorations, lesser blood transfusions and decreased rates of renal complications. Also total duration of ICU and hospital stay was shorter in the ECMO group [89]. Moreover, ECMO allows for gradual incremental reperfusion with insidious weaning from ECS, thereby overcoming reperfusion injury and accompanying haemodynamic instability. ECMO can also be continued in the postoperative period in cases of unsuccessful weaning from ventilatory support due to poor graft function. Conversely an absence of reservoir in the ECMO circuit mandates adequate maintenance of intravascular volume status. Total intravenous mode of anesthesia should be started during ECMO use as there is little pulmonary blood flow.

17.27 Primary Graft Dysfunction

Primary Graft Dysfunction (PGD) encompasses the previously described terms of ischaemia reperfusion injury, early graft dysfunction and reimplantation edema. Pathognomonic feature comprises poor oxygenation, alveolar damage and radiological presence of diffuse pulmonary opacities within 72 h of lung transplantation [92]. The severity of PGD is graded on the basis of PaO_2/FiO_2 ratio akin to acute lung injury. Positive radiographic infiltrates along with PaO_2/FiO_2 ratio >300, 200–300 and <200 are given a grade of 1, 2 and 3, respectively. In the absence of any radiological infiltrates, a grade 0 is assigned [93]. PGD is seen to occur in about 30% of overall cases with incidence of severe PGD grade 3 up to 20%, which contributes significantly towards early mortality. Several risk factors for grade 3 PGD have been identified: donor related (history of smoking), recipient related (obesity with BMI >30, preoperative sarcoidosis, pulmonary artery hypertension) and operative (single lung transplant, high units of blood transfusion, use of CPB, high FiO_2 at reperfusion) [87].

The treatment for PGD is supportive with lung protective ventilation and optimal fluid management. Low tidal volume ventilation with 6 ml/kg and limiting plateau pressure to less than 30 cm of H_2O is likely to prevent volutrauma and barotraumas [94]. Patients developing PGD after single lung transplant will require synchronous differential lung ventilation by a double-lumen tube. Pharmacological treatment should be considered for patients unresponsive to lung protective ventilation. Inhaled [NO] 10–40 ppm causes selective pulmonary vasodilatation with improvement in hypoxia and reduction of mean arterial pressure [95]. Intravenous prostaglandin E1 (alprostadil) and inhaled prostaglandin I2 (epoprostenol) have also been used for treatment of PGD at some centres. ECMO (V-A) may act as a bridge to extubation for patients with severe PGD (PaO_2/FiO_2 <100) who fail maximal therapeutic interventions.

17.28 Pain Control

Inadequate pain relief reduces the patient's ability for spontaneous deep breathing and coughing thereby hampering sputum clearance. Thoracic epidural analgesia (TEA) forms the mainstay of postoperative pain control after lung transplantation. Although institutional practices vary, it is reasonable to site an epidural in ICU prior to extubation and preoperative placement be avoided. Emergent nature of the surgery may not provide sufficient time for thoracic epidural insertion which itself requires expertise and can unexpectedly prove to be time consuming. In addition patients require intraoperative heparinisation for ECS and develop coagulopathy. Epidural insertion also can be an exercise in futility if the surgery is cancelled or the epidural was never activated due to severe haemodynamic instability. In addition to TEA, other opioid or nonopioid analgesia should be used as a part of multimodal analgesia regimen. Recently successful use of paravertebral catheter for adequate pain relief after lung transplant has been demonstrated [96].

17.28.1 Other Anesthetic Concerns

During implantation ice cold saline is circulated in the thoracic cavity along with placement of a cooling jacket to minimise warm ischaemia. Hypothermia can cause worsening of coagulopathy and pulmonary hypertension. Temperature monitoring with active warming of patient with in-line fluid warmer and forced air heating blankets is recommended. Multiple factors like intraoperative blood loss, hilar manipulation, right ventricular dysfunction, cardiac compression and post-reperfusion period unfailingly lead to hypotension. It is not uncommon for the patient to be on inotropic support with multiple drugs. Norepinephrine, phenylephrine and vasopressin are the most frequently used intraoperative inotropes. Vasopressin is particularly attractive as it can maintain systemic blood pressure without concomitant increase in pulmonary vascular resistance [97]. Two grams $MgSO_4$ is routinely infused in a bid to prevent arrhythmias. At the end of surgery DLT if in place is changed to single-lumen tube. Due to the ensuing airway edema during the course of surgery it is advisable to change DLT over an airway exchange catheter under direct or videolaryngoscopic examination. During transport of patient to intensive care unit, the anesthesiologist needs to be vigilant of haemodynamic and ventilator parameters. The perfusionist is also required to accompany if there is ongoing ECMO support. If used intraoperatively for worsening pulmonary hypertension or PGD, inhaled NO should be continued during transportation as a sudden withdrawal can lead to catastrophic rebound hypertension [98].

17.29 Conclusion

Lung transplant is now an accepted modality of treatment for patients suffering from end-stage pulmonary disease. The number of procedures performed every year is steadily increasing with a continually improving 5 year post-transplant survival. Due to inherent complexity of the procedure a successful outcome depends upon a close coordination between the various specialities of medical science. EVLP has the potential to revolutionise the organ availability with the possibility to heal injured donor lungs making them suitable for transplantation.

References

1. Vock DM, Durheim MT, Tsuang WM, et al. Survival benefit of lung transplantation in the modern era of lung allocation. Ann Am Thorac Soc. 2017;14(2):172–81.
2. Singer JP, Katz PP, Soong A, et al. Effect of lung transplantation on health-related quality of life in the era of the lung allocation score: a U.S. prospective cohort study. Am J Transplant. 2017;17(5):1334–45.
3. Kugler C, Gottlieb J, Warnecke G, et al. Health-related quality of life after solid organ transplantation: a prospective, multiorgan cohort study. Transplantation. 2013;96(3):316–23.
4. Chambers DC, Yusen RD, Cherikh WS, et al. The registry of the international society for heart and lung transplantation: thirty-fourth adult lung and heart-lung transplantation report-2017; focus theme: allograft ischemic time. J Heart Lung Transplant. 2017;36(10):1047–59.
5. Aryal S, Nathan SD. Single vs bilateral lung transplantation: when and why. Curr Opin Organ Transplant. 2018;23(3):316–23.
6. Hardy JD, Webb WR, Dalton ML Jr, et al. Lung homotransplantations in man. JAMA. 1963;186:1065–74.
7. Toronto Lung Transplant Group. Unilateral lung transplantation for pulmonary fibrosis. N Engl J Med. 1986;314:1140–5.
8. Weill D, Benden C, Corris PA, et al. A consensus document for the selection of lung transplant candidates: 2014-an update from the Pulmonary Transplantation Council of the International Society for Heart and Lung Transplantation. J Heart Lung Transplant. 2015;34(1):1–15.
9. Egan TM, Murray S, Bustami RT, et al. Development of the new lung allocation system in the United States. Am J Transplant. 2006;6:1212–27.
10. McCurry KR, Shearon TH, Edwards LB, et al. Lung transplantation in the United States, 1998–2007. Am J transplant. 2009;9(Part 2):942–58.

11. Egan TM, Edwards LB. Effect of lung allocation score on lung transplantation in the United States. J Heart Lung Transplant. 2016;35(4):433–9.
12. Rosengard BR, Feng S, Alfrey EJ, et al. Report of the crystal city meeting to maximise the use of organs recovered from the cadaver donor. Am J Transplant. 2002;2:701–11.
13. Rosendale JD, Kauffman HM, Mcbride MA, et al. Aggressive pharmacological donor management results in more transplanted organs. Transplantation. 2003;75:482–7.
14. Abdelnour T, Rieke S. Relationship of hormonal resuscitation therapy and central venous pressure on increasing organs for transplant. J Heart Lung Transplant. 2009;28(5):480–5.
15. Mascia L, Pasero D, Slutsky AS, et al. Effect of a lung protective strategy for organ donors on eligibility and availability of lungs for transplantation: a randomized controlled trial. JAMA. 304(23):2620–7.
16. Soluri-Martins A, Sutherasan Y, Silva PL, et al. How to minimise ventilator-induced lung injury in transplanted lungs: the role of protective ventilation and other strategies. Eur J Anaesthesiol. 2015;32(12):828–36.
17. Kirschbaum CE, Hudson S. Increasing organ yield through a lung management protocol. Prog Transplant. 2010;20(1):28–32.
18. Botha P, Rostron AJ, Fisher AJ, et al. Current strategies in donor selection and management. Semin Thorac Cardiovasc Surg. 2008;20:143–51.
19. Courtwright A, Cantu E. Evaluation and management of the potential lung donor. Clin Chest Med. 2017;38(4):751–9.
20. Reyes KG, Mason DP, Thuita L, et al. Guidelines for donor lung selection: time for revision? Ann Thorac Surg. 2010;89(06):1756–65.
21. Chaney J, Suzuki Y, Cantu E III, et al. Lung donor selection criteria. J Thorac Dis. 2014;6(8):1032–8.
22. Moreno P, Alvarez A, Santos F, et al. Extended recipients but not extended donors are associated with poor outcomes following lung transplantation. Eur J Cardio Thorac Surg. 2014;45:1040–7.
23. Puri V, Patterson GA. Adult lung transplantation: technical considerations. Semin Thorac Cardiovasc Surg. 2008;20(2):152–64.
24. de Perrot M, Fischer S, Liu M, et al. Prostaglandin E1 protects lung transplants from ischemia-reperfusion injury: a shift from pro-to anti-inflammatory cytokines. Transplantation. 2001;72(9):1505–12.
25. Müller C, Fürst H, Reichenspurner H, et al. Lung procurement by low-potassium dextran and the effect on preservation injury. Munich Lung Transplant Group. Transplantation. 1999;68(8):1139–43.
26. DeCampos KN, Keshavjee S, Liu M, et al. Optimal inflation volume for hypothermic preservation of rat lungs. J Heart Lung Transplant. 1998;17(6):599–607.
27. Van Raemdonck D, Neyrinck A, Verleden GM, et al. Lung donor selection and management. Proc Am Thorac Soc. 2009;6(1):28–38.
28. Okazaki M, Date H, Inokawa H, et al. Optimal time for post-mortem heparinization in canine lung transplantation with non-heart-beating donors. J Heart Lung Transplant. 2006;25(4):454–60.
29. Gomez-de-Antonio D, Campo-Cañaveral JL, Crowley S, et al. Clinical lung transplantation from uncontrolled non-heart-beating donors revisited. J Heart Lung Transplant. 2012;31(4):349–53.
30. Rabanal JM, Ibañez AM, Mons R, et al. Influence of preservation solution on early lung function (Euro-Collins vs Perfadex). Transplant Proc 2003. 2003;35(5):1938–9.
31. Munshi L, Keshavjee S, Cypel M. Donor management and lung preservation for lung transplantation. Lancet Respir Med. 2013;1(4):318–28.
32. Yamazaki F, Yokomise H, Keshavjee SH, et al. The superiority of an extracellular fluid solution over Euro-Collins solution for pulmonary preservation. Transplantation. 1990;49(4):690–4.
33. Sasaki S, McCully JD, Alessandrini F, et al. Impact of initial flush potassium concentration on the adequacy of lung preservation. J Thorac Cardiovasc Surg. 1995;109(6):1090–6.
34. Maccherini M, Keshavjee SH, Slutsky AS, et al. The effect of low-potassium-dextran versus Euro-Collins solution for preservation of isolated type II pneumocytes. Transplantation. 1991;52(4):621–6.
35. Fiser SM, Kron IL, Long SM, et al. Influence of graft ischemic time on outcomes following lung transplantation. J Heart Lung Transplant. 2001;20(12):1291–6.
36. Mason DP, Brizzio ME, Alster JM, et al. Lung transplantation for idiopathic pulmonary fibrosis. Ann Thorac Surg. 2007;84(4):1121–8.
37. Meyers BF, Lynch JP, Trulock EP, et al. Single versus bilateral lung transplantation for idiopathic pulmonary fibrosis: a ten-year institutional experience. J Thorac Cardiovasc Surg. 2000;120(1):99–107.
38. Schaffer JM, Singh SK, Reitz BA, et al. Single-vs double-lung transplantation in patients with chronic obstructive pulmonary disease and idiopathic pulmonary fibrosis since the implementation of lung allocation based on medical need. JAMA. 2015;313(9):936–48.
39. Gadre S, Turowski J, Budev M. Overview of lung transplantation, heart-lung transplantation, liver-lung transplantation, and combined hematopoietic stem cell transplantation and lung transplantation. Clin Chest Med. 2017;38(4):623–40.
40. Whited WM, Henley P, Schumer EM, et al. Does donor age and double versus single lung transplant affect survival of young recipients? Ann Thorac Surg. 105(1):235–41.
41. Avlonitis VS, Fisher AJ, Kirby JA, et al. Pulmonary transplantation: the role of brain death in donor lung injury. Transplantation. 2003;75(12):1928–33.
42. Wigfield C. Donation after cardiac death for lung transplantation: a review of current clinical practice. Curr Opin Organ Transplant. 2014;19(5):455–9.
43. Costa J, Shah L, Robbins H, et al. Use of lung allografts from donation after cardiac death donors:

a single-center experience. Ann Thorac Surg. 2018;105(1):271–8.
44. Cypel M, Yeung JC, Keshavjee S. Novel approaches to expanding the lung donor pool: donation after cardiac death and ex vivo conditioning. Clin Chest Med. 2011;32(2):233–44.
45. Reeb J, Keshavjee S, Cypel M. Expanding the lung donor pool: advancements and emerging pathways. Curr Opin Organ Transplant. 2015;20(5):498–505.
46. Mariani AW, Pêgo-Fernandes PM, Abdalla LG, et al. Ex vivo lung reconditioning: a new era for lung transplantation. J Bras Pneumol. 2012;38(6):776–85.
47. Cypel M, Yeung JC, Machuca T, et al. Experience with the first 50 ex vivo lung perfusions in clinical transplantation. J Thorac Cardiovasc Surg. 2012;144(5):1200–6.
48. Wallinder A, Riise GC, Ricksten SE, et al. Transplantation after ex vivo lung perfusion: a midterm follow-up. J Heart Lung Transplant. 2016;35(11):1303–10.
49. Machuca TN, Hsin MK, Ott HC, et al. Injury-specific ex vivo treatment of the donor lung: pulmonary thrombolysis followed by successful lung transplantation. Am J Respir Crit Care Med. 2013;188:878–80.
50. Nakajima D, Cypel M, Bonato R, et al. Ex vivo perfusion treatment of infection in human donor lungs. Am J Transplant. 2016;16:1229–37.
51. Nakajima D, Liu M, Ohsumi A, et al. Lung lavage and surfactant replacement during ex vivo lung perfusion for treatment of gastric acid aspiration-induced donor lung injury. J Heart Lung Transplant. 2017;36:577–85.
52. Date H. Living-related lung transplantation. J Thorac Dis. 2017;9(9):3362–71.
53. Date H, Sato M, Aoyama A, et al. Living-donor lobar lung transplantation provides similar survival to cadaveric lung transplantation even for very ill patients. Eur J Cardiothorac Surg. 2015;47:967–73.
54. Marasco SF, Than S, Keating D, et al. Cadaveric lobar lung transplantation: technical aspects. Ann Thorac Surg. 2012;93(6):1836–42.
55. Slama A, Ghanim B, Klikovits T, et al. Lobar lung transplantation—is it comparable with standard lung transplantation? Transpl Int. 2014;27(9):909–16.
56. Crotti S, Lissoni A. ECMO as a bridge to transplant. In: Sangall F, Patroniti N, Pesenti A, editors. ECMO-extracorporeal life support in adults. Milan: Springer; 2014. p. 293–302.
57. Reeb J, Olland A, Renaud S, et al. Vascular access for extracorporeal life support: tips and tricks. J Thorac Dis. 2016;8(Suppl 4):S353–63.
58. Chiumello D, Coppola S, Froio S, et al. Extracorporeal life support as bridge to lung transplantation: a systematic review. Crit Care. 2015;19:19.
59. Girgis RE, Khaghani A. A global perspective of lung transplantation: part 1-recipient selection and choice of procedure. Glob Cardiol Sci Pract. 2016;5.A.
60. Moser B, Jaksch P, Taghavi S, et al. Lung transplantation for idiopathic pulmonary arterial hypertension on intraoperative and postoperatively prolonged extracorporeal membrane oxygenation provides optimally controlled reperfusion and excellent outcome. Eur J Cardiothorac Surg. 2018;53(1):178–85.
61. Ius F, Sommer W, Tudorache I, et al. Five-year experience with intraoperative extracorporeal membrane oxygenation in lung transplantation: indications and midterm results. J Heart Lung Transplant. 2016;35(1):49–58.
62. Razvi S, Quittell L, Sewall A, et al. Respiratory microbiology of patients with cystic fibrosis in the United States, 1995 to 2005. Chest. 2009;136(6):1554–60.
63. Chaparro C, Maurer J, Gutierrez C, et al. Infection with *Burkholderia cepacia* in cystic fibrosis: outcome following lung transplantation. Am J Respir Crit Care Med. 2001;163(1):43–8.
64. Leung JM, Olivier KN. Nontuberculous mycobacteria in patients with cystic fibrosis. Semin Respir Crit Care Med. 2013;34(1):124–34.
65. Bridges N, Rowe R, Holt RIG. Unique challenges of cystic fibrosis-related diabetes. Diabet Med. 2018;35:1181–8.
66. Gelfond D, Borowitz D. Gastrointestinal complications of cystic fibrosis. Clin Gastroenterol Hepatol. 2013;11(4):333–42.
67. Hayanga AJ, Aboagye JK, Hayanga HE, et al. Contemporary analysis of early outcomes after lung transplantation in the elderly using a national registry. J Heart Lung Transplant. 2015;34(2):182–8.
68. Sherman W, Rabkin DG, Ross D, et al. Lung transplantation and coronary artery disease. Ann Thorac Surg. 2011;92(1):303–8.
69. Furuya Y, Jayarajan SN, Taghavi S, et al. The impact of alemtuzumab and basiliximab induction on patient survival and time to bronchiolitis obliterans syndrome in double lung transplantation recipients. Am J Transplant. 2016;16(8):2334–41.
70. Benveuto LJ, Anderson MR, Arcasoy SM. New frontiers in immunosuppression. J Thorac Dis. 2018;10(5):3141–55.
71. Hayanga JW, D'Cunha J. The surgical technique of bilateral sequential lung transplantation. J Thorac Dis. 2014;6(8):1063–9.
72. Nicoara A, Anderson-Dam J. Anaesthesia for lung transplantation. Anesthesiol Clin. 2017;35(3):473–89.
73. Marseu K, Slinger P, de Perrot M, et al. Dynamic hyperinflation and cardiac arrest during one-lung ventilation: a case report. Can J Anesth. 2011;58(4):396–400.
74. Myles PS. Pulmonary transplantation. In: Kaplan JA, Slinger PD, editors. Thoracic anaesthesia. 3rd ed. Philadelphia: Churchill Livingstone; 2003. p. 295–314.
75. Sheybani S, Attar AS, Golshan S, et al. Effect of propofol and isoflurane on gas exchange parameters following one-lung ventilation in thoracic surgery: a double-blinded randomized controlled clinical trial. Electron Phys. 2018;10(2):6346–53.
76. Módolo NS, Módolo MP, Marton MA, et al. Intravenous versus inhalation anaesthesia for one-lung ventilation. Cochrane Database Syst Rev. 2013;7:CD006313.

77. Schilling T, Kozian A, Senturk M, et al. Effects of volatile and intravenous anaesthesia on the alveolar and systemic inflammatory response in thoracic surgical patients. Anesthesiology. 2011;115(1):65–74.
78. Guth S, Prüfer D, Thorsten Kramm T, et al. Length of pressure-controlled reperfusion is critical for reducing ischaemia-reperfusion injury in an isolated rabbit lung model. J Cardiothorac Surg. 2007;2:54.
79. Barnes L, Reed RM, Parekh RK, et al. Mechanical ventilation for the lung transplant recipient. Curr Pulmonol Rep. 2015;4(2):88–96.
80. Thys DM, Brooker RF, Cahalan MK, et al. Practice guidelines for perioperative transesophageal echocardiography. An updated report by the American Society of Anesthesiologists and the Society of Cardiovascular Anesthesiologists Task Force on transesophageal echocardiography. Anesthesiology. 2010;112:1084–96.
81. Evans A, Dwarakanath S, Hogue C, et al. Intraoperative echocardiography for patients undergoing lung transplantation. Anesth Analg. 2014;118(4):725–30.
82. Gorcsan J 3rd, Reddy SC, Armitage JM, et al. Acquired right ventricular outflow tract obstruction after lung transplantation: diagnosis by transesophageal echocardiography. J Am Soc Echocardiogr. 1993;6(3 Pt 1):324–6.
83. Huppert LA, Matthay MA. Alveolar fluid clearance in pathologically relevant conditions: *in vitro* and *in vivo* models of acute respiratory distress syndrome. Front Immunol. 2017;8:371.
84. Sugita M, Ferraro P, Dagenais A, et al. Alveolar liquid clearance and sodium channel expression are decreased in transplanted canine lungs. Am J Respir Crit Care Med. 2003;167(10):1440–50.
85. Pilcher DV, Scheinkestel CD, Snell GI, et al. High central venous pressure is associated with prolonged mechanical ventilation and increased mortality after lung transplantation. J Thorac Cardiovasc Surg. 2005;129(4):912–8.
86. Geube MA, Perez-Protto SE, McGrath TL, et al. Increased intraoperative fluid administration is associated with severe primary graft dysfunction after lung transplantation. Anesth Analg. 2016;122(4):1081–8.
87. Diamond JM, Lee JC, Kawut SM, et al. Clinical risk factors for primary graft dysfunction after lung transplantation. Am J Respir Crit Care Med. 2013;187(5):527–34.
88. Weber D, Cottini SR, Locher P, et al. Association of intraoperative transfusion of blood products with mortality in lung transplant recipients. Perioper Med (Lond). 2013;2(1):20.
89. Machuca TN, Collaud S, Mercier O, et al. Outcomes of intraoperative extracorporeal membrane oxygenation versus cardiopulmonary bypass for lung transplantation. J Thorac Cardiovasc Surg. 2015;149(4):1152–7.
90. Ius F, Kuehn C, Tudorache I, et al. Lung transplantation on cardiopulmonary support: venoarterial extracorporeal membrane oxygenation outperformed cardiopulmonary bypass. J Thorac Cardiovasc Surg. 2012;144(6):1510–6.
91. Pettenuzzo T, Faggi G, Di Gregorio G, et al. Blood products transfusion and mid-term outcomes of lung transplanted patients under extracorporeal membrane oxygenation support. Prog Transplant. 2018;28(4):314–21.
92. Christie JD, Carby M, Bag R, et al. Report of the ISHLT working group on primary lung graft dysfunction part II: definition. A consensus statement of the International Society for Heart and Lung Transplantation. J Heart Lung Transplant. 2005;24(10):1454–9.
93. Snell GI, Yusen RD, Weill D, et al. Report of the ISHLT working group on primary lung graft dysfunction, part I: Definition and grading-A 2016 consensus group statement of the International Society for Heart and Lung Transplantation. J Heart Lung Transplant. 2017;36(10):1097–103.
94. Fan E, Del Sorbo L, Goligher EC, et al. An official American Thoracic Society/European Society of Intensive Care Medicine/Society of Critical Care Medicine Clinical Practice guideline: mechanical ventilation in adult patients with acute respiratory distress syndrome. Am J Respir Crit Care Med. 2017;195(9):1253–63.
95. Van Raemdonck D, Hartwig MG, Hertz MI, et al. Report of the ISHLT working group on primary lung graft dysfunction part IV: prevention and treatment: a 2016 consensus group statement of the International Society for Heart and Lung Transplantation. J Heart Lung Transplant. 2017;36(10):1121–36.
96. Hutchins J, Apostolidou I, Shumway S, et al. Paravertebral catheter use for postoperative pain control in patients after lung transplant surgery: a prospective observational study. J Cardiothorac Vasc Anesth. 2017;31(1):142–6.
97. Augoustides JG, Savino JS. Vasopressin: the perioperative gift that keeps on giving. Anesthesiology. 2014;121(5):914–5.
98. Atz AM, Adatia I, Wessel DL. Rebound pulmonary hypertension after inhalation of nitric oxide. Ann Thorac Surg. 1996;62(6):1759–64.

Pediatric Thoracic Anesthesia and Challenges

18

Deepanjali Pant and Archna Koul

18.1 Introduction

Safe intraoperative management of thoracic surgical procedures in children is challenging. During the course of thoracic surgery, airway and respiratory complications are the most common causes of morbidity [1]. One-third of all perioperative cardiac arrests in pediatric anesthesia are associated with complications related to respiratory system [2]. Therefore, thorough understanding of respiratory physiology and its clinical implications is necessary in these patients, when planning for a thoracic surgical procedure (Table 18.1).

Thoracic surgery in children is performed for a number of congenital, infectious, traumatic or neoplastic lesions involving [6, 7]:

Table 18.1 Clinical implications of respiratory characteristics in children

Physiological parameters	Clinical implications
Immature respiratory control system	Increased risk of apnea
Higher metabolic rate and oxygen consumption	Lower FRC (27–30 ml/kg), increased oxygen consumption (7–9 ml/kg/min) and increased alveolar ventilation (100–150 ml/kg/min) [3]
Less lung volume in relation to body size, so less surface area for gas exchange	Rapid desaturation with hypoventilation or apnea
Poorly developed lungs with fewer alveoli, lesser accessory interalveolar communications and poorly developed elastin tissue in alveolar septa [4]	Increased risk of alveolar collapse during expiration causing atelectasis
Horizontal rib alignment Absence of type I respiratory muscles	Reduced efficacy of intercostal muscles with increased work of breathing which may lead to early fatigue of respiratory muscles
Extremely compliant thorax	Airway closure during normal tidal ventilation causing atelectasis and V/Q imbalance
Small airway diameter (tracheal diameter 4.3 mm in neonates compared to 14 mm at 15 years of age) [5]	High airway resistance (19–28 cm H_2O/L/s in newborn) vs. less than 2 cm H_2O/L/s in an adult) [6]

D. Pant · A. Koul (✉)
Institute of Anaesthesiology, Pain and Perioperative Medicine, Sir Ganga Ram Hospital, New Delhi, India

- Lungs, conducting airway or pleura
  - Congenital lung cysts like congenital cystic adenomatoid malformation, bronchogenic cysts
  - Congenital lobar emphysema
  - Pulmonary sequestration
  - Lung abscess
  - Bronchiectasis
  - Congenital diaphragmatic hernia
  - Tracheo-esophageal fistula
  - Tumours (primary or secondary)
  - Foreign body
  - Trauma
- Mediastinum
  - Tumours or masses like lymphoma, cystic hygroma, thymoma, neuroblastoma, duplication cysts
- Chest wall
  - Deformities like pectus excavatum or chest wall masses
- Oesophagus
  - Trauma, esophageal atresia
- Spine
  - Scoliosis

18.2 Physiology of One Lung Ventilation (OLV) in Children

In an awake spontaneously breathing pediatric patient, except for infants, the dependent lung segment receives greater ventilation as well as perfusion, so V/Q ratios are well matched. However, after induction of general anesthesia with controlled ventilation, V/Q mismatch is introduced, as ventilation to the dependent lung is reduced. This is due to muscle paralysis, IPPV and compression of the dependent lung by the mediastinum and abdominal contents [8]. During thoracic surgery, lateral decubitus position may further increase compression of the dependent lung. The V/Q mismatch may be further increased by institution of OLV causing collapse of the operative lung and inhibition of hypoxic pulmonary vasoconstriction (HPV) by inhalational agents.

In the lateral decubitus position, there is more V/Q mismatching in children as compared to adults because the easily compressible rib cage in the pediatric age group is less efficient in supporting the dependent ventilated lung, resulting in atelectasis. The functional advantage of the doming effect of the diaphragm on the dependent lung is also lost in infants due to the much reduced transabdominal hydrostatic pressure gradient because of their small size. The lesser difference in the hydrostatic pressure gradient between the dependent and non-dependent lung also leads to a smaller increase in perfusion of the dependent ventilated lung [9].

So infants have a higher risk of desaturation during surgery in the lateral decubitus position with the healthy lung being dependent, as compared to adults who maintain better V/Q [10].

18.3 Challenges in Preoperative Evaluation

Age appropriate evaluation of the pediatric patient for thoracic surgical procedures is mandatory.

Investigations like spirometry, lung function tests and cardiopulmonary exercise testing cannot be conducted in neonates, infants and small uncooperative children.

As this may be the first anesthesia exposure of the patient, ruling out the presence of other associated congenital anomalies and any history of malignant hyperthermia in the family is important.

Although older children present with dyspnea, cyanosis, wheezing and cough, infants present with less specific signs such as poor feeding, irritability or change in sleep habits. Thus it is challenging to detect pulmonary dysfunction, as children become symptomatic only in the later stages of the disease. The presence of dyspnea or diminished exercise tolerance is ominous [11].

It is very difficult to evaluate functional capacity in children of varying ages. Difficulty in feeding, sweating or cyanosis during feeds in neonates and inability to run, play or keep pace with the peers is an indicators of decreased functional capacity.

Physical examination of the airway can also be complex as markers of difficult airway in adults cannot be applied to children. So, assessment of the airway should focus on any evidence of retrognathia, micrognathia or high arched palate [12].

In children markers of respiratory distress are tachypnea, nasal flaring, use of accessory muscles, grunting, and the presence of peripheral cyanosis. Identification of these markers is very important.

18.4 One Lung Ventilation in Pediatric Patients

A number of surgical procedures in children can be done by retraction of the operative lung. If surgical exposure is inadequate or there is fear of contamination of healthy lung then lung isolation should be considered. OLV is also beneficial for control of distribution of ventilation in a large bronchopleural fistula (BPF), bronchial injuries and during thoracoscopic procedures.

According to Slinger, the ABCD's of the pediatric lung isolation should be kept in mind when anesthetizing children for thoracic surgery [12]. These are:

A. Anatomy: The small size of the pediatric airway precludes the use of DLT in infants and small children, and so measures to be taken for lung isolation according to the airway anatomy should be planned well in advance.
B. Bronchoscopy: The anesthesiologist should be ready with the appropriate size fiberoptic bronchoscope (FOB) which can negotiate the tracheobronchial tree and still ventilate the trachea. For insertion, the outer diameter of the bronchoscope needs to be less than 90% of the inner diameter of the tracheal tube. However, to allow ventilation during bronchoscopy, cross-sectional area of the bronchoscope should not be more than 50% of the cross-sectional area of tracheal tube.
C. Chest imaging: Chest imaging such as X-ray or computed tomography (CT) can help predicting the appropriate size of the tracheal tube. Airway ultrasound can also help in selecting the right size of the tracheal tube [13].
D. Diameter of airway: Since the transverse diameter of the trachea is more than the anteroposterior diameter and the shape of trachea is elliptical, the size of the endotracheal tube should be in accordance with the anteroposterior diameter [14].

Options for Lung Isolation

A. *Single lumen endotracheal tube*: It is the simplest method of lung isolation and most commonly used in neonates and infants. In this technique the endotracheal tube is advanced into the main stem bronchus on the non-operative side until the breath sounds on the operable side disappear [15]. Right main stem endobronchial intubation is easier, while the left main stem bronchus is difficult to intubate as the left main stem bronchus is more horizontal than the right main stem bronchus; it takes off at angle of 40–50° with respect to the trachea. It is longer but smaller in diameter than the right. The right bronchus is wider, shorter and more vertical. For intubating the left main stem bronchus, the bevel of the ETT should be rotated 90–180° to the left and the patient's head turned to the right; and the concavity of ETT should be on the left instead of right [16]. A flexible FOB may be passed through or along the side of the endotracheal tube to either confirm or guide the placement of the cuffed ETT. The distance from the tip of the tube to the distal cuff must be less than the length of the bronchus so that the ETT does not occlude the right upper lobe bronchus. This method of lung isolation is simple and quick, requires no additional equipment and can be life-saving in an emergency situation, like airway haemorrhage. However, there is a risk of contamination of the normal lung or inadequate collapse of the diseased lung if an undersized tube is used. There is also a risk of hypoxemia, in case of obstruction of the right upper lobe bronchus. Another disadvantage of a single lumen ETT is that it is not possible to suction or provide CPAP to the operative lung, and it is inconvenient to withdraw the tube at the end of the surgical procedure for two lung ventilation.

Tobias [17] suggested using a tracheal tube one half to one size smaller than otherwise indicated, because of the smaller diameter of the main stem bronchus as compared to the trachea.

When OLV with right main stem bronchial intubation is needed, Oh et al. suggested leaving the cuff of the ETT mainly in the trachea using the usual size ETT on the basis of patient age [18]. David Cohen [19] suggested using a Magill (non -Murphy eye) tube for endobronchial intubation to prevent gas leaking into the operative lung especially in the presence of a short main stem bronchus. They have also reported the use of fluoroscopy to assess the adequacy of endobronchial intubation.

B. *Bronchial Blockers (BB)*: All these devices have a balloon at the end which, when inflated, occludes the main stem bronchus to allow lung collapse distal to the occlusion [20]. These are useful in patients between 3 months and 9 years of age and can be placed either through the endotracheal tube (coaxial method) or along the endotracheal tube (parallel method).

Bronchial blockers used in paediatric patients include:

- Vascular balloon catheters like the Fogarty arterial embolectomy catheter (FAEC)
- Arndt endobronchial blocker
- Uniblockers

Fogarty Arterial Embolectomy Catheter (FAEC): Although a vascular tool, its use has been described in many types of thoracic procedures (Fig. 18.1) [21]. It consists of a hollow tube with an inflatable balloon attached to its tip. Except for 2F and 3F catheters, all other catheter sizes have removable a guide wire that allows angulation of the tip towards the desired bronchus with the help of its stylet (Table 18.2). Open tip catheters are preferred over closed tip, to facilitate suction and oxygen insufflation. In patients between 6 months and 2 years of age the catheter is placed outside the endotracheal tube. Following laryngoscopy, the catheter is advanced through the vocal cords and then rotated 90° towards the desired side into the main stem bronchus. Subsequently, normal endotracheal intubation is done. Position of bronchial blockers is confirmed by FOB before inflating the balloon tip [15].

In patients between 2 and 8 years of age, the catheter is placed within the endotracheal tube. Endobronchial intubation into the desired bronchus is done, 15 mm adaptor is removed followed by insertion of the FAEC through the tube into the bronchus. The endotracheal tube is then withdrawn into the carina, FOB is done, followed by inflation of the balloon.

Advantages

An FAEC provides good operating conditions as it causes predictable lung collapse on inflation and allows rapid re-expansion of the operative

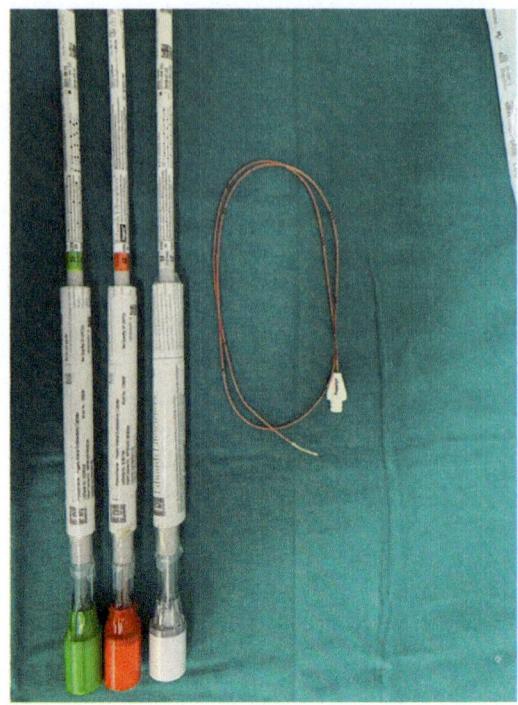

Fig. 18.1 Balloon-tipped embolectomy catheter

Table 18.2 Balloon wedge catheters

Size (F)	Length (cm)	Maximum inflating volume (mL)	Inflated balloon diameter (mm)	Guidewire size (inches)
5	60	0.75	8	0.025
6	60	1.0	10	0.035
7	110	1.25	11	0.038
8	110	1.25	11	0.038

lung on deflation. These catheters can be used in very small infants as well. They can also be used in critically ill intubated patients requiring OLV, tracheostomised patients and in patients with difficult airways [22].

Disadvantages

- If placed within the ETT, they can interfere with ventilation because of the decrease in the internal diameter of the tube.
- The balloon exerts low volume, high pressure on the bronchial mucosa which can cause airway trauma.
- Migration or displacement of the catheter can cause obstruction of both lungs, if the balloon turns back into the trachea.
- Bronchial blockers require longer time for correct placement.
- Bronchial blockers have the potential for inclusion in the stapling line.
- Cannot be used in children with latex allergy [23].

Arndt Endobronchial Blocker: this the wire-guided endobronchial blocker, is a balloon tipped catheter with a 2 ml cuff present at the distal end which has low pressure, high volume characteristics. It has a central lumen through which a wire with a looped end has been passed from proximal to distal end. Arndt pediatric blocker is available in 5F and 7F size for tracheal tubes 4.5–5.5 mm and 6.0–7.0 mm internal diameter, respectively. It is provided with a multiport adaptor which has three ports (Fig. 18.2) [24, 25]:

- For attachment of breathing circuit via standard 15 mm adaptor allowing uninterrupted ventilation during insertion of the blocker
- Port for the bronchial blocker, provided with a Tuohy Borst connector that locks the catheter in place and provides an airtight seal
- FOB port that has a plastic sealing cap

It can be either passed through the ETT (coaxial technique) or outside the ETT (parallel technique).

For coaxial technique, it is important to remember that the outer diameter of the bronchial blocker plus the outer diameter of the FOB together should be less than 90% of the inner diameter of the ETT. The smallest bronchial blocker (5F) has outer diameter of 2.2 mm and the smallest SLT that can be used is 4.5 mm, which is feasible in patients as young as 2 years.

In patients less than 2 years of age the blocker should be placed outside the ETT in parallel with the FOB inside the lumen [5].

The coaxial technique: Standard ETT intubation is done and the tip of the SLT is kept above the carina. A multiport adaptor is attached to the ETT and the breathing circuit connected for ventilation. The bronchial blocker is passed through the appropriate port of the adaptor and placed at the entrance of the ETT until the guide loop is within the body of the adaptor; the bronchoscope is now passed through its port and then through the wire loop of the blocker. The coupled FOB and the BB are advanced to the appropriate side. Wald et al.

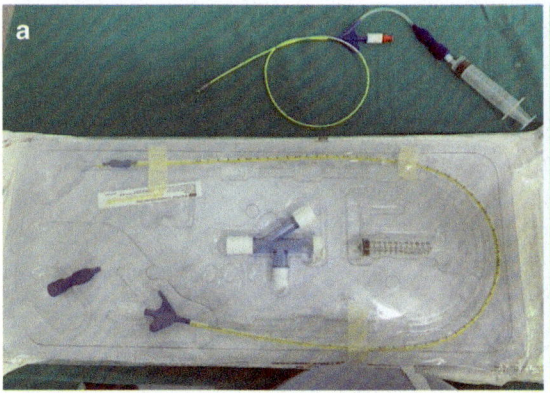 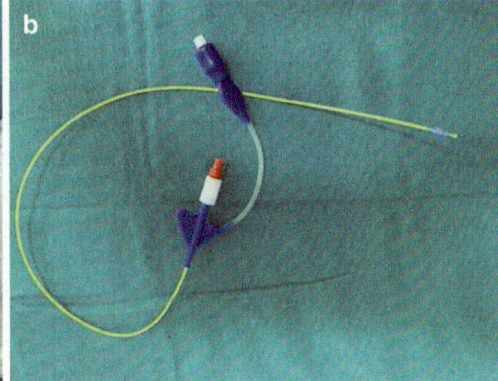

Fig. 18.2 (a) Arndt bronchial blocker; (b) Inflated tip

[25] performed the coupling of the bronchoscope to the loop of the BB outside the multiport adaptor before connecting to the ETT.

After insertion into the bronchus and confirmation, the cuff is inflated under FOB visualization with 1–2 ml air till total bronchial blockade is achieved. The blocker is decoupled from the bronchoscope. The wire loop is left protruding beyond the tip of the BB to allow recoupling and repositioning if required. Once the nylon guide is removed, it cannot be repositioned if the blocker gets misplaced.

The wire loop is then removed to enable lung deflation, to give CPAP or for suctioning.

The Parallel technique is the same as that for the Fogarty embolectomy catheter.

Disadvantages: The blockers are prone to displacement [26]. The Arndt blocker is more liable to get displaced as compared to a double lumen tube (DLT). In the lateral decubitus position the outer surface of the bronchial balloon should be at least 5 mm below the tracheal carina.

Wald et al. [25] reported the use of Arndt 5F endobronchial blocker in a series of 24 patients for thoracotomy or thoracoscopy. He remarked that since the fiberoptic port is larger than the bronchoscope, there is significant air leak during positive pressure ventilation and suggested slight tightening of the blocker's port during fiberoptic advancement.

Blockade of the right upper lobe bronchus may be difficult with the BB because of the early take off of the RUL bronchus. Arndt BB has the advantage that it can be used in very small children, can be placed easily if a single lumen tube is already in place, is simpler to use in patients with difficult airways and also there is no need to change the ETT for postoperative ventilation as in case of a DLT [27].

The Uniblocker Tube (5F Fuji Uniblocker tube) is suitable for children up to 8 years of age. It has a stiff shaft with an angled tip, no central lumen and comes with a swivel connector. It cannot provide CPAP and no suctioning can be done.

C. *The Univent Tube* is suitable and a preferred method of SLV in children between 6 and 8 years of age. Introduced by Inoue in 1982 [28], it is a silastic single lumen endotracheal tube containing an additional channel within the wall of the tube which has a cuffed bronchial blocker that can be advanced into the desired bronchus (Fig. 18.3). Univent tubes are available in sizes 3.5 and 4.5 mm internal diameter having 7.5–8.0 mm and 8.5–9 mm outer diameter, respectively, which can be used in children more than 6 years of age (Table 18.3). The blocker balloon has low volume, high pressure characteristics which can cause mucosal injury following inflation. There is disparity between the internal

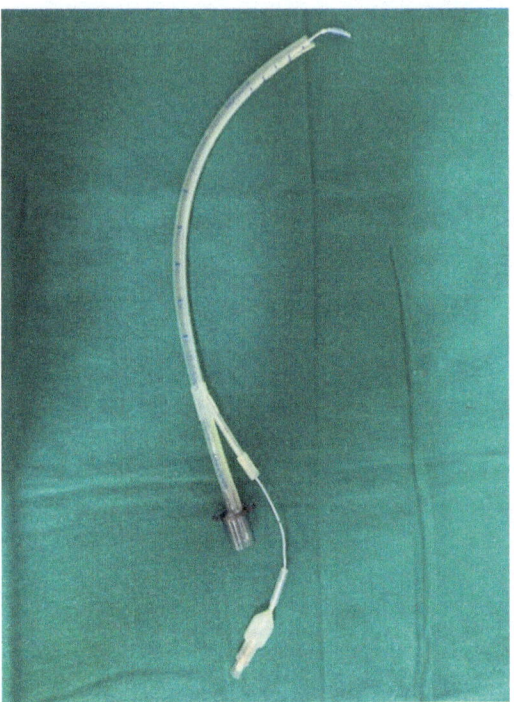

Fig. 18.3 Univent tube

Table 18.3 Univent tube

Size-ID in mm	OD (sagittal/transverse) in mm
3.5	7.5/8.0
4.5	8.5/9.0
6	10.0/11.0
6.5	10.5/11.5
7.0	11.0/12.0
7.5	11.5/12.5
8.0	12.0/13.0
8.5	12.5/13.5
9.0	13.0/14.0

diameter of endotracheal tube and the total outer diameter of the entire Univent tube causing high resistance to gas flow. In Univent tubes smaller than 6.5 mm ID, the blocker does not have a lumen to allow deflation of the lung, oxygen insufflation or CPAP.

Before insertion, the blocker tip is retracted into the blocker chamber. Laryngoscopy is done, the tube is inserted keeping the tracheal cuff just distal to cords then rotating it 90° so that the blocker lumen faces the desired side and therefore it becomes easy to manipulate the blocker in the appropriate direction. A fiberoptic bronchoscope should be used to position the bronchial blocker. The second method is FOB assisted, where the shaft of the blocker is pushed into position under direct vision.

There is, however, a high incidence of intraoperative malposition [29].

Compared to other bronchial blockers, the chances of blocker displacement are less as it is attached to the main tube; however, it leads to increased airway resistance, more so in small children and the bronchial balloon with low volume high pressure is more liable to cause mucosal ischaemia in the larynx.

D. *Double Lumen Tube*: It is the most preferred method used for lung isolation in children between 8 and 18 years of age. The basic design of the tube and the method of insertion and confirmation is same as in adults (Fig. 18.4).

The smallest size of the DLT that is available is 26F which has an outer diameter of 9.3 mm equivalent to 6.5 mm ID ETT [24], and may be used in children as young as 8 years (Table 18.4).

One study suggested that 26F DLT may be considered in children as young as 8 years, of 30 kg and 130 cm height. At least two of these three parameters should be fulfilled, before deciding on the insertion of a 26F DLT [30].

DLT sizes 28F and 32F can be considered for children 10 years and older. Left sided DLTs are preferred in children because they are easier to place and there is no possibility of obstruction of the right upper lobe bronchus.

A DLT allows rapid and efficient separation of the lungs, permits suctioning of both the lungs, allows application of CPAP to the operative lung, and PEEP to the non-operative lung.

In patients with difficult airways, it is challenging to insert a DLT, since it has to be changed if postoperative ventilation is required; besides, a right sided DLT can cause obstruction to the right upper lobe bronchus, especially in a younger patient.

Precautions to be taken during DLT insertion are:

- Gentle insertion, avoid advancing the tube against resistance.
- Fiberoptic confirmation of both the tracheal and bronchial side.

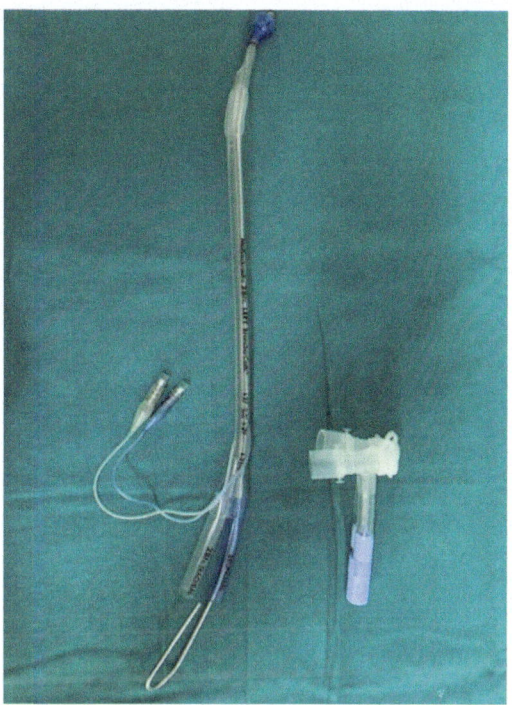

Fig. 18.4 Double lumen tube

Table 18.4 Double lumen tube

Size (F)	Main body OD (mm)	Bronchial lumen OD (mm)
26	9.3	5.1
28	10.2	6.9
32	11.2	8.1
35	13.5	9.7
37	14.0	

Table 18.5 Sizing of tubes used for single lung ventilation

Age (year)	Endotracheal tube; (internal diameter)	Bronchial blocker (French size)	Univent	DLT (French size)
0.5–1	3.5–4.0	5		
1–2	4.0–4.5	5		
2–4	4.5–5.0	5		
4–6	5.0–5.5	5		
6–8	5.5–6.0	6	3.5	
8–10	6.0 cuffed	6	3.5	26
10–12	6.5 cuffed	6	4.5	26–28
12–14	6.5–7.0 cuffed	6	4.5	32
14–16	7.0 cuffed	7	6.0	35
16–18	7.0–8.0 cuffed	7	7.0	35

DLT double lumen tube

- Avoid cuff inflation at the time of turning the patient.
- Avoiding overinflation of the tracheal and bronchial cuffs, the minimal volume necessary for cuff inflation is recommended.

The sizing of tubes used for single lung ventilation in Table 18.5.

18.5 Management of Hypoxia During OLV

1. Ventilate with 100% oxygen to increase the FiO$_2$ as this prevents hypoxia induced vasoconstriction and thus promotes perfusion of the dependent ventilated lung.
2. Rule out displacement of the airway device that may have occurred during positioning of the patient. In case of an increase in airway pressure, rule out blockage of the tube due to secretions.
3. Very high inspired concentrations of inhalational agents can cause inhibition of HPV and fall in cardiac output, so avoid high inspired concentration of inhalational agents.
4. Use of a lung protective ventilation strategy used in adult patients can be reasonably used in pediatric patients, which involves using low tidal volume, PEEP and permissive hypercapnia. Use of high frequency jet ventilation to the operative lung can also improve oxygenation. CPAP to the non-dependent lung and PEEP to the dependent ventilated lung also prevents atelectrauma.
5. Reinflation of the non-ventilated lung, if hypoxemia does not respond to the above measures.

18.6 Pain Management

Providing optimal analgesia in children undergoing thoracic surgery is the most challenging responsibility of the anesthesiologist. Small infants are more prone to pulmonary dysfunction due to thoracotomy, since the associated pain leads to complications like atelectasis and pneumonia. Good intraoperative and postoperative analgesia facilitates early deep breathing, coughing, early mobilization, extubation and early discharge. Inadequate pain management also leads to an augmented stress response that can alter neuronal plasticity and manifest as altered behavioral responses in later life. The various modalities that can be used are:

1. *Intravenous opioids*: Morphine 0.1 mg/kg intraoperatively and 0.01 mg/kg/h for the first 24 h followed by dose reduction and titration according to pain scores; or fentanyl 0.5–2 μg/kg intravenous bolus dose and 0.5 μg/kg/h infusion. However, with intravenous opioid use, there is an increased need of postoperative ventilation and intensive care due to opioid induced apneic spells and respiratory depression. There may be delayed feeding in the babies, nausea and vomiting because of the inhibitory effect of opioids on intestinal motility [31].

2. *Epidural analgesia*: In recent guidelines, regional anesthesia is accepted as the cornerstone of postoperative pain relief in children [32, 33].

Hindrances for regional analgesia in neonates and small infants are:

- Lack of availability of technical equipment
- Fear of complications
- Insufficient experience of pediatric regional analgesia practice by providers [34]

Considerations to be kept in mind when giving an epidural block in children are:

- The epidural catheter is placed after induction of general anesthesia. There is evidence that epidural catheterization under GA in pediatric patients is safe [31].
- Ideally the tip of the catheter should to be close to the dermatome associated with the surgical procedure. However, thoracic epidural puncture in very small children should be limited to cases involving extensive thoraco-abdominal surgery and should be performed by an experienced anesthesiologist [35–37].
- As the incidence of serious complications is low (<1:10,000) in young children, a catheter can be placed in the caudal space and advanced to the appropriate level [38], but there is an increased incidence of infection and malpositioning. The thoracic epidural catheter can be placed between T4 and T8 levels.
- Concentration of the local anesthetics should be less than 0.25% to avoid motor block. Local anesthetics have a greater volume of distribution, low clearance and a higher free fraction. Remember that the large volume of distribution limits peak plasma levels after a single dose, but the risk of accumulation is increased after continuous infusion [39].
- T-wave amplitude and changes in ST segment are the first indicators of systemic toxicity.
- The recommended maximum dose should be calculated in each child.
- Among local anesthetics, ropivacaine is relatively safe even in young children with a maximum dose of 0.2 mg/kg/h for continuous infusion.
- Technical difficulties to be kept in mind are very less distance between skin and epidural space, narrow epidural space, softer ligamentum flavum and large space occupied by the cord in thoracic region.

18.7 Other Modalities of Pain Relief

Those which can be used for supplementation of pain relief along with IV analgesics are intercostal blocks [40], intrapleural local anesthetic infusion [41], paravertebral block [42], IV or rectal paracetamol or diclofenac and local anesthetic infiltration.

Regional analgesia techniques have gained more favour in recent years. Di Pede et al. [31] reported that locoregional anesthesia is associated with better postoperative pain relief and earlier full feeding than systemic analgesia, in infants undergoing thoracotomy.

Intraoperative Fluids Basic principles:

1. The ultimate goal of perioperative fluid therapy is to maintain cardiovascular stability and ensure correct fluid and electrolyte balance [43].
2. Aim for replacement of fluid deficits, administration of maintenance fluids and replacement of losses.
3. Fasting fluid deficits should be minimized by allowing clear liquid orally till 2 h before surgery or give IV fluids to ensure good hydration.
4. All hypotonic fluids should be replaced by isotonic solutions, as hypotonic fluids can lead to potentially devastating neurological complications.
5. 1–2% dextrose in lactated Ringer is appropriate if glucose levels need to be built up in neonates and infants, otherwise glucose free isotonic solution is given.
6. Previously third space losses were replaced with crystalloids at a rate between 1 and 50 ml/kg/h depending on the type of surgical procedure. However, the concept of third space has been questioned and a more restrictive fluid protocol is associated with a better outcome.

7. In case of circulating instability or blood loss, volume replacement and blood transfusion are indicated after assessing maximum allowable blood loss. In neonates and infants blood transfusion is indicated if blood loss is more than 10% of SEQUELAE estimated blood volume.
8. Neonates and infants with congenital heart disease or respiratory distress syndrome should be transfused blood at a hemoglobin less than 12.0 g/dL, while neonates having hemoglobin less than 8 g/dL with symptoms of anemia require blood transfusion [44]. However, there is no single transfusion trigger given in any guideline; threshold for transfusion of red blood cells also depends on a patient's clinical status along with the blood loss.

In thoracic surgery, individualized goal directed fluid therapy is recommendation [45]. Stroke volume variation (SVV) guided fluid therapy in thoracic surgery does not result in pulmonary overload as previously thought [46].

There are some who propagate zero balance regimens which require concomitant administration of vasopressors and a limited amount of fluid to counteract vasodilatory effects of anesthetic agents.

Precaution should be taken so that no air bubbles enter the IV drip sets and infusion syringes so as to prevent occurrence of paradoxical air embolism through patent cardiac shunts.

Always administer warm fluids and calculate the volume accurately using either a burette set or a syringe pump [47].

Concern about the potential risk of postoperative lung injury mandates caution with liberal fluid administration [48], but younger patients require more volume replacements due to large ECF volumes and use of restrictive fluid therapy raises concern regarding hypovolemia, hypoperfusion and risk of acute kidney injury, so target euvolemia. "Do not drown the down lung" is a common dictum.

18.8 Challenges of Thoracoscopic Surgery in Pediatric Patients

Thoracoscopic procedures in children were initially done for evaluation of thoracic lesions or for biopsy purposes [49].

However, with advances in surgical technology and availability of high resolution cameras, shorter instruments and new energy sources, it has become an important tool for pediatric surgery. One of the most frequently performed thoracoscopic procedures in children is decortication for empyema. Inadequate working space and control of vascular structures is a challenge for the surgeons performing thoracoscopy in children.

The anesthesiologist also faces challenges. Institution of lung isolation to provide adequate exposure to facilitate visualization and prevent contamination of healthy lung can be challenging. Creation of capnothorax can cause increase in intrathoracic pressure. Although capnothorax facilitates lung collapse on the operative side, it can lead to decreased venous return and high ventricular afterload. Rapid insufflation of carbon dioxide (CO_2) can cause sudden mediastinal shift and CVS collapse.

- Slow insufflation should be done with flow rate 1 l/min and limitation of inflation pressure to 4–6 mmHg should be ensured [50].
- Younger children absorb proportionately more CO_2 than older children, leading to hypercarbia and acidosis [51].
- Management of hypoxemia, hypercapnia and aletectasis is mandatory.
- Children are prone to hypothermia during thoracoscopy with creation of capnothorax due to cold CO_2 gas insufflation, so temperature monitoring is important and corrective measures should be taken.
- Detection and treatment of arrhythmias is important.
- Aspiration prior to injection and slow creation of artificial pneumothorax will limit inadvertent CO_2 embolism.

18.9 Conclusion

It is vital for the pediatric thoracic anesthesiologist to have a thorough knowledge of the patient's anatomy and physiology in relation to age; there should be preplanning of airway management and one lung ventilation. Intraoperative vigilant monitoring of the patient's respiratory and cardiovascular parameters and effective perioperative analgesia regimen are important for the successful outcome of thoracic procedures in children.

References

1. Adewale L. Anatomy and assessment of the pediatric airway. Paediatr Anaesth. 2009;19(Suppl 1):1–8.
2. Bhananker SM, Ramamoorthy C, Geiduschek JM, et al. Anesthesia-related cardiac arrest in children: update from the pediatric perioperative cardiac arrest registry. Anesth Analg. 2007;105(2):344–50.
3. Miller RD, editor. Miller's anesthesia. Philadelphia: Churchill Livingstone; 2009. p. 3,084 (volumes 1 and 2 combined).
4. Neumann RP, von Ungern-Sternberg BS. The neonatal lung-physiology and ventilation. Paediatr Anaesth. 2014;24(1):10–21.
5. Letal M, Theam M. Paediatric lung isolation. BJA Educ. 2017;17:57–62.
6. Davis P, Cladis F, editors. Smith's anesthesia for infants and children. 9th ed: Elsevier; 2016. p. 1424.
7. Parikh DH, Crabbe D, Auldist A, et al. Pediatric thoracic surgery. London: Springer Science & Business Media; 2009.
8. Heaf DP, Helms P, Gordon I, et al. Postural effects on gas exchange in infants. N Engl J Med. 1983;308(25):1505–8.
9. Choudhary DK. Single-lung ventilation in paediatric anaesthesia. Anesthesiol Clin N Am. 2005;23:693–708.
10. Hammer GB. Single-lung ventilation in infants and children. Paediatr Anaesth. 2004;14(1):98–102.
11. Golianu B, Hammer GB. Pediatric thoracic anesthesia. Curr Opin Anaesthesiol. 2005;18(1):5–11.
12. Campos J. Lung isolation. In: Slinger P, editor. Principles and practice of anesthesia for thoracic surgery. New York: Springer; 2011.
13. Shibasaki M, Nakajima Y, Ishii S, et al. Prediction of pediatric endotracheal tube size by ultrasonography. Anesthesiology. 2010;113(4):819–24.
14. Griscom NT, Wohl ME. Dimensions of the growing trachea related to age and gender. AJR Am J Roentgenol. 1986;146(2):233–7.
15. Kubota H, Kubota Y, Toyoda Y, et al. Selective blind endobronchial intubation in children and adults. Anesthesiology. 1987;67(4):587–9.
16. Ho AMH, Flavin MP, Fleming ML, et al. Selective left mainstem bronchial intubation in the neonatal intensive care unit. Rev Bras Anestesiol. 2018;68(3):318–21.
17. Tobias JD. Thoracic surgery in children. Curr Opin Anaesthesiol. 2001;14:77–85.
18. Oh AY, Kwon WK, Kim KO, et al. Single-lung ventilation with a cuffed endotracheal tube in a child with a left mainstem bronchus disruption. Anesth Analg. 2003;96(3):696–7.
19. Cohen DE, McCloskey JJ, Motas D, et al. Fluoroscopic-assisted endobronchial intubation for single-lung ventilation in infants. Paediatr Anaesth. 2011;21(6):681–4.
20. Campos JH. Lung isolation tech. Anaesthesiol Clin North Am. 2001;19:455–74.
21. Chengod S, Chandrasekharan AP, Manoj P. Selective left bronchial intubation and left-lung isolation in infants and toddlers: analysis of a new technique. J Cardiothorac Vasc Anesth. 2005;19(5):636–41.
22. Borchardt RA, LaQuaglia MP, McDowall RH, et al. Bronchial injury during lung isolation in a pediatric patient. Anesth Analg. 1998;87(2):324–5.
23. Campos JH. An update on bronchial blockers during lung separation techniques in adults. Anesth Analg. 2003;97(5):1266–74. (Review. Erratum in: Anesth Analg. 2004 Jan;98(1):131)
24. Hammer GB, Fitzmaurice BG, Brodsky JB. Methods for single-lung ventilation in pediatric patients. Anesth Analg. 1999;89(6):1426–9.
25. Wald SH, Mahajan A, Kaplan MB, et al. Experience with the Arndt paediatric bronchial blocker. Br J Anaesth. 2005 Jan;94(1):92–4.
26. Campos JH, Kernstine KH. A comparison of a left-sided Broncho-Cath with the torque control blocker univent and the wire-guided blocker. Anesth Analg. 2003;96(1):283–9.
27. Campos JH. Which device should be considered the best for lung isolation: double-lumen endotracheal tube versus bronchial blockers. Curr Opin Anaesthesiol. 2007;20(1):27–31.
28. Inoue H, Shohtsu A, Ogawa J, et al. Endotracheal tube with movable blocker to prevent aspiration of intratracheal bleeding. Ann Thorac Surg. 1984;37(6):497–9.
29. Hammer GB, Brodsky JB, Redpath JH, et al. The Univent tube for single-lung ventilation in paediatric patients. Paediatr Anaesth. 1998;8(1):55–7.
30. Seefelder C. Use of the 26-French double-lumen tube for lung isolation in children. J Cardiothorac Vasc Anesth. 2014;28:e19–28.
31. Di Pede A, Morini F, Lombardi MH, et al. Comparison of regional vs. systemic analgesia for post-thoracotomy care in infants. Paediatr Anaesth. 2014;24(6):569–73.
32. Association of Paediatric Anaesthetists of Great Britain and Ireland. Good practice in postoperative and procedural pain management. 2nd ed. Paediatr Anaesth. 2012;22(Suppl 1):1–79.
33. Jöhr M. Regional anaesthesia in neonates, infants and children: an educational review. Eur J Anaesthesiol. 2015;32(5):289–97.
34. Bösenberg AT, Jöhr M, Wolf AR. Pro con debate: the use of regional vs systemic analgesia for neonatal surgery. Paediatr Anaesth. 2011;21(12):1247–58.
35. Allison CE, Aronson DC, Geukers VG, et al. Paraplegia after thoracotomy under combined

36. Kasai T, Yaegashi K, Hirose M, et al. Spinal cord injury in a child caused by an accidental dural puncture with a single-shot thoracic epidural needle. Anesth Analg. 2003;96(1):65–7.
37. Patel D. Epidural analgesia for children. Contin Educ Anaesth Crit Care Pain. 2006;6(2):63–6.
38. Bösenberg AT, Bland BA, Schulte-Steinberg O, et al. Thoracic epidural anesthesia via caudal route in infants. Anesthesiology. 1988;69(2):265–9.
39. Bösenberg AT, Thomas J, Cronje L, et al. Pharmacokinetics and efficacy of ropivacaine for continuous epidural infusion in neonates and infants. Paediatr Anaesth. 2005;15(9):739–49.
40. Cooper MG, Seaton HL. Intra-operative placement of intercostal catheter for post-thoracotomy pain relief in a child. Paediatr Anaesth. 1992;2:739–49.
41. Giaufré E, Bruguerolle B, Rastello C, et al. New regimen for interpleural block in children. Paediatr Anaesth. 1995;5(2):125–8.
42. Qi J, Du B, Gurnaney H, et al. A prospective randomized observer-blinded study to assess postoperative analgesia provided by an ultrasound-guided bilateral thoracic paravertebral block for children undergoing the Nuss procedure. Reg Anesth Pain Med. 2014;39(3):208–13.
43. Murat I, Dubois MC. Perioperative fluid therapy in pediatrics. Paediatr Anaesth. 2008;18(5):363–70.
44. Ali N. Red blood cell transfusion in infants and children – current perspectives. Pediatr Neonatol. 2018;59(3):227–30.
45. Chong MA, Wang Y, Berbenetz NM, et al. Does goal-directed haemodynamic and fluid therapy improve peri-operative outcomes?: a systematic review and meta-analysis. Eur J Anaesthesiol. 2018;35(7):469–83.
46. Haas S, Eichhorn V, Hasbach T, et al. Goal-directed fluid therapy using stroke volume variation does not result in pulmonary fluid overload in thoracic surgery requiring one-lung ventilation. Crit Care Res Pract. 2012;687018:8.
47. Assaad S, Popescu W, Perrino A. Fluid management in thoracic surgery. Curr Opin Anaesthesiol. 2013;26(1):31–9.
48. Feltracco P, Serra E, Barbieri S, et al. Postoperative care of patients undergoing lung resection. J Anesth Clin Res. 2012;4:288. https://doi.org/10.4172/2155-6148.1000288.
49. Engum SA. Minimal access thoracic surgery in the pediatric population. Semin Pediatr Surg. 2007;16(1):14–26.
50. Dave N, Fernandes S. Anaesthetic implications of paediatric thoracoscopy. J Minim Access Surg. 2005;1(1):8–14.
51. McHoney M, Corizia L, Eaton S, et al. Carbon dioxide elimination during laparoscopy in children is age dependent. J Pediatr Surg. 2003;38(1):105–10.

Anesthesia for Oesophageal Surgeries

19

Ajay Sirohi and Jayashree Sood

With the advancement of anesthesia techniques various surgical procedures have been developed for oesophageal diseases.

Oesophageal surgeries discussed in this chapter are:

- Hiatus hernia
- Oesophageal cancer
- Perforation and rupture
- Achalasia cardia
- Stricture of oesophagus
- Oesophago-respiratory tract fistula

19.1 Anatomy and Physiology

The oesophagus is a muscular tube conduit for food, that continues from the lower end of the pharynx, goes through the neck and thorax, and joins the upper end of the stomach in the abdomen. It is approximately 23–25 cm long in adults. It is behind the trachea and left recurrent laryngeal nerve in the superior mediastinum and anterior to the vertebral column (Fig. 19.1).

When it enters the posterior mediastinum, it lies behind the left mainstem bronchus. It continues down, going behind the pericardium and left atrium, anterior to descending aorta (Fig. 19.1).

In the thoracic cavity, the right edge of oesophagus is in relation to the mediastinal pleura of the right lung. The left edge is also in relation to the left lung and pleura, except in lower thoracic region, where the arch of aorta gives its two branches: common carotid and subclavian artery and continues into descending aorta, separating the oesophagus from the left lung.

The arterial supply of oesophagus comes from the inferior thyroid arteries in the neck, bronchial and intercostal arteries and the aorta in the thorax and left gastric artery in the abdomen.

The upper oesophagus drains into inferior thyroid veins, middle part into azygous veins and lower part into gastric veins. All these veins anastomose with one another, and form a portocaval anastomosis, where the portal drainage being gastric veins and the azygous veins being the vena caval system.

The oesophagus is innervated by both vagal and sympathetic nerves. The vagus nerves lie on either side of the oesophagus and form a rich plexus around the muscular tube.

The histology of oesophagus illustrates an outer covering called serosa, a muscular layer with outer longitudinal and inner circular layers, and an inner mucosa.

A peristaltic wave, which is predominantly under vagal control, takes 5–10 s to pass from the pharynx to the stomach [1].

When the stomach pressure rises, the lower oesophageal pressure also rises and thus the

---

A. Sirohi (✉) · J. Sood
Institute of Anaesthesiology, Pain and Perioperative Medicine, Sir Ganga Ram Hospital, New Delhi, India

© Springer Nature Singapore Pte Ltd. 2020
J. Sood, S. Sharma (eds.), *Clinical Thoracic Anesthesia*,
https://doi.org/10.1007/978-981-15-0746-5_19

barrier pressure remains unchanged. Medications that decrease lower oesophageal sphincter pressure are anticholinergics, tricyclic antidepressants and opioids [2]. Drugs that increase pressure in the lower oesophageal sphincter are anticholinesterases, metoclopramide, prochlorperazine and metoprolol (Table 19.1).

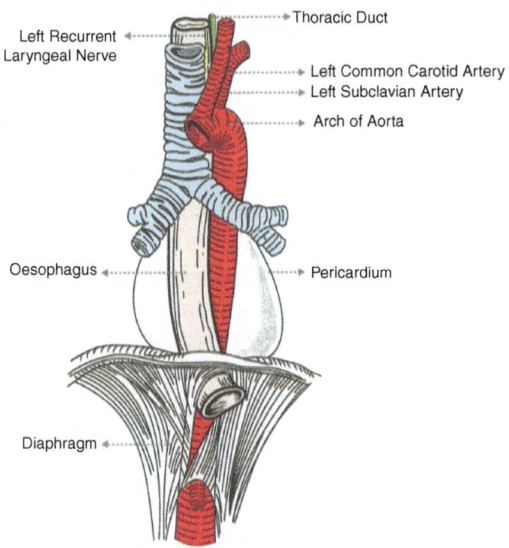

Fig. 19.1 Extent and relations of oesophagus. Source: Google image

Table 19.1 Effects of drugs on lower oesophageal sphincter pressure

Increase	Decrease	No change
Metoclopramide	Atropine	Propranolol
Domperidone	Glycopyrrolate	
Prochlorperazine	Dopamine	Cimetidine
Cyclizine	Sodium nitroprusside	Ranitidine
Edrophonium	Ganglion blockers	Atracurium
Neostigmine	Thiopental	Nitrous oxide
Histamine	Tricyclic antidepressants	
Succinylcholine	β-adrenergic agonists	
Pancuronium	Halothane	
Metoprolol	Enflurane	
α-adrenergic stimulants	Opioids	
Antacids	Nitrous oxide	

19.2 Surgical Diseases and Management

19.2.1 Hiatus Hernia

Hiatus hernia and gastroesophageal reflux may coexist or may be present independently.

It has been seen that significant reflux is not a finding in most of the patients with hiatus hernia [2], whereas most patients with reflux have a sliding hiatus hernia.

19.2.1.1 Types of Hiatus Hernia

Type 1—Sliding hernia (90%)—The oesophagogastric junction and fundus of stomach herniate axially into the thorax through the oesophageal hiatus [2]. In response to pressure changes in chest and abdomen the hernia may move cephalad and caudad. The term 'sliding' denotes the presence of a partial sac of parietal peritoneum and not the movement. Here the lower oesophageal sphincter may not respond appropriately to an increase in intra-abdominal pressure. Thus coughing or breathing leads to regurgitation due to decreased barrier pressure.

Type 2—Paraoesophageal hiatus hernia (10%)—Part of the stomach herniates into the thorax next to the oesophagus. The oesophageal junction is still located in abdomen in type 2 hernia. Gastric volvulus and anaemia due to blood loss are most common complications of type 2 hernia.

Hiatus hernia leads to decreased maximum breathing capacity, reduced total lung volume and increased residual volume.

A preoperative chest X-ray is important in patients presenting for oesophageal surgery. Evidence of aspiration or reduced lung volume can be seen in chest X-ray. Chest physiotherapy and antibiotics should be given in case of aspiration pneumonia. Pulmonary function tests are indicated in patients with coexisting lung disease and obesity.

Preoperative treatment to increase the gastric juice pH should be given to the patients with an incompetent lower oesophageal sphincter (Table 19.2).

Surgical repair like Nissen fundoplication is done to obtain the competence of the

Table 19.2 Drugs for increasing gastric pH

Name	Dose	Route	Effects	Side effects
Cimetidine	300 mg QID 400 mg BD 800 mg OD	Oral or intravenous	Increases the pH of gastric juice	Rapid intravenous injection can cause hypotension, bradycardia and heart block, confusion, agitation, seizures, metabolism of drugs with high hepatic extraction might be delayed
Ranitidine	150 mg BD 50 mg TDS	Oral Intravenous	Increases the pH of gastric juice	CNS side effects are less because of decreased ability to cross the blood–brain barrier
Omeprazole	20 mg	Oral, night before the surgery	Reduces acidity and volume of gastric contents	
Metoclopramide	10–20 mg	Intravenous (over a period of 3–5 min)	Increases lower oesophageal sphincter tone	

gastroesophageal junction. This can be done through thoracic or abdominal incision and entails wrapping the distal oesophagus with the fundus of the stomach.

Laparoscopic Nissen fundoplication can also be performed these days with the advantage of less postoperative pain, early postoperative recovery, although during the passage of oesophageal bougie oesophageal or gastric perforation can occur [3]. Open thoracotomy becomes necessary in such circumstances.

In children laparoscopic fundoplication is well tolerated.

19.2.2 Oesophageal Carcinoma

Oesophagus has the property of distensibility. Because of this quality it dilates proximal to the obstruction. Food in this dilated part does not come in contact with the acid milieu of stomach, so this gets infected and bacterial growth occurs. In patients with weak laryngeal reflexes regurgitated food can lead to aspiration pneumonitis and atelectasis. During induction of general anesthesia these patients are at risk of aspiration. Placing a large bore nasogastric tube and suctioning through it decreases the risk of aspiration significantly.

At the time of diagnosis, the disease is often in advanced stage so combined therapy with radiation and surgery is required. Most commonly used chemotherapeutic agents like bleomycin and doxorubicin are derived from antibiotics [4]. Doxorubicin can cause myelosuppression and cardiomyopathy. Cardiomyopathy is dose dependent and can be either acute or slowly progressive. Acute form of cardiomyopathy can present with decreased QRS voltage and nonspecific ST-T wave changes. Other signs like left axis deviation, cardiac conduction abnormalities, premature ventricular contractions and supraventricular tachyarrhythmias can appear [5]. Once treatment is discontinued, these changes reverse within 30–60 days. The slow onset of symptoms followed by rapidly progressive cardiac failure is the characteristic of the slow progressive form of cardiomyopathy.

Bleomycin causes minimal myelosuppression but pulmonary toxicity occurs in 5–8% patients resulting in 2% deaths. Cough, dyspnea and basilar rales develop first followed by severe form in the patients with bleomycin induced pulmonary toxicity [6].

Resting hypoxemia, fibrous appearance on chest X-ray and interstitial pneumonia occur in the severe forms.

Other drugs that can be used include cisplatinum, vinblastine and fluorouracil.

Effective treatment for squamous cell carcinoma is radiation. Complications of radiation are pericarditis, pneumonitis, myelitis and tracheoesophageal fistula [1].

Table 19.3 Surgical approaches for oesophagectomy and esophagogastrectomy

Surgery	Incisions	Anesthetic considerations
Laparotomy and right thoracotomy "Ivor Lewis" (lower and some middle-third esophageal lesion)	2 incisions: Upper Abdominal midline, then right thoracotomy approximately fifth, sixth intercostal spaces	One lung ventilation Repositioning supine to right-lateral intraoperatively
Transhiatal "Orringer" Lower third lesions may be used for mid thirds in some centers	2 incisions: Upper Abdominal midline then left neck	Hemodynamic instability from cardiac compression during blunt intra-thoracic dissection Possibility of occult perforation of tracheobronchial tree during blunt dissection (leave tracheal tube uncut in case of need to advance into bronchus) No vascular access in left neck
Left side thoraco-abdominal Lower esophageal lesions only	1 incision: left lateral thoracotomy extended to left upper lateral abdominal	One lung ventilation desirable
Combined chest, abdominal and neck ("three hole") ("upper oblique mid-esophageal lesion")	3 incisions: right thoracotomy then laparotomy, then left	One lung ventilation desirable repositioning lateral to supine intra-operatively No vascular access in left neck
Thoracoscopy plus laparotomy or combined with laparoscopy (upper/mid-esophgeal lesions)	1 or 2 incisions, plus video port access Thoracoscopy to avoid blunt dissection in chest Neck incision at end	One lung ventilation necessary Potentially prolonged surgery

Thoracic Anesthesia 3rd edition, James B. Eisenkraft, MD, Steven M. Neustein, MD Ch. 13 (Anesthesia for Esophageal and Mediastinal Surgery)

Surgical treatment of oesophageal cancer are (Table 19.3):

1. Oesophagogastrectomy
2. Replacement of the oesophagus with the colon
3. Oesophagectomy with gastric replacement

19.2.3 Benign Oesophageal Stricture

Benign stricture is most commonly caused by reflux of acidic gastric contents. Chronic reflux of acidic content may cause inflammation leading to ulceration and stricture formation in lower oesophagus. When the acidic contents stop coming in contact with oesophageal mucosa, pathological changes can get reversed.

It can be managed with medical treatment as well as with surgical treatment. Surgical treatment is indicated when medical treatment and dilatations are not successful.

There are two methods of surgical repair. For both, a left thoracoabdominal incision is given.

First is oesophageal dilatation followed by gastroplasty while the other is resection of stricture followed by creation of end-to-side oesophagogastrostomy via the thoracic route.

In the former method, fundus of stomach is put between oesophageal mucosa and acidic content, and the remaining fundus is stitched to lower oesophagus. This creates a valve-like effect [7]. Vagotomy and antrectomy are done to remove acidity of stomach while Roux-en Y gastric drainage helps to prevent alkaline reflux from intestine.

In second type of repair, end-to-end oesophagogastrostomy is created after resection of the stricture. Vagotomy and antrectomy are done to eliminate acidity of stomach and a Roux-en-Y gastric drainage can prevent alkaline reflux from intestine.

19.2.4 Intrathoracic Oesophageal Rupture and Perforation

Oesophageal rupture is bursting of oesophagus due to sudden increase in abdominal pressure with relaxed oesophageal sphincter and obstructed oesophageal inlet. Most common location of rupture is on the left side and within 2 cm of gastroesophageal junction [7]. Rupture often occurs due to uncoordinated vomiting, straining associated with weightlifting, parturition, defecation or crush injuries to chest and abdomen. When there is a ruptured stomach, the contents enter in mediastinum under high pressure and patient becomes symptomatic abruptly, whereas in perforation symptoms are not so abrupt.

Causes of oesophageal perforation are foreign bodies, endoscopy, bougies, traumatic tracheal intubation and oesophageal suction [7–11]. It is commonly caused by iatrogenic procedures like upper GI endoscopy. Other iatrogenic causes are endoesophageal intubation, oesophageal obturator airways, balloon tamponade and NG tubes [11]. Endoscopic perforations are more common at upper oesophageal sphincter, which is the narrowest site of oesophagus [2].

Perforation related to tracheal intubation usually occurs at cricopharyngeus muscle level [2]. At this level a cervical vertebra can compress oesophageal lumen [8]. Hyperextended neck may aggravate incidence of perforation during procedures.

Patients with rupture or perforation present with pain. They may develop diaphoresis, hypotension, tachypnea, cyanosis, emphysema, hydrothorax or hydropneumothorax.

Radiological signs may suggest subcutaneous emphysema, pneumomediastinum, widening of mediastinum, pleural effusion and pneumoperitoneum. Barium studies and iodinated water soluble contrast oesophagogram can locate the site. CT scan may indicate pneumomediastinum or pneumothorax [10].

Medical treatment should precede surgical treatment. These patients should be treated with antibiotics, IV fluids to replenish intravascular volume along with inotropic support if needed. Supplementary oxygen should be given. They may require invasive BP monitoring as well as CVP monitoring. Preoperative drainage of large hydrothorax or hydropneumothorax improves circulatory and respiratory function.

Surgery may be performed as primary closure or oesophagectomy in patients with malignancy. In hemodynamically unstable patients cervical oesophagostomy is done with feeding gastrostomy. Aim of surgery in perforation is drainage and prevention of contamination. Perforation or rupture is identified by oesophagoscopy [7]. When rupture is present in lower 1/3, right sided thoracotomy is performed [1]. Primary closure can be done if oesophageal wall is healthy. When lesion is present at lower end, it is repaired with stomach. Oesophagectomy is done in operable carcinoma cases.

19.2.5 Achalasia

Achalasia is an oesophageal dysmotility disorder resulting from absence of peristalsis and failure of relaxation of lower oesophageal sphincter with swallowing.

It has neurogenic aetiology characterised by either absence or degenerative Aurbach plexus ganglionic cells. Myentricus plexus is present in oesophageal wall. This nerve plexus consists of unmyelinated fibres and post-ganglionic autonomic cell bodies.

Patients develop symptoms of oesophageal distension, regurgitation and aspiration. As aetiology is not correctable, these patients are treated with oesophageal dilatation or surgery.

Surgical repair named Heller's myotomy is done by giving incision through circular muscle of oesophagogastric junction. It is usually done along with hiatus hernia repair. It helps in preventing reflux. It involves a thoracic approach or abdominal approach. Intraoperative endoscopy is done to check effectiveness of myotomy. Thoracic approach is performed for extension of myotomy proximally. Heller's myotomy can be performed laparoscopically. This approach has advantages like short hospital stay, less postoperative pain and better treatment of dysphagia.

The open approach may have complications like atelectasis and pneumothorax. To determine residual high pressure, manometry may also be performed. In surgically unfit patients or patients refusing surgery, oesophageal dilatation is performed to relieve dysphagia.

Failure of improvement of symptoms indicates inadequate myotomy. Recurrence of symptoms may occur due to re-apposition to severed muscle or stricture from post-myotomy gastroesophageal reflux [11].

A modified procedure named Dor operation can also be done. In this procedure a stent is placed in the muscular defect of myotomy. It helps in preventing muscular reapportion and dysphagia [11–13].

The latest therapy for achalasia is per-oral endoscopic myotomy (POEM). A tunnel is created in the submucosa until the gastric cardia by giving an incision in the mucosa in mid oesophagus. Then myotomy of circular fibres is done by using electrocautery. This technique is well tolerated, safe and effective [14–19].

19.2.6 Oesophageal Respiratory Tract Fistula

They have congenital or acquired aetiology. Acquired oesophageotracheal fistula, usually in adults, can be benign or malignancy related. Benign fistula is caused by tracheal tube related injury, trauma or inflammation [20]. Most common cause is malignancy [20, 21]. Eighty-five per cent of fistulas are secondary to oesophageal carcinoma. They can connect to any part of respiratory tract. They present with dysphagia, abdominal pain and cough.

In patients receiving radiotherapy and having poor prognosis, palliation is the preferred treatment. Palliative treatment by oesophageal bypass surgery has shown better long-term survival [22–27]. The aim of palliative procedure is to prevent entry of oesophageal contents into the respiratory tract and maintenance of continuity with gastrointestinal tract. In this procedure oesophagus is divided at two places—at cardia of stomach and proximally in neck. The proximal part of oesophagus is connected to the fundus of the stomach. The stomach, jejunum or colon is placed in presternal or retrosternal position and used as a connection. The other portion of oesophagus can be drained either externally or internally.

In patients with poor lung function, drainage of isolated oesophagus is advised as chronic aspiration may lead to hypoxemia, fever, sepsis, dyspnea and pneumothorax. These patients may develop aspiration because of RLN dysfunction due to tumour extension. Juxtapositioning of oesophagus and aorta may form a passage which results in bleeding on manipulation. So localisation of fistula should be done in preoperative period to avoid complications. The best method for identification of fistula is bronchoscopy but reported success rate is only 50–75% [28, 29].

19.2.7 Zenker's Diverticulum

It is a diverticulum of lower pharynx arising from a weakness at junction of thyropharyngeus and cricopharyngeus muscle just proximal to oesophagus. It is considered as an oesophageal lesion as its location is proximal to upper oesophagus. During swallowing there is failure of relaxation of upper oesophageal sphincter with an increase in pressure in lower pharynx, resulting in localised dilatations and diverticulum formation. Oral secretions filled in diverticulum are alkaline in nature, so aspiration of these contents is less dangerous than aspiration of stomach contents.

Patients present with nonspecific symptoms. Most common symptom is dysphagia. As diverticulum enlarges in size, patient may develop noisy swallowing, regurgitation and supine coughing spells. In advanced stage recurrent aspiration and pneumonia can develop [30].

Routine practice is to empty the diverticulum prior to induction of anesthesia as there is possibility of aspiration in intraoperative and postoperative period [31]. Cricoid pressure may increase chances of aspiration in these patients by emptying sac into pharynx (as most of the times diverticulum orifice is above the level of cricoid cartilage).

Treatment is excision of diverticulum by incision in left lower neck. Awake fiberoptic intubation is one of the safest methods to manage airway. Modified RSI without cricoid pressure should be performed in these patients in head up of 30° position. Placement of pack around endotracheal tube may decrease the chances of aspiration. Intraoperatively there are chances of perforation or injury of diverticulum by nasogastric tube or bougie.

19.3 Anesthetic Considerations for Oesophageal Surgery

19.3.1 Preoperative Evaluation and Preparation

A thorough preoperative evaluation should be done. These patients have poor nutritional status due to dysphagia and odynophagia for solids and liquids. Nutritional status should be improved before surgery to decrease morbidity and mortality [32, 33]. Poor preoperative respiratory status can be present due to chronic aspiration. Chest X-ray should be done to evaluate the condition of lungs. Pulmonary function tests are required in patients with chronic lung disease.

Cardiovascular system should be evaluated according to ACC/AHA guidelines [34, 35]. A 12-lead ECG is essential to rule out myocardial ischemia and arrhythmias and for perioperative comparison if there is any cardiac complication. Due to manipulation of heart and lungs during thoracotomy for oesophageal surgery, supraventricular tachyarrhythmias can occur very commonly. Arrhythmias can be decreased by giving digitalis in preoperative period although there are chances of digitalis toxicity because titration of the dose to clinical effect is not possible [36, 37].

19.3.2 Intraoperative Monitoring

Intraoperative monitoring depends on the nature of surgery, preoperative condition of the patient and comorbidities. Routine monitoring includes ECG, NIBP and pulse oximetry. Invasive monitoring may be required in patients with limited cardiovascular reserve, compromised respiratory system, major oesophageal surgeries, oesophageal trauma and perforation with sepsis component. Surgeries where transthoracic approach is used, continuous arterial blood pressure monitoring is indicated, as surgical intrathoracic manipulations can lead to arrhythmias and hypotension. In such cases central venous access is also required for central delivery of drugs to control arrhythmias. The procedures where one lung ventilation is required, arterial blood gas sampling gives information of arterial oxygenation along with electrolytes and acid-base status.

19.3.3 Pain Control

Adequate pain relief is important in patients receiving thoracotomy incision to avoid postoperative respiratory and cardiovascular complications. Analgesia required for endoscopic or laparoscopic surgeries is generally less compared to open thoracotomy. Thoracotomy incision given for transthoracic approach is very painful and requires multimodal approach for pain control.

Most commonly used multimodal approach for analgesia includes thoracic epidural analgesia along with intravenous analgesics. Thoracic epidural analgesia is considered to be gold standard analgesic technique [38, 39]. It is cost effective, safe component of multimodal analgesia with favourable outcome [40, 41]. It plays a significant role in reducing perioperative inflammatory response and provides better outcome [42, 43]. It provides better analgesia in comparison to parenteral opioid therapy alone.

Lumbar epidural analgesia technique can be used in patients who are not suitable candidates for thoracic epidural analgesia. But the quality of pain control is inferior to thoracic epidural analgesia.

Non-neuraxial techniques like intercostal, intrapleural and paravertebral approaches are in practise to provide postoperative analgesia. Studies suggest that paravertebral blocks are better alternative to thoracic epidural analgesia [44]. Limitation with paravertebral approach is that dermatomes at multiple levels need to be blocked to provide adequate analgesia.

Most commonly used analgesic technique is to place thoracic epidural catheter in preoperative period. A combination of opioid like fentanyl or morphine along with local anesthetic such as bupivacaine or ropivacaine can be given through epidural catheter as boluses or infusion. Epidural analgesia is continued in postoperative period in combination with other intravenous analgesics.

An epidural bolus of preservative free morphine provides neuraxial spread. It has synergistic action with local anesthetics but there are chances of delayed respiratory depression. Studies suggest that preoperative epidural analgesia provides better acute pain control [45–47].

19.3.4 Induction of Anesthesia

Choice of anesthesia for oesophageal surgery depends on patient-related factors as well as on surgery-related factors. Patient-related factors are respiratory and cardiovascular status, risk of aspiration pneumonitis, mediastinal lymphadenopathy or mass causing airway compression. Surgical factors include approach of surgery and duration of surgery.

Rapid sequence induction is indicated in patients for oesophageal surgeries as these patients have increased chances of aspiration. Awake tracheal intubation should be considered in patients with difficult airway, patients having mediastinal mass and in patients who are at highest risk of aspiration pneumonitis like in severe achalasia. Patients having mediastinal lymphadenopathy or mediastinal mass (posterior or superior mediastinal) might develop airway collapse and tracheal compression after receiving muscle relaxant. Tracheal tube must pass the obstruction for adequate ventilation.

In RSI force required for applying cricoid pressure is 30–40 newton. It has been reported that application of cricoid pressure decreases lower oesophageal sphincter tone, although it does not cause reflux clinically [48, 49].

Adequate compression and occlusion of oesophagus during RSI can be confirmed by real-time ultrasound of oesophagus also.

19.3.5 Choice of Tracheal Tube

Choice of tracheal tube depends on the approach of surgery. For lower oesophageal resection via left thoracoabdominal incision, single or double lumen endotracheal tube can be placed. When single lumen ETT is used, retraction of left lung provides surgical exposure. When thoracotomy approach is used, DLT is necessary to collapse the ipsilateral lung. Most common practice is to use left sided DLT irrespective of the side of thoracotomy. Right sided DLT is generally not used because it needs expertise for correct placement of the tube and little displacement intraoperatively can cause right upper lobe collapse, leading to desaturation, hypoxia and hemodynamic instability.

Other alternatives are Univent tubes and single lumen ETT with a blocker.

Univent tubes are bulky and difficult to pass through vocal cords and difficult to advance into mainstem bronchus. If postoperative ventilation is planned, Univent tube can be left after withdrawing the blocker completely into its channel. In difficult airway cases standard ETT can be placed along with Forgaty catheter under bronchoscopic guidance.

When bronchial blocker is used, smaller tidal volumes should be used to keep the airway pressures low and to prevent passage of gas beyond the blocker which can lead to lung inflation.

19.3.6 Intraoperative Considerations and Management

Most commonly used technique for maintenance of anesthesia involves use of intravenous opioids along with opioids and local anesthetics through an epidural for analgesia, nondepolarising muscle relaxant like atracurium or vecuronium for muscle relaxation and volatile inhalation agents like sevoflurane, isoflurane or desflurane.

Oesophageal surgeries can cause severe inflammatory response. Anesthetic agents decrease pulmonary and systemic inflammatory response associated with oesophageal surgery and one lung ventilation. Preconditioning of myocardium is dependent on quality of inhalation agents which saves myocardium from further ischemic insult.

These patients may develop hypotension due to either low intravascular volume status or surgical factors like IVC compression and surgical manipulation. Surgical trauma to trachea is another potential complication. In such a situation, bronchial lumen should be used for ventilation, provided bronchial lumen of DLT is placed in the bronchus of the lung being ventilated. If a single lumen endotracheal tube is used, it should be advanced beyond the tracheal injury into the bronchus [50]. Nitrous oxide should be avoided as it causes bowel distension, respiratory impairment and interference with surgical field. High inspired concentration of oxygen is required for conduction of one lung anesthesia. There are more chances of developing hypoxia during oesophageal surgery in patients with relatively normal lung function in comparison to patients undergoing lung surgery with compromised lung functions since patients presenting with lung disease for lung resection already have compromised blood flow to the diseased lung. So ventilation perfusion mismatch is further reduced during one lung ventilation.

For surgical repair the surgeon may request for placement of oropharyngeal bougie. Once repair is done, methylene blue is used to check for any leaks from anastomotic sites by injecting it through oroesophageal or nasoesophageal tube.

In postoperative period, in patients requiring postoperative ventilation, DLT is exchanged by single lumen tube. It is checked simultaneously to avoid oesophageal intubation or any manipulation with suture line.

19.4 Anesthetic Considerations for Robotic Oesophagectomy

- Access to the patient is very limited after robot docking.
- Limited access to the airway because robot chassis is just above the patient's head.
- Injury can occur due to collision of robotic arm with the patient's body.
- Nerve injuries like brachial plexus injury can occur due to extreme extension of arm for positioning.
- Position of bronchial blocker or DLT should be checked before docking of the robot.
- Proper vascular access with extension lines should be secured before positioning of robot.
- Carbon dioxide insufflation can cause hypercarbia, bradycardia and gas embolism.
- Hemodynamic and respiratory compromise can occur if there is surgical injury to the opposite pleura.

19.5 Anesthetic Considerations for Oesophageal Dilatation

Patients having achalasia, stricture and collagen diseases may require oesophageal dilatation. The appropriate method for induction of anesthesia is general anesthesia. Suction with wide bore tube should be done before induction. Current practise is to use propofol for induction along with short acting muscle relaxants. RSI with cricoid pressure or awake intubation if airway is difficult are preferred methods. Retching and bucking may aggravate incidence of oesophageal perforation and mediastinitis; therefore, short acting muscle relaxants are used. Atropine is avoided as it decreases LES tone. A good LES tone is necessary in these patients.

These patients have chances of aspiration in postoperative period and so trachea is extubated only when patient is fully awake and able to protect the airway.

19.6 Anesthetic Management of Oesophagorespiratory Tract Fistula Surgery

Spontaneous ventilation is necessary to be maintained until gentle ventilation is secured to achieve effective gas exchange as positive pressure ventilation results in loss of tidal volume and inspired gases, leading to inadequate ventilation. Chronic aspiration makes lung which is ipsilateral to the fistula, less compliant so it receives less tidal volume. Studies suggest that positive pressure ventilation should be avoided to decrease the incidence of abdominal distension, respiratory insufficiency and fatal complications like cardiac arrest [51, 52]. If positive pressure ventilation is necessary, preoperative gastrostomy is preferred but it does not reduce risk of leakage or mediastinitis.

Awake intubation or inhalation induction is preferred in these patients but it is slow as these patients have secretions and poor pulmonary reserve. High frequency ventilation (HFV), an alternative method is helpful to reduce gas loss through fistula.

DLT is preferred to protect opposite lung from contamination and allows ventilation without positive pressure application on fistula. It should be placed under fiberoptic guidance to avoid disruption of fistula. When fistula is present in distal trachea or in the left mainstem bronchus of left lung, a right sided DLT is used. Left sided DLT is used when fistula is present on right side.

Preoperative visualisation should be done to determine the site of fistula. If it is not visualised, right sided DLT should be placed and right sided ventilation should be secured. If there is gastric distension or loss of tidal volume suggestive of right sided fistula, left sided ventilation should be used. In case of two lung ventilation, there are chances of air leak and gastric distension, so NG tube should be placed. Drainage of excluded oesophageal portion is necessary against disruption of suture line.

In the postoperative period positive pressure ventilation may disrupt suture line in case of inadequate drainage of oesophageal segment. Other possible complications are loss of tidal volume, abdominal distension and disruption of fistula. So spontaneous ventilation is preferred in postoperative period. For early resumption of spontaneous ventilation, intraoperative suctioning, avoidance of deep sedation and good postoperative analgesia should be provided. HFV is an alternative in postoperative period as it applies minimum pressure.

19.7 Postoperative Management

These patients may develop hypotension in postoperative period due to hypovolemia, haemorrhage or dysrhythmias. Sympathectomy due to thoracic epidural analgesia can also cause hypotension. Hypovolemia can be differentiated from other causes by monitoring central venous pressure, urine output and other losses like drain output. Hypotension caused by sympathectomy due to epidural analgesia can be treated by intravenous fluids, decreasing the dose of local anesthetic or by replacing local anesthetic with opioid like morphine in epidural infusion. Patients receiving TPN develop hypoglycaemia or hyperosmolar coma and they may present with delayed awakening. TPN should be substituted with 10% dextrose or dose should be adjusted.

Patients having obesity and coexisting lung disease are at high risk to develop respiratory complications like aspiration pneumonia and deep vein thrombosis. Inadequate pain relief may also result in hypoventilation, hypoxemia and atelectasis; hence these patients must receive adequate pain relief.

Patients presenting with oesophageal rupture or perforation for thoracotomy and repair are prone to develop mediastinitis, severe septicaemia with anaerobic gram negative organism, hypotension due to blood loss, arrhythmias and respiratory impairment. To avoid all these circulatory and respiratory complications, trachea should be kept intubated in immediate postoperative period.

Thorough preoperative evaluation of cardiovascular system and thromboprophylaxis can significantly decrease cardiovascular complications like myocardial ischemia, dysrhythmias and congestive heart failure in postoperative period.

Patients who have undergone oesophageal respiratory tract fistula repair or oesophageal bypass may develop pneumothorax if pleural cavity is injured by surgeon performing retrosternal approach. During cervical dissection, RLN injury may cause aspiration.

19.8 Conclusion

Patients for oesophageal surgery are generally debilitated and prone to respiratory and cardiovascular complications. Thorough preoperative evaluation, optimisation of acute symptoms and selection of appropriate analgesic and anesthetic technique are the keys for early recovery and discharge from the hospital.

References

1. Greenhow DE. Oesophageal surgery. In: Marshall BE, Longnecker DE, Fairley HB, editors. Anaesthesia for thoracic procedure. Boston: Blackwell Scientific; 1988. p. 451.
2. Pairolero PC, Trastek VF, Payne WS. Oesophagus and diaphragmatic hernias. In: Schwartz SI, Shires GI, Spencer FL, editors. Principles of surgery. New York: McGraw-Hill; 1989. p. 1103.
3. Lowham AS, Filipi CJ, Hinder RA, et al. Mechanisms and avoidance of esophageal perforation by anesthesia personnel during laparoscopic foregut surgery. Surg Endosc. 1996;10(10):979–82.
4. Rao TLK, El-Str AA. Oesophageal and mediastinal surgery. In: Kaplan JA, editor. Thoracic anesthesia. New York: Churchill Livingstone; 1998.
5. Stoelting RK. Pharmacology and physiology in anesthetic practice. Philadelphia: JB Lippincott; 1987.
6. Crooke ST, Bradner WT. Bleomycin, a review. J Med. 1976;7(5):333–428.
7. Aitkenhead AR. Anesthesia for oesophageal surgery. In: Gothard JW, editor. Thoracic anesthesia. London: Biailliere-Tindall; 1987. p. 181.
8. Topsis J, Kinas HY, Kandall SR. Esophageal perforation—a complication of neonatal resuscitation. Anesth Analg. 1989;69(4):532–4.
9. Krasna IH, Rosenfeld D, Benjamin BG, et al. Esophageal perforation in the neonate: an emerging problem in the newborn nursery. J Pediatr Surg. 1987;22(8):784–90.
10. Sakurai H, McElhinney AJ. Perforation of the esophagus: experience at Bronx VA Hospital 1969-1984. Mt Sinai J Med. 1987;54(6):487–95.
11. O'Neill JE, Giffin JP, Cottrell JE. Pharyngeal and esophageal perforation following endotracheal intubation. Anesthesiology. 1984;60(5):487–8.
12. Dor J, Humbert P, Paoli JM, et al. Treatment of reflux by the so-called modified Heller-Nissen technic. Presse Med. 1967;75(50):2563–5.
13. Ali A, Pellegrini CA. Laparoscopic myotomy: technique and efficacy in treating achalasia. Gastrointest Endosc Clin N Am. 2001;11(2):347–58.
14. Testoni PA, Mazzoleni G, Testoni SG. Transoral incisionless fundoplication for gastro-esophageal reflux disease: techniques and outcomes. World J Gastrointest Pharmacol Ther. 2016;7(2):179–89.
15. Jain D, Singhal S. Transoral incisionless fundoplication for refractory gastroesophageal reflux disease: where do we stand? Clin Endosc. 2016;49(2):147–56.
16. Brar TS, Draganov PV, Yang D. Endoluminal therapy for gastroesophageal reflux disease: in between the pill and the knife? Dig Dis Sci. 2017;62(1):16–25.
17. Crespin OM, Liu LW, Parmar A, et al. Safety and efficacy of POEM for treatment of achalasia: a systematic review of the literature. Surg Endosc. 2017;31(5):2187–201.
18. Schneider AM, Louie BE, Warren HF, et al. A matched comparison of per oral endoscopic myotomy to laparoscopic Heller myotomy in the treatment of achalasia. J Gastrointest Surg. 2016;20(11):1789–96.
19. Marano L, Pallabazzer G, Solito B, et al. Surgery or peroral esophageal myotomy for achalasia: a systematic review and meta-analysis. Medicine (Baltimore). 2016;95(10):e3001.
20. Hindman BJ, Bert AA. Malignant esophago-respiratory tract fistulas: anesthetic considerations for exclusion procedures using esophageal bypass. J Cardiothorac Anesth. 1987;1(5):438–47.
21. Wesselhoeft CW Jr, Keshishian JM. Acquired nonmalignant esophagotracheal and esophagobronchial fistulas. Ann Thorac Surg. 1968;6(2):187–95.
22. Duranceau A, Jamieson GG. Malignant tracheoesophageal fistula. Ann Thorac Surg. 1984;37(4):346–54.
23. Angorn I. Intubation in the treatment of carcinoma of the esophagus. World J Surg. 1981;5:535–41.
24. Conlan AA, Nicolaou N, Delikaris PG, et al. Pessimism concerning palliative bypass procedures for established malignant esophagorespiratory fistulas: a report of 18 patients. Ann Thorac Surg. 1984;37(2):108–10.
25. Girardet RE, Ransdell HT Jr, Wheat MW Jr. Palliative intubation in the management of esophageal carcinoma. Ann Thorac Surg. 1974;18(4):417–30.
26. Symbas PN, McKeown PP, Hatcher CR Jr, et al. Tracheoesophageal fistula from carcinoma of the esophagus. Ann Thorac Surg. 1984;38(4):382–6.
27. Weaver RM, Matthews HR. Palliation and survival in malignant oesophago-respiratory fistula. Br J Surg. 1980;67(8):539–42.
28. Ong GB, Kwong KH. Management of malignant esophagobronchial fistula. Surgery. 1970;67(2):293–301.
29. Campion JP, Bourdelat D, Launois B. Surgical treatment of malignant esophagotracheal fistulas. Am J Surg. 1983;146(5):641–6.
30. Thiagarajah S, Lear E, Keh M. Anesthetic implications of Zenker's diverticulum. Anesth Analg. 1990;70(1):109–11.
31. Aouad MT, Berzina CE, Baraka AS. Aspiration pneumonia after anesthesia in a patient with a Zenker diverticulum. Anesthesiology. 2000;92(6):1837–9.
32. Moghissi K, Hornshaw J, Teasdale PR, et al. Parenteral nutrition in carcinoma of the oesophagus treated by surgery: nitrogen balance and clinical studies. Br J Surg. 1977;64(2):125–8.
33. Heatley RV, Williams RH, Lewis MH. Pre-operative intravenous feeding—a controlled trial. Postgrad Med J. 1979;55(646):541–5.
34. Fleisher LA, Fleischmann KE, Auerbach AD, et al. 2014 ACC/AHA guideline on perioperative cardiovascular evaluation and management of patients undergoing noncardiac surgery: a report of the American

College of Cardiology/American Heart Association task force on practice guidelines. J Am Coll Cardiol. 2014;64(22):e77–137.
35. Fleisher LA, Fleischmann KE, Auerbach AD, et al. 2014 ACC/ AHA guideline on perioperative cardiovascular evaluation and management of patients undergoing noncardiac surgery: a report of the American College of Cardiology/American Heart Association task force on practice guidelines. Circulation. 2014;130(24):e278–333.
36. Shields TW, Ujiki GT. Digitalization for prevention of arrhythmias following pulmonary surgery. Surg Gynecol Obstet. 1968;126(4):743–6.
37. Burman SO. The prophylactic use of digitalis before thoracotomy. Ann Thorac Surg. 1972 Oct;14(4):359–68.
38. Rudin A, Flisberg P, Johansson J, et al. Thoracic epidural analgesia or intravenous morphine analgesia after thoracoabdominal esophagectomy: a prospective follow-up of 201 patients. J Cardiothorac Vasc Anesth. 2005;19(3):350–7.
39. Flisberg P, Tornebrandt K, Walther B, et al. Pain relief after esophagectomy: thoracic epidural analgesia is better than parenteral opioids. J Cardiothorac Vasc Anesth. 2001;15(3):282–7.
40. Smedstad KG, Beattie WS, Blair WS, et al. Postoperative pain relief and hospital stay after total esophagectomy. Clin J Pain. 1992;8(2):149–53.
41. Tsui SL, Law S, Fok M, et al. Postoperative analgesia reduces mortality and morbidity after esophagectomy. Am J Surg. 1997;173(6):472–8.
42. Fares KM, Mohamed SA, Hamza HM, et al. Effect of thoracic epidural analgesia on pro-inflammatory cytokines in patients subjected to protective lung ventilation during Ivor Lewis esophagectomy. Pain Phys. 2014;17(4):305–15.
43. Li W, Li Y, Huang Q, et al. Short and long-term outcomes of epidural or intravenous analgesia after esophagectomy: a propensity-matched cohort study. PLoS One. 2016;11(4):e0154380.
44. Marret E, Bazelly B, Taylor G, et al. Paravertebral block with ropivacaine 0.5% versus systemic analgesia for pain relief after thoracotomy. Ann Thorac Surg. 2005;79(6):2109–13.
45. Yegin A, Erdogan A, Kayacan N, et al. Early postoperative pain management after thoracic surgery; pre- and postoperative versus postoperative epidural analgesia: a randomised study. Eur J Cardiothorac Surg. 2003;24(3):420–4.
46. Bong CL, Samuel M, Ng JM, et al. Effects of preemptive epidural analgesia on post-thoracotomy pain. J Cardiothorac Vasc Anesth. 2005;19(6):786–93.
47. Salengros JC, Huybrechts I, Ducart A, et al. Different anesthetic techniques associated with different incidences of chronic post-thoracotomy pain: low-dose remifentanil plus presurgical epidural analgesia is preferable to high-dose remifentanil with postsurgical epidural analgesia. J Cardiothorac Vasc Anesth. 2010;24(4):608–16.
48. Tournadre JP, Chassard D, Berrada KR, et al. Cricoid cartilage pressure decreases lower esophageal sphincter tone. Anesthesiology. 1997;86(1):7–9.
49. Skinner HJ, Bedforth NM, Girling KJ, et al. Effect of cricoid pressure on gastro-oesophageal reflux in awake subjects. Anaesthesia. 1999 Aug;54(8):798–800.
50. Sung HM, Nelems B. Tracheal tear during laryngopharyngectomy and transhiatal oesophagectomy: a case report. Can J Anaesth. 1989;36(3 Pt 1):333–5.
51. Calverley RK, Johnston AE. The anaesthetic management of tracheo-oesophageal fistula: a review of ten years' experience. Can Anaesth Soc J. 1972;19(3):270–82.
52. Grant DM, Thompson GE. Diagnosis of congenital tracheoesophageal fistula in the adolescent and adult. Anesthesiology. 1978;49(2):139–40.

Anesthetic Management of Thoracic Trauma

Sudeep Goyal and Bhuwan Chand Panday

20.1 Introduction

The thoracic cavity harbors the most important vital structure of the body. It is bounded by ribs which is a strong protective covering of organs of paramount importance. A great force is required to disrupt this wall and injure the underlying structures. Injury to thorax is related to a high incidence of morbidity and is the leading cause of death at young age (1–45 years) [1], and also the predominant cause of "years of life lost" before achieving 75 years of age [2]. These accounts for 25–50% of all trauma-related mortality [3, 4]. In majority (70%) of cases, this devastating injury to the chest is associated with multisystem injuries.

Majority of cases with thoracic trauma may be managed conservatively, but some cases (10%) require emergent thoracotomy and pose tremendous challenges to the anesthesiologists and intensivists. A quick, evaluation (e-FAST) (extended Focused Assessment with Sonography for Trauma) and intervention can lead to a fruitful outcome.

S. Goyal (✉) · B. C. Panday
Institute of Anaesthesiology, Pain and Perioperative Medicine, Sir Ganga Ram Hospital, New Delhi, India

20.2 Etiology

Chest trauma is caused either by penetrating or non-penetrating type of injury. Both of these may have a major impact with life-threatening complications.

Penetrating Injury
High-velocity objects (sharp and pointed objects like missiles, gunshot injuries) cause penetrating and most devastating injury due to these multifactorial impacts:

1. Puncturing the tissues
2. Direct energy transfer to the tissues
3. High temperature which causes burn injury

These fast-moving objects directly injure the skin, ribs, muscles and disrupt the underlying structures. This type of injury is caused by gunshots, stabs, arrows and high-velocity splinters. Direct trauma to the thorax leads to piercing injury to the chest wall, pleura, lung and blood vessels. These injuries cause major blood loss, pneumothorax, hemothorax and sometimes a combination of these injuries makes the condition more severe. Severe pain aggravates the situation as these patients are unable to generate adequate tidal volume to maintain oxygenation. These cases require multidisciplinary management (thoracic surgery, pain medications, critical care etc.) and robust monitoring for a successful outcome.

Non-penetrating Injury It is usually caused by blunt trauma or blast forces.

Blunt Injury It consists of two basic mechanisms of trauma either compression or direct energy transfer.

20.2.1 Compression Injury

High-pressure impact injury is due to its impact on the thoracic cage. Devastating injury of major vital structures occurs due to their crushing between anterior chest wall and posterior spine. Such injuries are mainly due to the impact of steering wheel and seatbelt on thorax. Higher the momentum of the vehicle, higher is the amplitude of the injury [5]. Major injury to these organs may have major impact on functioning of these vital organs, severely compromising hemodynamics and ventilation.

20.2.2 Direct Energy Transfer

The compression injury along with high-speed side impact crashes, is a significant cause of direct energy transfer injury to the intrathoracic organs. This causes drastic alteration in perfusion and oxygenation with high incidence of mortality if not intervened on time.

20.2.3 Blast Injury

Various mechanisms of blast injuries are described in the literature since centuries. Blast induced injuries commonly occur during military war and terrorist attack, but these explosives are also used for various reasons, e.g., breaking of hard rocks, mining and in some industries. There are four basic mechanisms which describe the blast injury.

Primary effects: Blast injury is followed by propagation of blast waves which are of two types: (a) stress waves and (b) shear waves.[R] Interaction of these destructive waves with body tissues leads to devastating changes due to over- and under-pressurization [6, 7]. Air filled structures are the most affected, which include tympanic membrane, lungs (including contusion, hemorrhage, pneumothorax, and hemothorax), and abdominal viscera, usually the rupture of colon is most common. *Secondary effects* are due to the fast-moving fragments that are part of the device.

Tertiary type of trauma is the result of persons/objects being thrown by the blast wind or from collapse of structures.

Quaternary effects are due to burn, asphyxia, and exposure to toxic substances.

20.3 Principles of Management

Mass causality during war or militant attack, where large population is injured, requires categorization of patients according to severity of injury. Hemodynamics, neurological evaluation, blood loss, oxygen saturation and various other parameters must be considered.

Essential steps for patients who have sustained thoracic injury include evaluation and categorization, thorough examination, diagnostic tests and if indicated surgical intervention. These steps have shown to improve the outcome.

20.4 Initial Assessment and Management

Initial evaluation of thoracic injury is done as per guidelines of the American College of Surgeons advanced trauma life support protocol [8]. During initial evaluation, 12 lethal or potentially lethal thoracic injuries were identified:

- Compromised airway
- Tension pneumothorax
- Open pneumothorax
- Large hemothorax
- Flail chest
- Cardiac tamponade

- Traumatic aortic disruption
- Tracheobronchial rupture
- Myocardial contusion
- Diaphragmatic rupture
- Oesophageal disruption
- Pulmonary injury

Management of these patients consists of the primary evaluation and resuscitation followed by secondary evaluation and later diagnostic evaluation for definitive treatment [9].

Primary evaluation is done to access airway and ventilation; tracheal intubation is indicated in an unconscious patient in shock. It is also important to maintain oxygenation and perfusion to avoid hypoxia-related injury. Cricothyroidotomy or tracheotomy is advocated in case of neck injury or bleeding to maintain oxygenation. Collapsed jugular veins are assumed to be a sign of severe hypovolemia. Large bore cannula is required to transfuse the fluid/blood rapidly and maintaining intravascular volume. But, contrary to this, a patient with distended neck veins along with decreased blood pressure is sign of myocardial injury, tension pneumothorax, air embolism or pericardial tamponade. Emergency pericardiocentesis and thoracotomy is the mainstay of treatment. Regular assessment of neurological status is essential to rule out any intracranial lesion in case of suspected head injury. The Glasgow Coma Scale plays an important role when there are associated head and neck injuries or suspicion of air in cerebral circulation.

20.5 Tracheal Tree Obstruction

Patient with tracheal trauma may present with cyanosis, stridor, subcutaneous emphysema and in severe cases apnea. The root cause may vary from avulsed teeth, thick secretions, increase in size of neck hematoma, Laryngeal or tracheal tears and in extreme cases, life-threatening tracheal transection. These cases require intubation and ventilation to maintain oxygenation.

20.6 Pneumothorax

Pneumothorax is not an uncommon entity during thoracic cage trauma but these patients may not have any signs or symptoms (occult, *simple* pneumothorax) or may present as overt respiratory failure and circulatory shock (*tension* pneumothorax). Pneumothorax can develop whenever there is disruption of the visceral pleura leading to one-way communication between lungs and pleural space. It results in the passage of air into the pleural space, typically through a "one-way valve" mechanism in which air enters the pleural space with inspiration and air gets trapped inside the pleural cavity and cannot be expelled out from the chest. Both injuries can result in sequestration of air and positive pressure in the ipsilateral hemithorax leading to lung collapse, tracheal deviation, jugular venous distension (JVD), hypotension, and mediastinal shift toward the contralateral hemithorax. Impedance to venous return by increased thoracic pressure and vena caval compression may result in hemodynamic embarrassment and compromised perfusion.

It is difficult to maintain ventilation and oxygenation due to loss of volume from the lung injury and mediastinal compression of the contralateral lung. The combination of these complications may lead to lethal outcome if not managed on time.

Clinical signs and symptoms of pneumothorax include chest pain, dyspnea, tachycardia, hypotension, subcutaneous emphysema, JVD, tracheal deviation to the opposite side, *hyperresonance* to percussion and absence of breath sounds or chest expansion on the impacted side. Radiological finding may reveal contralateral side deviation of trachea and mediastinum, inferior displacement of diaphragm, abnormally large intercostal spaces, and loss of bronchovascular markings on ipsilateral side.

A high degree of possibility of occult pneumothorax must be kept in mind in all trauma patients. This patient may develop tension pneumothorax after initiation of positive pressure ventilation. Placement of ICD prior to positive pressure ventilation avoids development of tension pneumothorax. It is difficult to diagnose tension pneumothorax during general anesthesia, but this can be suspected in case of unexplained hypotension, hypoxia, absent or diminished breath sounds on one side, or a sudden increase in airway pressure.

Patients with persistent air leak after tube thoracostomy require surgical intervention. The procedure may be conducted under video-assisted thoracic surgery (VATS) and needs one-lung ventilation. All precautions must be taken while positioning in patients with cervical spine trauma. Isolation of lungs can be achieved by various methods (e.g., double lumen tube, bronchial blocker). IPPV and nitrous oxide are avoided until definitive control is achieved. Invasive hemodynamic monitoring is advocated and restricted volume is administered for successful outcome.

20.7 Open Pneumothorax

Open pneumothorax is known to occur due to full-thickness injury in the chest wall without "one-way valve effect." Theoretically, if the diameter of the defect exceeds two-thirds of the tracheal diameter, the negative pleural pressure associated with inspiration will cause air trapping inside chest. Tension pneumothorax is unlikely in this case because the large size of the injury allows two-way gas exchange between the atmosphere and the pleural space; however, adequate ventilation and oxygenation will quickly become impossible, as air is no longer exchanged between the alveoli and the atmosphere.

Open pneumothorax is managed by chest wall closure and dressing. The other unsecured side allows air to exit the chest, but air will no longer preferentially enter the chest via low resistance pathway and will instead pass normally through the upper airway and trachea. Patients with an open pneumothorax can be safely intubated and placed on positive pressure ventilation prior to placement of a chest tube or surgical repair of the wound.

20.8 Tension Pneumothorax

Tension pneumothorax occurs due to entrapment of air in the pleural space. This air pressure then shifts the mediastinum and due to acute angulation of superior and inferior vena cava there is significant decrease in cardiac output. Patients may present with respiratory distress, unilateral breath sounds, neck vein distension, tracheal deviation, and in extreme cases cyanosis. Immediate needle decompression is advocated to decompress the chest cavity, followed by tube thoracostomy.

20.9 Hemothorax

A small hemothorax may be asymptomatic and blood in pleural cavity must be at least 200 ml to create blunting of the costophrenic angle on an upright chest film. A larger hemothorax on the other hand, may have similar signs and symptoms to a tension pneumothorax including varying degrees of respiratory failure and cardiovascular collapse. Physical findings of hemothorax include decreased or muffled breath sounds along with dullness on percussion to the affected side. Massive hemothorax is defined as the collection of more than 1500 ml fluid in pleural cavity. These are usually caused by large lacerations to pulmonary parenchyma or injury to the intercostal or great vessels. Thoracic cavity is so voluminous that it could accommodate up to 60% patient's blood volume in one side of the chest but results in profound hemodynamic instability.

Thoracotomy is usually indicated if the initial output from the thorax is 1500 mL or more after placing the chest tube or when there is continuous output of 200 ml blood for 2–3 consecutive hours. VATS is indicated in stable patients [10]. Common indications include retained hemothorax and entrapped lung where the surgeons perform VATS surgery after third day of trauma. Surgical evaluation is mandatory in cases of lung laceration, intercostal vessel bleeding, and great vessel injuries which are the cause in majority of the cases of hemothorax. The source of the hemorrhage will dictate the definitive treatment. If VATS or thoracotomy is required, the management may include considerations for lung isolation, whereas for embolization procedures, as in the case of intercostal arterial bleeding for example, conventional ventilation with a single-lumen endotracheal tube will probably be sufficient. Major trauma is associated with major hemorrhage, large bore intravenous cannula and invasive blood pressure monitoring should be obtained immediately. Central venous access and invasive hemodynamic monitoring may also be useful for the management of resuscitation in some cases, especially in the presence of severe coexisting cardiopulmonary disease. If available, consideration should be given to the use of autotransfusion techniques. Hemorrhagic shock should not be treated primarily with vasopressors, sodium bicarbonate, or continued crystalloid infusion, but with cross-matched packed red blood cells (PRBCs) or O-negative blood to maintain adequate oxygen-carrying capacity.

20.10 Cardiac Tamponade

Severe pressure on the heart leads to cardiac compromise, which is predominantly found in penetrating trauma while less commonly seen with blunt trauma. The pericardial sac is tough, fibrous, and even a volume of 75–100 ml may cause tamponade. The classic Beck's triad (JVD, hypotension and muffled heart sounds) are only present in one-third of the patients. While Kussmaul's sign (rise in central venous pressure with inspiration) is reliable, it is not practical in the trauma setting since few patients have a central line in place before the diagnosis is made. Diagnosis can be made in case of persistent hypotension without obvious blood loss. Rapid evaluation and instant diagnosis of trauma patient give advantage with e-FAST [11]. In a stable patient TEE evaluation [12] can also be conducted. Once the diagnosis is confirmed, aggressive fluid management is done until the definitive treatment is ensured. In case of myocardial injury, cardiopulmonary bypass may be required [13]. Though it is of great challenge to give heparin in bleeding cases, but it is mandatory to administer to avoid clot-related thromboembolism. Repair of moving myocardium is not easy, and to facilitate the repair, the myocardium can be made still for a very brief period with adenosine [14].

20.11 Chest Wall—Rib, Clavicle, and Sternum Injuries

Rib fractures are present in at least 10% patients who present with trauma, and in up to 94% of patients associated with serious injuries including pneumothorax, hemothorax, and lung contusion [15]. Injuries of multiple ribs, first and second rib fractures, and injuries of the clavicle and scapula are usually associated with high-energy mechanisms of injury and should raise awareness about the possibility of serious intra-abdominal and thoracic injuries, e.g., aortic transection and rupture of major vessels.

In the absence of flail chest physiology (see next section), the most significant consequences of rib and sternal fractures are usually related to severe pain and the associated effects on pulmonary function. Particularly in the elderly, inadequate pain control can lead to significant morbidity and mortality, usually from pneumonia because of impaired coughing and clearance of secretions.

20.12 Chest Wall—Flail Chest

A flail chest is the result of comminuted fractures of two or more adjacent ribs at two or more places, anteriorly and posteriorly. The fourth to ninth ribs are most commonly involved. The susceptibility to rib fracture increases with age and with the force of impact of trauma. The injured portion of the chest wall demonstrates paradoxical movement with inspiration which means the segment moves *inward with inspiration*, and *outward with exhalation*. This pattern of movement occurs due to the flail segment being mechanically separated from the chest wall and its movement becomes dependent upon the changes in pleural pressure during spontaneous respiration.

20.13 Clinical Features

Rib fracture is often a clinical diagnosis, when there is point tenderness, bony crepitus, ecchymosis, and muscle spasm over the injured rib. Also, bimanual compression of the thoracic cage away from the site of injury (barrel compression test) normally produces pain at the fracture site. Injury to the parenchyma may be detected by assessing the respiratory rate, oxyhemoglobin saturation, respiratory effort, effectiveness of ventilation, and pulmonary sounds.

Adverse Effects of Rib Fracture
- Tachypnoea, restlessness, air hunger
- Impaired cough and clearance of secretions
- Increased incidence of pneumonia and sepsis
- Atelectasis and hypoxia
- Reduced functional residual capacity
- Increased work of breathing due to chest wall instability
- Increased myocardial O_2 demand

Management of Pain Due to Rib Fracture
- Analgesics—NSAIDs/systemic opioids
- Intercostal nerve blocks
- Single-injection or continuous paravertebral blocks
- Intrapleural administration of local anesthetics
- Continuous epidural catheters

20.14 Analgesics

Adequate analgesia is important in all patients with thoracic trauma for good inspiration. Inadequate analgesia and fear of pain may cause atelectasis and other related problems.

NSAIDs The role of NSAID is limited due to their side effects, but may be use IV paracetamol. Diclofenac sodium injection administered in a dose of 1 mg/kg, may have long-term side effects like impaired renal function, inhibition of platelet aggregation and GI tract ulceration and perforation.

Opioids The main advantage of parenteral opioids in the management of rib fracture pain is absence of a need for regional analgesic intervention and the associated risks of bleeding, infection, or pneumothorax. However, the usual problems of respiratory and CNS depression related to their administration and the relative inferiority to regional techniques limit the utility of systemic opioids for the treatment of multiple rib fractures. If a regional technique is not feasible (coagulopathy, localized/systemic infection, limitation of patient positioning), patients can be managed adequately with an intravenous (IV) narcotic either as a continuous infusion, intermittent IV dosing, or in the form of a patient controlled analgesia (PCA) technique [16]. The PCA technique is superior to the other technique as pain threshold varies from patient to patient.

Intercostal Nerve Blocks (ICNB) It is a simple and universally practiced technique for the management of rib fractures. The main disadvantage of intercostal nerve blocks is higher blood levels of local anesthetics per block volume. There is also a risk of pneumothorax during the procedure and this block provides relief for a brief duration.

Continuous Thoracic Paravertebral Block (TPB) Is effective for unilateral analgesia and may be technically easier than a continuous epidural catheter. Continuous TPB may be associated with fewer hemodynamic changes, but increased serum levels of local anesthetic and systemic toxicity are possible. The infusion of a local anesthetic solution into the pleural space with a percutaneously placed catheter is also an effective technique [17].

The use of *intrapleural analgesia (IPA)* was described for patients' pain relief in multiple rib fractures [18]. The technique probably results in a unilateral, multilevel intercostal nerve block. There is also the concern that accumulation of the solution on the diaphragm could result in impaired diaphragmatic function and respiratory compromise. Further, there is the possibility of inadvertent removal of the solution by an ipsilateral chest tube that may be in place. IPA can result in high plasma concentrations of local anesthetics that could lead to systemic toxicity.

20.15 Continuous Thoracic Epidural Analgesia (TEA)

Although this modality of analgesia is superior to that achieved with systemic opioids and IPA, [19, 20] with the drawback that it is technically difficult and needs highly skilled personal and expertise. Local anesthetics with or without the addition of opioids may be used. TEA results in superior pulmonary function in terms of functional residual capacity, lung compliance, arterial PO_2, and airway resistance [21]. Patients treated with TEA helps in early weaning from mechanical ventilation, shorter ICU stays, and shorter hospitalization. The addition of opioids to the epidural solution can result in pruritus, nausea, vomiting, urinary retention, and rarely respiratory suppression but are less severe when compared with IV opioid administration.

The specific analgesic modality used in a given patient depends on many variables including the anesthesiologist's preference and skill, the preference of the thoracic or trauma surgeon, and the limitations of the institution's infrastructure and nursing capabilities. For any patient with acute pain resulting from chest wall injury, multimodal analgesia including the above methods with the addition of nonsteroidal anti-inflammatory drugs (NSAIDs), low-dose ketamine infusion, transcutaneous electrical nerve stimulation (TENS), anticonvulsant drugs, and pain specialist consultation should be considered early during the course of treatment.

20.16 Management of Flail Chest

Management of the flail chest thus no longer focuses primarily on surgical stabilization of the segment, but instead is concerned with the management of associated pain and lung injury which can result in decreased FRC and vital capacity (VC) and significant V/Q mismatch. Indeed, the management should be similar to that of any patient with multiple rib fractures assuming that the segment is not so large that its negative impact on spontaneous ventilation necessitates endotracheal intubation and mechanical ventilation. The management of the patient with flail chest may ultimately be determined by the extent and severity of coexisting injuries. In the setting of multiple severe intrathoracic or intracranial injuries, the patient will likely remain intubated and mechanically ventilated until these injuries are addressed or stabilized. Conversely, in the absence of other significant injuries, the patient may be successfully managed with parenteral narcotics or TEA, and the use of noninvasive positive pressure ventilation (NIPPV), which avoids the complications of endotracheal intubation and is showing promise for those patients who still require supportive ventilation. Historically, reduction and fixation for rib fractures have met with resistance and failure. Traditional management since the early trials of rib traction and wiring has yielded more complications and morbidity than success and relief. Newer devices attempt to be specific to ribs and even specific to rib size and side of the chest.

Rib stabilization is important for relief from intractable pain leading to failure to wean from mechanical ventilation, repeated trauma and chest wall instability leading to intubation, pneumonia, and failure to thrive. Newer techniques and devices have shown promise and several trauma centers have ongoing trials looking at length of stay (LOS), duration of mechanical ventilation, ICU stay, and amount of narcotic use. A few prospective studies have demonstrated significant improvement in LOS, and decreased duration of mechanical ventilation. Rib stabilization has appeared to improve patient comfort and decrease morbidity.

20.17 Conclusion

Patient with thoracic injury must be evaluated rapidly with quick diagnosis. Rapid intervention and adequate analgesia is the key to successful outcome.

References

1. Bergen G, Chen LH, Warner M, et al. Injury in the United States: 2007 Chartbook. Hyattsville, MD: National Center for Health Statistics; 2008.
2. Fingerhaut LA, Warner M. Injury Chartbook. Health, United States, 1996–1997. Hyattsville, MD: National Center for Health Statistics; 1998.
3. National Center for Injury Prevention and Control. Available from: http://webappa.cdc.gov/sasweb/ncipc/leadcaus10.html Atlanta, GA. Accessed 30 June 2009.
4. Moloney JT, Fowler SJ, Chang W. Anesthetic management of thoracic trauma. Curr Opin Anaesthesiol. 2008;21(1):41–6.
5. Orliaguet G, Ferjani M, Riou B. The heart in blunt trauma. Anesthesiology. 2001;95(2):544–8.
6. Gerhardt MA, Gravlee GP. Anesthesia considerations for cardiothoracic trauma. In: Smith CE, editor. Trauma anesthesia. Cambridge, New York: Cambridge University Press; 2008. p. 279–99.
7. DePalma RG, Burris DG, Champion HR, et al. Blast injuries. N Engl J Med. 2005;352(13):1335–42.
8. American College of Surgeons. Committee on Trauma. Advanced trauma life support program for doctors: ATLS. 7th ed. Chicago, IL: American College of Surgeons; 2004.
9. Herzig D, Biffl WL. Thoracic trauma. In: Fink MP, editor. Textbook of critical care. 5th ed. Philadelphia, PA: Elsevier Saunders; 2005. p. 2077–87.
10. Casos SR, Richardson JD. Role of thoracoscopy in acute management of chest injury. Curr Opin Crit Care. 2006;12(6):584–9.
11. Rozycki GS, Feliciano DV, Ochsner MG, et al. The role of ultrasound in patients with possible penetrating cardiac wounds: a prospective multicenter study. J Trauma. 1999;46:543–51.
12. Kirkpatrick AW, Ball CG, D'Armours SK, et al. Acute resuscitation of the unstable adult trauma patient: bedside diagnosis and therapy. Can J Surg. 2008;5(1):57–69.
13. Hakuba T, Minato N, Minematsu T, et al. Surgical management and treatment of traumatic right atrial rupture. Gen Thorac Cardiovasc Surg. 2008;56(11):551–4.
14. Lim R, Gill IS, Temes RT, et al. The use of adenosine for repair of penetrating cardiac injuries: a novel method. Ann Thorac Surg. 2001;71:1714–5.
15. Ziegler DW, Agarwal NN. The morbidity and mortality of rib fractures. J Trauma. 1994;37(6):975–9.
16. Karmakar MK, Ho AM. Acute pain management of patients with multiple fractured ribs. J Trauma. 2003;54(3):615–25.
17. Reiestad F, Kvalheim L. Continuous intercostal nerve block for postoperative pain relief. Tidsskr Nor Laegeforen. 1984;104(7):485–7.
18. Rocco A, Reiestad F, Gudman J, et al. Intrapleural administration of local anaesthetics for pain relief in patients with multiple rib fractures: preliminary report. Reg Anesth. 1987;12(1):10–4.
19. Moon MR, Luchette FA, Gibson SW, et al. Prospective, randomized comparison of epidural versus parenteral opioid analgesia in thoracic trauma. Ann Surg. 1999;229(5):684–91. Discussion 691–682
20. Luchette FA, Radafshar SM, Kaiser R, et al. Prospective evaluation of epidural versus intrapleural catheters for analgesia in chest wall trauma. J Trauma. 1994;36(6):865–9. Discussion 869–870
21. Dittmann M, Keller R, Wolff G. A rationale for epidural analgesia in the treatment of multiple rib fractures. Intensive Care Med. 1978;4(4):193–7.

Part III

Postoperative Management

General Principles of Postoperative Care

21

Bimla Sharma and Samia Kohli

21.1 Introduction

Postoperative care of patients undergoing thoracic surgery aims at early recovery and preventing pulmonary and other complications. The patients may be observed postoperatively in the post-anesthesia recovery room (PACU) to monitor the vital signs or else may be admitted to the high dependency unit (HDU) or an intensive care unit (ICU) for highly specialized therapeutic approach, necessitating cardiorespiratory and other organs support.

Patient, procedure-related risk factors, availability of equipment and personnel of the organization determine the ideal place for postoperative observation, monitoring or therapeutic intervention. However, this initial assessment may be modified by intraoperative complications. The need for intensive postoperative monitoring, postoperative risks and complications can be significantly reduced by maintaining high standards of care during anesthetic management. The current tendency is to keep many high-risk patients in HDUs or adequately staffed and equipped PACUs rather than the ICUs [1].

21.2 Post-anesthesia Care Unit

The tracheas of the majority of healthy patients are extubated in the operation theatre and then the patients are transferred to the PACU to recover from the effects of anesthesia and surgery. The PACU is an important area where timely recognition of any adverse event and its prompt treatment helps in preventing serious morbidity and mortality.

Here, patients are monitored for level of consciousness, spontaneous breathing rate and pattern, SpO_2, temperature, urine output and pain intensity. They are also counselled and encouraged to breathe deeply. Close attention should be paid to patients with hoarseness and whispering voice which may result from recurrent laryngeal nerve injury. In such cases, evaluation by direct laryngoscopy or fibrescopy is necessary, to rule out recurrent laryngeal nerve injury, as these patients are prone to aspiration postoperatively leading to multiorgan dysfunction and sepsis. Phrenic nerve injury may present as shortness of breath on exertion and impaired exercise tolerance. This may remain unnoticed and may not be detected in the early postoperative period [2].

The patients are transferred to the ward when they are haemodynamically stable and have adequate oxygenation with minimal oxygen requirement. They should also be able to cough out secretions, have unlaboured breathing and experience minimal or no postoperative pain.

B. Sharma (✉) · S. Kohli
Institute of Anaesthesiology, Pain and Perioperative Medicine, Sir Ganga Ram Hospital, New Delhi, India

21.2.1 Monitoring Patients with Respiratory Insufficiency

Meticulous monitoring is necessary to identify early warning of significant changes in a patient's condition so that therapeutic interventions can be applied as soon as possible. An ideal monitoring system is sensitive, accurate, reproducible and simple to apply; should be relevant and measure useful variables. Its use should be cost-effective and not be accompanied by any morbidity. Apart from SpO_2, ECG and BP monitoring, clinical observations such as respiratory rate and pattern, use of accessory muscles, respiratory distress and alterations in level of consciousness are all important indicators of respiratory function and are of great significance. Arterial blood gas analysis is another important tool as it provides a quantitative index of respiratory function.

21.3 High Dependency Unit (HDU) and Intensive Care Unit (ICU)

Patients undergoing major thoracic procedures, especially those subjected to extensive surgical resection, require stringent monitoring and cardiorespiratory support. They may, therefore, be shifted directly to HDU or an ICU where the emphasis is on rapid haemodynamic stabilization, complete relief of postoperative pain control and judicious fluid administration. Steps are taken to provide specific manoeuvers which increase lung volume, facilitate early mobilization and thus prevent postoperative pulmonary complications.

Routine extubation immediately after surgery is recommended in the current practice in thoracic surgery but a number of patients will still require postoperative management in an ICU. These are the patients that are not extubated in the operation theatre but are transferred to the ICU. This subset of patients are those that have preoperative comorbidities or critically reduced functional reserve that predict more intensive postoperative management or the extensive nature of surgical access demands it [3].

Efforts have been made to develop a risk score for patients undergoing major lung resection and requiring direct ICU admission post surgery. A multicenter investigation analyzed the risk factors for a patient scheduled for major lung resection. The factors included patients above the age of 65 and those scheduled for pneumonectomy. Other risks to be included were patients' cardiac comorbidity and those with predicted postoperative carbon monoxide capacity less than 50% and postoperative forced expiratory volume in 1 second of less than 65% [4]. In the ICU, these patients may require invasive or noninvasive postoperative ventilation, invasive monitoring and management of metabolic disturbances.

21.4 Preoperative Optimization

Age exceeding 75 years, BMI more than 30 kg/m^2, ASA physical status more than III, current smoking history, preoperative pulmonary function tests, cardiovascular comorbidity and chronic obstructive pulmonary disease (COPD) are some of the identified risk factors which cause postoperative pulmonary complications [5–9].

21.4.1 Smoking

Smoking should be stopped preoperatively since the period of cessation of smoking is directly related to reduction of the risk of developing postoperative pulmonary complications. There is a decrease in the concentration of carboxyhaemoglobin with stoppage of smoking for more than 12 hours [10]. Ceasing smoking for more than 4 weeks prior to surgery decreases postoperative pulmonary complications in patients undergoing thoracic surgery [11]. Even in those patients who were operated for lung neoplasms and had stopped smoking for less than 8 weeks prior to surgery, there was no increase in postoperative pulmonary complications [12]. Smoking in the postoperative period should also be avoided as it leads to prolonged tissue hypoxemia and affects wound healing.

21.4.2 Preoperative Rehabilitation (PR)

Prehabilitation (PR) is a process started preoperatively and is aimed at improving recovery and surgical outcomes. It incorporates education, exercise and physiotherapy. In patients with COPD, this process could improve the quality of life post lung volume reduction surgery or lung transplantation by improving exercise tolerance and symptoms of respiratory impairment and thus decrease the postoperative problems in these patients [13–15].

21.5 Enhanced Recovery After Surgery (ERAS) [16–18]

Enhanced recovery after surgery (ERAS) is an emerging concept in cardio-thoracic surgery [16, 17]. It is a goal-directed programme starting preoperatively and extending till the patient is discharged from the hospital. Apart from focussing on preoperative assessment, early mobilization management, prevention of postoperative pain, nausea and vomiting, early return to oral feeding and routine tasks; incorporating regional anesthetic techniques as an adjunct to anesthesia and surgical technique employing minimally invasive techniques (VATS) are important components of ERAS in thoracic surgery [17, 18]. It offers several benefits such as early postoperative recovery and discharge from hospital, and decreasing the occurrence of chronic pain following surgery. However, the effective protocols for its operation to obtain the preferred results are being developed.

21.6 Postoperative Care

21.6.1 Postoperative Nausea and Vomiting (PONV)

PONV has an overall incidence of 20–30%, in patients undergoing surgery under general anesthesia and it negatively affects patient satisfaction. This may invariably lead to complications like Boerhaave syndrome, airway compromise and emphysema [19]. Susceptibility to PONV is higher in females, young patients, non-smokers, patients with a history of motion sickness or PONV. Use of intraoperative volatile anesthetics or nitrous oxide, lengthy anesthesia and use of opioids postoperatively are the independent predictors of PONV. A multimodal approach is recommended for PONV prevention.

21.6.2 Postoperative Arrhythmias

Cardiac arrhythmias may occur postoperatively and are generally self-limiting and often under-reported. However, they may predispose the patients to increased perioperative morbidity and mortality. Major noncardiac thoracic surgeries may be associated with a 10–20% incidence of atrial arrhythmias. Advanced age, extensive surgical procedures, male gender, advanced tumours and intraoperative blood transfusions are predisposing factors for the development of AF [20, 21]. There is an increased incidence of AF with right-sided pneumonectomy and it is an independent risk factor for development of ventricular tachycardia [22].

Cardiac parasympathetic fibres may be injured during surgery with a resultant higher sympathetic tone leading to supraventricular arrhythmias. The right-sided heart pressures may also increase owing to a decline in pulmonary vascular bed volume and reactive pulmonary vasoconstriction [23, 24].

The majority of patients undergoing thoracic surgery probably do not receive pharmacologic prophylaxis for postoperative AF; however, digoxin, flecainide, verapamil, beta blockers, amiodarone and diltiazem have been used with mixed results [25].

21.6.3 Postoperative Analgesia

Thoracic surgical procedures result in severe pain, exemplified by a posterolateral incision thoracotomy. Postoperative pulmonary complications may follow inadequately treated pain, due to impaired sputum clearance and reduced ventilatory capacity [26]. Patients may also experience post-surgery chronic pain [27]. However, there has been a significant decline in postoperative complications like atelectasis, pneumonia and respiratory failure in the first three postoperative days with the provision of adequate pain relief in this period [28, 29].

Use of minimally invasive techniques like video-assisted thoracic surgery (VATS), muscle sparing incisions, reduction or abolition of rib spreading, minimal intercostal nerve compression and muscle retraction during open thoracotomies result in decreased pain scores and minimal use of postoperative analgesics [30, 31].

The major sensory afferent inputs following thoracic surgery are from the incision site, chest drains and ipsilateral shoulder, transmitted by intercostal nerves, vagus nerve, phrenic nerve and the brachial plexus, respectively [32]. Therefore, multimodal analgesia working at different sites with different mechanisms of action is required to produce effective pain relief. The choice of a particular technique will be governed by several factors such as the patient's choice, nature of surgery, availability of drugs, infrastructure and equipment.

Opioids, non-steroidal anti-inflammatory agents (NASIDs), paracetamol and local anesthetics are the most widely administered analgesics in the PACU [33]. Pregabalin and opioids are helpful in the management of post-thoracic surgery shoulder pain which may not respond to epidural analgesia [34, 35]. Dexmedetomidine and ketamine have also been tried recently.

Thoracic epidural at T4 to T8 levels is considered the gold standard for providing postoperative pain relief in patients undergoing thoracic surgery. However, local site infection and patients on anticoagulants are contraindications for administration of epidural analgesia. The most common side effects of epidural anesthesia are hypotension and urinary retention. Spinal hematoma is a rare but disastrous complication of epidural anesthesia.

Liposomal bupivacaine, is a new agent which when administered by the transcutaneous or intrathoracic routes along with regular bupivacaine and a non-narcotic oral pain regimen, offers several advantages over epidural analgesia. The surgeon can administer the drug intraoperatively without the need of a pain team or continuous catheter infusion in the postoperative period. The technique allows early ambulation with limited narcotic use. The analgesia provided by liposomal bupivacaine is better than that produced by shorter acting agents and comparable to thoracic epidural in a small number of patients [36, 37].

21.6.4 Fluid Management

Restricting intraoperative fluids to 6 mL/kg/hour reduces the risk of development of injury to the lung and complications like atelectasis, pneumonia and empyema. This is the outcome of a decrease in pulmonary hydrostatic pressure [38–41].

The benefits of conservative fluid over liberal fluid management have also been shown in mechanically ventilated patients who have acute lung injury (ALI) or acute respiratory distress syndrome (ARDS) in the form of superior oxygenation and earlier weaning from ventilator [42]. At present there is inconclusive RCT-based evidence to support the conservative or "zero-balance" approach [43].

Postoperatively, there is weight gain resulting from fluid administration and retention of salt and water, a consequence of ADH release and activation of the hypothalamo-sympathoadrenal axis and the renin-angiotensin-aldosterone system stimulated by surgical stress. Restrictive fluid strategy would limit this weight gain. The combination of restricted fluids and vasopressors is often necessary to achieve a "zero balance" and offset the vasodilatory actions of anesthesia and/thoracic epidural blockade, thus maintaining an equilibrium with stable haemodynamic variables and normovolemia. A euvolemic state is also aided by allowing the patient to take carbohydrate drinks up to 2 hours before commencing surgery [44].

Insensible fluid loss via the airways and from the exposed surgical field as well as urine output and losses from the gastrointestinal tract can be replaced by intraoperative balanced crystalloids restricted to 3–4 ml/kg/h. Blood and other losses may require blood transfusion or colloids [45]. The third space is a result of the infusion of excessive administration of salt containing crystalloids and as such needs no fluid therapy. Vasopressors will counter any relative hypovolemia consequent upon anesthesia vasorelaxation. A zero-balance fluid approach with balanced salt crystalloid can be a part of the enhanced recovery programme [46].

21.6.5 Chest Drainage System

An adequate chest drainage aims to drain fluid and air and restores the negative pleural pressure facilitating lung expansion in the postoperative thoracic surgical patient [47]. The introduction of an electronic drainage system has significantly contributed to the advancement of thoracic surgery, as it has facilitated standardized management of chest tubes by applying continuous suction and quantifying the drained fluid and/or air from the thoracic cavity [48]. It is important that chest tube management pathways be developed as postoperative clinical pathways. This has led to improved care in the postoperative period with associated shorter hospital stay. The following points are important in the management of this clinical pathway: role of chest X-ray in patients undergoing lung resection with chest drains, selecting fluid output threshold for safe removal of chest tubes, determining whether suction should be applied or not and choosing the safest method for chest tube removal.

21.6.6 Physiotherapy

It is essential to provide physiotherapy routinely in post-thoracotomy patients to prevent and treat pulmonary and musculoskeletal complications [49]. Oedema, infection and retained secretions may lead to postoperative insufficiency and subsequent post-pulmonary complications. Postoperative pulmonary complications cause patient discomfort, prolonged hospital stay and increase patient care cost. These complications can be decreased in COPD patients with preoperative commencement of intensive chest physiotherapy [50, 51].

Various modalities such as coughing, deep breathing, incentive spirometry, positive end-expiratory pressure (PEEP) and continuous positive airway pressure (CPAP) are available for chest physiotherapy; however, there is no established best method. Incentive spirometry compared to standard physiotherapy, breathing exercises and coughing has shown no additional benefit in the enhanced recovery programme [52].

During the preoperative assessment, care takers can be instructed to perform effective preoperative chest physiotherapy intended to benefit COPD patients with severe disease by improving exercise tolerance. COPD patients with excessive sputum will also be benefitted by chest physiotherapy. Early postoperative ambulation and physiotherapy reduces complications like atelectasis, pneumonia, empyema and DVT.

Regular medical and nursing care should embrace early and frequent patient position changes in bed, early ambulation and frequent pain assessment. This intervention should include deep breathing and it is imperative to remove secretions from the airway. Coughing exercises promote distention of lung tissue, assist ambulation and progressive shoulder and thoracic cage mobility programme.

The functional capacity of a patient with severe COPD can be improved by a multifaceted approach of pulmonary rehabilitation. This includes a combination of healthy food intake, physiotherapy, exercise and educating the concerned individuals to follow the path to optimizing or lessening the pulmonary dysfunction caused by COPD [53]. Since these rehabilitation programmes are long-lasting their use in patients with resections for malignancy is doubtful. However, those with nonmalignant resections in patients with severe COPD, the rehabilitation programme can play a useful role. The benefits of short-duration rehabilitation programmes before malignancy resection have not been fully evaluated.

There is a screening tool for physiotherapy treatment which includes criteria to grade the patients as: at the highest risk for developing PPC and those at low risk [54].

Potential high-risk patients on screening for PPCs should be assessed either on day 0 or day 1 postoperatively by a physiotherapist and can be mobilized within hours of their surgery [55]. Each patient has a standardized mobilization plan that requires a minimum of 60 m walk 4 times a day on day one, 80 m on day two, 100 m on day three and then increasing this as per the patient's ability throughout the rest of their admission. Patients are encouraged to mobilize at a pace where they achieve breathlessness of 3–4 on the Borg ten-point scale [56].

Portable suction drains are used as a standard of care as they allow the patients to be mobile. A standard component of each physiotherapy session is pain assessment to optimize the patient's analgesia requirement. The use of airway clearance and lung recruitment techniques are indicated, e.g., active cycle of breathing (ACBT), IPPV, cough assist, manual technique and forced expiratory time. At the time of discharge, patients should be checked for their return to baseline functional level and are independent with chest clearance technique, shoulder and postural exercises. They are also provided written information about exercise schedules to be followed at home [57].

21.6.7 Deep Venous Thrombosis Prophylaxis

Venous thromboembolism (VTE) is a leading cause of morbidity and mortality in thoracic surgical patients who are at moderate risk of developing VTE postoperatively [58]. However, consensus regarding the best practices to reduce VTE occurrence is lacking. The incidence of established deep vein thrombosis (DVT) is 10–40% in surgical and general medical patients and 40–60% after major orthopaedic surgery in absence of thromboprophylaxis [59]. Pulmonary embolism is the most common cause of preventable hospital death and is significantly reduced by thromboprophylaxis [59, 60].

Low-dose unfractionated heparin (UFH) or low-molecular-weight heparin (LMWH) is recommended by the American College of Chest Physicians (ACCP) for in-hospital perioperative VTE prevention [58]. The patients are advised to wear compression stockings and in addition sequential compression devices should be provided for high-risk patients [61].

Preoperative thromboprophylaxis is recommended by the American Society of Clinical Oncology (ASCO) in all patients subjected to major oncosurgery and continued for at least 7–10 days postoperatively and its duration extended for high-risk abdominopelvic surgical cases [62].

The Caprini and other risk assessment models (RAMs) developed outside of thoracic surgery recommend compression devices, chemoprophylaxis with unfractionated heparin and low-appropriate prophylactic measures such as early mobilization and inpatient mechanical compression devices and low molecular-weight heparin, among other anticoagulants.

Despite improvements achieved by implementing modified RAMs in thoracic surgery services at individual institutions, there are currently no field-specific guidelines to solidify practices nationwide. As a result, there remains considerable variability regarding patient screening, risk stratification and VTE chemoprophylaxis practices. As most postoperative VTE occur after patient discharge, field-specific guidelines surrounding extended courses of chemoprophylaxis are needed.

21.6.8 Hypothermia

Seventy per cent of patients admitted to the anesthetic recovery room (PACU) have been reported to suffer from hypothermia which may be accompanied by 3–4 times increase in oxygen consumption as it is accompanied by intense vasoconstriction which impairs peripheral perfusion leading to metabolic acidosis [63]. Intraoperative hypothermia predisposes the patients to a threefold greater risk for ischaemic cardiac events for instance cardiac arrest, unstable angina pectoris and myocardial infarction [64].

Not only does perioperative hypothermia delay wound healing and haemostasis but it also results in higher postoperative transfusion rates [65, 66].

Elderly and female patients, ASA physical status classes III or IV, surgery beyond 2 hours duration or temperature below 26 °C (78.8 °F), low body weight, history of chronic endocrine diseases and intravenous administration of cold fluids are some of the contributory factors for development of postoperative hypothermia [61].

Hypothermia in the postoperative period may follow excessive heat loss due to exposure of the body surface to cold surroundings, mostly during open procedures with large incisions and disturbance of normal thermoregulatory mechanisms due to the effects of general anesthetic agents or regional anesthesia (e.g., TEA). General as well as epidural anesthesia decreases the vasoconstriction and shivering threshold. Hence, a combination of epidural and general anesthesia can promote perioperative hypothermia [62, 63]. Other risk factors are the extent and the length of the surgical procedure [64, 65].

Hypothermia may be effectively treated by active warming, especially forced air warming [66]. Clonidine, dexmedetomidine, meperidine, tramadol, ondansetron, granisetron and parecoxib are some of the drugs which have been reported to reduce postoperative shivering [67, 68].

21.7 Conclusion

The thoracic surgical patients may have several problems owing to preceding comorbidities and varying impaired respiratory function in the postoperative period leading to poor outcome in high-risk individuals. Postoperatively, the patients may be observed and managed in the PACU, HDU or in an ICU depending on the patient, nature of surgery and accompanying complications. Preoperative prehabilitation comprising optimization of the patient's comorbidities, giving up smoking and physiotherapy can go a long way in significantly reducing postoperative morbidity and mortality.

References

1. Kreienbühl L, Cassina T, Licker M. Where should I send my patient after the operation? In: Şentürk M, Sungur MO, editors. Postoperative Care in Thoracic Surgery. Cham: Springer; 2017. https://doi.org/10.1007/978-3-319-19908-5_2.
2. Anand Iyer, Sumit Yadav. Postoperative care and complications after thoracic surgery, Principles and practice of cardiothoracic surgery, Michael S. Firstenberg, IntechOpen. 2013 12 June. https://doi.org/10.5772/55351. Available from https://www.intechopen.com/books/principles-and-practice-of-cardiothoracic-surgery/postoperative-care-and-complications-after-thoracic-surgery.
3. Feltracco P, Serra E, Barbieri S, et al. Postoperative care of patients undergoing lung resection. J Anesthe Clinic Res. 2012;4:288. https://doi.org/10.4172/2155-6148.1000288.
4. Brunelli A, Ferguson MK, Rocco G, et al. A scoring system predicting the risk for intensive care unit admission for complications after major lung resection: a multicenter analysis. Ann Thorac Surg. 2008;86:213–8.
5. Agostini P, Cieslik H, Rathinam S, et al. Postoperative pulmonary complications following thoracic surgery: are there any modifiable risk factors? Thorax. 2010;65:815–8.
6. Stéphan F, Boucheseiche S, Hollande J, et al. Pulmonary complications following lung resection: a comprehensive analysis of incidence and possible risk factors. Chest. 2000;118:1263–70.
7. Brunelli A, Al Refai M, Monteverde M, et al. Stair climbing test predicts cardiopulmonary complications after lung resection. Chest. 2002;121(4):1106–10.
8. Bernard A, Deschamps C, Allen MS, et al. Pneumonectomy for malignant disease: factors affecting early morbidity and mortality. J Thorac Cardiovasc Surg. 2001;121:1076e82.
9. Licker MJ, Widikker I, Robert J, et al. Operative mortality and respiratory complications after lung resection for cancer: impact of chronic obstructive pulmonary disease and time trends. Ann Thorac Surg. 2006;81:1830–7.
10. Akrawi W, Benumof JL. A pathophysiological basis for informed preoperative smoking cessation counseling. J Cardiothorac Vasc Anesth. 1997;11:629.
11. Vaporciyan AA, Merriman KW, Ece F, et al. Incidence of major pulmonary complications after pneumonectomy; association with timing of smoking cessation. Ann Thorac Surg. 2002;73:420.
12. Barrera R, Shi W, Amar D, et al. Smoking and timing of cessation: impact on pulmonary complications after thoracotomy. Chest. 2005;127:1977.
13. Cooper JD, Trulock EP, Triantafillou AN, et al. Bilateral pneumonectomy (volume reduction) for chronic obstructive pulmonary disease. J Thorac Cardiovasc Surg. 1995;109:106–16.

14. Ries AL, Make BJ, Lee SM, et al. The effects of pulmonary rehabilitation in the national emphysema treatment trial. Chest. 2005;128:3799–809.
15. Mujovic N, Mujovic N, Subotic D, et al. Preoperative pulmonary rehabilitation in patients with non-small cell lung cancer and chronic obstructive pulmonary disease. Arch Med Sci. 2014;10:68–75.
16. Brunelli A. Enhanced recovery after surgery in thoracic surgery: the past, the present and the future. Video-assist Thorac Surg. 2017;2:37.
17. Crumley, Stefan Schraag. The role of local anaesthetic techniques in ERAS protocols for thoracic surgery. Seamus. J Thorac Dis. 2018;10(3):1998–2004.
18. D'Andrilli A, Rendina EA. Enhanced recovery after surgery (ERAS) and fast-track in video-assisted thoracic surgery (VATS) lobectomy: preoperative optimisation and care-plans. J Vis Surg. 2018;4:4.
19. Jokinen J, Smith AF, Roewer N, et al. Management of postoperative nausea and vomiting: how to deal with refractory PONV. Anesthesiol Clin. 2012 Sep;30(3):481–93.
20. Onaitis M, D'Amico T, Zhao Y, et al. Risk factors for atrial fibrillation after lung cancer surgery: analysis of the society of thoracic surgeons general thoracic surgery database. Ann Thorac Surg. 2010;90:368–74.
21. Vaporciyan AA, Correa AM, Rice DC, et al. Risk factors associated with atrial fibrillation after noncardiac thoracic surgery: analysis of 2588 patients. J Thorac Cardiovasc Surg. 2004;127:779–86.
22. Amar D, Zhang H, Roistacher N. The incidence and outcome of ventricular arrhythmias after noncardiac thoracic surgery. Anesth Analg. 2002;95:537–43.
23. Asamura H, Naruke T, Tsuchiya R, et al. What are the risk factors for arrhythmias after thoracic operations? A retrospective multivariate analysis of 267 consecutive thoracic operations. J Thorac Cardiovasc Surg. 1993;106:1104–10.
24. Amar D, Roistacher N, Burt M, et al. Clinical and echocardiographic correlates of symptomatic tachydysrhythmias after noncardiac thoracic surgery. Chest. 1995;108:349–54.
25. Creswell LL. The problem of atrial arrhythmias after noncardiac thoracic surgery. J Thorac Cardiovasc Surg. 2004;127(3):629–30.
26. Wenk M, Schug SA. Perioperative pain management after thoracotomy. Curr Opin Anaesthesiol. 2011 Feb;24(1):8–12.
27. Khelemsky Y, Noto CJ. Preventing post-thoracotomy pain syndrome. Mt Sinai J Med. 2012;79(1):133–9.
28. Slinger PD, Johnston MR. Preoperative assessment: an anesthesiologist's perspective. Thorac Surg Clin. 2005 Feb;15(1):11–25.
29. Licker MJ, Widikker I, Robert J, et al. Operative mortality and respiratory complications after lung resection for cancer: impact of chronic obstructive pulmonary disease and time trends. Ann Thorac Surg. 2006 May;81(5):1830–7.
30. Popping DM, Elia N, Marret E, et al. Protective effects of epidural analgesia on pulmonary compications after abdominal and thoracic surgery: a meta-analysis. Arch Surg. 2008;143:990–9.
31. Nomori H, Horio H, Naruke T, et al. What is the advantage of a thoracoscopic lobectomy over a limited thoracotomy procedure for lung cancer surgery? Ann Thorac Surg. 2001;72:879–84.
32. Scawn ND, Pennefather SH, Soorae A, et al. Ipsilateral shoulder pain after thoracotomy with epidural analgesia: the influence of phrenic nerve infiltration with lidocaine. Anesth Analg. 2001 Aug;93(2):260–4.
33. Buvanendran A, Kroin JS. Multimodal analgesia for controlling acute postoperative pain. Curr Opin Anaesthesiol. 2009 Oct;22(5):588–93.
34. Bunchungmongkol N, Pipanmekaporn T, Paiboonworachat S, et al. Incidence and risk factors associated with ipsilateral shoulder pain after thoracic surgery. J Cardiothorac Vasc Anesth. 2014 Aug;28(4):979–82.
35. Imai Y, Imai K, Kimura T, et al. Evaluation of postoperative pregabalin for attenuation of postoperative shoulder pain after thoracotomy in patients with lung cancer, a preliminary result. Gen Thorac Cardiovasc Surg. 2015 Feb;63(2):99–104.
36. Jackson SM, Whitlark JD. Pain control with liposomal bupivacaine after Thoracoscopies/thoracotomies. Ann Thorac Surg. 2015 Dec;100(6):2414–5.
37. Rice DC, Cata JP, Mena GE, et al. Posterior intercostal nerve block with liposomal bupivacaine: an alternative to thoracic epidural analgesia. Ann Thorac Surg. 2015 Jun;99(6):1953–60.
38. Zeldin RA, Normandin D, Landtwing D, et al. Postpneumonectomy pulmonary edema. J Thorac Cardiovasc Surg. 1984 Mar;87(3):359–65.
39. Alam N, Park BJ, Wilton A, et al. Incidence and risk factors for lung injury after lung cancer resection. Ann Thorac Surg. 2007 Oct;84(4):1085–91.
40. Brandstrup B, Tønnesen H, Beier-Holgersen R, et al. Danish study group on perioperative fluid therapy. Effects of intravenous fluid restriction on postoperative complications: comparison of two perioperative fluid regimens: a randomized assessor-blinded multicenter trial. Ann Surg. 2003;238(5):641–8.
41. Arslantas MK, Kara HV, Tuncer BB, et al. Effect of the amount of intraoperative fluid administration on postoperative pulmonary complications following anatomic lung resections. J Thorac Cardiovasc Surg. 2015 Jan;149(1):314–20.
42. National Heart, Lung, and Blood Institute Acute Respiratory Distress Syndrome (ARDS) Clinical Trials Network, Wiedemann HP, Wheeler AP, Bernard GR, et al. Comparison of two fluid-management strategies in acute lung injury. N Engl J Med. 2006 Jun 15;354(24):2564–75.
43. Chappell D, Jacob M, Hofmann-Kiefer K, et al. A rational approach to perioperative fluid management. Anesthesiology. 2008 Oct;109(4):723–40.
44. Awad S, Varadhan KK, Ljungqvist O, et al. A meta-analysis of randomized controlled trials on preoperative oral carbohydrate treatment in elective surgery. Clin Nutr. 2013 Feb;32(1):34–44.

45. Yates DR, Davies SJ, Milner HE, et al. Crystalloid or colloid for goal-directed fluid therapy in colorectal surgery. Br J Anaesth. 2014 Feb;112(2):281–9.
46. Gupta R, Gan TJ. Peri-operative fluid management to enhance recovery. Anaesthesia. 2016 Jan;71(Suppl 1):40–5.
47. George RS, Papagiannopoulos K. Advances in chest drain management in thoracic disease. J Thorac Dis. 2016 Feb;8(Suppl 1):S55–64.
48. Bertolaccini L, Rizzardi G, Terzi A. A golden key can open any door of new protocol: the use of continuous digital measurement for postoperative air leak. Interact Cardiovasc Thorac Surg. 2011 Jan;12(1):31.
49. Reeve J, Denehy L, Stiller K. The physiotherapy management of patients undergoing thoracic surgery: a survey of current practice in Australia and New Zealand. Physiother Res Int. 2007 Jun;12(2):59–71.
50. Zehr KJ, Dawson PB, Yang SC, et al. Standardized clinical care pathways for major thoracic cases reduce hospital costs. Ann Thorac Surg. 1998 Sep;66(3):914–9.
51. Warner DO. Preventing postoperative pulmonary complications: the role of the anesthesiologist. Anesthesiology. 2000 May;92(5):1467–72.
52. Borg GA. Psychophysical bases of perceived exertion. Med Sci Sports Exerc. 1982;14(5):377–81.
53. Kesten S. Pulmonary rehabilitation and surgery for end-stage lung disease. Clin Chest Med. 1997;18:174.
54. Baddeley RA. Physiotherapy for enhanced recovery in thoracic surgery. J Thorac Dis. 2016;8(Suppl1):S107–10.
55. Kaneda H, Saito Y, Okamoto M, et al. Early postoperative mobilization with walking at 4 hours after lobectomy in lung cancer patients. Gen Thorac Cardiovasc Surg. 2007;55:493–8.
56. Agostini P, Naidu B, Cieslik H, et al. Effectiveness of incentive spirometry in patients following thoracotomy and lung resection including those at high risk for developing pulmonary complications. Thorax. 2013;68:580–5.
57. Reeve JC, Nicol K, Stiller K, et al. Does physiotherapy reduces the incidence of postoperative pulmonary complications following pulmonary resection via open thoracotomy? A preliminary randomised single-blind clinical trial. Eur J Cardiothorac Surg. 2010;37:1158–67.
58. Gould MK, Garcia DA, Wren SM. Prevention of VTE in nonorthopedic surgical patients: antithrombotic therapy and prevention of thrombosis, 9th ed: American College of Chest Physicians Evidence-Based Clinical Practice Guidelines. Chest. 2012;141:e227S–e77S.
59. Bergqvist D, Angelli G, Cohen A. Duration of prophylaxis against venous thromboembolism with enoxaparin after surgery for cancer. N Engl J Med. 2002;346:975–80. https://doi.org/10.1056/NEJMoa012385.
60. Geerts WH, Bergqvist D, Pineo GF, et al. Prevention of venous thromboembolism: American College of Chest Physicians Evidence-Based Clinical Practice Guidelines (8th edition). Chest. 2008;133:381S–453S.
61. National Institute for Health and Care Excellence. Venous thromboembolism: reducing the risk for patients in hospital, Clinical Guideline CG92. Updated June 2015. Available from https://www.nice.org.uk/guidance/cg92, on September 5, 2017.
62. Lyman GH, Bohlke K, Khorana AA, et al. Venous thromboembolism prophylaxis and treatment in patients with cancer: American Society of Clinical Oncology clinical practice guideline update 2014. J Clin Oncol. 2015;33:654–6.
63. National Institute for Health and Clinical Excellence Inadvertent perioperative hypothermia: the management of inadvertent perioperative hypothermia in adults having surgery [Internet]. [cited Apr. 2008; Last updated Dec. 2016]. Available from https://www.nice.org.uk/guidance/cg65/evidence. Accessed 8 October 2016.
64. Frank SM, Fleisher LA, Breslow MJ, et al. Perioperative maintenance of normothermia reduces the incidence of morbid cardiac events. A randomized clinical trial. JAMA. 1997;277:1127–34.
65. Valeri CR, Feingold H, Cassidy G, et al. Hypothermia-induced reversible platelet dysfunction. Ann Surg. 1987;205:175–81.
66. Rajagopalan S, Mascha E, Na J, et al. The effects of mild perioperative hypothermia on blood loss and transfusion requirement. Anesthesiology. 2008;108:71–7.
67. Kiekkas P, Poulopoulou M, Papahatzi A, et al. Effects of hypothermia and shivering on standard PACU monitoring of patients. AANA J. 2005 Feb;73(1):47–53.
68. Lau LL, Hung CT, Chan CK, et al. Anaesthetic clinical indicators in public hospitals providing anaesthetic care in Hong Kong: prospective study. Hong Kong Med J. 2001;7:251–60.

Postoperative Management of Thoracic Surgery Patients: A Surgeon's Perspective

Belal Bin Asaf, Harsh Vardhan Puri, and Arvind Kumar

Postoperative care of thoracic surgical patient is extremely important for ensuring consistently good outcomes as most of these patients have a unique set of issues that need to be addressed effectively. Many of these patients are elderly and have borderline lung functions with one or more comorbidities. Several factors that influence patient recovery after thoracic surgery have been discussed in this chapter:

- The extent of lung resection—Wedge, Segmentectomy, Lobectomy, or Pneumonectomy
- Pain associated with incisions
- Alteration in the respiratory mechanics
- Decreased mobility
- Poor nutrition in the postoperative period

These factors if not adequately addressed lead to poor outcomes and must be managed with utmost care. It must be remembered that the perioperative care of a patient undergoing thoracic surgery is a team approach. The team is usually led in by a thoracic surgeon who has all the necessary information about patient's preoperative status, the intraoperative findings and the procedure done and the implication of the procedure in the postoperative period. The team must include an anesthesiologist, pain management specialist, specialty nurses, dietician, and a dedicated respiratory and physical therapist.

22.1 Preoperative Counseling and Preparation

The more you sweat in peace, the less you bleed in war
Norman Schwarzkopf

Effective postoperative management begins in the preoperative period itself. As the above quote demonstrates, the key to a successful outcome is effective preparation. Direct extrapolation of this principle to thoracic surgical patients is the key to a patient going home safely after surgery and in sound health.

Patients and their caretakers need to be effectively counseled prior to surgery regarding the expected course of their hospital stay and any possible deviations. Cykert et al. have shown that patients are most concerned about their physical disability following surgery [1]. Typical questions are about the number of days they need to be confined to a bed, whether they will be able to use the restroom independently and how many days they will require any kind of assistance. Very few patients are worried about death. Hence, it becomes essential for the surgical team to allay these fears and answer the above questions satisfactorily.

B. B. Asaf (✉) · H. V. Puri · A. Kumar
Department of Thoracic Surgery, Sir Ganga Ram Hospital, New Delhi, India

Patients with comorbidities like chronic obstructive pulmonary disease (COPD), diabetes, and hypertension need to be medically optimized. Those with borderline pulmonary functions will benefit from preoperative rehabilitation program to increase the exercise tolerance and respiratory muscle strength. Preoperative pulmonary rehabilitation should be routinely employed for all patients undergoing lung volume reduction surgery [2, 3]. Preoperative counseling should also include smoking cessation, advice regarding diet, and also pre- and postoperative physical therapy.

22.2 Postoperative Management

Risk stratification is essential for good postoperative management. Even though there are no clear-cut criteria to define high-risk thoracic surgical patients, several scoring systems and their modifications have been applied by various studies. But these need to be validated on larger databases before being considered as standard. Factors such as age, comorbidities, type of procedure (pneumonectomy and three field esophagectomy are considered high risk), need for postoperative mechanical ventilation, and any intraoperative catastrophic event are taken into consideration to classify a patient as high risk. Low-risk patients are put into a fast track program and planned for early discharge.

22.2.1 Need for Intensive Care

In the earlier years nearly all patients undergoing a thoracic surgical procedure were shifted to an ICU in the immediate postoperative period. However, with advancement in the field of anesthesia and surgery, the requirement for ICU has reduced in the recent years. So, unlike a blanket rule of shifting all patients to ICU, a very selected group of patients require ICU. Most patients can be managed in a ward with adequate monitoring facilities. There is no need to shift all patients to ICU postoperatively, as this only increases costs and moreover it has been shown that shifting patients directly to a high dependency unit is safe and cost-effective [4].

As per the American College of Critical Care Medicine guidelines on selection criteria for admission to a High Dependency Unit (HDU) [5] and ICUs [6]:

- Admission to the HDU should be considered for hemodynamically stable patient after a major thoracic surgery who may require fluid resuscitation and monitoring by trained nurses.
- ICU admission is reserved for patients who require very close monitoring in view of hemodynamic instability or need for ventilatory support.

22.3 Medications in the Postoperative Period

Postoperative orders after a thoracic surgical procedure usually consist of analgesics, bronchodilators, antiemetics, proton pump inhibitors (PPI), and antibiotics when indicated.

22.3.1 Analgesics

Pain relief is an important aspect in thoracic surgical patients. Effective pain relief, apart from providing comfort to the patient, also ensures their participation in rehabilitation activities, which leads to better outcomes.

In patients who have undergone Video-Assisted Thoracic Surgery (VATS) and do not have an Epidural catheter in situ, we use Non-Steroidal Anti-Inflammatory Drugs (NSAIDs) round the clock for pain relief. In the initial 24 hours they are given intravenously and then converted to oral medications few days prior to discharge.

In patients who have undergone thoracotomy, an epidural catheter is used unless contraindicated. Epidural catheter is usually supplemented by NSAIDs to achieve total pain control.

A patient-controlled analgesia (PCA) pump is usually connected to the epidural catheter and the patients are counseled regarding their usage. The epidural catheter is usually removed by postoperative day 4.

Patients may sometimes develop ileus, constipation, and urinary retention, which may require premature removal of epidural catheter.

There are however a certain set of patients who do not achieve total pain relief with the above measures or in whom NSAIDs are contraindicated, in such patients we follow the WHO pain relief ladder and upgrade the analgesics as required. We usually upgrade to opioid-based medications such as tramadol and transdermal fentanyl patches.

Other methods of pain control include placing a paravertebral catheter intraoperatively to achieve a paravertebral block. Various authors have demonstrated that the paravertebral block avoids the side effects of an epidural catheter and gives equivalent pain relief [7].

As Savage and colleagues [8] have pointed out that there is no one standard rule for pain relief, the following factors must be considered before making any decision:

1. The physician's familiarity and experience with the particular method
2. The specific complication rate with the particular technique in the physician's hands
3. Presence of any contraindications to the particular method
4. The desired extent of pain control
5. Facilities available for monitoring and maintenance

Effective pain relief by whichever means necessary goes a long way in reducing the morbidity of thoracic surgery.

22.3.2 Antibiotics

As one of the largest chest surgical services in the Indian subcontinent, a fair proportion of our work is related to infectious diseases and hence our patients tend to already be on antibiotic therapy preoperatively.

Postoperatively the same antibiotics are continued till intraoperative culture reports are available and culture-specific therapy is started.

Antitubercular therapy is continued in the perioperative period. However, these drugs can cause severe gastritis and exacerbate the nausea and vomiting in the postoperative period, for which appropriate therapy is required and sometimes warrants modification of the antitubercular therapy in consultation with a chest physician. Regular monitoring of liver function test (LFT) is usually required for patients on ATT (antitubercular therapy).

In other patients, we strictly follow the guidelines issued by the Center for Disease Control (CDC), USA [9]. Usually a dose of prophylactic antibiotic (second-generation cephalosporin) is administered prior to induction and then stopped.

Antibiotics are restarted only when there is a clinical evidence of infection or sepsis and are strictly culture based.

22.3.3 Fluid Therapy

Thoracic surgical patients have been shown to be benefitted by having a Zero fluid balance [10]. In general giving too much fluids in postoperative patients has been shown to be associated with poor outcomes [11].

In patients who have undergone lung resections, giving 6–8 ml/kg/hr has been shown to have poor outcomes [12]. Not only does it lead to increased incidence of ALI/ARDS, but also associated with increased incidence of postoperative atelectasis and pneumonia [10].

Hence, it is advisable to individualize fluid therapy, based on the needs of the patient.

Pneumonectomy patients need special attention in this regard, as the possibility of developing post-pneumonectomy pulmonary edema is around 4% in most series [13]. Acute Respiratory Distress Syndrome (ARDS)/Postoperative Acute Lung Injury (PALI) can be life threatening with a reported mortality of >50% [14] and needs to be avoided at all costs. As per the recommendation based on a best evidence report, maintenance fluid administration should be kept restricted at 1–2 ml/kg/hour and a limit of 1.5 liter of positive balance must be ensured to prevent acute lung injury (ALI) and acute respiratory distress syndrome ARDS [15]. However, following a restrictive fluid approach can also be detrimental, it can sometimes lead to acute kidney injury, especially in patients whose renal functions are already compromised, and it can result in silent hypovolemia with impaired oxygen delivery [16]. In patients in whom this fluid limit is exceeded a high index of suspicion should be kept for ALI/ARDS and the patient should be shifted to HDU/ICU for close monitoring. If fluid restriction leads to symptoms of hypoperfusion in cases where the limit of fluid is reached, inotropic/vasopressor support should be considered [15].

22.3.4 DVT Prophylaxis

Death in hospitalized patients due to venous thrombo-embolism (VTE) is quite common and largely preventable. Higher age, presence of malignancy, and prolonged duration of surgery are the main risk factors for VTE. In a recent study by Mason et al., they demonstrated a DVT rate of 7.4% in patients undergoing Pneumonectomy [17]. Being a major surgery with most patients falling in high risk category for VTE, prophylaxis for thromboembolism should be used in all thoracic surgical patient.

As per American College of Chest Physician (ACCP) guidelines [18], all patients planned for pneumonectomy, extra-pleural pneumonectomy, or esophagectomy are at higher risk for VTE. It is recommended to use a Low Dose Un-Fractionated Heparin (LDUH)/Low Molecular Weight Heparin (LMWH) for patients who are at either moderate or high risk of VTE. In case of procedures with high risk of postoperative bleeding ACCP recommends use of mechanical prophylaxis over no prophylaxis till such time that the bleeding risk diminishes and pharmacological prophylaxis can be initiated.

In author's practice, a combination of mechanical prophylaxis and pharmacological methods are utilized for prevention of DVT. All patients receive a single dose of LMWH on the night before surgery and Intermittent Pneumatic Compression (IPC) during the surgery. All patients are encouraged for early ambulation. Postoperatively, low molecular weight heparin is continued till discharge.

22.4 Postoperative Rehabilitation/Physical Therapy

The importance of physiotherapy in thoracic surgical patients cannot be overemphasized enough. It constitutes the keystone to an early complication-free recovery and discharge.

With the application of Enhanced Recovery After Surgery (ERAS) protocols to thoracic surgical patients in recent times, there has been a trend toward early discharge of selected patients [19]. Usually these patients are made to ambulate 4–6 hours after surgery.

Aggressive physical therapy in the postoperative period has been conclusively shown to improve outcomes. In 2005 Varela and colleagues demonstrated that early ambulation, incentive spirometry, and assisted coughing techniques resulted in lower morbidity and early discharge from hospital [20].

Retention of secretions can cause atelectasis and pneumonia in patients who have undergone thoracic surgical procedures; this is commonly seen in patients who were smokers, elderly patients, and patients not able to cough due to pain [19]. Early ambulation has multiple beneficial effects; it gives a sense of confidence to the patient, prevents venous thromboembolism, and also assists in clearance of secretions from the airways [21].

The goal of our exercise program is for the patient to attain mild breathlessness. We subject our patients, under the supervision of a trained chest physiotherapist, to walk on the treadmill, if feasible on the day of surgery itself. In fragile patients, we follow a graded approach and slowly increase the intensity of the exercises over time.

We also teach them deep breathing techniques and assisted coughing to bring out the secretions. Usually, support is given at the incision site using a hard pillow and patient is asked to cough forcefully.

Active chest physiotherapy techniques such as manual percussions over the chest wall and positional drainage are employed in selected patients as and when required.

This exercise regimen is continued at home, after discharge also and patients are encouraged to continue exercising for as long as possible.

Based on our experience, this aggressive regimen has resulted in excellent postoperative outcomes.

22.5 Postoperative Nutrition

As we operate on a significant number of undernourished patients, especially patients who have been suffering from chronic forms of tuberculosis, we pay close and extra attention to their nutritional requirements.

Most of our patients, except patients who have undergone esophageal and tracheal procedures, are started on a normal diet, 6–8 hours postoperatively, if they are able to tolerate it. We recommend a high calorie–high protein diet.

A high protein and calorie intake ensures effective wound healing and is also able to effectively mitigate the stress of surgery, which tends to push the body into a catabolic phase in the immediate postoperative period [22].

Our dieticians individualize nutritional therapy for our patients, and provide them with a personalized diet chart, which needs to be strictly adhered to. In case patients are not able to adhere to the diet, either due to inability to take orally secondary to nausea or vomiting or due to severe loss of appetite, we do not hesitate to insert a nasogastric tube and start enteral feeds.

Total Parenteral Nutrition is rarely used in our patients; in exceptional cases, when the need arises, we use a central line with strict aseptic precautions and we try and use it for as short a period as possible.

22.6 Management of Chest Drainage Systems

The traditional underwater seal is a simple device and easy to manage and most of the hospital staff are trained to handle it. There are certain precautions to be taken, such as not to clamp the chest tube while shifting the patient and keeping the underwater seal bottle upright and below the waist level at all times. Daily output and presence or absence of air leak is noted.

Most of our patients, after lung resections, have their intercostal tubes connected to Digital Negative suction devices (Thopaz, Medela). These devices have the capability to maintain the thoracic cavity at a set negative pressure and also are able to quantify the air leak. These devices require special attention and care. The pressure to be set on the device is decided by the consulting physician, depending upon various factors, such as type of surgery performed, the need to achieve complete lung expansion, and the overall condition of the patient.

Use of these digital devices have shown to reduce the duration of chest tubes in patients with persistent air leak [23]. Removal of chest tubes generally occurs when there is complete lung expansion, no air leak for at least 24 hours and drainage is not hemorrhagic and less than 200 ml/day.

22.7 Management of Some Common Postoperative Complications

Postoperative Atelectasis/Pneumonia Effective chest physiotherapy results in prevention as well as resolution of atelectasis. But in certain susceptible patients, who are unable to clear their secretions a flexible fiberoptic bronchoscopy may be required for pulmonary toilet, which not only effectively clears secretions, but also acquires samples for culture.

Cardiac Arrythmias The commonest arrythmia seen after general thoracic surgery is atrial fibrillation and is more common in patients who have preexisting cardiovascular disease and in diabetics [24]. The Society of Thoracic Surgeons has issued guidelines in 2011 for management of perioperative atrial fibrillation [25]. The main recommendations have been summarized here.

Perioperative Prophylaxis
- In patients on beta blockers prior to surgery, it should be continued postoperatively to avoid beta blocker withdrawal.
- In cases with low serum magnesium levels supplementation with intra venous magnesium should be considered to prevent atrial fibrillation.
- Diltiazem in patients who are not on beta blockers should be considered in intermediate to high risk patients.
- Amiodarone used in the postoperative settings was deemed reasonable in intermediate and high-risk patients undergoing lung surgery or esophagectomy.

22.8 Management of Postoperative Atrial Fibrillation

- Catecholaminergic agents being used as inotropes should be reduced or stopped wherever possible.
- Normal fluid electrolyte balance should be ensured.
- Identification and correction of possible triggering factors like bleeding, pulmonary embolism, pneumothorax, cardiac ischemia or infection/sepsis.
- Electrical cardioversion is recommended for patients with hemodynamic instability or patients with myocardial infarction or ischemia.
- Hemodynamic instability includes those with hypotension, shock, or pulmonary edema.
- Anticoagulation should not be given prior to DC cardioversion, but should be initiated as soon as possible and continued for 4 weeks.
- The drug of choice is amiodarone infusion—for treatment of atrial fibrillation, it is usually given intravenously for a short period and then tapered off.
- Anticoagulation is mandatory in all patients who have developed an episode of postoperative atrial fibrillation, lasting 48 hours or more.
- Anticoagulation is usually continued for 4 weeks postoperatively.

Prolonged Air Leak Air leak lasting for more than 5 days is termed as persistent air leak as per the Ottawa Thoracic Morbidity and Mortality Classification [26] these patients require prolonged chest tube drainage attached to negative suction device. Most air leaks settle down with conservative management and rarely require any intervention.

22.9 Conclusion

Effective postoperative care requires coordination between team members and nursing staff in the ward. So, all channels of communication must be kept active. All team members must have a designated role in the management of the patient, there should be regular team meetings and audit to identify any failure or pitfalls in the system to ensure timely remedial measures.

References

1. Cykert S, Kissling G, Hansen CJ. Patient preferences regarding possible outcomes of lung resection: what outcomes should preoperative evaluations target? Chest. 2000;117:1551.
2. Ries AL, Make BJ, Lee SM, et al. The effects of pulmonary rehabilitation in the National Emphysema Treatment Trial. Chest. 2005;128:3799–809.
3. Bartels MN, Kim H, Whiteson JH, et al. Pulmonary rehabilitation in patients undergoing lung volume reduction surgery. Arch Phys Med Rehabil. 2006;87(3 Suppl. 1):s84–8.
4. Schweizer A, Khatchatourian G, Höhn L, et al. Opening of a new postanesthesia care unit: impact on critical care utilization and complications following major vascular and thoracic surgery. J Clin Anesth. 2002;14:486.

5. Nasraway SA, Cohen IL, Dennis RC, et al. Guidelines on admission and discharge for adult intermediate care units. American College of Critical Care Medicine of the Society of Critical Care Medicine. Crit Care Med. 1998;26:607.
6. Guidelines for intensive care unit admission, discharge, and triage. Task force of the American College of Critical Care Medicine, Society of Critical Care Medicine. Crit Care Med. 1999;27:633–8.
7. Richardson J, Sabanathan S, Jones J, et al. A prospective randomised comparison of preoperative and continuous balanced epidural or paravertebral bupivacaine on post thoracotomy pain, pulmonary function and stress responses. Br. J Anesthesia. 1999;83(3):387–92.
8. Savage C, McQuitty C, Wang D, et al. Post thoracotomy pain management. Chest Surg Clin North Am. 2002;12:251.
9. Mangram AJ, Horan TC, Pearson ML, et al. Guideline for prevention of surgical site infection 1999. Hospital infection control practices advisory committee. Infect Control Hosp Epidemiol. 1999;20:250.
10. Licker M, de Parrot M, Anastase S, et al. Risk factors for acute lung injury after thoracic surgery for lung cancer. Anesth Analg. 2003;97(6):1558–65.
11. Doherty M, Buggy DJ. Intraoperative fluids: how much is too much? Br J Anesthesia. 2012;109(1):69–79.
12. Alam N, Park BJ, Wilton A, et al. Incidence and risk factors for lung injury after lung cancer resection. Ann Thorac Surg. 2007;84(4):1085–91.
13. Shapira OM, Shahian MD. Post pneumonectomy pulmonary edema. Ann Thorac Surg. 1993;56(1):190–5.
14. Jordan S, Mitchell JA, Quinlan GJ, et al. The pathogenesis of lung injury following pulmonary resection. Eur Respir J. 2000;15:790–9.
15. Evans RG, Naidu B. Does a conservative fluid management strategy in the perioperative management of lung resection patients reduce the risk of acute lung injury? Interact Cardiovasc Thorac Surg. 2012 Sep;15(3):498–504.
16. Licker M, Cartier V, Robert J, et al. Risk factors of acute kidney injury according to RIFLE criteria after lung cancer surgery. Ann Thorac Surg. 2011;91:844–50.
17. Cerfolio RJ, Pickens A, Bass C, et al. Fast-tracking pulmonary resections. J Thorac Cardiovasc Surg. 2001;122:318.
18. Varela G, Ballesteros E, Jiménez MF, et al. Cost-effectiveness analysis of prophylactic respiratory physiotherapy in pulmonary lobectomy. Eur J Cardiothorac Surg. 2006;29:216.
19. Shields TW, Lo Cicero IIIJ, Reed EC, et al. General thoracic surgery. 7th ed. Philadelphia: Lippincott William and Wilkins; 2005. Chapter 41. p. 571–80.
20. Desborough JP. The stress response to trauma and surgery. Br J Anesthesia. 2000;85(1):109–17.
21. Brunelli A, Monteverde M, Borri A, et al. Comparison of water seal and suction after pulmonary lobectomy: a prospective randomised controlled trial. Ann Thorac Surg. 2004;77(6):1932–7.
22. Roselli EE, Murthy SC, Rice TW, et al. Atrial fibrillation complicating lung cancer resection. J Thorac Cardiovasc Surg. 2005 Aug;130(2):438–44.
23. Badhwar V, Rankin JS, Damiano RJ Jr, et al. The Society of Thoracic Surgeons 2017 clinical practice guidelines for the surgical treatment of atrial fibrillation. Ann Thorac Surg. 2017 Jan 1;103(1):329–41.
24. Seely AJE, Ivanovic J, Threader J, et al. Systematic classification of morbidity and mortality after thoracic surgery. Ann Thor Surg. 2010;90:936–42.
25. Mason DP, Quader MA, Blackstone EH, et al. Thromboembolism after pneumonectomy for malignancy: an independent marker of poor outcome. J Thorac Cardiovasc Surg. 2006;131:711.
26. Geerts WH, Pineo GF, Heit JA, et al. Prevention of venous thromboembolism: the seventh ACCP conference on antithrombotic and thrombolytic therapy. Chest. 2004;126:338S.

Enhanced Recovery After Thoracic Surgery

Samia Kohli and Jayashree Sood

Enhanced recovery after surgery (ERAS) pathways are protocolled collections of perioperative decisions designed to improve surgical outcomes [1]. The first ERAS protocol was developed nearly two decades ago in colorectal surgery which was preceded by fast-track pathway in other surgical specialties including cardiothoracic surgeries [2].

ERAS pathway is effective in reducing the duration of stay in hospital as well as decreasing postoperative complications. ERAS pathways for thoracic surgery have shown benefits like modest use of opioids, minimization of fluid overload, decreased hospital cost, and less postoperative cardiac and pulmonary complications [3].

23.1 Key Components for Enhanced Recovery After Thoracic Surgery (ERATS)

1. The overall goal of fluid therapy is to achieve euvolemia. Clear liquids should be allowed up to 2 hours preoperatively which can reduce the fluid deficit. Balanced intravenous fluids should be used. Enteral hydration should be started in postoperative period as soon as possible.
2. Lung protective ventilation.
3. Multimodal analgesia along with locoregional techniques.
4. The routine aspects such as venous thromboembolism (VTE), antibiotic prophylaxis, and active warming should be consistently employed [4].

23.2 Implementation of ERATS

Various pathways include:

1. *Preoperative information and counselling of the patient*

    Patients presenting for thoracic surgery have several comorbidities associated with pulmonary disease, thus preoperative counselling helps in decreasing the anxiety associated with surgery, anesthesia and postoperative pain. This leads to early recovery and discharge [5].

    The patient should receive information both in writing as well as verbally and both the patient and relatives should meet the entire team involved in the program, including the nursing staff [6].
2. *Preoperative Assessment*

    The American College of Chest Physicians recommends full evaluation of patients regardless of their age. Risk prediction is fundamental to informed consent, stratification, and resources allocation [7].

S. Kohli (✉) · J. Sood
Institute of Anaesthesiology, Pain and Perioperative Medicine, Sir Ganga Ram Hospital, New Delhi, India

Evaluation includes measurement of lung functions (forced expiratory volume in 1 second, diffusion capacity factor of lung for carbon monoxide and functional capacity via shuttle walk or cardiopulmonary exercise testing to determine the likelihood of postoperative dyspnea [8].

Recently the thoracic surgery scoring system (Thoracoscore) is widely used as a multidimensional tool consisting of nine variables with a correlation between the observed and expected mortality of 0.99 [9].

3. *Optimization before surgery*
   (a) *Preoperative Nutrition*: Involves preoperative fluid and carbohydrate loading, minimal fasting, and early intake of oral diet and nutritional supplements in postoperative period. Oral nutritional supplements (ONS) are recommended, as it improves patient's quality of life and muscle function [10].

   ONS if routinely administered both pre- and postoperatively improves patient's outcome by reducing weight loss and improving nutritional status and muscle strength of the patient post surgery thus decreasing postoperative complications [11].

   Routine nutritional screening should be done using various method like the Nutritional Risk Score (NRS), the Malnutrition Universal Screening Tool (MUST), and the Subjective Global Assessment Tool (SGA) [12].

   As per European Society for Clinical Nutrition and Metabolism (ESPEN) guidelines, surgery should be delayed in patients with at least one of the following criteria; weight loss >10–15% within 6 months, BMI < 18.5 kg/m^2 and serum albumin <30 g/l. [12]

   (b) *Cessation of Smoking*: Smoking leads to increased postoperative complications, though pulmonary effects can be reduced within 4 weeks of cessation [13]. With intensive preoperative physiotherapy, smoking causes minimal postoperative complications [14].

   All clinical guidelines recommend patients to stop smoking as soon as lung cancer is detected but the surgery should not be delayed to facilitate cessation of smoking preoperatively [15]. A study by Sihoe et al. found that the smokers were less likely to adhere to an ERAS pathway and had longer chest drainage duration and mean length of stay in hospital [16].

   If smoking is continued till the time of lung cancer surgery it further leads to poor quality of life in the postoperative period and also shortens the long-term survival in such patients.

   Various interventions like behavioral support, pharmacotherapy and nicotine replacement help in short-term cessation and long-term abstinence from smoking [17].

   (c) *Alcohol Withdrawal*: The long-term effects of alcohol in chronic alcoholics result in multiorgan disorders like cardiac dysfunction, bleeding disorders, and immunosuppression leading to increased morbidity, postoperative pulmonary complications, and mortality; therefore, it is recommended that alcohol should be avoided for at least 4 weeks before surgery [18].

   (d) *Anemia Management*: Anemia is a common finding in patients of lung cancer. The causes may be multifactorial including nutritional deficiency, in patients receiving chemotherapy or radiotherapy or malignancy itself [19]. The most common cause of anemia is iron deficiency, thus anemia should be identified and corrected before elective surgery.

   Recent guidelines have shown no benefit from preoperative blood transfusion and erythropoietin stimulating agents, rather it is associated with poorer outcome for cancer patients [20]. Preoperative blood transfusion does not reduce total transfusion requirement. The main aim should be on preventing further blood loss during intraoperative period.

(e) *Rehabilitation in patients undergoing lung surgery*

Preoperative physical conditioning enhances the functional and physiological capacity of an individual to overcome stressful events and helps in early mobilization postoperatively [21].

Various exercises include aerobic training with strength training, breathing exercises, relaxation, and educational sessions.

The minimum duration is 4 weeks with frequency of 5 sessions per week of moderate to high intensity as per patient's tolerance.

An inverse in peak oxygen consumption or functional capacity is observed with 6 min-walk test from baseline to postoperative period [22].

Prehabilitation (rehabilitation in the preoperative period) enhances postoperative recovery, reduces length of stay in hospital, and decreases overall morbidity and mortality [22].

4. *Preoperative Carbohydrate Loading*
   (a) Patients should be allowed intake of clear fluids until 2 hours before induction of anesthesia and surgery. This neither increases gastric content nor does it reduce the gastric pH.
   (b) Recent guidelines recommend preoperative fasting of 6 hours for solids [23].
   (c) Preoperative carbohydrate loading decreases postoperative insulin resistance and improves preoperative well-being and decreases anxiety.

5. *Premedication*

   Patients posted for thoracic surgery are usually elderly and have compromised pulmonary functions, thus the routine use of either short or long acting benzodiazepines is not recommended as they cause over-sedation resulting in airway obstruction and decreased postoperative cognitive function and delirium [24].

   One study showed that preoperative administration of melatonin 1–2 hours prior to surgery was equivalent to midazolam for reducing preoperative anxiety [25].

   Other non-pharmacological interventions include counselling and relaxation techniques like listening to music [26], preoperative carbohydrate loading, and avoiding starvation and dehydration [27].

6. *Prophylactic measures for Venous Thromboembolism (VTE)*

   Patients undergoing thoracic surgery for lung cancer are more prone to postoperative venous thromboembolism [28], risk being 3 times more for pulmonary embolism, resulting in increased 30-day mortality after cancer surgery [29].

   VTE prophylaxis guidelines are based on 2012 "American College of Chest Physicians" and 2010 "British National Institute for Health Care Excellence" [30].

   Methods include both pharmacological and mechanical prophylaxis.

Pharmacological	Mechanical
• Use of either LMWH or unfractionated heparin	• Antiembolism stocking • Intermittent pneumatic compression devices • Foot impulse devices

These practices should be started from the time of admission and continued till the patient has recovered full mobility in postoperative period [31].

The incidence is highest in first month after surgery while the incidence is highest 6–7 days post surgery in patients undergoing pneumonectomy in lung cancer [32].

7. *Antibiotic Prophylaxis*
   (a) Infection is not only associated with surgical site but may also present as empyema or pneumonia in postoperative period [33].
   (b) Approximately 10–38% develop postoperative infection with bacterial colonization of airways [34].
   (c) Administration of antibiotics 60 minutes prior to surgery decreases the incidence of surgical site infection after thoracic surgery [35].

- A single dose of antibiotic before incision is equivalent to 48 hours of postoperative prophylaxis in such cases. Extended postoperative antibiotic prophylaxis is not required [36].
- It is recommended to repeat the antibiotic dose if the duration of surgery is prolonged or there is excessive blood loss of more than 1500 ml [37].
- The choice of antibiotic depends on pattern of pulmonary flora and antibiotic resistance. Cephalosporins are considered as standard for prophylaxis due to their broad spectrum of action, low cost, and minimal allergic potential [38]. Amoxicillin–clavulanic acid, vancomycin and teicoplanin may be used in patients who are allergic to penicillin or cephalosporin.

8. *Skin preparation*

    Patients should be advised to take bath night before or morning of surgery, which is effective in reducing surgical site infection (SSI) [39]. Hair clipping just before surgery is associated with lower rates of SSI [40].

    Chlorhexidine alcohol should be used for skin preparation in place of povidone iodine as it is reported that chlorhexidine causes 40% reduction in SSI [41].

9. *Temperature Regulation and Monitoring*
    (a) ERATS guidelines recommend maintaining body temperature and active body warming because of significant heat loss due to large exposed surface area in thoracic surgery, involving the pleura and airway during open surgeries [42].
    (b) Intraoperative hypothermia (body temperature < 36 °C) results in inadequate metabolism of drugs, increased SSI, cardiovascular morbidity, coagulopathy, and increased oxygen consumption due to shivering can worsen postoperative outcomes [43].
    (c) Active warming reduces the risk of SSI as compared to conventional warming [43].
    (d) Convective prewarming in addition to intraoperative warming results in decreased postoperative hypothermia [44].
    (e) Various body warming techniques include forced air warming blankets, heating mattress, circulating water garment system, and use of warm intravenous and irrigation fluids [45, 46].
    (f) Other passive warming techniques include maintaining room temperature and covering exposed body surface [46].
    (g) Intraoperative core temperature monitoring using nasopharyngeal temperature probe.
    (h) Active warming should be continued till postoperative period to maintain core body temperature of 36 °C.

23.3 Anesthetic Management

1. *Perioperative Intravenous Fluid Management*
    (a) Avoidance of preoperative fasting and carbohydrate loading helps in avoiding dehydration in patients prior to induction of anesthesia [12].
    (b) In thoracic surgeries fluid management is very important and complex as patients undergoing lung resection are more prone to develop interstitial and pleural edema which can result in increased risk of ARDS postoperatively.
    (c) There may also be increased risk of atelectasis, pneumonia, empyema, and death [47].
    (d) ERATS recommend volume restricted fluid regime of 1–2 ml/kg/hr. for both intraoperative and postoperative fluid maintenance and also to maintain preoperative positive fluid balance of <1500 ml/20 ml/kg/24 hr. [48], resulting in decreasing the hydrostatic pressure in pulmonary capillaries [48].

        Intraoperative cardiac output monitoring can be done by various methods like:
        - Pulse contour analysis or doppler ultrasound.
        - Extravascular lung water by transpulmonary thermodilution.
        - Central venous oximetry.
        - Extreme fluid restriction can lead to organ dysfunction but it has been

observed that intravenous fluid administration at 2–3 ml/kg/h in patients undergoing lung resection does not result in AKI. Vasopressors can be used to avoid tissue hypoperfusion [49].

2. *Ventilation*

ERATS guidelines recommend protective lung ventilation using one lung ventilation technique and delivering tidal volume in the range of 4–6 ml/kg with an addition of positive and expiratory pressure (PEEP) 5 cm of H_2O that helps providing equivalent oxygenation to larger tidal volume strategies.

Most of the procedures including both open thoracotomies or minimally invasive techniques require lung isolation for adequate access into operative hemithorax. This is achieved by using DLTs or bronchial blockers. Fiber-optic bronchoscopy should be done for positioning the device in the airway and avoiding obstruction [50]. FiO_2 of 1.0 for ventilation prior to one lung ventilation increases the rate of collapse of the non-ventilated lung and improves surgical access [51].

Other techniques include awake fiber-optic intubation and non-intubated general anesthesia with spontaneous ventilation.

Regional anesthesia includes thoracic epidural or paravertebral combined with intravenous sedation.

Non-intubated surgical procedures include lobectomy, pneumonectomy, bullectomy, and lung volume reduction. These procedures have been observed with better outcomes and shorter hospital stay when compared to general anesthesia [52].

(a) *Intraoperative anesthesia technique*

Anesthesia should be accomplished by using combined regional and general anesthesia and use of short acting agents which allow early recovery and extubation.

Isoflurane, sevoflurane, and desflurane are considered weak inhibitors of hypoxic pulmonary vasoconstriction; whereas desflurane has been shown to increase the inflammatory markers [53] when compared to use of TIVA with propofol in ventilated lung, sevoflurane results in decreased inflammatory response in non-ventilated lung [54]. Recent studies have shown that intravenous dexmedetomidine enhances oxygenation and decreases the markers of oxidative stress during thoracic surgery [55].

(b) *Postoperative Nausea and Vomiting Prophylaxis*

Multiple risk factors have been identified for PONV. Most common are:

Patient related	Anesthetic related	Surgery related
Females	Use of volatile anesthetic agents	Longer duration of surgery or anesthesia
Non-smokers	Intraoperative or postoperative use of opioids	
Patients with H/O PONV		
H/O motion sickness		

PONV prophylaxis can be divided into two groups:

1. Pharmacological
2. Non-pharmacological

Pharmacological It involves administration of one or combination of antiemetic drugs.

Various antiemetics used are:	$5-HT_3$ receptor antagonists
	Corticosteroids
	Phenothiazines
	Anticholinergics

Single 8 mg preoperative dexamethasone reduces the incidence of PONV for first 24 hours and decreases the requirement of antiemetics for up to 72 hours [56].

High dose methylprednisolone reduces nausea for first 24 hours post VATS lobectomy [57].

Most commonly used drug is ondansetron, one dose prophylacticaly.

Guidelines recommend that PONV prophylaxis should be performed with drugs from different classes.

Non-pharmacological Apfel score is most commonly used for risk stratification of patients into low, medium, or high risk for PONV which allows use of multiple approaches to prevent PONV [58].

The non-pharmacological measures are:
(a) Preoperative carbohydrate loading—avoids fasting and dehydration, thus decreases the incidence of PONV.
(b) Intraoperative use of TIVA with propofol.
(c) Peripheral nerve blocks (intercostal or paravertebral) or use of epidural results in minimal use of intraoperative and postoperative opiates.
(d) More use of intraoperative NSAIDS has a known opioid sparing effect.
(e) Electrical stimulation of P6 point is very effective, done either pre- or postoperative.

23.4 Perioperative Multimodal Analgesia

- Pain following lung resection surgeries occurs primarily by two main mechanisms:
  – Activation of neuropathic pathway by damage of intercostal nerves
  – Activation of nociceptive pathway by surgical trauma due to various factors like rib retraction, fracture or dislocation of ribs, intercostal nerves or irritation of the pleura or intercostal bundles by chest tubes [59]
- Inadequate analgesia results in compromised respiratory status post thoracic surgery, which may further lead to respiratory failure secondary to splinting or pneumonia that may result due to inadequate cough and poor clearance of secretions.
- It can further lead to hypoxemia, hypercarbia, increased work of breathing, arrythmia, and ischemia.
- The enhanced recovery after lung surgery and the American Pain Society guidelines on postoperative pain management recommend the use of non-opioid analgesics combined with regional anesthesia to reduce postoperative opioid use [60]. Patient education along with it has shown better tolerance in patients in postoperative period.
  – *Preemptive analgesia*—aims to reduce the acute pain postoperatively and inhibits the development of chronic postoperative pain.
  – *Intraoperative regional analgesia*— Epidural analgesia is considered as the gold standard in many major thoracic surgeries for postoperative pain control. Adverse effects related to intraoperative epidural analgesia are urinary retention, hypotension, muscular weakness with increased risk in patients who are on anticoagulants or have renal failure [61].
- Other method is paravertebral analgesia which may result in unilateral somatic and sympathetic nerve block. It is considered to be more effective in decreasing respiratory complications when compared to TEA. It also decreases the risk of complications like PONV, pruritus, hypotension, and urinary retention [62, 63].
- Intercostal catheters are cost-effective and are usually placed by the surgeons during the end of surgery. They cause minimal postoperative complications [64].
- The most recent technique studied is the serratus anterior plane block used as rescue analgesia in surgeries like pleurectomy and decortication or in single port VATS [65, 66].
- Multilevel intercostal infiltration with liposomal bupivacaine provides intercostal nerve block lasting up to 96 hours [67].

3. *Postoperative Analgesia*: Multimodal analgesia should be employed with the aim to restrict use of postoperative opioids. This can be

achieved with a synergetic effect of different analgesics, which may include:
(a) *Acetaminophen*: This can be administered both i/v or orally. It has been observed that acetaminophen reduces morphine consumption by 20% in postoperative period [68]. It is also considered safe in patients with renal failure [69].
(b) *Nonsteroidal anti-inflammatory drugs*: NSAIDs in combination with acetaminophen is more effective in controlling post-thoracotomy pain, though it should be avoided in patients with preexisting renal failure and hypovolemic patients which are most common risk factors in patients undergoing thoracic surgery.
(c) *N-methyl-D-aspartate antagonists (NMDA) antagonists*: It has been observed that ketamine reduces overall morphine consumption and enhances early postoperative recovery. Low dose intravenous ketamine infusion along with TEA enhances post-thoracotomy analgesia [70].
(d) *Gabapentin*: It decreases early postoperative pain scores and opioid use. It has not been evidenced to reduce acute or chronic pain following thoracic surgery.
(e) *Glucocorticoids*: They have properties of analgesics, antiemetics, antipyretics, and anti-inflammation. Most commonly used glucocorticoids are dexamethasone and methylprednisolone. Dexamethasone produces dose-dependent opioid-sparing effect.

In recent trials it was observed that preoperative high dose methylprednisolone decreases postoperative pain, nausea, and fatigue without any complications [57].

Adverse effects are gastric irritation, impaired wound healing, impaired glucose homeostasis, and sodium retention.

23.4.1 Postoperative Management

1. *Prevention of atrial fibrillation*
    (a) Postoperative atrial fibrillation (POAF) is commonly observed after thoracic surgery.
    (b) Major risk factors are: old age, males, Caucasian race, hypertension, COPD, heart failure, valvular heart disease, pneumonectomy > lobectomy [71].
    (c) American Association of Thoracic Surgery guidelines 2014 recommendations for prevention of POAF [72]:
        - Continue β-blockers in patients who are on β-blocker therapy previously.
        - Intravenous magnesium in patient with low levels of serum magnesium.
        - Use of preoperative diltiazem in patients at high risk of developing POAF.
2. *Management of Intercostal Drainage System*
    Intercostal drain is important part of thoracic surgery.
    (a) *Suction or no suction*: Suction promotes pleural apposition, sealing of air leak and drainage of large air leaks. It increases the flow through chest tubes proportional to level of suction applied. It also reduces patient's mobility.

    No suctioning of the intercostal drains reduces the duration of air leak by decreasing the airflow, it may be ineffective in drawing larger air leaks resulting in complications like pneumonia and arrhythmia.
    (b) *Digital drainage system*: These devices are light weight, compact, and have inbuilt suction pump. These devices automatically quantify the amount of air leak and also are able to store the information and show various trends in air leak which helps in making invariable decisions regarding early chest tube removal. It has been observed that with digital drainage system there is early postoperative recovery and decreased length of stay in hospital after lung resection surgeries.
    (c) *Pleural fluid drainage*: The recommended cutoff value for pleural fluid drainage is 200 ml/day as it is the threshold below which it is safe to remove chest tube. The hourly conversion of pleural fluid is 0.2 ml/kg to its complete removal in 1 hour.

(d) *Chest tubes*: It is advisable to use single chest tube drainage after lung resection surgeries which both safe and effective and less painful as compared to use of two chest tube drains. It is associated with decreased duration of chest drainage and lesser volume of fluid which is drained. It has been observed that both dynamic and static pain scores have decreased by 40% and lung function increased by 13% after removal of chest tube following either VATS on open lobotomy [73].

3. Urinary catheterization: In patients with normal renal function urine output monitoring does not affect renal outcomes in AKI. Postoperative urinary retention (POUR) is related to delayed discharge and increased risk of UTI which may furthermore result in long-term bladder dysfunction:
   (a) There are multifactorial causes related to POUR including increasing age, male sex, diabetes mellitus, pain, and TEA.
   (b) Prolonged bladder catheterization inhibits early mobilization and is also associated with increased risk of UTI.
   (c) Early removal of catheters results in low incidence of POUR and UTI resulting in early recovery and discharge.

4. *Early mobilization and physiotherapy*
   Postoperative immobility is a significant risk factor in prolonging hospital length of stay due to physical deconditioning, reduced muscle mass, and increased pulmonary complications like atelectasis, pneumonia, and VTE.

23.5 Conclusion

Early mobilization is the most important component of ERATS to avoid complications and enhance postoperative recovery.

Thus chest tubes, urinary catheters, intravenous fluids, and inadequate pain control should be avoided to enhance early mobilization and shorter duration of hospital stay.

References

1. Semenkovich TR, Hudson JL, Subramanian M, et al. Enhanced recovery after surgery (ERAS) in thoracic surgery. Semin Thorac Cardiovasc Surg. 2018;30(3):342–9.
2. Ljungqvist O, Scott M, Fearon KC. Enhanced recovery after surgery: a review. JAMA Surg. 2017 Mar 1;152(3):292–8.
3. Rogers LJ, Bleetman D, Messenger DE, et al. The impact of enhanced recovery after surgery (ERAS) protocol compliance on morbidity from resection for primary lung cancer. J Thorac Cardiovasc Surg. 2018 Apr;155(4):1843–52.
4. Teeter EG, Kolarczyk LM, Popescu WM. Examination of the enhanced recovery guidelines in thoracic surgery. Curr Opin Anaesthesiol. 2019 Feb;32(1):10–6.
5. Egbert LD, Battit GE, Welch CE, et al. Reduction of postoperative pain by encouragement and instruction of patients. A study of doctor-patient rapport. N Engl J Med. 1964 Apr 16;270:825–7.
6. Barlési F, Barrau K, Loundou A, et al. Impact of information on quality of life and satisfaction of non-small cell lung cancer patients: a randomized study of standardized versus individualized information before thoracic surgery. J Thorac Oncol. 2008 Oct;3(10):1146–52.
7. Detterbeck FC, Lewis SZ, Diekemper R, et al. Executive summary: diagnosis and management of lung cancer, 3rd ed: American College of Chest Physicians evidence-based clinical practice guidelines. Chest. 2013 May;143(5 Suppl):7S–37S.
8. Wright CD, Gaissert HA, Grab JD, et al. Predictors of prolonged length of stay after lobectomy for lung cancer: a Society of Thoracic Surgeons general thoracic surgery database risk-adjustment model. Ann Thorac Surg. 2008 Jun;85(6):1857–65.
9. Falcoz PE, Conti M, Brouchet L, et al. The thoracic surgery scoring system (Thoracoscore): risk model for in-hospital death in 15,183 patients requiring thoracic surgery. J Thorac Cardiovasc Surg. 2007 Feb;133(2):325–32.
10. Collins PF, Elia M, Stratton RJ. Nutritional support and functional capacity in chronic obstructive pulmonary disease: a systematic review and meta-analysis. Respirology. 2013 May;18(4):616–29.
11. Awad S, Varadhan KK, Ljungqvist O, et al. A meta-analysis of randomized controlled trials on preoperative oral carbohydrate treatment in elective surgery. Clin Nutr. 2013 Feb;32(1):34–44.
12. Weimann A, Braga M, Carli F, et al. ESPEN guideline: clinical nutrition in surgery. Clin Nutr. 2017 Jun;36(3):623–50.
13. Sørensen LT. Wound healing and infection in surgery: the pathophysiological impact of smoking, smoking cessation, and nicotine replacement therapy: a systematic review. Ann Surg. 2012 Jun;255(6):1069–79.

14. Rodriguez M, Gómez-Hernandez MT, Novoa N, et al. Refraining from smoking shortly before lobectomy has no influence on the risk of pulmonary complications: a case-control study on a matched population. Eur J Cardiothorac Surg. 2017 Mar 1;51(3):498–503.
15. Lim E, Baldwin D, Beckles M, et al. Win T; British Thoracic Society; Society for Cardiothoracic Surgery in Great Britain and Ireland. Guidelines on the radical management of patients with lung cancer. Thorax. 2010 Oct;65(Suppl 3):iii1–27.
16. Sihoe AD, Yu PS, Kam TH, et al. Adherence to a clinical pathway for video-assisted thoracic surgery: predictors and clinical importance. Innovations (Phila). 2016 May-Jun;11(3):179–86.
17. Thomsen T, Villebro N, Møller AM. Interventions for preoperative smoking cessation. Cochrane Database Syst Rev. 2014 Mar 27;3:CD002294.
18. Oppedal K, Møller AM, Pedersen B, et al. Preoperative alcohol cessation prior to elective surgery. Cochrane Database Syst Rev. 2012 Jul 11;7:CD008343.
19. Kosmidis P. Krzakowski M; ECAS investigators. Anemia profiles in patients with lung cancer: what have we learned from the European cancer Anaemia survey (ECAS)? Lung Cancer. 2005 Dec;50(3):401–12.
20. Tonia T, Mettler A, Robert N, et al. Erythropoietin or darbepoetin for patients with cancer. Cochrane Database Syst Rev. 2012 Dec 12;12:CD003407.
21. Pouwels S, Hageman D, Gommans LN, et al. Preoperative exercise therapy in surgical care: a scoping review. J Clin Anesth. 2016;33:476–90.
22. Sebio Garcia R, Yáñez Brage MI, Giménez Moolhuyzen E, et al. Functional and postoperative outcomes after preoperative exercise training in patients with lung cancer: a systematic review and meta-analysis. Interact Cardiovasc Thorac Surg. 2016 Sep;23(3):486–97.
23. Smith I, Kranke P, Murat I, et al. in't veld B; European Society of Anaesthesiology. Perioperative fasting in adults and children: guidelines from the European Society of Anaesthesiology. Eur J Anaesthesiol. 2011 Aug;28(8):556–69.
24. Bilotta F, Lauretta MP, Borozdina A, et al. Postoperative delirium: risk factors, diagnosis and perioperative care. Minerva Anestesiol. 2013 Sep;79(9):1066–76.
25. Hansen MV, Halladin NL, Rosenberg J, et al. Melatonin for pre- and postoperative anxiety in adults. Cochrane Database Syst Rev. 2015;4:CD009861.
26. Bradt J, Dileo C, Shim M. Music interventions for preoperative anxiety. Cochrane Database Syst Rev. 2013;6:CD006908.
27. Hausel J, Nygren J, Thorell A, et al. Randomized clinical trial of the effects of oral preoperative carbohydrates on postoperative nausea and vomiting after laparoscopic cholecystectomy. Br J Surg. 2005;92:415–21.
28. Brunelli A. Deep vein thrombosis/pulmonary embolism: prophylaxis, diagnosis, and management. Thorac Surg Clin. 2012;22:25–8.
29. Merkow RP, Bilimoria KY, McCarter MD, et al. Post-discharge venous thromboembolism after cancer surgery: extending the case for extended prophylaxis. Ann Surg. 2011;254:131–7.
30. van Dongen CJ, MacGillavry MR, Prins MH. Once versus twice daily LMWH for the initial treatment of venous thromboembolism. Cochrane Database Syst Rev. 2005;5:CD003074.
31. Venous thromboembolism in over 16s: reducing the risk of hospitalacquired deep vein thrombosis or pulmonary embolism. NICE guideline 89. 2018. https://www.nice.org.uk/guidance/ng89. Accessed from 10 February 2019.
32. Raja S, Idrees JJ, Blackstone EH, et al. Routine venous thromboembolism screening after pneumonectomy: the more you look, the more you see. J Thorac Cardiovasc Surg. 2016;152:524–32.
33. Imperatori A, Nardecchia E, Dominioni L, et al. Surgical site infections after lung resection: a prospective study of risk factors in 1,091 consecutive patients. J Thorac Dis. 2017;9:3222–31.
34. D'Journo XB, Rolain JM, Doddoli C, et al. Airways colonizations in patients undergoing lung cancer surgery. Eur J Cardiothorac Surg. 2011;40:309–19.
35. Hawn MT, Richman JS, Vick CC, et al. Timing of surgical antibiotic prophylaxis and the risk of surgical site infection. JAMA Surg. 2013;148:649–57.
36. Mangram AJ, Horan TC, Pearson ML, et al. Guideline for prevention of surgical site infection, 1999. Centers for Disease Control and Prevention (CDC) hospital infection control practices advisory committee. Am J Infect Control. 1999;27:97–132.
37. Swoboda SM, Merz C, Kostuik J, et al. Does intraoperative blood loss affect antibiotic serum and tissue concentrations. Arch Surg. 1996;131:1165–71.
38. Chang SH, Krupnick AS. Perioperative antibiotics in thoracic surgery. Thorac Surg Clin. 2012;22: 35–45.
39. Berríos-Torres SI, Umscheid CA, Bratzler DW, et al. Centers for Disease Control and Prevention guideline for the prevention of surgical site infection, 2017. JAMA Surg. 2017;152:784–91.
40. Tanner J, Norrie P, Melen K. Preoperative hair removal to reduce surgical site infection. Cochrane Database Syst Rev. 2011;11:CD004122.
41. Darouiche RO, Wall MJ, Itani KM, et al. Chlorhexidine-alcohol versus povidone-iodine for surgical-site antisepsis. N Engl J Med. 2010;362:18–26.
42. Karalapillai D, Story D, Hart GK, et al. Postoperative hypothermia and patient outcomes after major elective non-cardiac surgery. Anaesthesia. 2013;68:605–11.
43. Scott EM, Buckland R. A systematic review of intraoperative warming to prevent postoperative complications. AORN J. 2006;83:1090–104. 1107
44. Emmert A, Franke R, Brandes IF, et al. Comparison of conductive and convective warming in patients undergoing video-assisted thoracic surgery: a prospective randomized clinical trial. Thorac Cardiovasc Surg. 2017;65:362–6.

45. Madrid E, Urrútia G, Roqué i Figuls M, et al. Active body surface warming systems for preventing complications caused by inadvertent perioperative hypothermia in adults. Cochrane Database Syst Rev. 2016;4:CD009016.
46. Campbell G, Alderson P, Smith AF, et al. Warming of intravenous and irrigation fluids for preventing inadvertent perioperative hypothermia. Cochrane Database Syst Rev. 2015;4:CD009891.
47. Arslantas MK, Kara HV, Tuncer BB, et al. Effect of the amount of intraoperative fluid administration on postoperative pulmonary complications following anatomic lung resections. J Thorac Cardiovasc Surg. 2015;149:314–20.321.e1
48. Evans RG, Naidu B. Does a conservative fluid management strategy in the perioperative management of lung resection patients reduce the risk of acute lung injury. Interact Cardiovasc Thorac Surg. 2012;15:498–504.
49. Chappell D, Jacob M, Hofmann-Kiefer K, et al. A rational approach to perioperative fluid management. Anesthesiology. 2008;109:723–40.
50. de Bellis M, Accardo R, Di Maio M, et al. Is flexible bronchoscopy necessary to confirm the position of double-lumen tubes before thoracic surgery. Eur J Cardiothorac Surg. 2011;40:912–6.
51. Ko R, McRae K, Darling G, et al. The use of air in the inspired gas mixture during two-lung ventilation delays lung collapse during one-lung ventilation. Anesth Analg. 2009;108:1092–6.
52. Tacconi F, Pompeo E. Non-intubated video-assisted thoracic surgery: where does evidence stand. J Thorac Dis. 2016;8:S364–75.
53. Schilling T, Kozian A, Kretzschmar M, et al. Effects of propofol and desflurane anaesthesia on the alveolar inflammatory response to one-lung ventilation. Br J Anaesth. 2007;99:368–75.
54. Lumb AB, Slinger P. Hypoxic pulmonary vasoconstriction: physiology and anesthetic implications. Anesthesiology. 2015;122:932–46.
55. Xia R, Xu J, Yin H, et al. Intravenous infusion of dexmedetomidine combined isoflurane inhalation reduces oxidative stress and potentiates hypoxia pulmonary vasoconstriction during one-lung ventilation in patients. Mediat Inflamm. 2015;2015:238041.
56. DREAMS Trial Collaborators and West Midlands Research Collaborative. Dexamethasone versus standard treatment for postoperative nausea and vomiting in gastrointestinal surgery: randomised controlled trial (DREAMS trial). BMJ. 2017;357:j1455.
57. Bjerregaard LS, Jensen PF, Bigler DR, et al. High-dose methylprednisolone in video-assisted thoracoscopic surgery lobectomy: a randomized controlled trial. Eur J Cardiothorac Surg. 2018;53:209–15.
58. Apfel CC, Läärä E, Koivuranta M, et al. A simplified risk score for predicting postoperative nausea and vomiting: conclusions from cross-validations between two centers. Anesthesiology. 1999;91:693–700.
59. Qiu R, Perrino AC Jr, Zurich H, et al. Effect of preoperative gabapentin and acetaminophen on opioid consumption in video-assisted thoracoscopic surgery: a retrospective study. Rom J Anaesth Intensive Care. 2018;25:43–8.
60. Chou R, Gordon DB, de Leon-Casasola OA, et al. Management of postoperative pain: a clinical practice guideline from the American pain society, the American Society of Regional Anesthesia and Pain Medicine, and the American Society of Anesthesiologists' committee on regional anesthesia, executive committee, and administrative council. J Pain. 2016;17:131–57.
61. Cook TM, Counsell D, Wildsmith JA, Royal College of Anaesthetists Third National Audit Project. Major complications of central neuraxial block: report on the third National Audit Project of the Royal College of Anaesthetists. Br J Anaesth. 2009;102:179–90.
62. Davies RG, Myles PS, Graham JM. A comparison of the analgesic efficacy and side-effects of paravertebral vs epidural blockade for thoracotomy– a systematic review and meta-analysis of randomized trials. Br J Anaesth. 2006;96:418–26.
63. Yeung JH, Gates S, Naidu BV, et al. Paravertebral block versus thoracic epidural for patients undergoing thoracotomy. Cochrane Database Syst Rev. 2016;2:CD009121.
64. Luketich JD, Land SR, Sullivan EA, et al. Thoracic epidural versus intercostal nerve catheter plus patient-controlled analgesia: a randomized study. Ann Thorac Surg. 2005;79:1845–9. Discussion 1849
65. Blanco R, Parras T, McDonnell JG, et al. Serratus plane block: a novel ultrasound-guided thoracic wall nerve block. Anaesthesia. 2013;68:1107–13.
66. Khalil AE, Abdallah NM, Bashandy GM, et al. Ultrasound-guided serratus anterior plane block versus thoracic epidural analgesia for thoracotomy pain. J Cardiothorac Vasc Anesth. 2017;31:152–8.
67. Khalil KG, Boutrous ML, Irani AD, et al. Operative intercostal nerve blocks with long-acting bupivacaine liposome for pain control after thoracotomy. Ann Thorac Surg. 2015;100:2013–8.
68. Cook TM, Riley RH. Analgesia following thoracotomy: a survey of Australian practice. Anaesth Intensive Care. 1997;25:520–4.
69. Dahl V, Raeder JC. Non-opioid postoperative analgesia. Acta Anaesthesiol Scand. 2000;44:1191–203.
70. Suzuki M, Haraguti S, Sugimoto K, et al. Low-dose intravenous ketamine potentiates epidural analgesia after thoracotomy. Anesthesiology. 2006;105:111–9.

71. Giambrone GP, Wu X, Gaber-Baylis LK, et al. Incidence and implications of postoperative supraventricular tachycardia after pulmonary lobectomy. J Thorac Cardiovasc Surg. 2016;151:982–8.
72. Frendl G, Sodickson AC, Chung MK, et al. 2014 AATS guidelines for the prevention and management of perioperative atrial fibrillation and flutter for thoracic surgical procedures. J Thorac Cardiovasc Surg. 2014;148:e153–93.
73. Refai M, Brunelli A, Salati M, et al. The impact of chest tube removal on pain and pulmonary function after pulmonary resection. Eur J Cardiothorac Surg. 2012;41:820–2.

Postoperative Complications Following Thoracic Surgery

24

Anjeleena Kumar Gupta

24.1 Introduction

Thoracic surgical procedures present challenges to the surgeon and the anesthesiologist. Rapid physiological changes make the patients prone to surgical and anesthetic complications in the perioperative period.

Injury during intubation, surgical procedure, or disease process itself could be the causative factor. Type of surgical procedure and the preoperative medical status determines the type and severity of the complications.

Complications may present in the immediate postoperative period in the post-anesthesia care unit (PACU), intensive care unit (ICU), or the surgical wards. Complications range from minor atelectasis to life-threatening lobar torsion. Incidence varies between hospitals, higher complication rates in hospitals with lower workload [1]. Complication rates have been variedly reported between 5–80% [2].

Five independent risk factors have been associated with the development of postoperative pulmonary complications (PPCs): age > 75 years, BMI > 30 kg/m^2, ASA physical status > 3, current smoking history, and chronic obstructive pulmonary disease (COPD) [3]. Abstinence of smoking for atleast 1 month is required to reduce the frequency of perioperative complications [4]. PPCs is a major contributory factor in deaths occurring post lung resection.

Extubation of the trachea is mostly performed in the operating room after the surgical procedure, but sometimes postoperative mechanical ventilation may be required depending on the preexisting disease process. Lateral thoracotomy results in reduced forced vital capacity and functional residual capacity (FRC) as much as <60% of preoperative values on postoperative day 1 (POD1). This may normalize to preoperative values by up to 2 weeks. Decreased FRC results in hypoxemia requiring postoperative mechanical ventilation.

24.2 Risk Stratification

Risk stratification helps in identification of the 'at risk' patients. Every patient should undergo a detailed anesthetic assessment (medical history, medications, upper airway evaluation) and 'three legged stool' of respiratory assessment [5] (medical function, pulmonary parenchymal function, and cardiorespiratory reserve) prior to thoracic surgery. Risk stratification should take into consideration the state of non-operative lung whether normal or diseased, presence of obstructive or restrictive lung disease, infective or malignant state, pre-surgery radiotherapy, and preoperative serum albumin levels [6]. Preoperative screening

A. K. Gupta (✉)
Institute of Anaesthesiology, Pain and Perioperative Medicine, Sir Ganga Ram Hospital, New Delhi, India

© Springer Nature Singapore Pte Ltd. 2020
J. Sood, S. Sharma (eds.), *Clinical Thoracic Anesthesia*,
https://doi.org/10.1007/978-981-15-0746-5_24

and adequate preoperative preparation are the key factors in prevention of postoperative crisis. Risk stratification and risk classification following thoracic and abdominal surgical procedures have been developed by Shapiro et al. [7]. Each of the five categories is evaluated based on the points ascribed to: spirometric variables (0–3), arterial blood gases (0–1), comorbidities of cardiovascular (0–1) and nervous system (0–1) and postoperative ambulation (0–1). Point given to each category is summed to achieve a total score from 0 to 7. The total score of points indicates the degree of risk: low risk—0 point, moderate risk—1 to 2 points, and high risk—3 or more points [6, 7]. Low risk patients may or may not need oxygen therapy after discharge from PACU. Moderate risk patients require observation in ICU or high dependency unit (HDU). High risk patients need monitoring and interventions in ICU [6, 7].

Complications can be grouped into general complications or specific complications: respiratory, cardiovascular, and neurological (Table 24.1).

Table 24.1 Complications of thoracic surgical procedures

I. General complications
(a) Airway injury
(b) Bronchospasm
(c) Hemorrhage
(d) Atelectasis
(e) Deep vein thrombosis and pulmonary embolism
(f) Acute kidney injury
(g) Injury to surrounding structures
(i) Vocal cord palsy
(ii) Phrenic nerve injury
(iii) Chylothorax
(iv) Horner's syndrome
II. Specific complications
(a) Respiratory problems
(i) Pulmonary edema
(ii) Air leak
(iii) Post-pneumonectomy syndrome
(iv) Lobar torsion
(v) Mediastinal emphysema
(vi) Pleural effusion and empyema
(vii) Bronchopleural fistula
(viii) Pneumonia
(b) Cardiac problems
(i) Arrhythmia
(ii) Interatrial shunt
(iii) Cardiac herniation
(iv) Cardiac tamponade
(c) Neurological problems
(i) Cerebral infarction

24.3 General Complications

24.3.1 Airway Injury

Thoracic surgery involves insertion of double lumen endotracheal tube (DLT) for selective ventilation of one lung. DLT has a large diameter and by virtue of this, increases the chances of trauma to the airway. Both anesthesia and surgical interventions contribute to be a cause of airway injury. Sore throat, vocal cord injury, laryngeal trauma, bronchial injury, glottic edema, erythema, tracheobronchial lacerations, and tracheal rupture are known to occur.

24.3.2 Bronchospasm

Patients undergoing thoracic surgical procedures often have respiratory embarrassment. Bronchospasm may occur in intraoperative or postoperative period. Aspiration of gastric contents, histamine releasing drugs (morphine, atracurium), increased reactivity of the airway, or an allergic manifestation of drugs can result in bronchospasm. Acute exacerbation of asthma or COPD, tracheal handling in the form of endotracheal intubation, suctioning of the trachea, and extubation of the trachea with inadequate depth of anesthetic are known to provoke bronchospasm. In the intraoperative period, bronchospasm may present as an increase in the mean airway pressure. Blood gas analysis demonstrates hypercapnia. Dyspnea, tightness in chest, or wheezing may be the presenting features in the postoperative period. Expiratory time is often prolonged. Treatment involves increasing the depth of anesthesia, inhaled β_2 agonists, and inhaled anticholinergic agents (ipratropium bromide). In the absence of improvement after 2 doses of inhaled bronchodilators, systemic glucocorticoids should be supplemented. Role of methylxanthines and systemic β_2 agonists is controversial [8].

24.3.3 Hemorrhage

Minor injuries to lip, dentition, oropharyngeal mucosa, or tracheobronchial tree secondary to tracheal intubation can lead to bleeding from these sites. It is usually self-limiting in nature. Incidence of bleeding after video-assisted thoracoscopic surgery (VATS) is less than 2% as opposed to 1–3% with open surgery [9–11].

Bleeding can occur from vessels in the chest wall, mediastinum, or azygos veins (Fig. 24.1). One can expect some blood loss into the pleural cavity but it generally does not exceed 100–200 ml/h [12]. Catastrophic bleeding from pulmonary arteries and veins can be life threatening. Hemorrhage from surgical site or from chest drains may be a result of surgical bleeding or secondary to coagulopathy. In presence of chest tube output exceeding 1000 ml/h, assessment for coagulopathy should be undertaken. Serial drainage of blood exceeding 200 ml/h for 2–3 h despite correction of coagulopathy points toward surgical cause of bleeding and warrants re-exploration [13]. Postoperative hemoptysis signifies bleeding into the tracheobronchial tree. It is imperative to maintain a clear airway and adequate ventilation. Isolate the healthy lung with DLT till bleeding is controlled. One may need replacement of smaller size DLT with a larger size airway tube to accomplish suctioning. Rigid bronchoscopy should be done to remove clots and tamponade the bleeding site. Emergency thoracotomy may have to be considered. In presence of excessive bleeding, antiplatelet drugs (aspirin) and warfarin should be withheld in the postoperative period. Herbs like garlic, ginseng that prolong bleeding time should be stopped 2 weeks prior to lung resection as per the recommendations [14].

Lymphatic leak can also be a cause of high output from chest drain. It can be ruled out by estimating the hematocrit of the chest tube drainage. However, in a hemodynamically unstable patient absence of chest tube output may signify a thrombosed chest tube. Chest X-ray (CXR) film then shows radio opacity of the operative side with thrombosed chest tubes [13]. Treatment option includes VATS or open exploration to evacuate hematoma, thereby preventing respiratory embarrassment and empyema.

24.3.4 Atelectasis

It is the commonest postoperative pulmonary complication following thoracic surgery. Factors responsible for atelectasis are inadequate pain relief, decreased lung compliance, impaired regional ventilation, inadequate cough, and retained secretions post surgery [15]. It usually manifests as breathlessness, tachypnea, tachycardia, or arrhythmia. Hypoxemia is observed as soon as the patient leaves the PACU and tends to worsen from second to fourth postoperative day [16, 17].

After left upper lobectomy, there is a risk of kinking of the left bronchus as it passes under the aortic arch. This occurs due to the rise of the left lower lobe in order to fill the hemithorax. After right upper lobectomy, middle lobe bronchus is vulnerable to kinking as the horizontal fissure rises and rotates to a more perpendicular position (Fig. 24.2) [9].

Mainstay of treatment is re-expansion of the collapsed lung with continuous positive airway

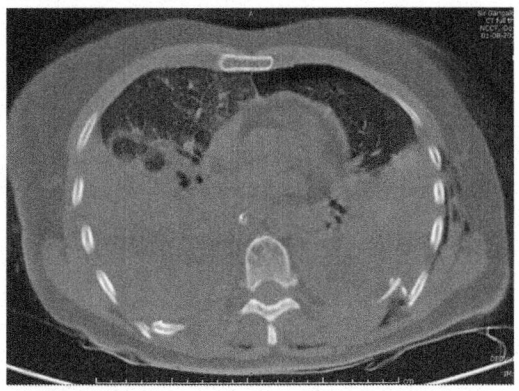

Fig. 24.1 CT thorax showing hemopneumothorax

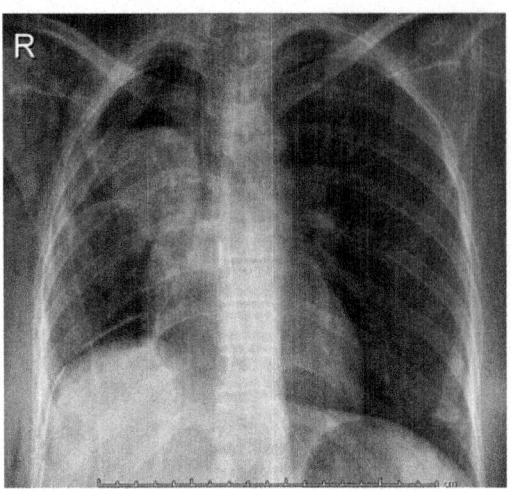

Fig. 24.2 Chest X-ray showing atelectasis

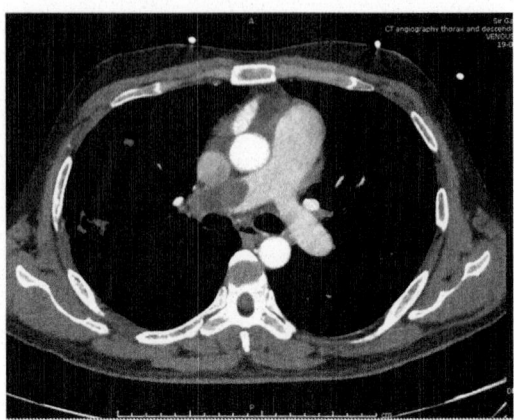

Fig. 24.3 CT angiogram thorax showing pulmonary artery thrombus

pressure. This is useful for patients with marginal or low volume of secretions. In presence of copious secretions, chest physiotherapy and bronchial toileting is warranted. Role of flexible bronchoscopy is uncertain but can be an option in cases unresponsive to tracheobronchial suctioning and chest physiotherapy [18, 19]. Closely watch for the need of intubation. Role of N-acetylcysteine to improve or prevent postoperative atelectasis is unconvincing, without much benefit [20].

24.3.5 Deep Vein Thrombosis and Pulmonary Embolism

Thromboembolism is a potentially fatal condition with an incidence of 1.7% following thoracic surgery [21]. Presence of malignancy and prolonged surgical times are the known risk factors. Small embolic events are often undiagnosed and can only be detected on autopsy but large embolus produces hemodynamic imbalance. High index of suspicion is needed for diagnosis. Initial CXR films are normal. Fleischner sign (enlarged pulmonary artery), Hampton hump (peripheral wedge of airspace opacity), and Westermark's sign (regional oligemia and pleural effusion) are characteristic findings described on plain CXR [22]. In late stages, large pulmonary embolus produces characteristic changes on electrocardiogram (ECG) described as $S_1 Q_{III} T_{III}$ pattern (deep S wave in lead I, Q wave and inverted T wave in lead III). However, gold standard diagnostic test for pulmonary embolism is pulmonary angiography. Computed tomography (CT) angiogram, easily performed, less invasive procedure, currently used demonstrates filling defects in the pulmonary vasculature (Fig. 24.3). Ventilation perfusion scan demonstrating unmatched segmental perfusion defects are indicative of pulmonary embolism [23]. These are difficult to interpret, hence, rarely performed. In presence of hemodynamic compromise, right ventricular dilatation and strain pattern are observed on echocardiography.

Treatment depends on the size and location of embolus and the hemodynamic status of the patient. Surgical options are to be considered in presence of hemodynamic embarrassment. Catheter embolectomy, operative embolectomy, systemic anticoagulation, and thrombolytic administration are different treatment modalities to be considered [24].

24.3.6 Acute Kidney Injury

Postoperative acute kidney injury (AKI) is a devastating problem. It is associated with an increased incidence of morbidity and mortality. Renal dysfunction in the postoperative period has a reported incidence at 4% [25]. This is an underestimated value due to nonconformity in the definition of AKI. The risk factors for AKI post lung surgery are similar to those after other surgical procedures. Assessment of AKI post lung surgery has been done by RIFLE classification: R—risk, I—injury, F—failure, L—loss of function, and E—end stage kidney disease. It was adopted by Acute Dialysis Quality Initiative Workgroup in 2004 [26].

Identifiable risk factors are ASA grade III and IV, forced expiratory volume in 1 s (FEV_1), use of vasopressors, and anesthetic duration [27]. Incidence of AKI is less following thoracoscopic procedures. Ishikawa S demonstrated independent association between postoperative AKI with hypertension, peripheral vascular disease, low glomerular filtration rate or preoperative use of angiotensin II receptor blockers [28]. Perioperative management involving intraoperative synthetic colloid use has also been reported to potentiate AKI [28]. Early postoperative AKI is a common reason for re-intubation, postoperative mechanical ventilation, cause of readmission to hospital and prolonged hospital stay secondary to cardiorespiratory embarrassment. Treatment of AKI consists of maintenance of tissue oxygenation, sepsis control, nutritional support, dialysis, or hemofiltration.

24.3.7 Injury to Surrounding Structures

24.3.7.1 Vocal Cord Palsy
Surgeries like mediastinoscopy, esophagectomy, and pulmonary resection predispose to a high risk of vocal cord palsy with a reported incidence of 1–6, 5–22, and 30% respectively [29]. Injury to recurrent laryngeal nerve can be secondary to poor intubating conditions, use of larger size DLT, proximal airway traction in anterior mediastinum [29], or direct nerve trauma. It should be suspected in patients with weak voices, hoarseness of throat, and weak cough. Hoarse voice is however, relatively common after endotracheal intubation. Unilateral palsy may present with a voice change but unlikely to result in airway obstruction. Bilateral vocal cord palsy, although rare after thoracic surgery has been reported following lung resection [30]. It can be associated with dyspnea, stridor, pulmonary aspiration of gastric contents secondary to glottic incompetence. Prompt recognition in the extubated patient is critical to avoid life-threatening complication. On suspicion, safest approach is prompt re-intubation. Examination of vocal cords prior to extubation should be considered. Use of latest advancements of videolaryngoscopes allows visualization of vocal cords without much discomfort to the patient. Flexible fiberoptic laryngoscopy can also be considered in cases with high clinical suspicion of injury to vocal cords [30]. There would be a demonstrable lack of movement of affected cord with phonation. It is imperative to determine if the dysfunction is temporary or permanent.

In case of mild symptoms, consider conservative treatment with oxygen via facemask, steroids, and racemic epinephrine [21]. Heliox, a mixture of 70% helium and 30% oxygen offers instant advantage of reduced effort of breathing due to it being less viscous than air [21]. Mostly, heliox has been used in pediatric population. In cases of permanent damage, consider chest physiotherapy, withhold oral feed, change to nasogastric or parenteral feeding and surgical intervention [9]. Vocal cord injection of collagen or laryngeal framework surgery to medialize the cord to re-establish competent glottis can also be considered [31].

24.3.7.2 Phrenic Nerve Injury
Thoracic surgical procedures like anterior mediastinal tumor excision, resection of superior sulcus tumors, or repair of thoracic outlet syndrome could result in phrenic nerve injury [13]. During lobectomy, there is a high risk of injury to the nerve at the time of mediastinal lymph node dissection or during pericardial adhesiolysis. Injury is mostly secondary to mechanical trauma resulting in diaphragmatic dysfunction.

In the absence of significant pulmonary disease, unilateral diaphragmatic dysfunction is well tolerated [32]. Patient may complain of shortness of breath on exertion. Thoracic surgical patients often have poor lung functions and inability to wean them off the ventilator may be

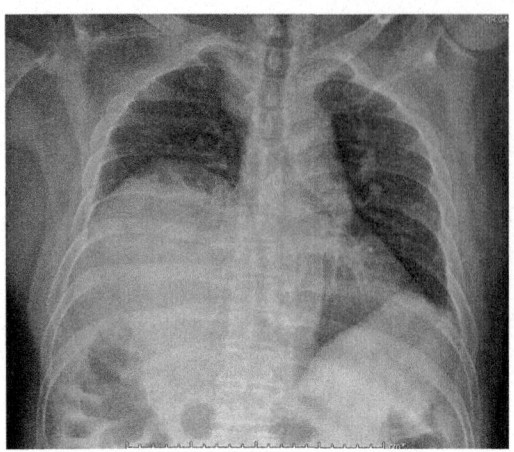

Fig. 24.4 Chest X-ray showing right phrenic nerve palsy

the first sign of injury to the phrenic nerve. CXR would demonstrate an elevated hemidiaphragm (Fig. 24.4). Electromyography, ultrasound, or fluoroscopic sniff test demonstrating paradoxical movement of diaphragm on the side of injury can also be used for diagnostic confirmation [33]. Postoperative abnormal diaphragmatic movement can result in diminished lung volumes and reduced exercise capacity. Depending on the severity of respiratory embarrassment, expectant treatment or surgical option should be considered. In severe cases with inability to maintain quality of life due to breathlessness, diaphragmatic plication is indicated [33].

24.3.7.3 Chylothorax

Injury to thoracic duct during pulmonary resection is known to occur with a reported incidence of 0.7–2% [34]. Extensive dissection of mediastinal lymph nodes, incomplete thoracic duct ligation, or direct injury to thoracic duct are the causative factors [33]. Chylothorax presents as difficulty in breathing, not associated with pleuritic pain. It may present within days or weeks postoperatively. It is associated with nutritional deficiency secondary to loss of calories, proteins, and vitamins more than fats. Dehydration and immunologic dysfunction may ensue. Prolonged chylothorax may result in respiratory embarrassment [13] which is affected by volume and rate of loss of chyle.

Lecithin and fatty acids present in chyle are bacteriostatic in nature. Therefore, sterile chyle does not cause inflammation and fibrosis. However, empyema is a rare occurrence.

Diagnosis is based on the examination of effusion fluid. Triglyceride level >110 mg/dl and lymphocyte count >90% are diagnostic [33]. Electrophoresis shows presence of Sudan 3 stain and chylomicrons. Total protein content of effusion approaches that of plasma [13].

Conservative management involving replacement of nutrients and chest tube drainage of chylothoraces to improve chest expansion is the initial modality of treatment. Nil by mouth or administration of medium chain triglycerides is advised. Medium chain triglycerides are directly absorbed into the portal system without passing through the intestinal lymphatic system thereby decreasing flow of chyle into the thoracic duct. This gives time for thoracic duct to heal [35]. If the flow of chyle does not decrease, then consider total parenteral nutrition [35, 36]. Reduction of chyle production by somatostatin and octreotide can be considered [37]. Conservative treatment can be continued for 5–7 days if drainage decreases and nutritional status is maintained. However, consider surgical options, if despite conservative treatment; (1) drainage of chyle is: >1.5 L/day (adult), >100 ml/kg/day (child), 1 L/day for 5 days, persistent flow for >2 weeks. (2) rapid decline in nutritional status.

Ligation of thoracic duct by thoracotomy or VATs procedure is the mainstay of treatment [38, 39].

High success rate is achieved if ligation is done as low as possible, preferably just above the right diaphragm. This has the added advantage of preventing flow from any unidentified accessory ducts.

Pleural decortication along with pleurodesis should be considered for localized or complicated chylothorax. If the patient is too sick to undergo surgical procedure then chemical pleurodesis with talcum powder is an alternative option [37].

24.3.7.4 Horner's Syndrome

Horner's syndrome can occur following thoracic surgery or thoracic trauma. Kaya et al. have reported an incidence of 1.3% of its occurrence [40]. Injury to the three neuron oculosympathetic pathway results in pupillary miosis, ptosis, enophthalmos and facial anhidrosis on ipsilateral face [41].

The thoracic apex has a thin endothoracic fascia between the parietal pleura and the stellate ganglion. Localized ischemia by the malpositioned chest tube is proposed to cause neuropraxia of the second neuronal pathway.

Apical cauterization damaging the second-order neuron [40] and malposition of the chest tube are the etiological factors during thoracic surgery, apart from invasion of the thoracic chain by the malignant tumor. Rib fracture, by virtue of direct effect of fracture of the bone or localized hematoma has also been proposed as an etiological factor [42]. Diagnosis is based on the clinical features. Mostly anisocoria is observed. Clinical confirmation is obtained by "cocaine test" [40]. Cocaine, a noradrenergic reuptake blocker induces mydriasis after topical administration in presence of intact oculosympathetic pathway. In suspected Horner's syndrome, pupillary dilatation is less or absent with respect to the other eye. Time period of pressure is an important factor for recovery. Hence, early repositioning of the chest tube, pulling out 2–3 cm back as soon as possible, post radiological confirmation results in good recovery. Recovery of ptosis has been reported to be earlier than miosis [40].

24.4 Specific Complications

24.4.1 Respiratory Problems

Respiratory complications are the major cause of perioperative morbidity and mortality. Thoracic surgery impairs postoperative respiratory function.

24.4.1.1 Pulmonary Edema

Pulmonary edema post lung resection is a life-threatening condition with an incidence of 2.5–5% in literature [43, 44]. The term "post pneumonectomy pulmonary edema (PPO)" was coined by Zeldin et al. [45]. Causative mechanism is thought to be an excessive fluid perfusion exceeding the drainage capacity of the remaining lymphatic tissue, in absence of left ventricular failure or infection. Other proposed theories are ischemia reperfusion injury [46] and reactive oxygen species [47]. PPO presents as severe respiratory failure with clinical symptoms appearing within 48–72 h postoperatively. Despite this association with excess intraoperative fluid administration, the pulmonary artery occlusion pressure is low [6].

There is a greater incidence of PPO after right pneumonectomy than the left. Predisposing factors are fluid overload, transfusion of fresh frozen plasma, arrhythmia, increased permeability of alveolocapillary membrane, high intraoperative ventilatory pressure, abnormal preoperative lung function, marked postsurgical diuresis, low serum colloid osmotic pressure, and previous radiotherapy [43, 48, 49].

PPO is primarily a diagnosis of exclusion. There should be absence of clinical or radiologic evidence of pulmonary aspiration, bacterial pneumonia, heart failure, sepsis, pulmonary thromboembolism, bronchopleural fistula, or other causes of acute respiratory distress syndrome (ARDS) [44]. CXR finding of PPO is an increased lung parenchymal opacity similar to that of ARDS. Other features are Kerley lines, peribronchial cuffing and poorly defined vessels. Most of the features resolve in few days signifying mild form of disorder [50].

Pulmonary edema may occur post lobectomy but the incidence is low [51]. Treatment is largely supportive including diuretics, fluid restriction, nutritional support, high dose corticosteroids, pulmonary artery vasodilators [inhaled nitric oxide (10–20 ppm)] [52], or extracorporeal support [53].

24.4.1.2 Air Leak

Postoperative air leak is defined as the escape of air from lung parenchyma to the pleural space. Air leaks are common after lung resection surgery with a reported incidence around 50% [54]. Majority of these get resolved on their own within hours or days without the need for any specific intervention. However, some air leaks may occur for a number of days postoperatively referred to as prolonged air leak (PAL). Society of Thoracic Surgeons defines PAL as that air leak that extends beyond fifth postoperative day. Incidence of PAL varies between 18 and 26% [55, 56], with significant morbidity, prolonged hospital stay, and increased costs.

Significant risk factors for air leak are:

- $FEV_1 < 80\%$ [54]
- Low predicted postoperative FEV_1 (ppo FEV_1) [54]
- Age > 65 years [54]
- Upper lobe disease [57]
- Presence of pleural adhesions [57]
- Incomplete or fused fissures [58]
- Emphysema [59]
- Infectious conditions: tuberculosis [60], aspergillosis [61], cystic fibrosis [62]
- Body mass index <25.5 kg/m² [63]

Predictors of air leak on POD 1 [64]:

- Low FEV_1/FVC ratio
- Advanced RV/TLC ratio
- Increased RV
- Increased FRC

Common treatment option is to apply suction of -20 cm H_2O to chest tube till no further evidence of air leak and then convert to plain water seal. However, this suction pressure has been found to prolong air leak in patients undergoing lung volume reduction surgery (LVRS) [65]. Increased air flow prevents leaks from sealing and creates new tears in emphysematous lungs of patients of LVRS. In these cases, use water seal without suction [66]. This should also be used if $FEV_1 < 40\%$ of predicted value.

Expert consensus suggests water seal or, if needed, low amount of suction not exceeding -10 cm H_2O to be applied in the following situations:

- Absence of large, symptomatic growing pneumothorax
- Progressive subcutaneous emphysema
- Clinical deterioration

In absence of emphysema, a short period of suction followed by water seal only or 'alternate suction' are safe [67]. If water seal only protocol is used, a CXR should be done to detect pneumothorax and then apply suction of atleast -10 cm H_2O. Avoid the water seal protocol, and use suction in presence of highly restrictive lung disease or substantial risk of bleeding [54].

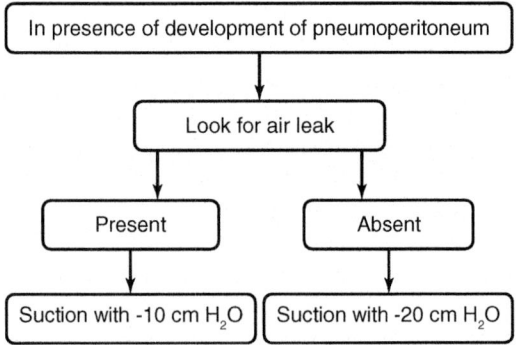

If large leak is present and water seal cannot be tolerated then mechanically seal site of leak. Consider chemical pleurodesis (tetracycline, doxycycline, silver nitrate, or talcum powder) with instillation via thoracostomy tube [66]. Another effective management option is autologous blood patch but it carries the risk of intrathoracic infection [66].

Other conservative management options are:

- Prolonged chest tube drainage
- Provocative chest tube clamping
- Permissive chest tube removal
- Physiotherapy
- Outpatient management with chest tube and Heimlich valve (one way valve) [54]

Surgical options are [54]:

1. VATS to accomplish pleural symphysis with sclerosing agents, pleural abrasion, or pleurectomy
2. Pleural tenting
3. Prophylactic intraoperative pneumoperitoneum
4. Sealing of the lung
5. Buttressing of staple lines

24.4.1.3 Post-pneumonectomy Syndrome

It is a delayed and a rare complication which is known to occur in children and young adults within a year post-pneumonectomy. It was first diagnosed in 1979 after right pneumonectomy by Wasserman et al. [68, 69]. Later, in 1991 left post pneumonectomy syndrome was coined by Quillin and Shackelford [70].

Characteristic feature of the post-pneumonectomy syndrome is the mediastinal shift towards the side of the resected lung by the negative pressure created on that side. Herniation of the overexpanded contralateral lung occurs towards that side. In case of right pneumonectomy, heart descends in the hemithorax and rotates counterclockwise along its main axis. Trachea displaces towards the right causing stretching of the left main bronchus which is compressed between the left main pulmonary artery anteriorly and vertebral column posteriorly [69]. Tracheobronchomalacia in children compounds the bronchial compression.

Increased elasticity and compliance of lung and mediastinum is thought to be the causes for its increased incidence in children and women compared to older patients and men [45, 69, 70].

Presenting complains are exertional dyspnea, stridor and recurrent pulmonary infection ensuing gradually over a year after pneumonectomy. Esophageal compression may result in dysphagia and heartburn [71]. High index of suspicion is helpful in diagnosis. Confirmation is done by bronchoscopy, pulmonary function tests, and CT. CXR demonstrates displacement of the heart and trachea towards the operated hemithorax. CT scan gives information of status of post-pulmonary space, position of mediastinal blood vessels, bronchi and thoracic spine, and specific site of bronchial narrowing [72].

Treatment modalities include mediastinal repositioning with expandable saline prosthesis [73]. Breast silicone implants have been used in children to prevent rotational shifting [69, 73].

24.4.1.4 Lobar Torsion

Lobar torsion is a fatal complication following thoracic surgery with a rare occurrence (0.09–0.4%) [74]. Torsion refers to the twisting of the lobe over the bronchovascular pedicle resulting in obstruction to the bronchial and vascular structures. Right middle lobe is more prone to torsion (70%) compared to the left (15%) [75].

Torsion can result in gangrene if not untwisted promptly. Risk factors for torsion are lack of pleural adhesions, airless lobe, long slim lobar pedicle, incision of inferior pulmonary ligament, complete fissure, or complete mobilization of remaining lung [76, 77].

Presenting symptoms are high grade fever, severe chest pain, massive hemoptysis, sudden unexplained dyspnea, and copious secretions. Pulmonary venous thrombosis may result following prolonged torsion. Diagnosis is based on high index of clinical suspicion or radiological manifestation of sudden opacity of the previously expanded lobe.

Bronchoscopy demonstrates fish mouth appearance of compressed lobar bronchus [78]. Contrast enhanced CT of the chest shows distorted bronchi. Transesophageal echocardiography may show right heart strain, turbulent flow secondary to occluded vascular structure, or presence of thrombus in pulmonary vein. Pulmonary angiography may demonstrate tapered pulmonary artery [76].

Treatment involves de-torsion or pulmonary resection. Prompt diagnosis and de-torsion done within few hours of primary surgery have an improved patient outcome. Best to staple or suture [13] the lobe to the adjacent lobe to prevent further torsion. Essential to rule out presence of pulmonary venous thrombosis prior to de-torsion to avoid risk of stroke [79]. Completion lobectomy is necessitated if ischemic necrosis occurs.

24.4.1.5 Mediastinal Emphysema

Mediastinal emphysema or pneumomediastinum is an entity wherein air accumulates in the mediastinal cavity. It was first described in 1819 by René Laennec [80, 81]. It can result from alveolar, esophageal rupture or following thoracic surgery. In rare circumstances, spontaneous occurrence can even occur [82].

Patient presents with severe central chest pain, labored breathing, voice distortion, subcutaneous emphysema affecting face, neck and chest [9, 83]. Symptoms mimic cardiac tamponade, 'crunching' sound timed with cardiac cycle may be recognized on chest auscultation. CXR demonstrates a radiolucent outline around the heart and mediastinum. Diagnosis is confirmed by CXR and CT scan of the thorax (Fig. 24.5). Treatment is mostly conservative, allowing slow reabsorption of air in the cavity. If lung collapse occurs, then individual is advised to lie on the side of collapse to allow inflation of unaffected lung. Presence of pneumothorax warrants chest tube drainage. In the event of esophageal rupture, surgical repair or esophageal stenting is to be considered [21].

24.4.1.6 Pleural Effusion and Empyema

Small pleural effusions may be seen postoperatively which resolve spontaneously without any specific treatment or intervention. However, in presence of atypical presentation further diagnostic evaluation of pleural exudate should be considered.

Empyema is the collection of purulent material in the post-pneumonectomy space. It is a rare but potentially fatal complication carrying significant morbidity and mortality [84] with a reported incidence of 2–16% in literature [85]. It may be simple or complicated type. Presence of fistula commonly bronchopleural fistula (BPF) is an association in the complicated type. Tumor recurrence and invasion can also result in fistula formation [86]. Early onset empyema manifests in early postoperative period, secondary to intraoperative contamination or presence of preoperative pleural infection. Late onset empyema is generally seen months or several years post surgery [87]. Development of empyema is associated with several risk factors viz completion pneumonectomy, right pneumonectomy, mediastinal lymph node dissection, contaminated pleura, surgery-related sepsis, postoperative mechanical ventilation, prolonged chest tube drainage, long bronchial stumps (>2 cm), tumor recurrence, disrupted bronchial blood supply, poor nutritional status, anemia, preoperative local radiotherapy, chemotherapy, steroid therapy, diabetes, ongoing sepsis, etc. [88, 89].

Clinical features: Initial signs are low grade pyrexia and general expectoration of serosanguinous fluid or pus. Contralateral aspiration, pneumonitis, and auscultation of high pitched sound during Valsalva maneuver is observed in the presence of BPF [90].

Diagnosis: Leukocytosis is seen and C-reactive protein (CRP) levels are often raised which act as a diagnostic indicator for empyema. CRP levels more than 100 mg/l have been reported to have 100% sensitivity and 91.4% specificity for empyema [91]. CXR demonstrates shift of mediastinum towards the remaining lung rather than towards the post-pneumonectomy space (PPS) (Fig. 24.6). There could be a decrease in the air fluid level in PPS along with the presence of communication to outside through bronchus or skin. Replacement of pleural fluid in the hemithorax by air also points toward the presence of BPF or a gas forming organism [92]. CT imaging is superior to radiography in absence of change in

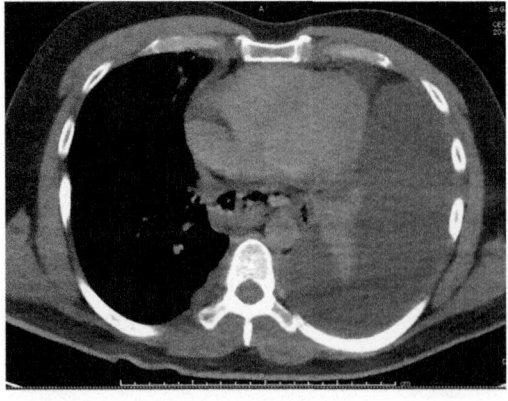

Fig. 24.5 CT thorax showing mediastinal emphysema secondary to esophageal perforation

air fluid level. PPS expansion with mass effect is revealed on CT images. Normal concave border of PPS becomes convex or straightens out. Residual parietal pleura thickens irregularly (Fig. 24.7). BPF or esophagopleural fistula may even be observed [93].

Thoracocentesis involves the risk of introducing infection into the pleural cavity and is therefore not used as a diagnostic indicator. Empyema is best diagnosed based on the clinical findings.

Management: Chest tube drainage is the definitive treatment option. However, consider bronchoscopy to identify presence of BPF, its size, tumor recurrence, and assessment of bronchial stump length. Identification of BPF is difficult if the size is small and slough encases the bronchial stump end. Bubbling or expulsion of fluid at stump end during Valsalva maneuver or coughing during bronchoscopy, points toward the presence of BPF [90]. Specimen of bronchial aspirate should be sent for routine microscopic, cytology, and culture. Commonest organisms are *staphylococcus aureus* and *pseudomonas aeruginosa* [94]. It is vital to control infection, prevent soiling of contralateral lung, optimize functioning of residual lung, provide ventilatory and nutritional support, obliterate pleural space, and close BPF if it exists [90]. This often requires multidisciplinary team approach.

24.4.1.7 Bronchopleural Fistula

Bronchopleural fistula (BPF) is a potentially fatal condition, with a reported incidence from 0–9% [95] and associated mortality rate of 16–23% [96]. Aspiration pneumonitis with resultant ARDS is the commonest cause of death. Bronchial erosion by carcinoma, chronic inflammatory conditions or rupture of lung abscess, bronchus, bulla, cyst or parenchymal tissue into the pleural space can result in BPF.

Bronchial stump dehiscence post lung resection can result in leakage during the first week due to poor primary closure while in the second or third week is often a result of failure of healing by secondary intention. Predisposing risk factors are [97]:

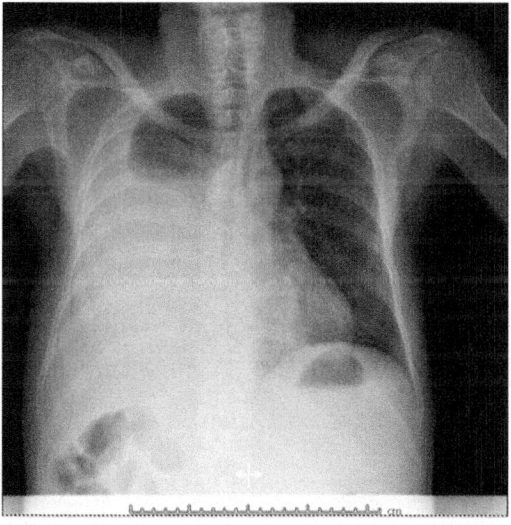

Fig. 24.6 Chest X-ray showing empyema on the right side of the chest

1. Bronchial ischemia from long stump
2. Diameter of bronchial stump [98]
3. Too proximal ligation of bronchial arteries
4. Disruption of tracheobronchial blood supply during lymph node dissection
5. Preoperative pleuropulmonary infection
6. Poor healing after preoperative radiation therapy
7. Malnutrition
8. Steroid therapy
9. Resection through tumor or infection
10. Postoperative positive pressure ventilation for greater than 24 h [99]

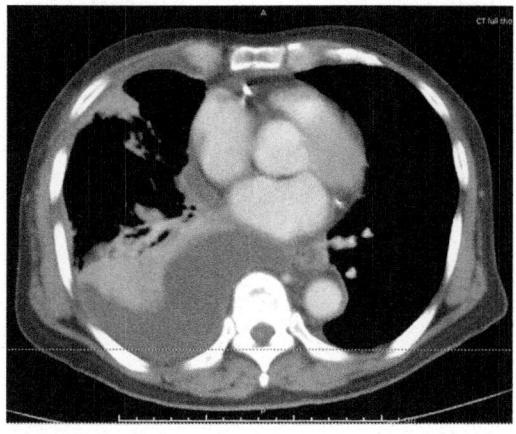

Fig. 24.7 CT thorax showing empyema

Occurrence of BPF after right pneumonectomy is more likely due to shorter stump length, less effective concealment of bronchial stump, and single bronchial artery increasing the vulnerability to ischemia [95, 100].

Presenting features of BPF post pneumonectomy are sudden onset of dyspnea, subcutaneous emphysema, contralateral deviation of trachea, and decrease in fluid level on serial radiographs. However, post lobectomy persistent air leak, drainage and expectoration of purulent material also points toward the presence of BPF. Patients have respiratory embarrassment and hemodynamic instability.

CXR findings corroborative of BPF post pneumonectomy are [92, 96]:

- Failure of PPS to fill with fluid
- In presence of adequate chest drainage, continued or progressive pneumothorax or reappearance of air in previously opaque PPS
- Progressive subcutaneous or mediastinal emphysema
- Consolidation of remaining lung secondary to transbronchial spillage and aspiration
- A 2 cm drop in air fluid level with mediastinal shift to contralateral side during inspiration
- Drop in air fluid level through incision or rent in diaphragm
- ≥1.5 cm decrease in the height of fluid level. A decrease <1.5 cm can be due to difference in posture or in the degree of inspiration unless accompanied by contralateral mediastinal shift

Therefore, cardinal signs of BPF are increased air and decreased fluid level on CXR.

Management: In presence of hemodynamic and respiratory instability, secure the airway with either a DLT or single lumen endotracheal tube placed into the main stem bronchus. Margin of safety is more on the left side. It is usual to extubate the patient immediately post pneumonectomy [21] as spontaneous respiration is desirable but if postoperative positive pressure ventilation is deemed necessary, low inspiratory pressures should be aimed for [21].

24.4.1.8 Pneumonia

There is an increased risk of pneumonia of the remaining lung post pneumonectomy. The incidence varies from 2 to 15% with a reported mortality rate of 25% [101]. Atelectasis of the lung can be attributed to poor postoperative pain control, poor cough, impaired baseline pulmonary functions or anatomical variations viz. chest wall or diaphragmatic dysfunction [33]. Bacterial colonization of the atelectatic lung and silent or overt aspiration of gastric secretions are the most likely causes of pneumonia. Aspiration can be secondary to continued postoperative mechanical ventilation of lungs. Diagnosis should be based on clinical manifestations (cough, fever, leukocytosis) as radiographic appearances are often late. Send blood and sputum for microscopic examination and culture. CXR may reveal foci of increased opacity, air bronchogram, or lobar consolidation (Fig. 24.8). Abscess formation may be evident in case of infection of aspirated material [102]. CT evidence of transbronchial spill in presence of BPF and direct depiction of fistula aids diagnosis (Fig. 24.9).

Emphasis should be on prevention strategies viz preoperative cessation of smoking,

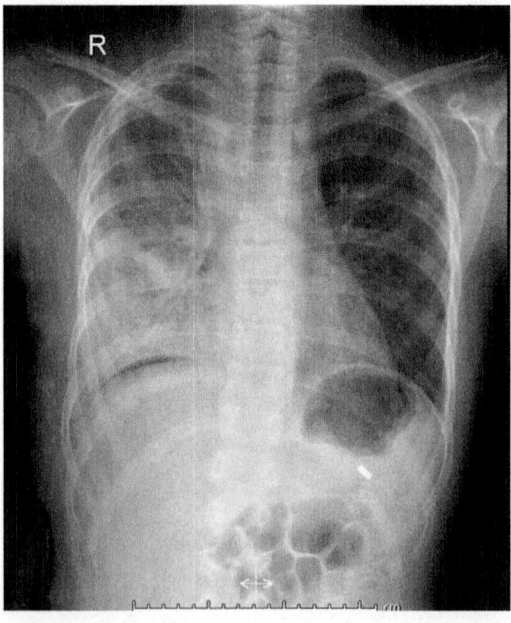

Fig. 24.8 Chest X-ray showing right sided lobar consolidation

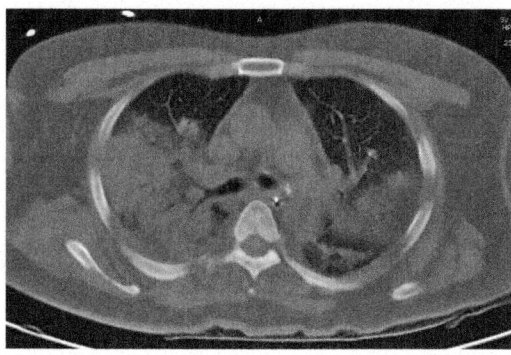

Fig. 24.9 CT thorax showing broncho-pleural fistula

postoperative early extubation and return to spontaneous respiration, chest physiotherapy, coughing, chest percussion, incentive spirometry, early ambulation, inhaled mucolytics, and adequate postoperative pain control [33].

Aggressive chest physiotherapy and antibiotics are the mainstay of treatment. Bronchoalveolar lavage is the most effective way to obtain sputum sample for culture. Antibiotics sensitive to isolated organism should be started. In presence of severe infection, ventilatory support may be required for adequate gas exchange.

24.4.2 Cardiac Problems

24.4.2.1 Arrhythmia

Arrhythmia is common after thoracic surgery in the recovery period or 2–3 days after surgery. Most commonly occurring arrhythmia is atrial fibrillation (AF), accounting for 10–20% post lobectomy and 40% post pneumonectomy [103, 104]. During thoracotomy, association of supraventricular tachycardia with adverse patient outcome or development of myocardial infarction is not clear [105].

Multiple risk factors are known to exist during thoracic surgical procedures leading to arrhythmia. These could be related to [103, 104, 106]:

1. Patient factors:
   (a) Age > 70 years
   (b) Male gender
   (c) Preexisting cardiac disorder
   (d) Postural change
   (e) Extent of pulmonary reserve
   (f) Previous episode of congestive heart failure (CHF)/arrhythmia
2. Surgical factors:
   (a) Amount of lung resected
   (b) Intrapericardial/extrapleural pneumonectomy
   (c) Massive bleeding and need for blood transfusion
3. Anesthetic factors:
   (a) Inhalational agents
   (b) Dyselectrolemia
4. Treatment factors:
   (a) Previous intrathoracic radiotherapy

Prevention strategies are best to avoid perioperative occurrence of AF. Fluid management, electrolyte balance and drugs (β blockers, calcium channel blockers, and amiodarone) have been considered for its prevention. Continuation of preoperative β blockers into the postoperative period can be used as a preventive strategy. Amiodarone and diltiazem can also be considered for prophylaxis in those not taking preoperative β blockers. Flecainide and digoxin do not have a preventive role [107].

Onset of AF in perioperative period is well established but its management depends on the patient's hemodynamic state. AF developing post surgery is often transient and self-limiting but heralds other respiratory complications or infection [108]. In the presence of hemodynamic instability, consider electrical cardioversion. However, if the patient is hemodynamically stable, initially rate controlling agents should be considered for 24 h. This resolves AF within a day of hospital discharge. β blockers can however precipitate bronchospasm, so selective β1 blockers (metoprolol) are first-line drugs to be considered in patients with COPD. In presence of moderate to severe COPD or bronchospasm, diltiazem should be given [107]. β blockers are better than calcium channel blockers in treating AF during thoracic surgery. Oral metoprolol has shown to decrease AF from 40 to 6.7% when given in the perioperative period (pre-, intra-, and postoperative) [109]. Digoxin should not be used for rate control but has a role along with β blockers or calcium channel blockers.

Magnesium has a role in controlling AF if started on the day of lung resection. It has been reported to decrease the incidence of AF from 26.7 to 10.7% [110]. Oral anticoagulation therapy (warfarin) should be considered in presence of risk factors for stroke, recurrent AF, or AF persisting for >48 h. In presence of contraindication to warfarin, aspirin 325 mg daily is recommended [107].

24.4.2.2 Interatrial Shunt

Interatrial shutting of blood from the right to the left side of the heart is a rare occurrence after major thoracic surgery. It occurs secondary to a patent foramen ovale or asymptomatic atrial septal defect. 20–25% adults are known to have a patent foramen ovale [111]. Right pneumonectomy increases the shunting and results in more dramatic presentation than that after left pneumonectomy.

Symptoms can occur immediately in the postoperative period or even a month later. Common presenting symptoms are dyspnea, increase in oxygen consumption, and platypnea–orthodeoxia. Neurological symptoms secondary to paradoxical embolism have also been reported in literature [112].

Pathophysiology of interatrial shunting and presentation of symptoms is poorly understood. Early presentation of symptoms is attributed to increase in resistance of pulmonary vasculature and decreased compliance of right ventricle [113]. Perioperative fluid administration impairs the right heart function and further worsens the symptoms. Mediastinal shift post pneumonectomy distorts the relative relation of the two atria. Pleural fluid accumulated after right pneumonectomy compresses the right atria. Pressure gradient is created between the right and the left atria. Procedures done on the right side relax and elevate the right hemidiaphragm causing distortion of the cardiac axis thereby patent foramen ovale preferentially receives inferior vena caval flow.

Late presentation of symptoms is therefore secondary to distortion of interatrial septum. Posture-dependent hypoxia occurs as the lateral decubitus and upright position (platypnea) decreases right ventricular compliance with resultant increase in shunt fraction. Other predisposing factors for shunting are pulmonary emboli, right ventricular infection, hypovolemia, increased intrathoracic pressure, COPD, and positive pressure ventilation [114].

Diagnosis is predominately made by echocardiogram. Arterial blood gas analysis, nuclear lung perfusion scanning, MRI, and cardiac catheterization have a role in diagnosis [13].

Mostly the symptoms disappear by conservative management. Surgical repair is the standard treatment. Intravascular occlusion of septal defect has been successful. Transcatheter percutaneous closure has a high success rate [13]. High risk of embolic stroke can be devastating. Hence, prompt cardiac investigation and management should be considered.

24.4.2.3 Cardiac Herniation

Cardiac herniation is a potentially fatal complication. The onset is generally in the immediate postsurgical period or within 24 h post intrapericardial pneumonectomy but late onset with gradual development has also been reported [115]. Its occurrence is rare with a reported mortality rate of 40–50% [116]. Surgical exposure during pneumonectomy or lobectomy requires creating a defect in the pericardium through which the heart muscle prolapses which is referred to as cardiac herniation [115].

Presenting features: Sudden hypotension, cyanosis, and circulatory distress. Right sided herniation impairs the venous drainage of superior vena cava resulting in raised jugular venous pulse, cyanosis of face and neck, obstructive shock secondary to impaired cardiac filling. Ventricular strangulation by pericardial edges in case of left sided herniation results in myocardial ischemia and arrhythmia. Ventricular fibrillation is known to occur.

Triggering factors are [97]:

- Positive intrathoracic pressure secondary to coughing and mechanical ventilation
- Negative pressure suction on chest tube drainage
- Change in patient's position

Diagnosis: Prompt diagnosis is critical, based on CXR or echocardiogram. Right side herniation is easier to diagnose on CXR.

Radiographic findings are:

Right sided herniation
- Displacement of cardiac apex to right hemithorax in lateral costophrenic sulcus. Occasionally, it may be seen in posterior costophrenic sulcus [117], if counterclockwise rotation has occurred.

Left sided herniation
- Gas-filled pericardial sac may be present in the left hemithorax.
- Bulge in the cardiac contour with sharp demarcation by constricting pericardial edge [97].

Management: Emergency thoracotomy for immediate repositioning of the herniated heart is crucial in maintaining hemodynamic stability. Pericardial defect is repaired either by suturing cut edges of pericardium to the epicardium or patching the defect. Bovine pericardial patch, PTFE patch, or parietal pleura can be used for repairing the defect [118]. In cases of right pneumonectomy intrapericardial defect should be surgically repaired while the defect should be sufficiently enlarged during left pneumonectomy in order to prevent strangulation, should herniation occur.

24.4.2.4 Cardiac Tamponade

Although rare, cardiac tamponade can occur even with minor retraction and dissection during thoracic surgery. Repeated episodes of hypotension with venodilator therapy points to the possibility of pericardiac tamponade. Symptomatology is those of low cardiac output state. Hypotension, raised jugular venous pulse, and muffled heart sound form the Beck's triad, diagnostic of cardiac tamponade [13]. Diagnosis is based on high index of suspicion.

Echocardiography demonstrates impaired filling of the right ventricle. Treatment involves urgent pericardiocentesis to prevent fatal adverse outcome. Definite management requires surgical exploration either by reopening the thoracotomy wound or formal median sternotomy.

24.4.3 Neurological Problem

24.4.3.1 Cerebral Infarction

Cardiogenic thrombus is the commonest cause of cerebral infarction. Post-lobectomy thrombus formation in the pulmonary vein occurs with a reported incidence of 3.3–3.6% with a particularly higher incidence after left upper lung lobectomy (13.5–17.9%) [119].

The long length of left superior pulmonary vein compared to other vessels makes it prone to blood stasis creating turbulence in its stump resulting in thrombus formation. This propensity of thrombosis is further exaggerated by the structural position of this vessel and the left atrium. New onset atrial fibrillation post lobectomy with a high incidence of 10.8–11.8% [120] is also an embolic risk factor. Cerebral infarction can occur within days or years after lung surgery. There have also been reports of some idiopathic causes of stroke. However, the overall reports of cerebral infarction post-thoracotomy are rare.

24.5 Conclusion

Advancement in surgical procedures has increased the number of thoracic operations performed in recent years. Preoperative disease process, dynamic changes in respiratory physiology in the intraoperative and postoperative period results in a number of complications post thoracic surgery. Risk stratification enables the identification of 'at risk' patients. Added attention to postoperative strategies, vigilance, and immediate intervention can circumvent the potentially lethal complications.

References

1. Dimick JB, Pronovost PJ, Cowan JA, et al. Variation in postoperative complication rates after high-risk surgery in the United States. Surgery. 2003;134:534–40.
2. Fisher BW, Majumdar SR, McAlister FA. Predicting pulmonary complications after nonthoracic surgery: a systematic review of blinded studies. Am J Med. 2002;112:219–25.

3. Agostini P, Cieslik H, Rathinam S, et al. Postoperative pulmonary complications following thoracic surgery: are there any modifiable risk factors? Thorax. 2010;65:815–8.
4. Nakagawa M, Tanaka H, Tsukuma H, et al. Relationship between the duration of the preoperative smoke-free period and the incidence of postoperative pulmonary complications after pulmonary surgery. Chest. 2001;120:705–10.
5. Slinger P, Darling G. Preanesthetic assessment for thoracic surgery. In: Slinger P, editor. Principles and practice of anesthesia for thoracic surgery. New York: Springer; 2011. p. 19.
6. Sengupta S. Post-operative pulmonary complications after thoracotomy. Indian J Anaesth. 2015;59:618–26.
7. Shapiro BA, Harrison RA, Kacmarek RM, et al. Clinical application of respiratory care. 3rd ed. Chicago: Year Book; 1985.
8. Nair P, Milan SJ, Rowe BH. Addition of intravenous aminophylline to inhaled beta (2)-agonists in adults with acute asthma. Cochrane Database Syst Rev. 2012;12:CD002742.
9. Ahmed ST. General postoperative management. In: Searl CP, Ahmed ST, editors. Core topics in thoracic anesthesia. Cambridge Books Online ©. Cambridge: Cambridge University Press; 2009.
10. Sirbu H, Busch T, Aleksic I, et al. Chest re-exploration for complications after lung surgery. Thorac Cardiovasc Surg. 1999;47:73–6.
11. Krasna MJ, Deshmukh S, McLaughlin JS. Complications of thoracoscopy. Ann Thorc Surg. 1996;61:1066–9.
12. Yim AP, Liu HP. Complications and failures of video-assisted thoracic surgery: experience from two centers in Asia. Ann Thorac Surg. 1996;61:538–41.
13. Iyer A, Yadav S. Postoperative care and complications after thoracic surgery, principles and practice of cardiothoracic surgery. Intech Open. 2013. https://doi.org/10.5772/55351. https://www.intechopen.com/books/principles-and-practice-of-cardiothoracic-surgery/postoperative-care-and-complications-after-thoracic-surgery
14. Litle VR, Swanson SJ. Postoperative bleeding: coagulopathy, bleeding, hemothorax. Thorac Surg Clin. 2006;16:203–7.
15. Wahba RM. Airway closure and intraoperative hypoxaemia: twenty-five years later. Can J Anaesth. 1996;43:1144–9.
16. Rosenberg J, Ullstad T, Rasmussen J, et al. Time course of postoperative hypoxaemia. Eur J Surg. 1994;160:137–43.
17. Powell JF, Menon DK, Jones JG. The effects of hypoxaemia and recommendations for postoperative oxygen therapy. Anaesthesia. 1996;51:769–72.
18. Marini JJ, Pierson DJ, Hudson LD. Acute lobar atelectasis: a prospective comparison of fiberoptic bronchoscopy and respiratory therapy. Am Rev Respir Dis. 1979;119:971–8.
19. Feldman NT, Huber GL. Fiberoptic bronchoscopy in the intensive care unit. Int Anesthesiol Clin. 1976;14:31–42.
20. Jepsen S, Nielsen PH, Klaerke A, et al. Peroral N-acetylcysteine as prophylaxis against bronchopulmonary complications of pulmonary surgery. Scand J Thorac Cardiovasc Surg. 1989;23:185–8.
21. Raiten JM, Blank RS. Anesthetic management of post-thoracotomy complication. In: Slinger P, editor. Principles and practice of anesthesia for thoracic surgery. New York: Springer; 2011. p. 601–8.
22. Worsley DF, Alavi A, Aronchick JM, et al. Chest radiographic findings in patients with acute pulmonary embolism: observations from the PIOPED study. Radiology. 1993;189:133–6.
23. Stein PD, Woodard PK, Weg JG, et al. Diagnostic pathways in acute pulmonary embolism: recommendations of the PIOPED II investigators. Radiology. 2007;242:15–21.
24. Chen Q, Tang AT, Tsang GM. Acute pulmonary thromboembolism complicating pneumonectomy: successful operative management. Eur J Cardiothorac Surg. 2001;19:223–5.
25. Schweizer A, Khatchatourian G, Hohn L, et al. Opening of a new postanesthesia care unit: impact on critical care utilization and complications following major vascular and thoracic surgery. J Clin Anesth. 2002;14:486–93.
26. Bellomo R, Ronco C, Kellum JA, et al. Acute renal failure—definition, outcome measures, animal models, fluid therapy and information technology needs: the second international consensus conference of the acute dialysis quality initiative (ADQI) group. Crit Care. 2004;8:R204–R12.
27. Licker M, Cartier V, Robert J, et al. Risk factors of acute kidney injury according to RIFLE criteria after lung cancer surgery. Ann Thorac Surg. 2011;91:844–50.
28. Ishikawa S, Griesdale DE, Lohser J. Acute kidney injury after lung resection surgery: incidence and perioperative risk factors. Anesth Analg. 2012;114:1256–62.
29. Roberts J, Wadsworth J. Recurrent laryngeal nerve monitoring during mediastinoscopy: predictors of injury. Ann Thorac Surg. 2007;83:388–92.
30. Sagawa M, Donjo T, Isobe T, et al. Bilateral vocal cord paralysis after lung cancer surgery with a double-lumen endotracheal tube: a life-threatening complication. J Cardiothorac Vasc Anesth. 2006;20:225–6.
31. Bhattacharyya N, Batirel H, Swanson SJ. Improved outcomes with early vocal fold medicalization for vocal fold paralysis after thoracic surgery. Auris Nasus Larynx. 2003;30:71–5.
32. Haithcock BE, Feins RH. Complications of pulmonary resection. In: Shields MD, Thomas W, LoCicero J, Reed CE, Feins RH, editors. General thoracic surgery. 7th ed. Philadelphia: Lippincott Williams & Wilkins; 2009. p. 558.
33. Ziarnik E, Grogan EL. Post lobectomy early complications. Thorac Surg Clin. 2015;25:355–64.

34. Kutlu CA, Sayar A, Olgac G, et al. Chylothorax: a complication following lung resection in patients with NSCLC: chylothorax following lung resection. Thorac Cardiovasc Surg. 2003;51:342–5.
35. de Beer HG, Mol MJ, Janssen JP. Chylothorax. Neth J Med. 2000;56:25–31.
36. Fernandez Alvarez JR, Kalache KD, Grauel EL. Management of spontaneous congenital chylothorax: oral medium-chain triglycerides versus total parenteral nutrition. Am J Perinatol. 1999;16:415–20.
37. Emmet EM, Zoe B, Paul BA. Chylothorax: aetiology, diagnosis and therapeutic options. Respir Med. 2010;104:1–8.
38. Graham DD, McGrahren ED, Tribble CG, et al. Use of video-assisted thoracic surgery in the treatment of chylothorax. Ann Thorac Surg. 1994;57:1507–11.
39. Kent RB 3rd, Pinson TW. Thoracoscopic ligation of the thoracic duct. Surg Endosc. 1993;7:52–3.
40. Kaya SO, Liman ST, Bir LS, et al. Horner's syndrome as a complication in thoracic surgical practice. Eur J Cardiothorac Surg. 2003;24:1025–8.
41. Ors Kaya S, Cakan A, Yuncu G, et al. Horner's syndrome. An unusual complication. Minerva Pneumol. 2001;40:49–51.
42. Hassan AN, Ballester J, Slater N. Bilateral first rib fractures associated with Horner's syndrome. Injury. 2000;31:273–4.
43. Turnage WS, Lunn JJ. Postpneumonectomy pulmonary edema: a retrospective analysis of associated variables. Chest. 1993;103:1646–50.
44. Deslauriers J, Aucoin A, Grégoire J. Postpneumonectomy pulmonary edema. Chest Surg Clin N Am. 1998;8:611–31.
45. Zeldin RA, Normandin D, Landtwing D, et al. Postpneumonectomy pulmonary edema. J Thorac Cardiovasc Surg. 1984;87:359–65.
46. Hamvas A, Palazzo R, Kaiser L, et al. Inflammation and oxygen free radical formation during pulmonary ischemia–reperfusion injury. J Appl Physiol. 1992;72:621–8.
47. Halliwell B. Reactive oxygen species in living systems: source, biochemistry, and role in human disease. Am J Med. 1991;91:14S–22S.
48. van der Werff YD, van der Houwen HK, Heijmans PJ, et al. Postpneumonectomy pulmonary edema. A retrospective analysis of incidence and possible risk factors. Chest. 1997;111:1278–84.
49. Parquin F, Marchal M, Mehiri S, et al. Post pneumonectomy pulmonary edema: analysis and risk factors. Eur J Cardiothorac Surg. 1996;10:929–32.
50. Gluecker T, Capasso P, Schnyder P, et al. Clinical and radiologic features of pulmonary edema. Radiographics. 1999;19:1507–31.
51. Slinger P. Post pneumonectomy pulmonary edema: is anesthesia to blame? Curr Opin Anaesthesiol. 1999;12:49–54.
52. Samano MN, Sancho LM, Beyruti R, et al. Postpneumonectomy pulmonary edema. J Bras Pneumol. 2005;31:69–75.
53. Alvarez JM, Bairstow BM, Tang C, et al. Post-lung resection pulmonary edema: a case for aggressive management. J Cardiothorac Vasc Anesth. 1998;12:199–205.
54. Mueller MR, Marzluf BA. The anticipation and management of air leaks and residual spaces post lung resection. J Thorac Dis. 2014;6:271–84.
55. Stéphan F, Boucheseiche S, Hollande J, et al. Pulmonary complications following lung resection: a comprehensive analysis of incidence and possible risk factors. Chest. 2000;118:1263–70.
56. Abolhoda A, Liu D, Brooks A, et al. Prolonged air leak following radical upper lobectomy: an analysis of incidence and possible risk factors. Chest. 1998;113:1507–10.
57. DeCamp MM, Blackstone EH, Naunheim KS, et al. Patient and surgical factors influencing air leak after lung volume reduction surgery: lessons learned from the National Emphysema Treatment Trial. Ann Thorac Surg. 2006;82:197–206.
58. Gómez-Caro A, Calvo MJ, Lanzas JT, et al. The approach of fused fissures with fissureless technique decreases the incidence of persistent air leak after lobectomy. Eur J Cardiothorac Surg. 2007;31:203–8.
59. Keller CA. Lasers, staples, bovine pericardium, talc, glue and suction cylinders? Tools of the trade to avoid air leaks in lung volume reduction surgery. Chest. 2004;125:361–3.
60. Mohsen T, Zeid AA, Haj-Yahia S. Lobectomy or pneumonectomy for multidrug-resistant pulmonary tuberculosis can be performed with acceptable morbidity and mortality: a seven-year review of a single institution's experience. J Thorac Cardiovasc Surg. 2007;134:194–8.
61. Csekeo A, Agócs L, Egerváry M, et al. Surgery for pulmonary aspergillosis. Eur J Cardiothorac Surg. 1997;12:876–9.
62. Amin R, Noone PG, Ratjen F. Chemical pleurodesis versus surgical intervention for persistent and recurrent pneumothoraces in cystic fibrosis. Cochrane Database Syst Rev. 2009;2:CD007481.
63. Brunelli A, Varela G, Refai M, et al. A scoring system to predict the risk of prolonged air leak after lobectomy. Ann Thorac Surg. 2010;90:204–9.
64. Cerfolio RJ, Tummala RP, Holman WL, et al. A prospective algorithm for the management of air leaks after pulmonary resection. Ann Thorac Surg. 1998;66:1726–31.
65. Cooper JD, Patterson GA, Sundaresan RS, et al. Results of 150 consecutive bilateral lung volume reduction procedures in patients with severe emphysema. J Thorac Cardiovasc Surg. 1996;112:1319–29.
66. Burt BM, Shrager JB. Prevention and management of postoperative air leaks. Ann Cardiothorac Surg. 2014;3:216–8.
67. Brunelli A, Sabbatini A, Xiumé F, et al. Alternate suction reduces prolonged air leak after pulmonary lobectomy: a randomized comparison versus water seal. Ann Thorac Surg. 2005;80:1052–5.

68. Wasserman K, Jamplis RW, Lash H, et al. Post pneumonectomy syndrome. Surgical correction using silastic implants. Chest. 1979;75:78–81.
69. Mehran RJ, Deslauriers J. Late complications. Postpneumonectomy syndrome. Chest Surg Clin N Am. 1999;9:655–73.
70. Quillin SP, Shackelford GD. Postpneumonectomy syndrome after left lung resection. Radiology. 1991;179:100–2.
71. Soll C, Hahnloser D, Frauenfelder T, et al. The postpneumonectomy syndrome: clinical presentation and treatment. Eur J Cardiothorac Surg. 2009;35:319–24.
72. Kim EA, Lee KS, Shim YM, et al. Radiographic and CT findings in complications following pulmonary resection. Radiographics. 2002;22:67–86.
73. Ng T, Ryder BA, Maziak DE, et al. Thoracoscopic approach for the treatment of postpneumonectomy syndrome. Ann Thorac Surg. 2009;88:1015–8.
74. Apostolakis E, Koletsis EN, Panagopoulos N, et al. Fatal stroke after completion pneumonectomy for torsion of left upper lobe following left lower lobectomy. J Cardiothorac Surg. 2006;1:25.
75. Wagner RB, Nesbitt JC. Pulmonary torsion and gangrene. Chest Surg Clin N Am. 1992;2:839–52.
76. Cable DG, Deschamps C, Allen MS, et al. Lobar torsion after pulmonary resection: presentation and outcome. J Thorac Cardiovasc Surg. 2001;122:1091–3.
77. Jones JM, Paxton LD, Graham AN. Acute postoperative lobar torsion associated with pulmonary arterial rupture. J Thorac Cardiovasc Surg. 2003;126:303.
78. Schamaun M. Postoperative pulmonary torsion: report of a case and survey of the literature including spontaneous and posttraumatic torsion. Thorac Cardiovasc Surg. 1994;42:116–21.
79. Burri E, Duwe J, Kull C, et al. Pulmonary vein thrombosis after lower lobectomy of the left lung. J Cardiovasc Surg. 2006;47:609–12.
80. Laënnec RTH. De l'auscultation médiate ou Traité du diagnostic des maladies des Poumon et du Coeur. 1st ed. Paris: Brosson & Chaudé; 1819.
81. Roguin A. Rene Theophile Hyacinthe Laënnec (1781–1826): the man behind the stethoscope. Clin Med Res. 2006;4:230–5.
82. Yellin A, Gapany-Gapanavicius M, Lieberman Y. Spontaneous pneumomediastinum: is it a rare cause of chest pain? Thorax. 1983;38:383–5.
83. Quresi SA, Tilyard A. Unusual presentation of spontaneous mediastinum: a case report. Cases J. 2008;1:349.
84. Puskas JD, Mathisen DJ, Grillo HC, et al. Treatment strategies for bronchopleural fistula. J Thorac Cardiovasc Surg. 1995;109:989–95.
85. Darling GE, Abdurahman A, Yi QL, et al. Risk of a right pneumonectomy: role of bronchopleural fistula. Ann Thorac Surg. 2005;79:433–7.
86. Oliaro A, Filosso PL, Casadio C, et al. Right post pneumonectomy pleural empyema caused by an esophagopleural fistula due to an esophageal carcinoma. J Cardiovasc Surg. 1995;36:607–9.
87. Kirsh MM, Rotman H, Behrendt DM, et al. Complications of pulmonary resection. Ann Thorac Surg. 1975;20:215–36.
88. Asamura H, Naruke T, Tsuchiya R, et al. Bronchopleural fistulas associated with lung cancer operations. Univariate and multivariate analysis of risk factors, management, and outcome. J Thorac Cardiovasc Surg. 1992;104:1456–64.
89. Algar FJ, Alvarez A, Aranda JL, et al. Prediction of early bronchopleural fistula after pneumonectomy: a multivariate analysis. Ann Thorac Surg. 2001;72:1662–7.
90. Ng CS, Wan S, Lee TW, et al. Post-pneumonectomy empyema: current management strategies. ANZ J Surg. 2005;75:597–602.
91. Icard P, Fleury JP, Regnard JF, et al. Utility of C-reactive protein measurements for empyema diagnosis after pneumonectomy. Ann Thorac Surg. 1994;57:933–6.
92. Goodman LR. Postoperative chest radiograph. II. Alterations after major intrathoracic surgery. AJR Am J Roentgenol. 1980;134:803–13.
93. Choe DH, Lee JH, Lee BH, et al. Postpneumonectomy empyema: CT findings in six patients. Clin Imaging. 2001;25:28–31.
94. Deschamps C, Allen MS, Trastek VF, et al. Empyema following pulmonary resection. Chest Surg Clin N Am. 1994;4:583–92.
95. Hubaut JJ, Baron O, Al Habash O, et al. Closure of the bronchial stump by manual suture and incidence of bronchopleural fistula in a series of 209 pneumonectomies for lung cancer. Eur J Cardiothorac Surg. 1999;16:418–23.
96. Lauckner ME, Beggs I, Armstrong RF. The radiological characteristics of bronchopleural fistula following pneumonectomy. Anaesthesia. 1983;38:452–6.
97. Tsukada G, Stark P. Postpneumonectomy complications: pictorial essay. AJR. 1997;169:1363–71.
98. Hollaus PH, Setinek U, Lax F, et al. Risk factors for bronchopleural fistula after pneumonectomy: stump size does matter. Thorac Cardiovasc Surg. 2003;51:162–6.
99. Javadpour H, Sidhu P, Luke D. Bronchopleural fistula after pneumonectomy. Ir J Med Sci. 2003;172:13–5.
100. Lams P. Radiographic signs in post-pneumonectomy bronchopleural fistula. J Can Assoc Radiol. 1980;31:178–80.
101. Nagasaki F, Flehinger BJ, Martini N. Complications of surgery in the treatment of carcinoma of the lung. Chest. 1982;82:25–9.
102. Franquet T, Giménez A, Rosón N, et al. Aspiration diseases: findings, pitfalls, and differential diagnosis. Radiographics. 2000;20:673–85.
103. Amar D. Cardiac arrhythmias. Chest Surg Clin N Am. 1998;8:479–93.
104. Amar D, Zhang H, Roistacher N. The incidence and outcome of ventricular arrhythmias after noncardiac thoracic surgery. Anesth Analg. 2002;95:537–43.
105. Groves J, Edwards ND, Carr B, et al. Perioperative myocardial ischaemia, heart rate and arrhythmia in

patients undergoing thoracotomy: an observational study. Br J Anaesth. 1999;83:850–4.
106. Asamura H, Naruke T, Tsuchiya R, et al. What are the risk factors for arrhythmias after thoracic operations? A retrospective multivariate analysis of 267 consecutive thoracic operations. J Thorac Cardiovasc Surg. 1993;106:1104–10.
107. Fernando HC, Jaklitsch MT, Walsh GL, et al. The STS practice guideline on the prophylaxis and management of atrial fibrillation associated with general thoracic surgery: an executive summary. Ann Thorac Surg. 2011;92:1144–52.
108. Roselli EE, Murthy SC, Rice TW, et al. Atrial fibrillation complicating lung cancer resection. J Thorac Cardiovasc Surg. 2005;130:438–44.
109. Jakobsen CJ, Bille S, Ahlburg P, et al. Perioperative metoprolol reduces the frequency of atrial fibrillation after thoracotomy for lung resection. J Cardiothorac Vasc Anesth. 1997;11:746–51.
110. Terazi A, Furlan G, Chiavacci P, et al. Prevention of atrial tachyarrhythmias after non-cardiac thoracic surgery by infusion of magnesium sulfate. Thorac Cardiovasc Surg. 1996;44:300–3.
111. Hagen PT, Scholz DG, Edwards WD. Incidence and size of patent foramen ovale during the first 10 decades of life: an autopsy study of 965 normal hearts. Mayo Clin Proc. 1984;59:17–20.
112. Ng SY, Sugarbaker DJ, Frend G. Interatrial shunting after major thoracic surgery: a rare but clinically significant event. Ann Thorac Surg. 2012;93:1647–51.
113. Bakris NC, Siddiqi AJ, Fraser CD Jr, et al. Right to left interatrial shunt after pneumonectomy. Ann Thorac Surg. 1997;63:198–201.
114. Karamichalis JM, Putnam JB Jr, Lambright ES. Cardiovascular complications after lung surgery. Thorac Surg Clin. 2006;16:253–60.
115. Asamura H. Early complications: cardiac complications. Chest Surg Clin N Am. 1999;9:527–41.
116. Dippel WF, Ehrenhaft JL. Herniation of the heart after pneumonectomy. J Thorac Cardiovasc Surg. 1973;65:207–9.
117. Gurney JW, Arnold S, Goodman LR. Impending cardiac herniation: the snow cone sign. Radiology. 1986;161:653–5.
118. Papsin BC, Gorenstein LA, Goldberg M. Delayed myocardial laceration after intrapericardial pneumonectomy. Ann Thorac Surg. 1993;55:756–7.
119. Ohtaka K, Hida Y, Kaga K, et al. Thrombosis in the pulmonary vein stump after left upper lobectomy as a possible cause of cerebral infarction. Ann Thorac Surg. 2013;95:1924–8.
120. Xin Y, Hida Y, Kaga K, et al. Left lobectomy might be a risk factor for atrial fibrillation following pulmonary lobectomy. Eur J Cardiothorac Surg. 2014;45:247–50.

Pain Management in Thoracic Surgery

Manish Kohli and Pradeep Jain

25.1 Introduction

Pulmonary dysfunction of variable intensity occurs in post-thoracotomy patients. The severity of dysfunction depends not only on the sequelae or complex etiopathogenesis of the disease process for which thoracic surgery was done, but also on the severity of pain which the patient experiences after thoracic surgery. In such case scenarios, pain is the only factor that is manageable. Post-thoracotomy pain, when left untreated, is associated with exaggerated pulmonary as well as extra pulmonary complications. This affects the quality of life and satisfaction levels of the patients, thereby resulting in longer hospital stay, which in turn incurs increased costs [1]. Acute post-thoracotomy pain, when left unattended, may lead to an even worse situation: chronic post-thoracotomy pain (CPTP) [2, 3]. This type of pain is neuropathic in nature and is generally less detrimental to respiration, but it can be severely incapacitating, making daily activities impossible.

Inspiration is extremely painful after thoracotomy as it results in stretching of the surgical incision. If there is inadequate pain control, the patient reflexly contracts the expiratory muscles to limit stretch of incision or injured structures. Splinting of injured hemithorax occurs and passive respiration is converted to an active one. Thus, there is a failure to inspire adequately or deeply before forceful expiration. The functional residual capacity (FRC) (Table 25.1) decreases and cough is ineffective, which causes retention of secretions. Sputum clearance is also affected. At a stage where FRC falls below the closing capacity, airway closure starts and resultant atelectasis develops with ventilation–perfusion mismatch [4, 5]. There is a resultant decrease in diaphragmatic function due to surgery, along with reduced forced expiratory volume in 1 s (FEV1) and forced vital capacity (FVC). Early tracheal extubation is practiced for thoracotomy patients to prevent respiratory infection and to decrease the risk of barotrauma, like "blow out" of bronchial sutures. Inadequate pain relief causes hypoxemia, hypercarbia, and the potential

Table 25.1 Pulmonary dysfunction in post-thoracotomy

Partial or complete resection of lung
Lobar collapse due to bronchial architecture distortion
Impaired airway resistance and mucociliary clearance
Altered pulmonary pressures due to physiological and mechanical factors
Liberal fluid therapy
Altered thoracic cage mechanics due to pain
Diaphragmatic dysfunction
Residual lung tissue edema
Postoperative hemorrhage
Abdominal distension
Residual anesthetic agents

M. Kohli (✉) · P. Jain
Institute of Anaesthesiology, Pain and Perioperative Medicine, Sir Ganga Ram Hospital, New Delhi, India

for tracheal re-intubation in the postoperative period for the purpose of pulmonary toileting. Adequate pain control increases the ability of patients to cooperate for postoperative physiotherapy and early remobilization [6].

Pain triggers the stress response which, in turn, causes an increase in the sympathetic tone along with a rise in circulating catecholamine or lactate levels and catabolic hormones resulting in tachycardia, hypertension, and hyperglycemia [7, 8]. The amalgamation of these factors leads to an enhanced risk of myocardial ischemia in a respiratory compromised patient. Effective perioperative analgesia can prevent many of these catastrophic events and the onus of providing optimum analgesia lies on the anesthesiologists [9].

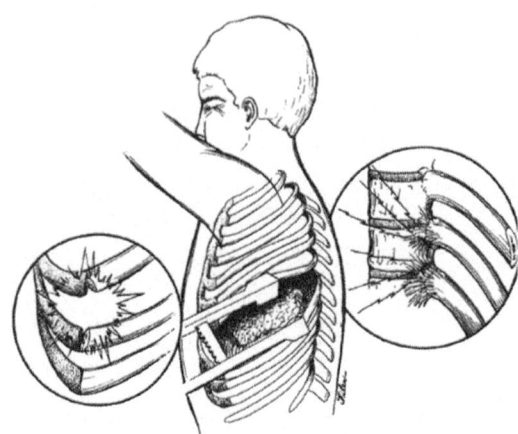

Fig. 25.1 Ribs with intercostal joints and neurovascular bundles get damaged during thoracotomy. Source: Landreneau RJ, Mack MJ, Hazelrigg SR, Naunheim K, Dowling RD, Ritter P, et al. Prevalence of chronic pain after pulmonary resection by thoracotomy or video-assisted thoracic surgery. J Thorac Cardiovasc Surg. 1994;107(4):1079–85. discussion 85–6

25.2 Pathogenesis of Post-thoracotomy Pain

The pathogenesis of pain in post-thoracotomy patients is complex, involving stimulation of peripheral nociceptive receptors and the sympathetic and parasympathetic systems as well. Perioperative mechanisms contributing to the stimulation of nociceptors include [5] (Table 25.2 and Fig. 25.1):

- Skin incision
- Muscle retraction
- Rib retraction, dislocation, and sometimes fractures
- Ligament stretching or injury
- Dislocation of costochondral joints
- Intercostal nerve injury
- Inflammatory process activation due to incision of pleura, residual blood in pleura and chest drains
- Diaphragmatic irritation and positioning, leading to ipsilateral shoulder pain

Transmission of sensory pain stimulus in post-thoracotomy patients [10, 11]

These multiple nociceptive signals when transmitted centrally, synergistically amplify pain perception. Perception of pain is thus altered through central sensitization [12].

Table 25.2 Transmission of sensory pain stimuli in post-thoracotomy patients [10, 11]

Transmitting Nerve	Region of Sensory stimulus
Intercostal nerves	Chest wall, costal pleura, peripheral diaphragmatic pleura
Phrenic nerve	The mediastinal pleura, diaphragmatic dome pleura, the parietal layer of the serous pericardium, fibrous pericardium
Vagus nerve	Somatic and visceral afferent nerve fibers
Sympathetic nerves	Lung and mediastinum

25.3 Factors Influencing Pain After Thoracotomy

- Sex
- Age
- Preoperative education and enhanced recovery after surgery (ERAS) protocol. ERAS is a multimodal pathway designed for early recovery in the postoperative period in patients undergoing major surgery
- Opioid tolerance

- Psychological factor
- Preemptive analgesia
- Surgical approach
  - Sternotomy
  - Video-assisted thoracoscopic surgery
  - Open thoracotomy
    o Posterolateral incision
    o Muscle-sparing incision
    o Anterior incision
    o Transverse sternothoracotomy

25.3.1 Sex

Female patients experience more frequent, diffuse, and severe pain than males with similar disease patterns, but the results are not consistent [20]. It is further stated that this alteration of pain perception decreases with age. No recommendations have, however, been made and management needs to be individualized.

25.3.2 Age

Young patients experience more pain postoperatively. There is blunting of peripheral nociceptors with age [21], but practically pain severity does not decrease much. Analgesic drug doses need to be calibrated and individualized with increasing age as pharmacokinetics or sensitivity of drugs is altered. Even epidural spread is more in elderly patients requiring about 40% less epidural dose [22, 23].

25.3.3 Preoperative Education

Perioperative pain management should be initiated preoperatively. During preoperative counselling, all the preexisting pain issues should be addressed. Patients should be educated well regarding favorable surgical outcomes and on issues regarding expectations from pain control methods. Adequate psychological support, anxiety control, and motivating patients to express their feelings and concerns greatly help in establishing faith and good pain control postoperatively. Each patient's therapy has to be individualized and all pertinent issues should be meticulously documented [13]. The postoperative nursing staff should know each patient individually and be aware of the importance of good pain control for patient recovery. In this enhanced recovery program, a multidisciplinary team of anesthesiologists, nurses, thoracic surgeons, and a pain physician significantly lowers the amount of analgesic consumption [14, 15]. This preoperative program may vary among institutes, depending on available resources and expertise of staff and doctors. This not only improves patient satisfaction and stay in hospital but is also beneficial for the institution.

25.3.4 Opioid Tolerance

Postoperative opioid therapy for analgesia, even for 2 weeks, can lead to opioid consumption [16]. This overconsumption is also augmented in patients who are previous substance abusers or those receiving opioid therapy for malignant or nonmalignant disease, or on opioids for chronic pain management. These patients have higher pain scores and readmission rates [17].

25.3.5 Psychological Factors

IASP has defined pain as "an unpleasant sensory and emotional experience associated with actual or potential tissue damage, or described in terms of such damage." Neuroticism, depression, and anxiety are shown to be predictors of severe pain postoperatively. Preoperative anxiety lowers the pain threshold [24–26]. Good preoperative communication, reassurance, and anxiolytics reduce anxiety. Depression is found to be a risk factor for conversion to chronic pain. Altered cognitive functions enhance pain perception and lead to multidimensional sequelae of helplessness and suicidal tendencies. Cognitive behavioral therapy should be part of an enhanced recovery program [24].

Suicidal tendencies, however, can also develop with both uncontrolled and chronic pain [27].

25.3.6 Preemptive Analgesia

Crile [18] has suggested that pain therapy, if initiated before the generation of a pain stimulus, results in decreased postoperative pain scores for prolonged periods, and also inhibits the transformation of acute to chronic pain. For thoracic surgery patients preemptive analgesia can be given via pharmacological agents and regional analgesia techniques. Though the results are conflicting it is a widely accepted concept. However, a systemic review in 2005 concluded that incidence of chronic post-thoracotomy pain does not decrease with preemptive epidural analgesia [19].

25.3.7 Surgical Approaches for Thoracic Surgery

25.3.7.1 Sternotomy

Sternotomy closure includes fixing the sternum internally with steel wire. This reduces the movement of the raw bony edges leading to comparatively less pain in the postoperative period. However, sternotomy may cause severe pain when there is a major distraction of the sternum leading either to sternal fractures or to a major strain over the anterior or posterior intercostal articulations.

25.3.7.2 Video-Assisted Thoracoscopic Surgery (VATS)

Early postoperative pain or respiratory complications are less after VATS as compared to thoracotomy since the surgical incision is small [28]. Incidence of chronic postsurgical pain is also less. On the other hand, VATS becomes more painful with the use of multiple ports and larger diameter instruments. Excessive twisting of instruments in inexperienced hands can cause rib fractures and damage to the intercostal nerves.

25.3.7.3 Open Thoracotomy

Posterolateral Incision
This is the most painful surgical incision as it involves incising major chest wall muscles. This incision gives a better surgical exposure and can be extended if required. As in sternotomy closure the internal fixation of the divided ribs can lessen the postoperative pain [29].

Muscle-Sparing Incision
Axillary muscle sparing incision is the commonest. With this incision, the subcostal neurovascular bundle is dissected free to avoid injury, and the ribs are widely retracted for better exposure. Incidence of chronic pain is comparatively less with this incision [30]. However, post-thoracotomy pain can worsen, due to increased stretching of the posterior costovertebral joints, rib fractures, and occasionally injury to the intercostal nerves [31].

Anterior Incision
Anterior incisions are as painful as classical posterolateral thoracotomy as these incisions require multiple rib resections. This incision is given for anterior mediastinal masses and some cardiac procedures. Intercostal nerve blocks are effective for postoperative pain relief with this approach, as territory of the posterior cutaneous nerves is not involved.

25.3.8 Transverse (Clamshell) Sternothoracotomy

Pain control is particularly challenging, with the clamshell incision as shown in Fig. 25.2. It causes significant postoperative pain. This incision is used for lung transplantation, mediastinal tumors, or complex cardiopulmonary surgery [32].

25.4 Analgesic Modalities

As discussed in the pathogenesis of post-thoracotomy pain, there are multiple pain generators and multiple afferent pain pathways for pain

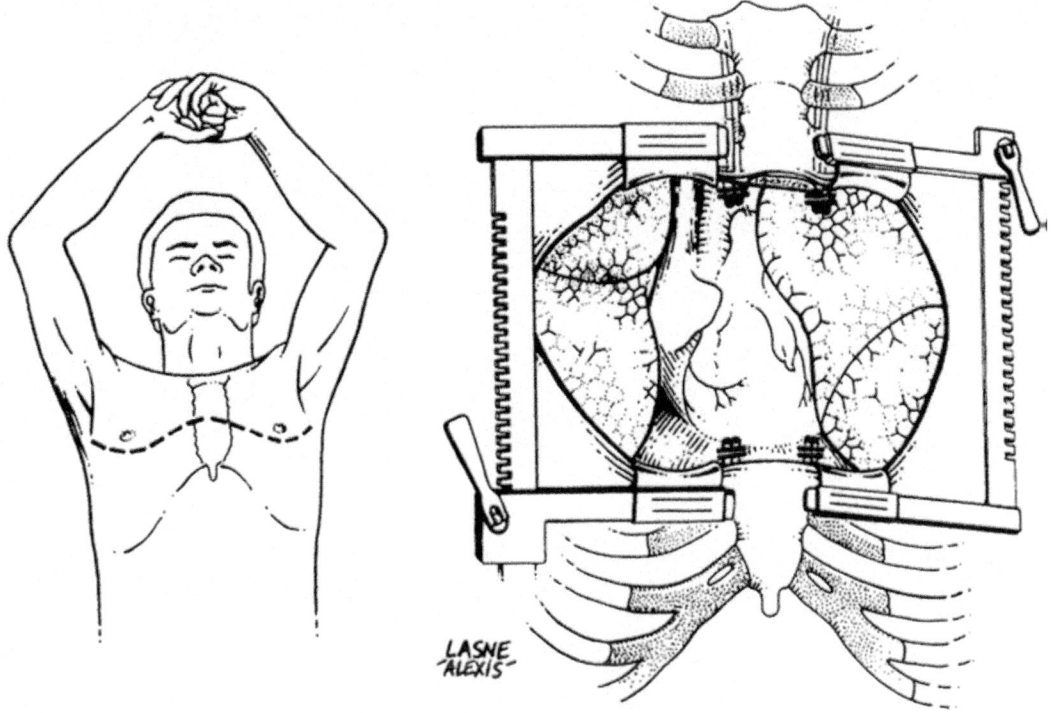

Fig. 25.2 Clamshell incision. Source: Macchiarini P, Ladurie FL, Cerrina J, Fadel E, Chapelier A, Dartevelle P. Clamshell or sternotomy for double lung or heart-lung transplantation? Eur J Cardiothorac Surg. 1999;15(3):333–9

impulse transmission during thoracic surgery in both VATS and thoracotomy. Perception of pain is therefore complex. More than one potential pain pathway should be blocked simultaneously for a synergistic and qualitative effect. We recommend a safe multimodal approach (Figs. 25.3 and 25.4) using regional analgesia techniques along with systemic opioids or non-opioid analgesics and supplementing them with other adjuvants when required.

25.4.1 Non-opioid Pharmacological Methods

25.4.1.1 Nonsteroidal Anti-Inflammatory Drugs (NSAIDs)

The synthesis of prostaglandins, which reduces the inflammatory response to surgical insult, is blocked by NSAIDs by inhibiting cyclooxygenase (COX). These drugs act peripherally as well as centrally in the spinal cord by suppressing prostaglandin synthesis. Out of the many isoenzymes of the COX enzyme, like COX-1, COX-2, and COX-3, the COX-2 isoenzyme has primary anti-inflammatory actions whereas COX-1 has mostly physiological functions [33, 34].

COX-2 inhibitors have comparatively less platelet inhibitory function and upper gastrointestinal side effects. However, they have a detrimental effect on bone growth. Some COX-2 inhibitors like rofecoxib and valdecoxib, when taken for longer periods, are known to cause cardiovascular thrombotic complications because of associated vasoconstrictive and prothrombotic effects along with reduced prostacyclin production [35, 36]. The cardiovascular risk profile with diclofenac is more than with

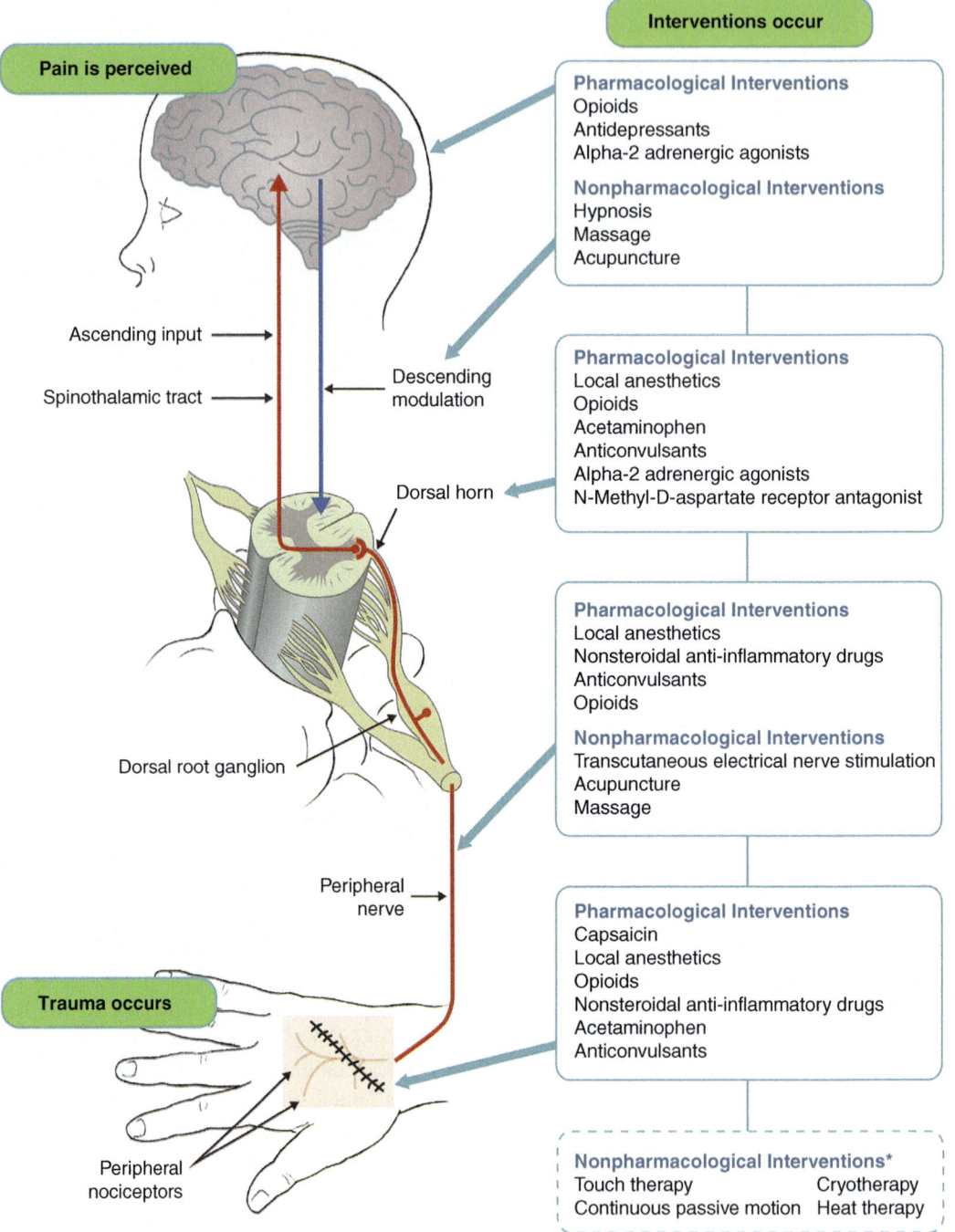

Fig. 25.3 Action of analgesics at various sites of the pain pathway. Source: Manworren RC. Multimodal pain management and the future of a personalized medicine approach to pain. AORN J. 2015 Mar;101(3):308–14; quiz 315–8

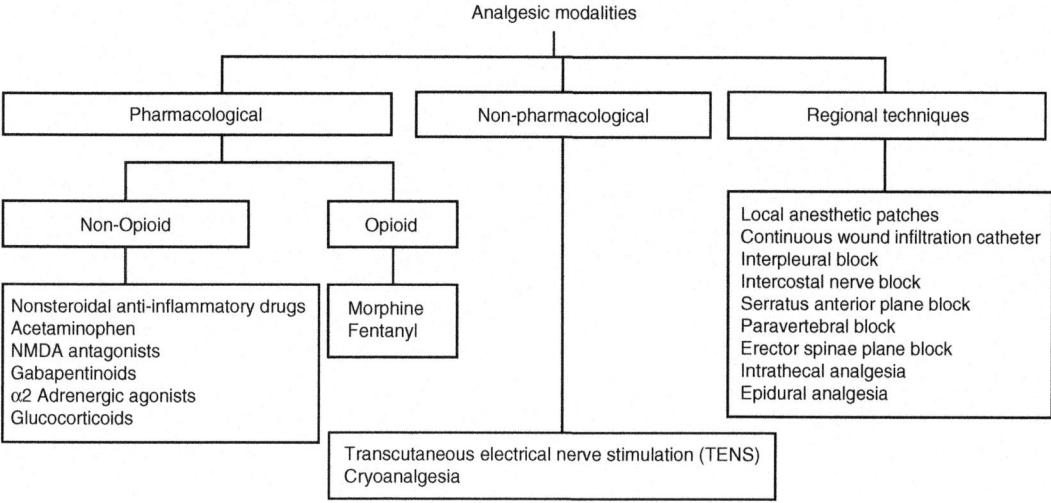

Fig. 25.4 Multimodal analgesia

naproxen. The incidence of renal injury with NSAIDs is between 1:1000 and 1:10,000 in normal adults. The risk is more in elderly, hypovolemic patients and in patients having preexisting renal insult because these patients are relying upon prostaglandins for their vasodilatory effects to maintain adequate renal perfusion pressure. NSAIDs used perioperatively may render pleurodesis surgery less efficacious by reducing inflammation [37].

Perioperative NSAIDs reduce the use of systemic opioids and are very helpful in treating post-thoracotomy ipsilateral shoulder pain. Perioperative use of parecoxib 40 mg for 3 days reduces the dose of drugs during patient-controlled epidural analgesia (PCEA) or continuous paravertebral analgesia. NSAIDs reduce the pain scores at rest or during coughing, along with a reduced incidence of chronic pain [38].

25.4.1.2 Acetaminophen

Acetaminophen works centrally, via the modulation of the serotoninergic system by suppressing COX-2 and COX, thereby inhibiting prostaglandin synthesis. Its peripheral actions include anti-inflammatory effects. Paracetamol, a prodrug, is hydrolyzed by plasma esterases to acetaminophen. The effects of acetaminophen and NSAIDs are additive. It is safe in renal failure and has few side effects or contraindications [39]. It is a very effective adjuvant with perioperative opioids or other regional anesthesia techniques [40, 41]. The clinical efficacy of intravenously or orally administered acetaminophen is the same in terms of pain score.

25.4.1.3 N-Methyl-D-Aspartate (NMDA) Antagonists

Ketamine is a noncompetitive antagonist of the phencyclidine site of the N-methyl-D-aspartate (NMDA) receptor, an anesthetic with analgesic properties. It also has mild anti-hyperalgesic and anti-inflammatory potential. A small dose of ketamine when used as an adjuvant to intravenous or epidural patient-controlled analgesia (PCA) reduces opioid consumption [42], enhances opioid-induced analgesia, limits opioid-induced hyperalgesia and progression to opioid tolerance. In our experience, ketamine is useful, particularly in patients on chronic high doses of opioids [43, 44]. Some common side effects reported are dysphoria, hallucinations, and increased secretions, but these are well tolerated in low doses. The conversion from acute to chronic post-thoracotomy pain is another important aspect in which ketamine can help, by blocking the cascade of central sensitization. Glutamate is an excitatory neurotransmitter acting via the NMDA receptor and is widely linked in the pathogenesis of chronic painful conditions like hyperalgesia and allodynia, which is also known as "wind up phenomenon" [45]. The role of the NMDA glutamate receptor blockade with drugs like ketamine is implicated in progress to central sensitization.

25.4.1.4 Gabapentinoids

An anticonvulsant, gabapentin (1-(aminomethyl) cyclohexane acetic acid), attaches to the α2δ subunit of voltage-dependent calcium channels. It is a sedative as well as anxiolytic [46]. It has been studied in different doses as an adjunct to PCA for varied acute as well as chronic pain conditions [47]. It has been postulated that a single preoperative dose has little effect but a slightly higher dose of 1200 mg preoperatively, followed by 600 mg 12-hourly, leads to decreased analgesic requirement and an improvement in pulmonary function as well [48–50]. No significant reduction in shoulder pain was found [51].

Pregabalin is structurally similar to ϒ-aminobutyric acid, with a similar mechanism of action, but more potent than gabapentin [52]. It is anti-hyperalgesic, anticonvulsant, and anxiolytic. Postoperative pain score is found to be reduced in some studies, but no clear cut recommendations are postulated [53–55]. Further studies are required to establish its role for perioperative use.

25.4.1.5 α2 Adrenergic Agonists

Clonidine and dexmedetomidine reduce sympathetically mediated pain without any respiratory side effects [56]. They can cause hypotension, bradycardia, and sedation (clonidine to a greater degree than dexmedetomidine). As an adjuvant to intravenous PCA, it reduces opioid requirement [57] and increases patient satisfaction, especially for patients in whom regional analgesia cannot be given. However, sedation should be taken into consideration during perioperative care.

25.4.1.6 Glucocorticoids

During thoracotomy, circulating pro-inflammatory mediators such as IL-6 and IL-8 are released [58]. Glucocorticoids reduce prostaglandin production by inhibiting COX-2 isoenzymes and other phospholipases. This leads to a decrease in the presynaptic release of neurotransmitters and increased production of kynurenic acid, an NMDA antagonist [59, 60]. Thus the glucocorticoids are analgesic, antiemetic, anti-inflammatory, and antipyretic. Dexamethasone has a dose-dependent opioid-sparing effect. The onset of analgesia is slow and long-lasting, lasting up to 7 days. Dexamethasone is an excellent adjunct for prolonging peripheral regional blocks [61, 62]. Glucocorticoids can cause gastric irritation, sodium retention, impaired wound healing, and can impair glucose homeostasis. In our experience, a single 4–8 mg dose of dexamethasone is not associated with adverse effects.

25.4.2 Opioid-Based Pharmacological Methods

Opioids are the most effective analgesics for post-thoracotomy pain. The opioids most commonly used are morphine, fentanyl, and tramadol. The other commonly used agents are paracetamol, NSAIDs, ketamine, dexmedetomidine, or the combination of one or more drugs.

Morphine is the most widely and commonly used opioid for postoperative thoracotomy pain. The intravenous dose of morphine is 0.03–0.15 mg/kg. Morphine is metabolized in the body into morphine-6-glucuronide which is a pharmacologically active metabolite and morphine 3 glucuronide, the accumulation of which causes restlessness, excitement, and even convulsions. Morphine is used cautiously in hepatorenal compromised individuals.

Fentanyl is a synthetic opioid with a short duration of action. As compared to morphine it causes less histamine release, the metabolites are normative, less incidence of nausea, vomiting and the residual psychokinetic effects are minimized with the use of fentanyl.

The IV dose of fentanyl is 0.5–2 μg/kg.

25.4.2.1 Patient Controlled Analgesia (PCA)

It is the self-administration of small doses of analgesics by patients when they experience pain. It is the major development in postoperative pain management and is considered the therapeutic standard for postoperative pain management [63]. It overcomes the wide variation in patient analgesic requirements and allows patients to balance their own comfort without any major side effects of the patient-controlled epidural analgesia (PCEA) regime [64].

In this, the epidural route is used for the drug delivery by PCA.

Pain relief by the neuraxial route as compared to PCA by IV route provides more intense analgesia, blunting the stress response to surgery, associated with early ambulation and dynamic pain relief.

PCEA via a thoracic epidural, using a combination of opioid and local anesthetic, is considered the standard of core for post-thoracotomy pain.

Patient controlled analgesia

	Strength
Morphine	0.5–1 mg/ml
Fentanyl	5–10 µg/ml
Dexmedetomidine	0.5–1 µg/ml
Tramadol	2.5 mg/ml

BASAL DOSE: 1–4 ml/h
DEMAND DOSE: 2–4 ml
LOCKOUT INTERVAL: 5–8 min

If background infusion is used, the inherent safety of this technique is jeopardized and the major concern is respiratory depression.

Patient controlled epidural analgesic

	Strength
Morphine	0.05 mg/ml
Fentanyl 0.125%	2.5–5 µg/ml
Bupivacaine	0.0625%
Ropivacaine	0.1%

BASAL DOSE: 3–5 ml/h
DEMAND DOSE: 2–6 ml
LOCK OUT INTERVAL: 15–20 min

If background infusion is used, the bolus dose should be used and lockout period increased.

25.4.3 Non-pharmacological Methods

25.4.3.1 Cryoanalgesia

The intercostal nerves are blocked using a cryoprobe once the chest is open. The block may be effective from 1 to 4 days, or even for up to 6 months. Cryoanalgesia is not practiced since the quality of analgesia is poor [65] and it is associated with chronic post-thoracotomy pain [66].

25.4.3.2 Transcutaneous Nerve Stimulation

Transcutaneous nerve stimulation (TENS) is based on the gate control theory of pain [67]. TENS modulates nociceptive impulses from the spinal cord and releases endogenous opioids [68], leading to a reduction in the levels of circulating inflammatory cytokines IL-6, IL-8, and TNFα [69]. In a recent meta-analysis, TENS appears to be an effective and safe technique when combined with other methods [70].

25.4.4 Regional Techniques

Until the early 1980s, systemic opioids were used widely for post-thoracotomy analgesia. Gradually thoracic epidurals became the gold standard [71]. Till date, numerous other peripheral regional analgesic techniques have been developed, but each technique has its own advantages and pitfalls. The paravertebral block has, however, established its acceptance in terms of comparable quality of analgesia and minimal side effects with respect to thoracic epidurals [72–76].

No single regional analgesia technique is effective and safe or completely applicable to all patients. The onus of this can be given to the complex pathophysiology of post-thoracotomy pain, multiple afferent pathways involved, high-risk patients with associated comorbidities, the disease pattern itself, available resources in hospital, and expertise of anesthesiologists. Hence, the methodology of effective care is "the multimodal analgesia" incorporating and titrating different available modalities for the maximum benefit of patients.

25.4.4.1 Local Anesthetic Patch

Its use in post-thoracotomy patients is controversial in terms of efficacy [77, 78]. The lidocaine 5% patch has 700 mg in an aqueous base over a soft adhesive tape. It is applied over the skin near the incision. The amount of drug absorbed depends upon the total skin area covered and duration for which the patch is applied.

25.4.4.2 Continuous Wound Infiltration Catheter

This catheter is positioned safely at the end of surgery near the intercostal nerve, between the serratus muscle and the pericostal sutures. These catheters are normally used as an adjunct to IV-PCA or when any regional analgesia technique cannot be given. Their use has been shown to reduce postoperative opioid consumption [79, 80], wound edema, improve recovery of FEV1 and FVC, and improve resting as well as dynamic pain scores [79]. This technique is unnecessary for patients receiving continuous paravertebral block or thoracic epidural analgesia. There is the potential risk for local anesthetic toxicity when two regional techniques are combined. These catheters are particularly helpful in surgeries like pleurectomy or chest wall resection, where a paravertebral catheter cannot be placed. Bupivacaine 0.1% is given at a rate of 4 ml/hr. and 6 ml bolus as and when required. Since these catheters are expensive, their cost–benefit ratio has to be ascertained.

Liposomal Bupivacaine

Encapsulating bupivacaine (Fig. 25.5) with multivesicular biodegradable liposomes using DepoFoam technology gives an extended release form which is effective for approximately

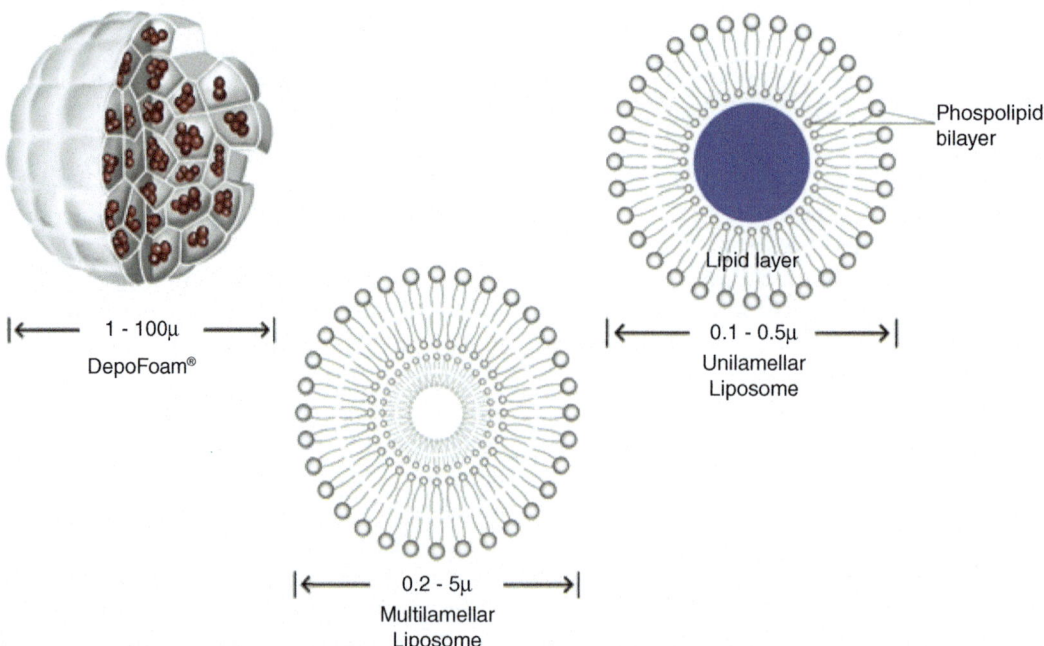

Fig. 25.5 Multivesicular liposome structure vs. uni- and multilamellar liposomes. Source: Coppens SJR, Zawodny Z, Dewinter G, Neyrinck A, Balocco AL, Rex S. In search of the Holy Grail: Poisons and extended release local anesthetics. Best Pract Res Clin Anaesthesiol. 2019 Mar;33(1):3–21

2–3 days [81–84]. The encapsulated drug is released in a controlled manner, thereby avoiding systemic toxicity and having a longer duration of action. Commercially the encapsulated form of bupivacaine is available as 20 ml of 1.3% solution containing 266 mg of free base bupivacaine, which is the molar equivalent of 300 mg of bupivacaine. This potent formulation can provide significantly prolonged analgesia when administered either subcutaneously or around nerves. To avoid direct cardiotoxicity, frequent aspirations are of vital importance while administering liposomal bupivacaine.

25.4.4.3 Interpleural Block

Kvalheim and Reiestad [85], in 1984 described a technique where local anesthetic is deposited between visceral and parietal pleura, blocking multiple ipsilateral thoracic dermatomes. This is the interpleural block or pleural block [86, 87]. Normally the two layers of pleura, separated by a distance of 10–20 μm, have a space between them with a surface area of about 0.2. This space contains approximately 10 ml of pleural fluid [88], and local anesthetic deposited within this area, spreads evenly and widely by surface tension forces. This block is ineffective in patients for thoracic surgery, since the continuity of pleural layers is not maintained after surgery [89]. Post-thoracotomy patients have a larger volume of pleural space and contains air and blood, rendering surface tension forces ineffective. Further, the local anesthetic agents are lost to drains via gravity, limiting its duration of action [90, 91]. The inter-pleural space is quite vascular. Administering a large dose by this route in order to make it effective always carries the risk of local anesthetic toxicity and ipsilateral diaphragm function may also get impaired. Consequently, it is not an appropriate block for a post-thoracotomy patient.

25.4.4.4 Erector Spinae Plane Block

At the level of the T5 transverse process, erector spinae plane (ESP) block is given with ultrasound guidance, either in sitting or lateral position. The needle tip is seen contacting the transverse process on ultrasound. Twenty milliliters of local anesthetic solution (e.g., 0.2% ropivacaine) is injected into the fascial plane deep to the erector spinae muscle (Fig. 25.6). A catheter can also be passed another 5 cm in the same plane and an infusion of 5–8 ml/h is started. Adequate pain relief is achieved from C7 to T8 levels [92]. Practically, the ESP block is a safe and easy variant of the paravertebral block with similar clinical effects. This block can be given for acute and chronic post-thoracotomy pain, failed epidurals, and even in a patient receiving prophylactic anticoagulation [93]. This can be given as a single shot or as a continuous infusion unilaterally or bilaterally. There are some case reports of using bilateral, continuous ESP block in open sternotomy and thoracotomy surgeries for perioperative analgesia. This block in our experience is giving promising results but further studies need to be done for establishing its efficacy. The results are not so comparable in posterolateral thoracotomies.

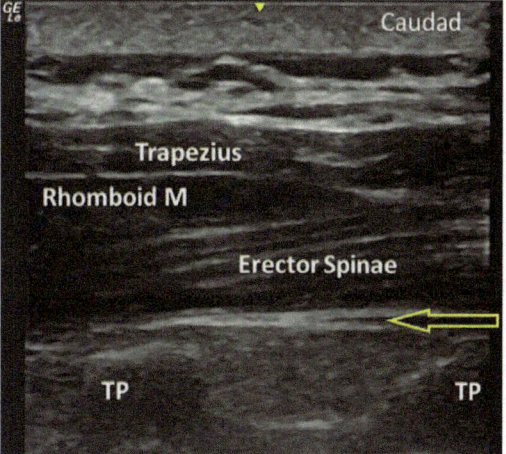

Fig. 25.6 Ultrasound image of the erector spinae plane with the transducer placed in a longitudinal parasagittal orientation. TP indicates transverse process. Source: Forero M, Rajarathinam M, Adhikary S, Chin KJ. Continuous Erector Spinae Plane Block for Rescue Analgesia in Thoracotomy After Epidural Failure: A Case Report. A A Case Rep. 2017 May 15;8(10):254–256

25.4.4.5 Intrathecal Analgesia

Opioids when administered in the subarachnoid space are 100 times more potent than the equivalent intravenous dose [94, 95]. Although used in the mid-1990s intrathecal analgesia for postthoracotomy patients has not gained much popularity. Side effects of intrathecal opioids include urinary retention, nausea, pruritus, vomiting, delayed respiratory depression (0.2–1%), and decreased peristalsis.

25.4.4.6 Intercostal Nerve Block

Intercostal nerves are a continuation of the ventral rami of the upper 11 thoracic spinal roots. They run forward in the intercostal spaces of respective ribs and lie in a plane between the internal and innermost intercostal muscles. The intercostal nerves are blocked much more medial to the posterior axillary line, as the lateral cutaneous nerve branch for chest wall originates proximally before emerging subcutaneously. The dorsal rami of the intercostal nerve which give cutaneous supply to the mid back are not blocked by an intercostal nerve block. Therefore, it is not used for posterolateral thoracotomies (Fig. 25.7).

Better results for intercostal nerve block can be obtained without difficulty (under direct vision) while the chest is still open for VATS, or percutaneously using ultrasound guidance (Fig. 25.8). The intercostal space is highly vascular and therefore the effect of local anesthetics is short lived. A dose of 2–5 ml bolus of local anesthetic is sufficient for a single intercostal nerve. Three to five levels of intercostal nerves need to be blocked for providing analgesia for a particular thoracotomy incision. When larger doses are given, it either spreads to the adjacent intercostal space or to the paravertebral space medially, but this spread is highly variable. Perioperative analgesic requirement is reduced significantly after intercostal blocks [96].

25.4.4.7 Serratus Anterior Plane Block

In 2013, Blanco and colleagues [97], with the help of ultrasound, deposited local anesthetic in a

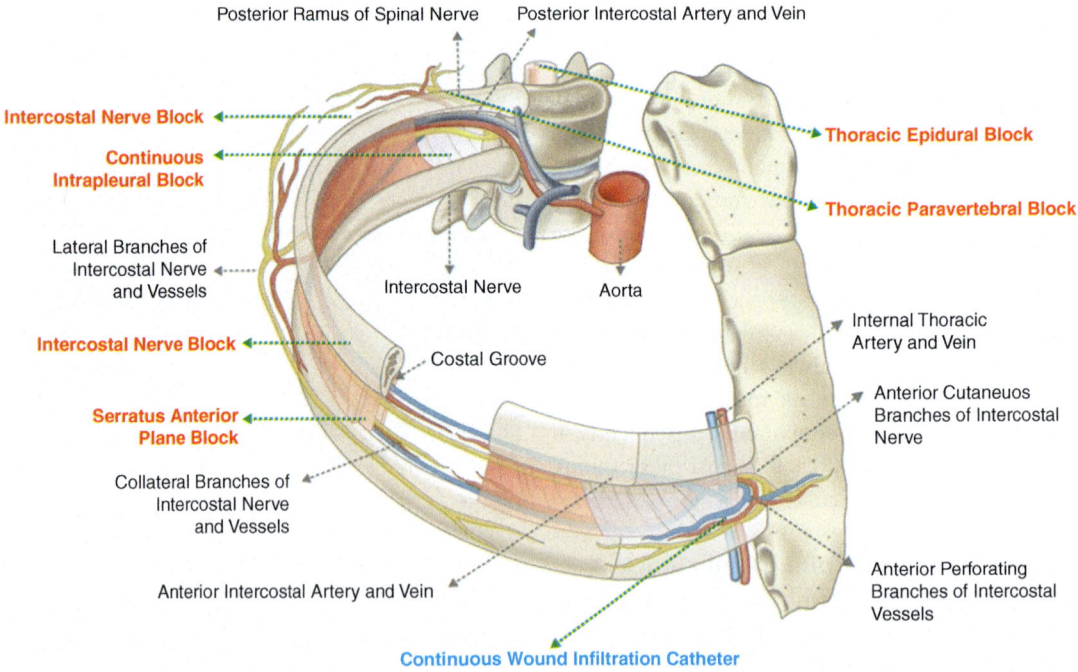

Fig. 25.7 Nerve supply of thoracic cage and approximate site of USG guided blocks

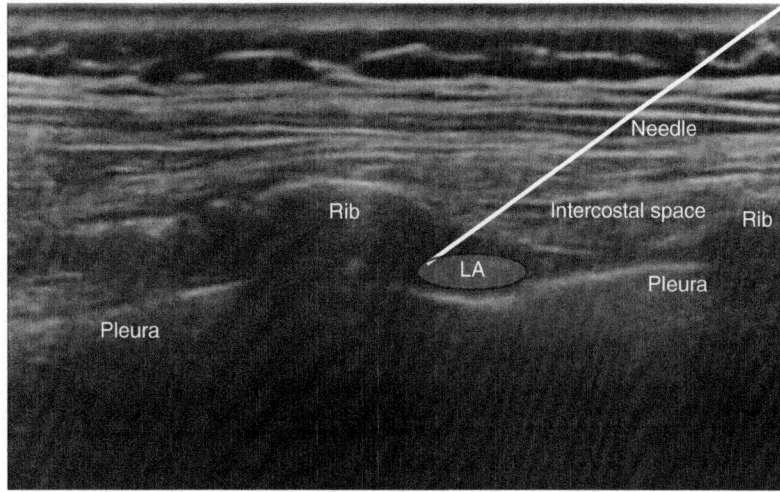

Fig. 25.8 Sonogram of the intercostal interspace, needle placement is shown. Pleural depression from local anesthetic (LA) can be appreciated

plane above and below the serratus anterior muscle for pain relief to the lateral chest wall. This technique blocks T2–T9 dermatomes by blocking the long thoracic nerve and thoracodorsal nerve. Serratus anterior plane injection, when given superficial to the serratus anterior spreads more dorsally, while an injection given deep to the serratus muscle will spread in the dorsal as well as ventral directions with the patient in the supine position. The duration of the block is longer when the injection is given superficial to the serratus muscle [98].

This block can be given in the supine, sitting, or lateral position with the help of a linear transducer. The ultrasound transducer is placed in the mid-axillary line (Fig. 25.9), at the level of the fifth rib in the vertical plane. The serratus anterior muscle is sandwiched between the ribs inferiorly and the latissimus dorsi muscle lying superiorly. The intercostal space and pleura are identified in between the ribs. The needle is inserted either in-plane or out-of-plane, depending upon operator choice, 20 ml of either 0.25% bupivacaine or 0.2% ropivacaine is sufficient for the desired effect. Efficacy of this block is being studied in breast surgery, rib fractures or in those patients where the thoracic epidural space cannot be secured because of hypotension or other reasons. This block is showing promising results in reducing perioperative opioid consumption [99]. However, this block is not useful where the incision extends posterolaterally beyond the mid-axillary line.

25.4.4.8 Paravertebral Block

The thoracic paravertebral space is a potential wedge-shaped area which on one side communicates with the epidural space medially via the intervertebral foramen, whereas laterally it continues with the intercostal neurovascular space. Anatomically the medial boundary is made up of the vertebral bodies and discs, while posteriorly lie the costotransverse ligaments, transverse processes and necks of the ribs, whereas the parietal pleura lies anteriorly [100] (Fig. 25.10). The psoas major muscle forms the caudal boundary. The adjacent paravertebral spaces are continuous with each other (Fig. 25.11). The endothoracic fascia [101], which is the deep fascia of the thorax, divides the thoracic paravertebral space. The subpleural paravertebral compartment lies anteriorly while the sub-endothoracic paravertebral compartment lies posteriorly. The paravertebral space contains the sympathetic chain, dorsal and ventral rami of the spinal nerves plus the gray and white rami communicantes. This block is given at T6/T7 vertebra or lower for lower lobe surgery and at T5/T6 for upper/middle lobe surgery as the trocars are placed more cephalad [102]. It is performed with the patient either sitting while awake or in lateral decubitus position (with the side to be blocked uppermost), when the patient is anesthetized.

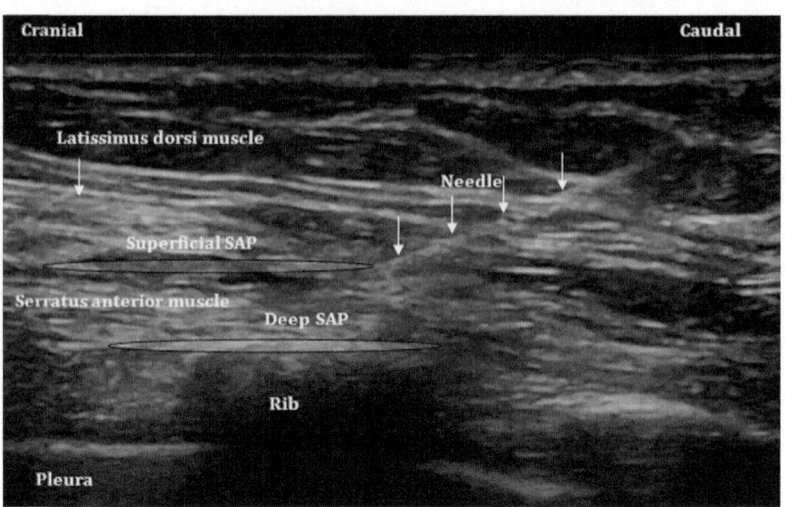

Fig. 25.9 USG image of superficial and deep serratus anterior plain (SAP) block

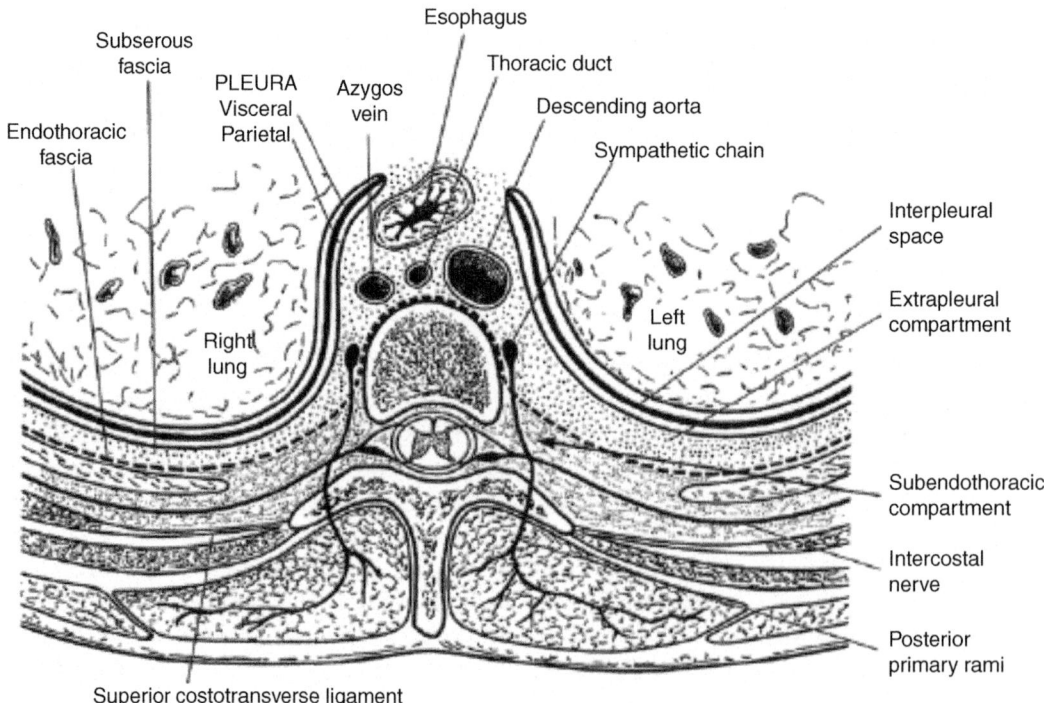

Fig. 25.10 Anatomy of the thoracic paravertebral space. Source: Karmakar MK. Thoracic paravertebral block. Anesthesiology. 2001;95(3):771–80

Continuous thoracic paravertebral blocks can provide good post-thoracotomy analgesia comparable to thoracic epidurals, with fewer side effects like urinary retention, pruritis, hypotension, nausea, vomiting, and with less perioperative hemodynamic instability [103–106]. The incidence of complications is low. The reported complications are inadvertent pleural puncture, dural puncture, pulmonary hemorrhage, ipsilateral Horner's syndrome, and occasional hypotension, apart from local anesthetic toxicity.

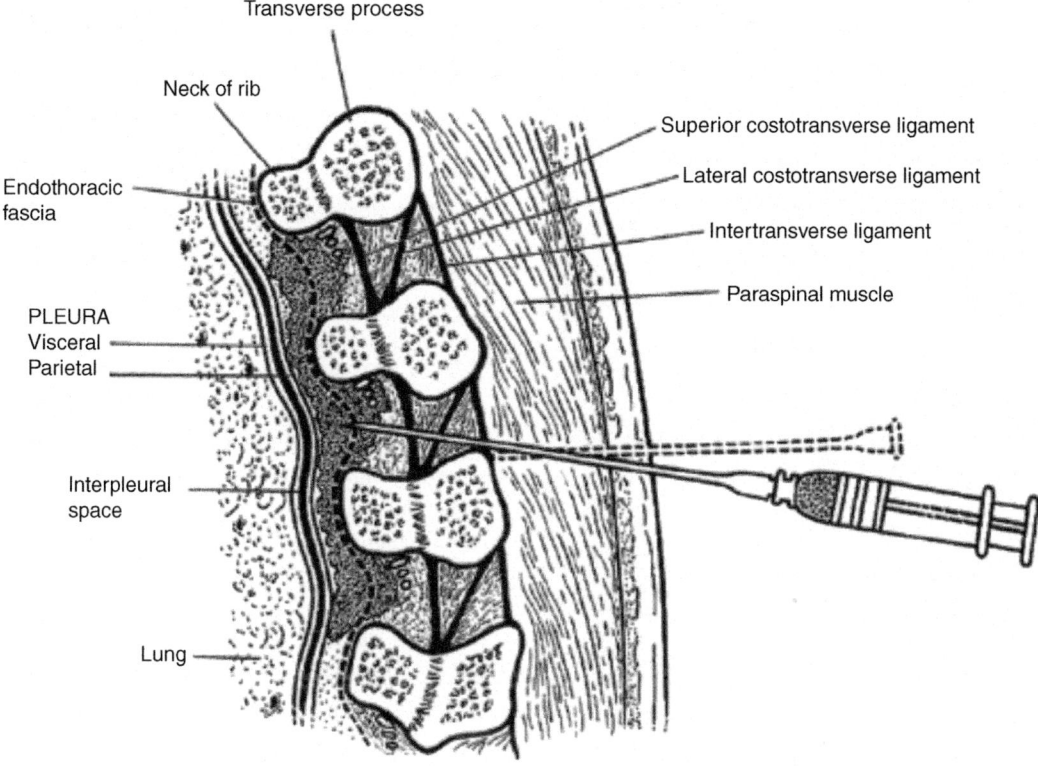

Fig. 25.11 Sagittal section through the paravertebral space showing a needle that has been walked off the transverse process. Source: Karmakar MK. Thoracic paravertebral block. Anesthesiology. 2001;95(3):771–80

Methods of Performing Paravertebral Blocks
- Landmark technique
- Under direct vision
  Ultrasound-guided techniques

Landmark Technique
Eason and Wyatt [107] described the loss of resistance technique while "walking off" a transverse process at thoracic levels. At a point 3 cm lateral to the spinous process of the corresponding vertebra, a Tuohy needle is inserted perpendicular to the skin and advanced slowly to contact the transverse process. The needle first touches the transverse process and is then withdrawn slightly. It is then redirected or walked off the transverse process and advanced blindly for not more than 1–1.5 cm or till there is a subtle click or loss of resistance of the costotransverse ligament. Sudden loss of resistance means that the costotransverse ligament has been pierced and the needle is in the paravertebral space. If the transverse process cannot be appreciated at an estimated depth, then the needle is withdrawn and redirected to a sagittal plane for a palpable contact with the transverse process. Twenty milliliters of 0.25% bupivacaine or other local anesthetic is given after negative aspiration in adults. For placing a catheter, the initial injection bolus of local anesthetic is given for adequate hydrodissection of the paravertebral space. A colored dye can be used for visually confirming spread during thoracoscopy or thoracotomy.

Under Direct Vision (Fig. 25.12)
In open surgical methods, catheters are inserted percutaneously into the paravertebral space and the position is checked directly under vision while the chest is still open. For this procedure, however, not only should the posterior extent of the incision be limited to give space to catheter placement and insertion, but also enough pleura

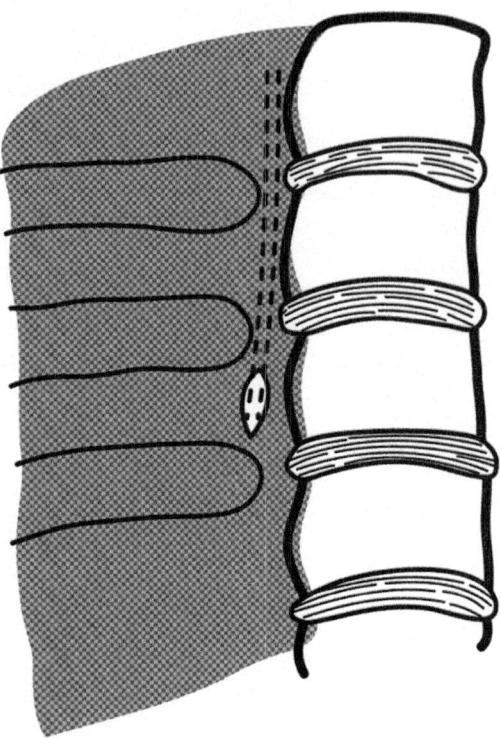

Fig. 25.12 Technique for performing paravertebral blocks. The endothoracic fascia (stippled) is exposed by raising the parietal pleura from the posterior chest wall. A catheter is inserted deep to the endothoracic fascia through a small hole created in the fascia. Source: Berrisford RG, Sabanathan SS. Direct access to the paravertebral space at thoracotomy. Ann Thorac Surg. 1990;49(5):854

the catheter is then secured by tunneling. In a randomized study the quality of analgesia at rest or while coughing by surgically placed paravertebral catheter is superior to thoracic epidurals. Results are also comparable for FEV1 and even oxygen saturation in ambient air. This open method of inserting a paravertebral catheter is safe and can be performed in a coagulopathic patient or where VATS surgery is converted into open thoracotomy.

The catheter in the paravertebral space can be kept for 3–7 days. An initial bolus of 0.3 ml/kg of 0.25% bupivacaine is given for adequate analgesic effect. This can be continued via infusion at the rate of 0.1 ml/kg/h of 0.25% bupivacaine. Early postoperative pain relief may be poor as sufficient local anesthetic spread may take time. To provide effective analgesia in post-thoracotomy patients with paravertebral blocks, the drug needs to cover up to ten dermatomal segments [109, 110]. Clinically the effect of a single-shot paravertebral injection is better than surgically administered intercostal nerve block and the effect has been shown to last between 6 and 24 h. Some adjuvants like dexmedetomidine, dexamethasone, or clonidine were used to increase the duration of block. Requirement for opioids decreased significantly perioperatively and hence the related side effects.

should be preserved posteriorly for adequate effect. It is done during closure of the thoracotomy incision. A slight modification of a technique as given by Sabanathan et al. [108] is where the catheter is inserted percutaneously via a Tuohy needle, just medial and slightly proximal to the posterior margin of the thoracotomy incision so that it exits from a space between the angle of the ribs and rests in the chest cavity. The endothoracic fascia and intercostal nerves are visible when the parietal pleura is lifted away medially. Next the catheter is advanced in the sub-endothoracic paravertebral space, via a little incision made in the endothoracic fascia. Subsequently the catheter is advanced and directed cranially via blunt dissection to a few more centimeters. The endothoracic fascia is sutured and the cutaneous end of

Absolute Contraindications
- Local infection
- Local anesthetic allergy
- Tumor at injection site

Relative Contraindications
- Impaired coagulopathy
- Severe respiratory compromise, patient using accessory muscles of respiration
- Diaphragmatic paresis on the same side
- Severe spinal deformities such as kyphosis or scoliosis

Dilated intercostal vessels as in coarctation of the aorta or thoracic aneurysm

Ultrasound-Guided Methods

We can be more specific with ultrasound-guidance for performing a thoracic paravertebral block. For this, any ultrasound probe, linear, convex, or micro-convex can be used for both out-of-plane and in-plane techniques. The approach can either be transverse or sagittal (Fig. 25.13). This block can be given in the supine or lateral position. In both approaches, the spinous and transverse processes are round, hyperechoic structures with zones of acoustic shadowing (Fig. 25.14).

Technique A: In-plane, saggital approach [111, 112]

This view uses a simple anatomical fact that the paravertebral space continues with the intercostal spaces laterally. In this approach, the probe is first oriented transversely over the spinous process of the desired thoracic level. It is then moved slowly and more laterally to identify the transverse process. Now, the probe is gradually angulated either in caudad or cephalad direction to attain a view between two adjacent ribs. The pleura is visualized as a moving hyperechoic line. After orientation the transducer is moved caudally and tilted medially till the paravertebral space is visualized clearly. The needle is inserted from a lateral to medial direction with its tip visualized throughout under the ultrasound beam.

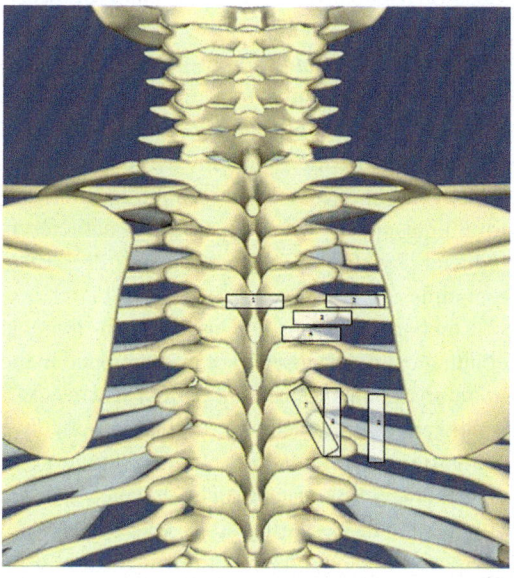

Fig. 25.13 Sequence of transverse scan for thoracic paravertebral space (1, 2, 3, 4) and sequence of paramedian sagittal scan (5, 6, 7)

Technique B: Out-of-plane, saggital approach

The paravertebral space is identified in the same way as the "in-plane" technique. Needle insertion is from a point 1 cm caudal to the ultrasound transducer in a craniocaudal angulation. The needle tip is visualized and the local anesthetic is injected under direct vision which causes a distinctive depression of the pleura.

Technique C: In-plane, transverse approach (Fig.25.14b) [112]

The transducer is kept in the sagittal plane approximately 5 cm from the midline. It is then moved medially while scanning the intercostal space. The ribs and moving pleura are visualized. In this view, the paravertebral space is bound anteriorly by the pleura and intercostalis intimus muscle; by the external intercostal muscle and intercostal membrane posteriorly; membrane of the intercostalis intimus muscle lies medially; and laterally, the costotransverse joint. The target is the space lying between the internal intercostal muscle and the pleura and the needle is directed to this from the caudal to cephalad direction. In our experience, this block requires considerable expertise and should not be performed by beginners.

Technique D: In-plane, oblique transverse approach [113]

As described in the abovementioned approach, after identification of the intercostal space, the transducer is moved medially till the transverse processes and the costotransverse joint (approximately 3–4 cm from the midline) are seen. In this view, it is difficult to insert needle. However, the needle insertion is facilitated by simply rotating the probe slightly to a cephalomedial/caudolateral orientation so that superior end of probe lies over transverse process and inferior end of probe lies over rib. The needle is inserted from a point caudal to the transducer and passed through the superior costotransverse ligament into the paravertebral space (Fig.25.14b). The movement of pleura anteriorly is taken as a confirmatory sign for correct needle position [114].

Krediet et al. [112] found that the size of paravertebral space is 2–2.5 in diameter at 1–2 cm from the midline and approximately 0.5 cm in diameter laterally at 4–5 cm. Chances of

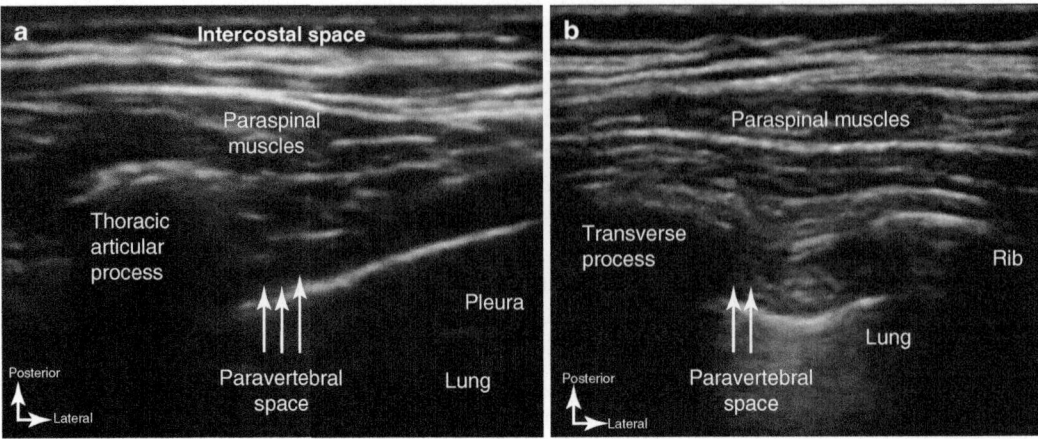

Fig. 25.14 USG image of paramedian transverse scan (**a**), USG image of paramedian oblique sagittal scan (**b**)

accidental pleural puncture increase with more medial approaches. When a catheter is inserted for continuous infusions, it is recommended that it should not be passed more than 2–3 cm beyond the tip of the needle to avoid migration into the epidural space.

Cowie et al. [111] compared a single-injection of 20 ml contrast dye vs. dual-injection of 10 ml in the paravertebral space of cadavers. Dye spread was equal in both techniques. A single paravertebral injection at T6 produced comparable results with multiple injections at five levels from T4 to T8 [115–117]. The risk of complications was more with multiple paravertebral injections.

25.4.4.9 Epidural Analgesia

Since 1970, thoracic epidural is used extensively for perioperative analgesia in thoracotomy patients as it is reliable, effective and reduces postoperative pulmonary complications. Though thoracic epidural analgesia is considered a "gold standard" for patients undergoing thoracic surgery [118, 119], it is associated with side effects. The sympathetic nerve fibers to the heart are also blocked. It is useful in refractory angina, decreases chances of perioperative supraventricular arrhythmias and thromboembolic events. Thoracic epidural increases FRC, improves diaphragmatic function and mucociliary clearance, and reduces chances of sedation and nausea.

Accessing the thoracic epidural space is technically more challenging than the lumbar epidural space, as the obliquity of the thoracic vertebral spinous processes means that the tips of the spinous process lie at the level of the intervertebral space of the lower vertebrae. The ligamentum flavum is thin and resistance to needle insertion is less. Several techniques to confirm epidural space are described, like the "loss-of resistance" technique, "hanging-drop" technique and recently "pressure waveform analysis" by attaching the proximal hub of the needle to a pressure transducer [120, 121]. Epidural catheters at thoracic levels are kept at 5–6 cm within the space to avoid accidental dislodgement or to avoid migration to the transforaminal space. Migration of the catheter is reduced by fixing with adhesive dressings, tunneling, or suturing.

Lumbar epidurals are used when thoracic epidural cannot be inserted or as mentioned in the literature, in an anesthetized patient where VATS is converted to thoracotomy. Achieving effective analgesia is difficult with lumbar epidural in post-thoracotomy patients [122], since a large volume of local anesthetic is required for an adequate effect and hence more chances of drug toxicity and hemodynamic instability.

Techniques of Thoracic Epidural Catheter Insertion

Position
- Sitting
- Lateral

Approach
- Midline
- Paramedian

Midline Approach
Following palpation of the apex of the lower spinous process, the Tuohy needle is inserted in the midline or interspinous space immediately above the palpable tip. The needle is advanced cephalad at an oblique angle, which is adjusted depending on the obliquity of the spinous process.

Paramedian Approach
The needle is inserted at a point 1 cm lateral to the palpable tip of appropriate spinous process and angulated to about 45° cephalad and approximately 10° medial toward the epidural space. When the lamina is contacted, the needle is withdrawn and re-angulated to hit the inter-laminar space.

Dose and Regimens of Epidural Solution
We advocate the use of a mixture of local anesthetics and opioids acting in synergism, to minimize concentration and consequently individual side effects. High concentrations of local anesthetics provide good analgesia but cause hypotension, while opioids can cause constipation and pruritus. At our hospital we use an epidural mixture of 0.0625% bupivacaine plus 2 μg/ml of fentanyl. Levobupivacaine and ropivacaine the relatively recent local anesthetic agents are less toxic than bupivacaine with comparable results. Different adjuvants have been tried in various doses, to further potentiate this synergistic combination, but none have been shown to deliver the best risk–benefit ratio. Among effective adjuvants is epinephrine but it is found to have the potential for cord ischemia. Clonidine [123–125] and magnesium have sedative side effects. Out of the many factors affecting the spread of drugs in the epidural space, age is found to be an independent factor, approximately 40% less volume of the local anesthetic injected in the epidural space being sufficient for the elderly.

Adverse Effects

Urinary Retention
Inhibiting sacral parasympathetic outflow [126] and pontine micturition center [127] cause the adverse effects of epidural opioid. It was seen that when naloxone was given to reverse these effects, the analgesic effects of epidurally given drugs were also reversed, without any significant reduction in the need for urinary catheterization.

Gastric Emptying
Thoracic epidurals can cause delayed gastric emptying by blocking the T6–T10 sympathetic nerves which innervate the stomach. Gastric emptying was found to be delayed for >48 h in post-thoracotomy patients receiving fentanyl plus bupivacaine epidurally. However, gastric emptying is better with epidurally administered opioids as compared to intravenously administered opioid via IV-PCA [128, 129]. Dexmedetomidine has shown to be a suitable adjuvant when used epidurally [130].

Hypotension
The systemic vasodilatation that can occur during lumbar epidural analgesia reduces cardiac preload and afterload and this leads to hypotension [131]. Thoracic epidurals may cause blockade of the cardiac sympathetic supply, thereby decreasing contractility [132]. Drugs such as β-adrenergic or a mixed agonist (e.g., ephedrine, dopamine, etc.) increase contractility and maintain the cardiac output.

25.5 Techniques for Specific Situations

25.5.1 Sternotomy

Post sternotomy, the sternum is closed with wire, which restricts bone movement and hence limits pain. In our practice, thoracic epidural analgesia is the first choice for analgesia at a higher level (T3/T4) [133]. Second choice is intravenous PCA along with regional analgesia techniques like bilateral erector spinae block or parasternal local anesthetic infiltration [134] or continuous wound infiltration catheters [135] and non-opioid analgesics.

25.5.2 Video-Assisted Surgery

Comparable pain scores were demonstrated with either thoracic epidural or paravertebral block perioperatively. There are studies which advocate the less invasive paravertebral blocks, considering the side effects of epidural block. For minimally invasive surgeries like pleural [136] biopsy, sympathetectomies or small lung resections, the paravertebral block is a good option and for surgeries like esophagectomies or posterior pleurodesis, thoracic epidural is a better option [137].

25.5.3 Open Thoracotomy

Regional anesthetic techniques in open thoracotomies should be used as part of a multimodal analgesia plan. The thoracic epidural [118, 119, 121, 138, 139] remains the gold standard, followed by the paravertebral blocks. Other effective options can be intercostal nerve blocks, lumbar epidural analgesia and intrathecal opioids [140–142].

25.5.4 Esophageal Surgery

The first choice for pain relief here is thoracic epidural analgesia [143, 144] followed by intravenous patient controlled anesthesia, bilateral paravertebral blocks, and non-opioid analgesics.

25.5.5 Shoulder Pain

The incidence of ipsilateral post-thoracotomy pain can be reduced 2–3 times [145–147] by simply infiltrating local anesthetic intraoperatively around the phrenic nerve [148] at the diaphragmatic level. Care has to be taken in patients with poor diaphragmatic or pulmonary function. Other effective options are acetaminophen [149], nonsteroidal anti-inflammatory agents, indirect postoperative phrenic nerve blocks, and interscalene nerve block [150]. Previous studies with suprascapular nerve block and stellate ganglion block [151] did not provide promising results.

25.6 Chronic Post-thoracotomy Pain (CPTP)

CPTP is defined as pain that recurs or persists along a thoracotomy scar at least 2 months following the surgical procedure [152]. It represents one of the highest risk procedures for the development of chronic pain due to inevitable neurological injury affecting one half of the patients undergoing this operative procedure.

Uncontrolled pain in the perioperative period consistently predicts the development of chronic pain [153].

Strategies that emphasize preemptive analgesia may provide protection against this chronic pain syndrome, with some evidence suggesting as high as a 50% reduction in the incidence of chronic pain syndromes at 1 year after thoracotomy [154].

25.6.1 Prevalence of Post-thoracotomy Pain

The incidence of post-thoracotomy pain has been reported to be 80% at 3 months, 75% at 6 months and 61% at 1 year after surgery. The most severe pain is experienced by 3–5% and in about 50% of patients the pain following thoracotomy which interferes with normal life [155].

The rate of long-term persistent pain (3–18 months) has been found to be same for thoracotomy and thoracoscopy procedures [2, 156].

The incidence of post-thoracotomy pain has been to be less with video-assisted thoracoscopic procedures as compared to thoracotomy [5, 157].

25.6.2 Mechanism of Post-thoracotomy Pain

The mechanism of CPTP is not fully understood. Initially there is primary sensitization as mediators released from damaged tissue decrease the pain threshold by increasing the activity of nociceptors. The release of substance P calcitonin gene-related peptide, and glutamate causes activation of NMDA receptors due to continuation of postoperative nociceptive stimulation. This leads to the development of secondary sensitization and CPTP.

The costal retraction causing damage to intercostal nerve, costochondral and subsequently costovertebral injuries, and muscle and pleural injures are the major causes of CPTP. Other case are parenchymal injuries and irritation at site due to drainage tubes.

25.6.3 Predisposing Factors for the Development of Post-thoracotomy Pain

A relationship between preoperative pain and CPTP has been demonstrated [158, 159].

Recently a variant of the catecholamine-o-methyltransferase (COMT) gene has been implicated in the development of CPTP [160].

The incidence of CPTP has been reported to be 40–80% particularly after thoracotomy and 20–40% after VATs [3]. Hence the severity of pain is related to location and length of surgical incision.

Postoperative pain management by epidural analgesia decreases the incidence of CPTP [3].

25.6.4 Signs and Symptoms

The CPTP can be localized, radicular, burning, or aching in nature. The pleuritic component of pain can be exacerbated by movement of ipsilateral shoulder.

The patient may develop signs and symptoms of CRPS. The other causes of pain generators post thoracotomy may include bony instability, retained foreign bodies, chest wall lesion, and myofascial pain.

25.6.5 Management

After comprehensive evaluation an individualized plan should be made with multimodal pharmacological, interventional, and behavioral therapy (Fig. 25.15) [161].

Acute postoperative pain has been identified as a factor in the development of CPTP. A recent Cochrane review of pharmacotherapy for prevention of chronic pain after surgery reported that the use of ketamine, gabapentin, pregabalin, and parecoxib may be beneficial in the prevention of CPTP.

Good postoperative pain control by multimodal analgesia and management of concurrent conditions like depression, anxiety, sleep disturbances are important factors in preventing CPTP.

Postoperative rehabilitation therapy like breathing exercises and ambulation prevent the development of CPTP [162].

The pharmacological treatment includes tricycle antidepressants anticonvulsants, selective serotonin non-adrenaline reuptake inhibitors, topical lignocaine, NSAIDs, tramadol, and opioids.

In the interventional methods the neurologic block of intercostal nerves, paravertebral block, pulse radiofrequency of dorsal root ganglion, thoracic epidural and the spinal cord stimulation can be done.

Other methods include TENS, acupuncture, and botulinum toxin application.

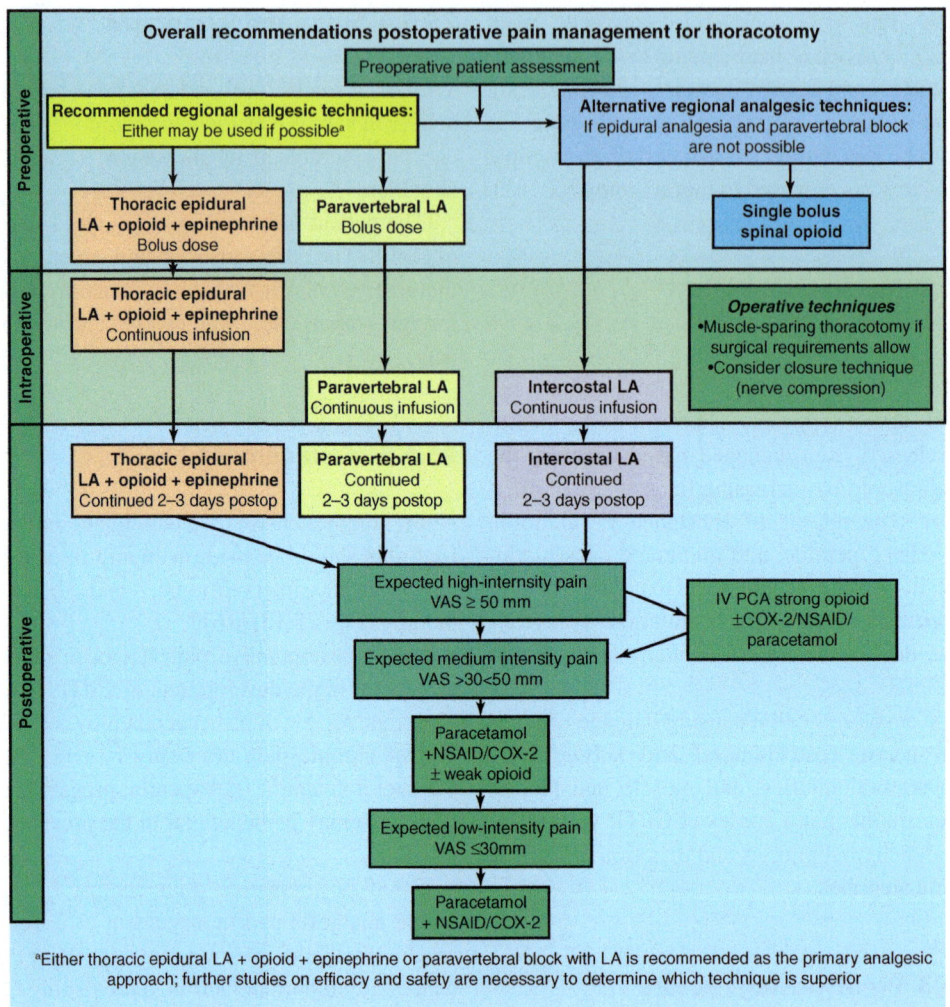

Fig. 25.15 Recommendation for postoperative pain management for thoracotomy. Source: Kehlet H, Wilkinson RC, Fischer HB, Camu F; Prospect Working Group. PROSPECT: evidence-based, procedure-specific postoperative pain management. Best Pract Res Clin Anaesthesiol. 2007 Mar;21(1):149–59 (Done) (permission to be taken)

25.7 Conclusion

Multimodal analgesia is recommended for managing post-thoracotomy painful conditions. More often regional analgesia techniques are supplemented with other parenterally administered agents for maximum benefit. The doses, duration, and choice of modality used should always be individualized and titrated to achieve a synergistic effect and to reduce side effects.

References

1. Stadler M, Schlander M, Braeckman M, et al. A cost-utility and cost-effectiveness analysis of an acute pain service. J Clin Anesth. 2004;16(3):159–67.
2. Maguire MF, Ravenscroft A, Beggs D, et al. A questionnaire study investigating the prevalence of the neuropathic component of chronic pain after thoracic surgery. Eur J Cardiothorac Surg. 2006;29(5):800–5.
3. Steegers MAH, Snik DM, Verhagen AF, et al. Only half of the chronic pain after thoracic surgery shows a neuropathic component. J Pain. 2008;9(10):955–61.

4. Nosotti M, Baisi A, Mendogni P, et al. Muscle sparing versus posterolateral thoracotomy for pulmonary lobectomy: randomised controlled trial. Interact Cardiovasc Thorac Surg. 2010;11(4):415–9.
5. Landreneau RJ, Mack MJ, Hazelrigg SR, et al. Prevalence of chronic pain after pulmonary resection by thoracotomy or video-assisted thoracic surgery. J Thorac Cardiovasc Surg. 1994;107(4):1079–85; discussion 85–6.
6. Holte K, Kehlet H. Effect of postoperative epidural analgesia on surgical outcome. Minerva Anestesiol. 2002;68(4):157–61.
7. Kehlet H. Effect of pain relief on the surgical stress response. Reg Anesth. 1996;21(6 Suppl):35–7.
8. Sorkin LS, Wallace MS. Acute pain mechanisms. Surg Clin North Am. 1999;79(2):213–29.
9. Liu S, Carpenter RL, Neal JM. Epidural anesthesia and analgesia. Their role in postoperative outcome. Anesthesiology. 1995;82(6):1474–506.
10. Macintosh RR, Mushin WW. Anaesthetics research in wartime. Med Times. 1945:253–5.
11. Mark JB, Brodsky JB. Ipsilateral shoulder pain following thoracic operations. Anesthesiology. 1993;79(1):192.
12. Pennefather SH, Russell GN. Postthoracotomy analgesia. In: Slinger PD, editor. Progress in thoracic anesthesia a society of cardiovascular anesthesiologists monograph. Philadelphia: Lippincott Williams and Wilkins; 2004.
13. Kol E, Alpar SE, Erdogan A. Preoperative education and use of analgesic before onset of pain routinely for post-thoracotomy pain control can reduce pain effect and total amount of analgesics administered postoperatively. Pain Manag Nurs. 2014;15(1):331–9.
14. Doan LV, Augustus J, Androphy R, et al. Mitigating the impact of acute and chronic post-thoracotomy pain. J Cardiothorac Vasc Anesth. 2014;28(4):1048–56.
15. Scarci M, Solli P, Bedetti B. Enhanced recovery pathway for thoracic surgery in the UK. J Thorac Dis. 2016;8(Suppl 1):S78–83.
16. Twycross RG. Choice of strong analgesic in terminal cancer: diamorphine or morphine? Pain. 1977;3(2):93–104.
17. Gulur P, Williams L, Chaudhary S, et al. Opioid tolerance—a predictor of increased length of stay and higher readmission rates. Pain Physician. 2014;17(4):E503–7.
18. Crile GW. The kinetic theory of shock and its prevention through anoci-association (shockless operation). Lancet. 1913;182(4688):7–16.
19. Bong CL, Samuel M, Ng JM, et al. Effects of preemptive epidural analgesia on post-thoracotomy pain. J Cardiothorac Vasc Anesth. 2005;19(6):786–93.
20. Hurley RW, Adams MC. Sex, gender, and pain: an overview of a complex field. Anesth Analg. 2008;107(1):309–17.
21. Perry F, Parker RK, White PF, et al. Role of psychological factors in postoperative pain control and recovery with patient-controlled analgesia. Clin J Pain. 1994;10(1):57–63; discussion 82–5.
22. Yokoyama M, Hanazaki M, Fujii H, et al. Correlation between the distribution of contrast medium and the extent of blockade during epidural anesthesia. Anesthesiology. 2004;100(6):1504–10.
23. Hirabayashi Y, Shimizu R. Effect of age on extradural dose requirement in thoracic extradural anaesthesia. Br J Anaesth. 1993;71(3):445–6.
24. Ip HY, Abrishami A, Peng PW, et al. Predictors of postoperative pain and analgesic consumption: a qualitative systematic review. Anesthesiology. 2009;111(3):657–77.
25. Bachiocco V, Morselli-Labate AM, Rusticali AG, et al. Intensity, latency and duration of post-thoracotomy pain: relationship to personality traits. Funct Neurol. 1990;5(4):321–32.
26. Caumo W, Schmidt AP, Schneider CN, et al. Preoperative predictors of moderate to intense acute postoperative pain in patients undergoing abdominal surgery. Acta Anaesthesiol Scand. 2002;46(10):1265–71.
27. Racine M, Sanchez-Rodriguez E, Galan S, et al. Factors associated with suicidal ideation in patient with chronic non-cancer pain. Pain Med. 2017;18:283–93.
28. Landreneau RJ, Hazelrigg SR, Mack MJ, et al. Postoperative pain-related morbidity: video-assisted thoracic surgery versus thoracotomy. Ann Thorac Surg. 1993;56(6):1285–9.
29. Iwasaki A, Hamatake D, Shirakusa T. Biosorbable poly-L-lactide rib-connecting pins may reduce acute pain after thoracotomy. Thorac Cardiovasc Surg. 2004;52(1):49–53.
30. Benedetti F, Vighetti S, Ricco C, et al. Neurophysiologic assessment of nerve impairment in posterolateral and muscle-sparing thoracotomy. J Thorac Cardiovasc Surg. 1998;115(4):841–7.
31. Ochroch EA, Gottschalk A, Augoustides JG, et al. Pain and physical function are similar following axillary, muscle-sparing vs posterolateral thoracotomy. Chest. 2005;128(4):2664–70.
32. Macchiarini P, Ladurie FL, Cerrina J, et al. Clamshell or sternotomy for double lung or heart-lung transplantation? Eur J Cardiothorac Surg. 1999;15(3):333–9.
33. Romsing J, Moiniche S, Ostergaard D, et al. Local infiltration with NSAIDs for postoperative analgesia: evidence for a peripheral analgesic action. Acta Anaesthesiol Scand. 2000;44(6):672–83.
34. Goppelt-Struebe M. Regulation of prostaglandin endoperoxide synthase (cyclooxygenase) isozyme expression. Prostaglandins Leukot Essent Fatty Acids. 1995;52(4):213–22.
35. Graham DJ, Campen D, Hui R, et al. Risk of acute myocardial infarction and sudden cardiac death in patients treated with cyclo-oxygenase 2 selective and non-selective non-steroidal anti-inflammatory drugs: nested case-control study. Lancet. 2005;365(9458):475–81.

36. Hippisley-Cox J, Coupland C. Risk of myocardial infarction in patients taking cyclo-oxygenase-2 inhibitors or conventional non-steroidal anti-inflammatory drugs: population based nested case-control analysis. BMJ. 2005;330(7504):1366.
37. Glassman SD, Rose SM, Dimar JR, et al. The effect of postoperative nonsteroidal anti-inflammatory drug administration on spinal fusion. Spine (Phila Pa 1976). 1998;23(7):834–8.
38. Ling XM, Fang F, Zhang XG, et al. Effect of parecoxib combined with thoracic epidural analgesia on pain after thoracotomy. J Thorac Dis. 2016;8(5):880–7.
39. Dahl V, Raeder JC. Non-opioid postoperative analgesia. Acta Anaesthesiol Scand. 2000;44(10):1191–203.
40. McNicol ED, Ferguson MC, Haroutounian S, et al. Single dose intravenous paracetamol or intravenous propacetamol for postoperative pain. Cochrane Database Syst Rev. 2016;5:CD007126.
41. Remy C, Marret E, Bonnet F. Effects of acetaminophen on morphine side-effects and consumption after major surgery: meta-analysis of randomized controlled trials. Br J Anaesth. 2005;94(4):505–13.
42. Mathews TJ, Churchhouse AM, Housden T, et al. Does adding ketamine to morphine patient-controlled analgesia safely improve post-thoracotomy pain? Interact Cardiovasc Thorac Surg. 2012;14(2):194–9.
43. Mao J, Price DD, Mayer DJ. Mechanisms of hyperalgesia and morphine tolerance: a current view of their possible interactions. Pain. 1995;62(3):259–74.
44. Michelet P, Guervilly C, Helaine A, et al. Adding ketamine to morphine for patient-controlled analgesia after thoracic surgery: influence on morphine consumption, respiratory function, and nocturnal desaturation. Br J Anaesth. 2007;99(3):396–403.
45. Moyse DW, Kaye AD, Diaz JH, et al. Perioperative ketamine administration for thoracotomy pain. Pain Physician. 2017;20(3):173–84.
46. Menigaux C, Adam F, Guignard B, et al. Preoperative gabapentin decreases anxiety and improves early functional recovery from knee surgery. Anesth Analg. 2005;100(5):1394–9.
47. Serpell MG, Neuropathic Pain Study Group. Gabapentin in neuropathic pain syndromes: a randomised, double-blind, placebo-controlled trial. Pain. 2002;99(3):557–66.
48. Chang CY, Challa CK, Shah J, et al. Gabapentin in acute postoperative pain management. Biomed Res Int. 2014;2014:631756.
49. Zakkar M, Frazer S, Hunt I. Is there a role for gabapentin in preventing or treating pain following thoracic surgery? Interact Cardiovasc Thorac Surg. 2013;17(4):716–9.
50. Omran AF, Mohamed AER. A randomized study of the effects of gabapentin versus placebo on post-thoracotomy pain and pulmonary function. Egypt J Anaesth. 2005;21:277–81.
51. Huot MP, Chouinard P, Girard F, et al. Gabapentin does not reduce post-thoracotomy shoulder pain: a randomized, double-blind placebo-controlled study. Can J Anaesth. 2008;55(6):337–43.
52. Zhang J, Ho KY, Wang Y. Efficacy of pregabalin in acute postoperative pain: a meta-analysis. Br J Anaesth. 2011;106(4):454–62.
53. Mishriky BM, Waldron NH, Habib AS. Impact of pregabalin on acute and persistent postoperative pain: a systematic review and meta-analysis. Br J Anaesth. 2015;114(1):10–31.
54. Baidya DK, Agarwal A, Khanna P, et al. Pregabalin in acute and chronic pain. J Anaesthesiol Clin Pharmacol. 2011;27(3):307–14.
55. Singla NK, Chelly JE, Lionberger DR, et al. Pregabalin for the treatment of postoperative pain: results from three controlled trials using different surgical models. J Pain Res. 2015;8:9–20.
56. Wahlander S, Frumento RJ, Wagener G, et al. A prospective, double-blind, randomized, placebo-controlled study of dexmedetomidine as an adjunct to epidural analgesia after thoracic surgery. J Cardiothorac Vasc Anesth. 2005;19(5):630–5.
57. Dong CS, Zhang J, Lu Q, et al. Effect of dexmedetomidine combined with sufentanil for post-thoracotomy intravenous analgesia:a randomized, controlled clinical study. BMC Anesthesiol. 2017;17(1):33.
58. Talbot RM, McCarthy KF, McCrory C. Central and systemic inflammatory responses to thoracotomy—potential implications for acute and chronic postsurgical pain. J Neuroimmunol. 2015;285:147–9.
59. Hong D, Byers MR, Oswald RJ. Dexamethasone treatment reduces sensory neuropeptides and nerve sprouting reactions in injured teeth. Pain. 1993;55(2):171–81.
60. Marek P, Ben-Eliyahu S, Vaccarino AL, et al. Delayed application of MK-801 attenuates development of morphine tolerance in rats. Brain Res. 1991;558(1):163–5.
61. Rasmussen SB, Saied NN, Bowens C Jr, et al. Duration of upper and lower extremity peripheral nerve blockade is prolonged with dexamethasone when added to ropivacaine: a retrospective database analysis. Pain Med. 2013;14(8):1239–47.
62. Tomar GS, Ganguly S, Cherian G. Effect of perineural dexamethasone with bupivacaine in single space paravertebral block for postoperative analgesia in elective nephrectomy cases: a double-blind placebo-controlled trial. Am J Ther. 2017;24:e713–7.
63. Ballantyne JC, Carr DB, deFerranti S, et al. The comparative effects of postoperative analgesic therapies on pulmonary outcome: cumulative meta-analyses of randomized, controlled trials. Anesth Analg. 1998;86(3):598–612.
64. Bauer C, Hentz JG, Ducrocq X, et al. Lung function after lobectomy: a randomized, double-blinded trial comparing thoracic epidural ropivacaine/sufentanil and intravenous morphine for patient-controlled analgesia. Anesth Analg. 2007;105(1):238–44.

65. Gough JD, Williams AB, Vaughan RS, et al. The control of post-thoracotomy pain. A comparative evaluation of thoracic epidural fentanyl infusions and cryo-analgesia. Anaesthesia. 1988;43(9):780–3.
66. Muller LC, Salzer GM, Ransmayr G, et al. Intraoperative cryoanalgesia for postthoracotomy pain relief. Ann Thorac Surg. 1989;48(1):15–8.
67. Melzack R, Wall PD. Pain mechanisms: a new theory. Science. 1965;150(3699):971–9.
68. Rodriguez-Aldrete D, Candiotti KA, Janakiraman R, et al. Trends and new evidence in the management of acute and chronic post-thoracotomy pain-an overview of the literature from 2005 to 2015. J Cardiothorac Vasc Anesth. 2016;30(3):762–72.
69. Fiorelli A, Morgillo F, Milione R, et al. Control of post-thoracotomy pain by transcutaneous electrical nerve stimulation: effect on serum cytokine levels, visual analogue scale, pulmonary function and medication. Eur J Cardiothorac Surg. 2012;41(4):861–8.
70. Sbruzzi G, Silveira SA, Silva DV, et al. Transcutaneous electrical nerve stimulation after thoracic surgery: systematic review and meta-analysis of 11 randomized trials. Rev Bras Cir Cardiovasc. 2012;27(1):75–87.
71. Cook TM, Eaton JM. Epidural analgesia after thoracotomy: United Kingdom practice. Eur J Anaesthesiol. 1997;14(1):108–11.
72. Yeung JH, Gates S, Naidu BV, et al. Paravertebral block versus thoracic epidural for patients undergoing thoracotomy. Cochrane Database Syst Rev. 2016;2:CD009121.
73. Cook TM, Counsell D, Wildsmith JA, Royal College of Anaesthetists Third National Audit Project. Major complications of central neuraxial block: report on the Third National Audit Project of the Royal College of Anaesthetists. Br J Anaesth. 2009;102(2):179–90.
74. Counsell D. Complications after perioperative central neuraxial blocks. The Third National Audit Project (NAP3), editor. Major complications of central neuraxial blocks in the United Kingdom. London: Royal College of Anaesthetists; 2009. pp. 101–11.
75. Scarci M, Joshi A, Attia R. In patients undergoing thoracic surgery is paravertebral block as effective as epidural analgesia for pain management? Interact Cardiovasc Thorac Surg. 2010;10(1):92–6.
76. Daly DJ, Myles PS. Update on the role of paravertebral blocks for thoracic surgery: are they worth it? Curr Opin Anaesthesiol. 2009;22(1):38–43.
77. Bai Y, Miller T, Tan M, et al. Lidocaine patch for acute pain management: a meta-analysis of prospective controlled trials. Curr Med Res Opin. 2015;31(3):575–81.
78. Vrooman B, Kapural L, Sarwar S, et al. Lidocaine 5% patch for treatment of acute pain after robotic cardiac surgery and prevention of persistent incisional pain: a randomized, placebo-controlled. Double-Blind Trial Pain Med. 2015;16(8):1610–21.
79. Fiorelli A, Izzo AC, Frongillo EM, et al. Efficacy of wound analgesia for controlling post-thoracotomy pain: a randomized double-blind studydagger. Eur J Cardiothorac Surg. 2016;49(1):339–47.
80. Liu SS, Richman JM, Thirlby RC, et al. Efficacy of continuous wound catheters delivering local anesthetic for postoperative analgesia: a quantitative and qualitative systematic review of randomized controlled trials. J Am Coll Surg. 2006;203(6):914–32.
81. Angst MS, Drover DR. Pharmacology of drugs formulated with DepoFoam®: a sustained release drug delivery system for parenteraladministration using multivesicular liposome technology. Clin Pharmacokinet. 2006;45(12):1153–76.
82. Lambert WJ, Los K. DepoFoam® multivesicular liposomes for the sustained release of macromolecules. In: Rathbone MJ, et al., editors. Modified-releasedrug delivery technology, vol. 2. 2nd ed. New York: Informa Healthcare; 2008. p. 207–14.
83. Bergese S, Onel E, Portillo J. Evaluation of DepoFoam® bupivacainefor the treatment of postsurgical pain. Pain Manag. 2011;1(6):539–47.
84. Chahar P, Cummings KC III. Liposomal bupivacaine: a review of anew bupivacaine formulation. J Pain Res. 2012;5:257–64.
85. Kvalheim LR, Reiestad F. Intrapleural catheter in the management of postoperative pain. Anesthesiology. 1984;61:A231.
86. Miguel R, Smith R. Intrapleural, not interpleural, analgesia. Reg Anesth. 1991;16(5):299.
87. Baumgarten RK. Intrapleural, interpleural, or pleural block? Simpler may be better. Reg Anesth. 1992;17(2):116.
88. Dravid RM, Paul RE. Interpleural block—part 1. Anaesthesia. 2007;62(10):1039–49.
89. Pennefather SH, Akrofi ME, Kendall JB, et al. Double-blind comparison of intrapleural saline and 0.25% bupivacaine for ipsilateral shoulder pain after thoracotomy in patients receiving thoracic epidural analgesia. Br J Anaesth. 2005;94(2):234–8.
90. Kambam JR, Hammon J, Parris WC, et al. Intrapleural analgesia for post-thoracotomy pain and blood levels of bupivacaine following intrapleural injection. Can J Anaesth. 1989;36(2):106–9.
91. Broome IJ, Sherry KM, Reilly CS. A combined chest drain and intrapleural catheter for post-thoracotomy pain relief. Anaesthesia. 1993;48(8):724–6.
92. Chin KJ, Malhas L, Perlas A. The erector spinae plane block provides visceral abdominal analgesia in bariatric surgery, a report of 3 cases. Reg Anesth Pain Med. 2017;42(3):372–6.
93. Forero M, Rajarathinam M, Adhikary S, et al. Continuous erector spinae plane block for rescue analgesia in thoracotomy after epidural failure: a case report. A&A Case Rep. 2017;8:254–6.
94. Gustafsson LL, Wiesenfeld-Hallin Z. Spinal opioid analgesia. A critical update. Drugs. 1988;35(6):597–603.
95. Cousins MJ, Mather LE. Intrathecal and epidural administration of opioids. Anesthesiology. 1984;61(3):276–310.

96. Dryden CM, McMenemin I, Duthie DJ. Efficacy of continuous intercostal bupivacaine for pain relief after thoracotomy. Br J Anaesth. 1993;70(5):508–10.
97. Blanco R, Parras T, McDonnell JG, et al. Serratus plane block: a novel ultrasound-guided thoracic wall nerve block. Anaesthesia. 2013;68(11):1107–13.
98. Okmen K, Okmen BM. The efficacy of serratus anterior plane block in analgesia for thoracotomy: a retrospective study. J Anesth. 2017;31(4):579–85.
99. Madabushi R, Tewari S, Gautam SK, et al. Serratus anterior plane block: a new analgesic technique for post-thoracotomy pain. Pain Physician. 2015;18(3):E421–4.
100. Lonnqvist PA, Hildingsson U. The caudal boundary of the thoracic paravertebral space. A study in human cadavers. Anaesthesia. 1992;47(12):1051–2.
101. Karmakar MK. Thoracic paravertebral block. Anesthesiology. 2001;95(3):771–80.
102. Hutchins J, Sanchez J, Andrade R, et al. Ultrasound-guided paravertebral catheter versus intercostals blocks for postoperative pain control in video-assisted thoracoscopic surgery: a prospective randomized trial. J Cardiothorac Vasc Anesth. 2017;31(2):458–63.
103. Davies RG, Myles PS, Graham JM. A comparison of the analgesic efficacy and side-effects of paravertebral vs epidural blockade for thoracotomy—a systematic review and meta-analysis of randomized trials. Br J Anaesth. 2006;96(4):418–26.
104. Ding X, Jin S, Niu X, et al. A comparison of the analgesia efficacy and side effects of paravertebral compared with epidural blockade for thoracotomy: an updated meta-analysis. PLoS One. 2014;9(5):e96233.
105. Baidya DK, Khanna P, Maitra S. Analgesic efficacy and safety of thoracic paravertebral and epidural analgesia for thoracic surgery: a systematic review and meta-analysis. Interact Cardiovasc Thorac Surg. 2014;18(5):626–35.
106. Okajima H, Tanaka O, Ushio M, et al. Ultrasound-guided continuous thoracic paravertebral block provides comparable analgesia and fewer episodes of hypotension than continuous epidural block after lung surgery. J Anesth. 2015;29(3):373–8.
107. Eason MJ, Wyatt R. Paravertebral thoracic block-a reappraisal. Anaesthesia. 1979;34(7):638–42.
108. Sabanathan S, Smith PJ, Pradhan GN, et al. Continuous intercostal nerve block for pain relief after thoracotomy. Ann Thorac Surg. 1988;46(4):425–6.
109. Soni AK, Conacher ID, Waller DA, et al. Video-assisted thoracoscopic placement of paravertebral catheters: a technique for postoperative analgesia for bilateral thoracoscopic surgery. Br J Anaesth. 1994;72(4):462–4.
110. Yamauchi Y, Isaka M, Ando K, et al. Continuous paravertebral block using a thoracoscopic catheter-insertion technique for postoperative pain after thoracotomy: a retrospective case-control study. J Cardiothorac Surg. 2017;12(1):5.
111. Cowie B, McGlade D, Ivanusic J, et al. Ultrasound-guided thoracic paravertebral blockade: a cadaveric study. Anesth Analg. 2010;110(6):1735–9.
112. Krediet AC, Moayeri N, van Geffen GJ, et al. Different approaches to ultrasound-guided thoracic paravertebral block: an illustrated review. Anesthesiology. 2015;123(2):459–74.
113. Riain SCO, Donnell BO, Cuffe T, et al. Thoracic paravertebral block using real-time ultrasound guidance. Anesth Analg. 2010;110(1):248–51.
114. Taketa Y, Fujitani T, Irisawa Y, et al. Ultrasound-guided thoracic paravertebral block by the paralaminar in-plane approach using a microconvex array transducer: methodological utility based on anatomical structures. J Anesth. 2017;31(2):271–7.
115. Kaya FN, Turker G, Mogol EB, et al. Thoracic paravertebral block for video-assisted thoracoscopic surgery: single injection versus multiple injections. J Cardiothorac Vasc Anesth. 2012;26(1):90–4.
116. Vogt A, Stieger DS, Theurillat C, et al. Single-injection thoracic paravertebral block for postoperative pain treatment after thoracoscopic surgery. Br J Anaesth. 2005;95(6):816–21.
117. Fibla JJ, Molins L, Mier JM, et al. A randomized prospective study of analgesic quality after thoracotomy: paravertebral block with bolus versus continuous infusion with an elastomeric pump. Eur J Cardiothorac Surg. 2015;47(4):631–5.
118. Griffiths DP, Diamond AW, Cameron JD. Postoperative extradural analgesia following thoracic surgery: a feasibility study. Br J Anaesth. 1975;47(1):48–55.
119. Shuman RL, Peters RM. Epidural anesthesia following thoracotomy in patients with chronic obstructive airway disease. J Thorac Cardiovasc Surg. 1976;71(1):82–8.
120. Hoffmann VL, Vercauteren MP, Vreugde JP, et al. Posterior epidural space depth: safety of the loss of resistance and hanging drop techniques. Br J Anaesth. 1999;83:807–9.
121. Leurcharusmee P, Arnuntasupakul V, Chora De La Garza D, et al. Reliabilty of waveform analysis as an adjunct to loss of resistance for thoracic epidural blocks. Reg Anesth Pain Med. 2015;40:694–7.
122. Pennefather SH, Gilby S, Danecki A, et al. The changing practice of thoracic epidural analgesia in the United Kingdom: 1997–2004. Anaesthesia. 2006;61(4):363–9.
123. Eisenach JC, De Kock M, Klimscha W. Alpha(2)-adrenergic agonists for regional anesthesia. A clinical review of clonidine (1984–1995). Anesthesiology. 1996;85(3):655–74.
124. Neil MJ. Clonidine: clinical pharmacology and therapeutic use in pain management. Curr Clin Pharmacol. 2011;6(4):280–7.
125. Mohammad W, Mir SA, Mohammad K, et al. A randomized double-blind study to evaluate efficacy and safety of epidural magnesium sulfate and clonidine

as adjuvants to bupivacaine for postthoracotomy pain relief. Anesth Essays Res. 2015;9(1):15–20.
126. Bromage PR, Camporesi EM, Durant PA, et al. Nonrespiratory side effects of epidural morphine. Anesth Analg. 1982;61(6):490–5.
127. Yaksh TL. Spinal opiate analgesia: characteristics and principles of action. Pain. 1981;11(3):293–346.
128. Bonica JJ. Autonomic innervation of the viscera in relation to nerve block. Anesthesiology. 1968;29(4):793–813.
129. Jorgensen H, Wetterslev J, Moiniche S, et al. Epidural local anaesthetics versus opioid-based analgesic regimens on postoperative gastrointestinal paralysis, PONV and pain after abdominal surgery. Cochrane Database Syst Rev. 2000;4:CD001893.
130. Zeng XZ, Lu ZF, Lv XQ, et al. Epidural Co-administration of dexmedetomidine and levobupivacaine improves the gastrointestinal motility function after colonic resection in comparison to co-administration of morphine and levobupivacaine. PLoS One. 2016;11(1):e0146215.
131. Lundberg JF, Martner J, Raner C, et al. Dopamine or norepinephrine infusion during thoracic epidural anesthesia? Differences in hemodynamic effects and plasma catecholamine levels. Acta Anaesthesiol Scand. 2005;49(7):962–8.
132. Li XQ, Tan WF, Wang J, et al. The effects of thoracic epidural analgesia on oxygenation and pulmonary shunt fraction during one-lung ventilation: an meta-analysis. BMC Anesthesiol. 2015;15:166.
133. Magnano D, Montalbano R, Lamarra M, et al. Ineffectiveness of local wound anesthesia to reduce postoperative pain after median sternotomy. J Card Surg. 2005;20(4):314–8.
134. McDonald SB, Jacobsohn E, Kopacz DJ, et al. Parasternal block and local anesthetic infiltration with levobupivacaine after cardiac surgery with desflurane: the effect on postoperative pain, pulmonary function, and tracheal extubation times. Anesth Analg. 2005;100(1):25–32.
135. Ziyaeifard M, Azarfarin R, Golzari SE. A review of current analgesic techniques in cardiac surgery. Is epidural worth it? J Cardiovasc Thorac Res. 2014;6(3):133–40.
136. Steinthorsdottir KJ, Wildgaard L, Hansen HJ, et al. Regional analgesia for video-assisted thoracic surgery: a systematic review. Eur J Cardiothorac Surg. 2014;45(6):959–66.
137. Zingg U, McQuinn A, DiValentino D, et al. Minimally invasive versus open esophagectomy for patients with esophageal cancer. Ann Thorac Surg. 2009;87(3):911–9.
138. Mahon SV, Berry PD, Jackson M, et al. Thoracic epidural infusions for post-thoracotomy pain: a comparison of fentanyl-bupivacaine mixtures vs. fentanyl alone. Anaesthesia. 1999;54(7):641–6.
139. Tan CN, Guha A, Scawn ND, et al. Optimal concentration of epidural fentanyl in bupivacaine 0.1% after thoracotomy. Br J Anaesth. 2004;92(5):670–4.
140. Samii K, Feret J, Harari A, et al. Selective spinal analgesia. Lancet. 1979;1(8126):1142.
141. Neustein SM, Cohen E. Intrathecal morphine during thoracotomy, Part II: effect on postoperative meperidine requirements and pulmonary function tests. J Cardiothorac Vasc Anesth. 1993;7(2):157–9.
142. Liu M, Rock P, Grass JA, et al. Double-blind randomized evaluation of intercostal nerve blocks as an adjuvant to subarachnoid administered morphine for post-thoracotomy analgesia. Reg Anesth. 1995;20(5):418–25.
143. Cense HA, Lagarde SM, de Jong K, et al. Association of no epidural analgesia with postoperative morbidity and mortality after transthoracic esophageal cancer resection. J Am Coll Surg. 2006;202(3):395–400.
144. Li W, Li Y, Huang Q, et al. Short and long-term outcomes of epidural or intravenous analgesia after esophagectomy: a propensity-matched cohort study. PLoS One. 2016;11(4):e0154380.
145. Scawn ND, Pennefather SH, Soorae A, et al. Ipsilateral shoulder pain after thoracotomy with epidural analgesia: the influence of phrenic nerve infiltration with lidocaine. Anesth Analg. 2001;93(2):260–4.
146. Tan N, Agnew NM, Scawn ND, et al. Suprascapular nerve block for ipsilateral shoulder pain after thoracotomy with thoracic epidural analgesia: a double-blind comparison of 0.5% bupivacaine and 0.9% saline. Anesth Analg. 2002;94(1):199–202.
147. Blichfeldt-Eckhardt MR, Andersen C, Ording H, et al. Shoulder pain after thoracic surgery: type and time course, a prospective cohort study. J Cardiothorac Vasc Anesth. 2017;31(1):147–51.
148. Danelli G, Berti M, Casati A, et al. Ipsilateral shoulder pain after thoracotomy surgery: a prospective, randomized, double-blind, placebo-controlled evaluation of the efficacy of infiltrating the phrenic nerve with 0.2%wt/volropivacaine. Eur J Anaesthesiol. 2007;24(7):596–601.
149. Mac TB, Girard F, Chouinard P, et al. Acetaminophen decreases early post-thoracotomy ipsilateral shoulder pain in patients with thoracic epidural analgesia: a double-blind placebo-controlled study. J Cardiothorac Vasc Anesth. 2005;19(4):475–8.
150. Urmey WF, McDonald M. Hemidiaphragmatic paresis during interscalene brachial plexus block: effects on pulmonary function and chest wall mechanics. Anesth Analg. 1992;74(3):352–7.
151. Garner L, Coats RR. Ipsilateral stellate ganglion block effective for treating shoulder pain after thoracotomy. Anesth Analg. 1994;78(6):1195–6.
152. Classification of chronic pain. Descriptions of chronic pain syndromes and definitions of pain terms. Prepared by the International Association for the Study of Pain, Subcommittee on Taxonomy. Pain Suppl. 1986;3:S1–226.
153. Katz J, Jackson M, Kavanagh BP, et al. Acute pain after thoracic surgery predicts long-term post-thoracotomy pain. Clin J Pain. 1996;12(1):50–5.

154. Gottschalk A, Cohen SP, Yang S, et al. Preventing and treating pain after thoracic surgery. Anesthesiology. 2006;104(3):594–600.
155. Perttunen K, Tasmuth T, Kalso E. Chronic pain after thoracic surgery: a follow-up study. Acta Anaesthesiol Scand. 1999;43(5):563–7.
156. Furrer M, Rechsteiner R, Eigenmann V, et al. Thoracotomy and thoracoscopy: postoperative pulmonary function, pain and chest wall complaints. Eur J Cardiothorac Surg. 1997;12(1):82–7.
157. Forster R, Storck M, Schafer JR, et al. Thoracoscopy versus thoracotomy: a prospective comparison of trauma and quality of life. Langenbeck's Arch Surg. 2002;387(1):32–6.
158. Hetmann F, Kongsgaard UE, Sandvik L, et al. Post-thoracotomy pain syndrome and sensory disturbances following thoracotomy at 6- and 12-month follow-ups. J Pain Res. 2017;10:663–8.
159. Hetmann F, Kongsgaard UE, Sandvik L, et al. Prevalence and predictors of persistent post-surgical pain 12 months after thoracotomy. Acta Anaesthesiol Scand. 2015;59(6):740–8.
160. Hoofwijk DM, van Reij RR, Rutten BP, et al. Genetic polymorphisms and their association with the prevalence and severity of chronic post-surgical pain: a systematic review. Br J Anaesth. 2016;117(6):708–19.
161. Kehlet H, Wilkinson RC, Fischer HB, et al. Prospect Working Group. PROSPECT: evidence-based, procedure-specific postoperative pain management. Best Pract Res Clin Anaesthesiol. 2007;21(1):149–59.
162. Mishra A, Nar AS, Bawa A, et al. Pregabalin in chronic post-thoracotomy pain. J Clin Diagn Res. 2013;7:1659–61.

The manufacturer's authorised representative in the EU is Springer Nature Customer Service Centre GmbH, Europaplatz 3, 69115 Heidelberg, Germany. If you have any concerns regarding our products, please contact ProductSafety@springernature.com

Printed and bound by CPI Group (UK) Ltd, Croydon, CR0 4YY

25/03/2026

02078177-0019